Dr. M. R. C. Greenwood
Columbia University
Julius & Armand Hammer Health Sciences Center
Institute of Human Nutrition
701 West 168th Street, 7th Floor
New York, N.Y. 10032   8/4/8

NUTRITION AND DRUG INTERRELATIONS

THE NUTRITION FOUNDATION

A Monograph Series

HORACE L. SIPPLE AND KRISTEN W. MCNUTT, EDS.: *Sugars in Nutrition,* 1974

ROBERT E. OLSON, ED.: *Protein-Calorie Malnutrition,* 1975

ANANDA S. PRASAD, ED.: *Trace Elements in Human Health and Disease, Volume I, Zinc and Copper, 1976; Volume II, Essential and Toxic Elements,* 1976

MORLEY R. KARE AND OWEN MALLER, EDS.: *The Chemical Senses and Nutrition,* 1977

JOHN N. HATHCOCK AND JULIUS COON, EDS.: *Nutrition and Drug Interrelations,* 1978

NUTRITION AND DRUG INTERRELATIONS

Edited by

John N. Hathcock

Department of Food and Nutrition
Iowa State University
Ames, Iowa

Julius Coon

Department of Pharmacology
Thomas Jefferson University
Philadelphia, Pennsylvania

ACADEMIC PRESS   New York   San Francisco   London   1978

A Subsidiary of Harcourt Brace Jovanovich, Publishers

ACADEMIC PRESS, INC.
111 Fifth Avenue, New York, New York 10003

United Kingdom Edition published by
ACADEMIC PRESS, INC. (LONDON) LTD.
24/28 Oval Road, London NW1 7DX

Library of Congress Cataloging in Publication Data

International Symposium on Nutrition and Drug Inter-
    relations, Iowa State University, 1976.
    Nutrition and drug interrelations.

    (Nutritional Foundation monograph series)
    "Based on papers presented at the International
Symposium on Nutrition and Drug Interrelations held at
Iowa State University, August 4-6, 1976."
    Includes bibliographies and index.
    1.   Drugs—Physiological effect—Congresses.
2.   Nutrition—Congresses.   3.   Diet therapy—Congresses.
4.   Medicated feeds—Congresses.   I.   Hathcock, John N.
II.   Coon, Julius.   III.   Title.   IV.   Series: Nutrition
Foundation, New York.Nutrition Foundation monograph
series.
RM300.I56 1976   615'.73   77-82413
ISBN 0-12-332550-1

Contents

SECTION II / NUTRITIONAL EFFECTS ON DRUG METABOLISM AND ACTION

12   Ascorbic Acid and Drug Metabolism
V. G. ZANNONI, P. H. SATO, AND L. E. RIKANS

13   Dietary Minerals and Drug Metabolism
GEORGE C. BECKING

14   Drug Metabolism and Infantile Undernutrition
FERNANDO MÖNCKEBERG, MARÍA BRAVO, AND ONOFRE GONZÁLEZ

15   Effects of Dietary Protein on Drug Metabolism
T. COLIN CAMPBELL

SECTION III / USE OF DRUGS IN ANIMAL FEEDS

20   The Role of Antibiotics in Efficient Livestock Production
VIRGIL W. HAYS

21   Physiological Effects of Estrogens in Animal Feeds with Emphasis on Growth of Ruminants
ALLEN TRENKLE AND WISE BURROUGHS

22   Distribution and Fate of Growth-Promoting Drugs Used in Animal Production
P. W. ASCHBACHER

23   Antibiotics in Animal Feeds: An Assessment of the Animal and Public Health Aspects
RICHARD P. SILVER AND H. DWIGHT MERCER

SECTION IV / USE OF NUTRIENTS AND FOODS AS DRUGS

24 Some Aspects of Pharmacologic Use and Abuse of Water-Soluble Vitamins
WILLIAM B. BEAN

25 Uses and Function of Vitamin K
WALTER H. SEEGERS

26 Vitamin D: Metabolism, Drug Interactions, and Therapeutic Applications in Humans
MARK R. HAUSSLER

27 Toxic Effects of Megadoses of Fat-Soluble Vitamins
LOTTE ARNRICH

List of Contributors

Numbers in parentheses indicate the pages on which the authors' contributions begin.

LOTTE ARNRICH (751), Department of Food and Nutrition, Iowa State University, Ames, Iowa

P. W. ASCHBACHER (613), Metabolism and Radiation Research Laboratory, Agricultural Research Service, U.S. Department of Agriculture, State University Station, Fargo, North Dakota

JAMES A. BARROWMAN (113), Faculty of Medicine, Memorial University of Newfoundland, St. John's, Newfoundland, Canada

WILLIAM B. BEAN (667), Institute for Medical Humanities, University of Texas Medical Branch, Galveston, Texas

GEORGE C. BECKING (371), Department of National Health and Welfare, Health Protection Branch, Bureau of Chemical Hazards, Environmental Health Directorate, Ottawa, Canada

MARÍA BRAVO (399), Instituto de Nutricion y Tecnologia de los Alimentos, Universidad de Chile, Santiago, Chile

MYRON BRIN (131), Department of Biochemical Nutrition, Roche Research Center, Hoffmann-La Roche Inc., Nutley, New Jersey

WISE BURROUGHS (577), Department of Animal Science, Iowa State University, Ames, Iowa

T. COLIN CAMPBELL (409), Division of Nutritional Sciences, Cornell University, Ithaca, New York

LORRAINE CHENG (21), Department of Scientific Literature, Roche Research Center, Hoffmann-La Roche Inc., Nutley, New Jersey

RAJENDRA S. CHHABRA (253), Laboratory of Pharmacology, National Institute of Environmental Health Sciences, Research Triangle Park, North Carolina

MICHAEL A. DORATO (423), Department of Inhalation Toxicology, Huntingdon Research Center, New City, New York

JENET S. EVANS (475), Department of Pharmacology, School of Pharmacy, University of Georgia, Athens, Georgia

JOHN E. FLETCHER (447), Laboratory of Applied Studies, Division of Computer Research and Technology, National Institutes of Health, Bethesda, Maryland

ONOFRE GONZÁLEZ (399), Departmento Medicina Experimental Unidad Microbiologia, Facultad de Medicina Sede Sur, Universidad de Chile, Santiago, Chile

CHARLES H. HALSTED (83), Department of Internal Medicine, University of California, School of Medicine, Davis, California

MARK R. HAUSSLER (717), Department of Biochemistry, Health Sciences Center, University of Arizona, Tucson, Arizona

VIRGIL W. HAYS (545), Department of Animal Sciences, University of Kentucky, Lexington, Kentucky

KEVIN J. IVEY (279), Harry S Truman Memorial Veterans Hospitals, Columbia, Missouri, and University of Missouri Medical Center, Columbia, Missouri

ROBERT M. KARK (821), Department of Medicine, Rush Medical College and Presbyterian-St. Luke's Hospital, Chicago, Illinois

H. DWIGHT MERCER (649), Division of Veterinary Medical Research, Bureau of Veterinary Medicine, Food and Drug Administration, Beltsville, Maryland

FERNANDO MÖNCKEBERG (399), Instituto de Nutricion y Tecnologia de los Alimentos, Universidad de Chile, Santiago, Chile

WILLIAM P. NORRED (475), Pharmacology Research Laboratory, Richard B. Russell Agricultural Research Center, Agricultual Research Services, U.S. Department of Agriculture, Athens, Georgia

R. A. PRINS * (189), Laboratory of Veterinary Biochemistry, State University of Utrecht, Utrecht, The Netherlands

L. E. RIKANS (347), Department of Pharmacology, The University of Michigan Medical School, Ann Arbor, Michigan

DAPHNE A. ROE (319), Division of Nutritional Sciences, Cornell University, Ithaca, New York

ADRIANNE E. ROGERS (505), Department of Nutrition and Food Science, Massachusetts Institute of Technology, Cambridge, Massachusetts

DAVID P. ROSE (151), Division of Clinical Oncology, Wisconsin Clinical Cancer Center, University of Wisconsin, Madison, Wisconsin

P. H. SATO (347), Department of Pharmacology, The University of Michigan Medical School, Ann Arbor, Michigan

GUSTAV SCHONFELD (773), Lipid Research Center, Washington University School of Medicine, St. Louis, Missouri

WALTER H. SEEGERS (687), Department of Physiology, Wayne State University, School of Medicine, Detroit, Michigan

RICHARD P. SILVER (649), Division of Veterinary Medical Research, Bureau of Veterinary Medicine, Food and Drug Administration, Beltsville, Maryland

ARTHUR A. SPECTOR (447), Departments of Biochemistry and Medicine, University of Iowa, Iowa City, Iowa

ANN C. SULLIVAN (21), Department of Biochemical Nutrition, Roche Research Center, Hoffmann-La Roche Inc., Nutley, New Jersey

J. MICHAEL TREDGER† (253), Laboratory of Pharmacology, National Institute of Environmental Health Sciences, Research Triangle Park, North Carolina

ALLEN TRENKLE (577), Department of Animal Science, Iowa State University, Ames, Iowa

ADELBERT E. WADE (475), Department of Pharmacology, School of Pharmacy, University of Georgia, Athens, Georgia

CHARLES O. WARD (423), Department of Toxicology, Medical Division, Gulf Science and Technology Company, Pittsburgh, Pennsylvania

* Present address: Laboratory of Animal Nutrition, Practicumgebouw, Utrecht, The Netherlands

† Present address: Liver Unit, Kings College Hospital Medical School, Denmark Hill, London, England

R. T. WILLIAMS* (303), Department of Biochemistry, St. Mary's Hospital Medical School, London, England

JOSEPH L. WITZTUM (773), Lipid Research Center, Washington University School of Medicine, St. Louis, Missouri

JAMES HARVEY YOUNG (1), Department of History, Emory University, Atlanta, Georgia

V. G. ZANNONI (347), Department of Pharmacology, The University of Michigan Medical School, Ann Arbor, Michigan

* Present address: Department of Biochemical and Experimental Pharmacology, St. Mary's Hospital Medical School, London, England

Foreword

The Nutrition Foundation Monograph Series provides systematic coverage of new, important areas of nutritional knowledge. The content of each monograph is planned to consolidate subject material of fundamental importance and broad significance. The texts not only review recent advances, but provide a perspective derived from historical and multidisciplinary viewpoints. The international authors identify areas in which additional useful research should be pursued and address the application of research findings for the benefit of man.

The numerous interrelationships between nutrition and the metabolism and effects of drugs are underscored by the expanding number of therapeutic agents that now are regularly and repeatedly used over long periods of time. Certain of these interrelationships are beneficial; others have potential ill effects. Several established beneficial actions are utilized not only in human medicine, but in animal husbandry and veterinary medicine as well. These aspects are brought together in the present volume.

The Nutrition Foundation is indebted to the authors of this work for their participation in its preparation and to the editors, Dr. John N. Hathcock and Dr. Julius Coon, whose skill has provided the uniformity of coverage desirable for a maximally useful monograph. We are further indebted to the Iowa State University Nutritional Sciences Council, the planning committee of which selected the content and authors of the chapters.

William J. Darby
President
The Nutrition Foundation, Inc.
New York and Washington, D.C.

Preface

The interrelations between nutrition and drugs have historical and current importance. While some drugs were first discovered in foods, modern increases in diversity and use of drugs have led to numerous interactions with nutrients and diet. These interrelations are important in research, medicine, dietetics, and animal production. The title "Nutrition and Drug Interrelations" was chosen for this monograph and the corresponding symposium because it denotes a wider, more extensive affiliation than the more usual term of "drug–nutrient interactions." The wider scope was intended and, we believe, suitably accomplished.

The chapter titles represent only a fraction of the total subjects which could have been included appropriately under the symposium title. They are organized into four major sections. The section titled Drug Effects on Nutrient Intake, Function, and Requirement gives some important examples of the impacts of drugs on the processes of nutrition. Many of these influences are harmless under optimal nutritional circumstances but may be deleterious when nutritional intake or function is inadequate. The section on Nutritional Effects on Drug Metabolism and Action illustrates several of the numerous influences nutritional condition has on biochemical competence to cope with xenobiotics, including drugs. With ever-increasing use of drugs, food additives, and other substances, increased understanding of the effects of nutrition on their metabolism and elimination is imperative. The section on the Use of Drugs in Animal Feeds gives some examples of the important uses pharmacological agents have in food production, and expresses concern about subsequent effects in the food chain. The last section, Use of Nutrients and Foods as Drugs, demonstrates that the boundary between dietetic and pharmacological treatment is by no means sharp. This overlap is clearly illustrated by the pharmacological (nutritional?) use of vitamin D derivatives to effectively treat certain familial diseases, and by the widespread use of megavitamin treatments of doubtful benefit. These sections represent a functional relationship categorization. It is difficult to imagine a nutrition and drug interrelation which would not fit aptly into one of these sections. Some chapters are wide enough in coverage to fit possibly into more than one section. Although the perspective and focus of the chapters differ from one section to another and between chapters within sections, we believe the section titles give a subject matter organization that is both informative and useful.

The specific topics and authors were chosen to provide expert information selection and perspective in what we believe are timely subjects in terms of state of knowledge, research activity, and professional interest. Each author was asked to provide the best combination of "state-of-the-art" comprehensive review and "frontiers-of-research" detailed new information in their subject. The ways they interpreted this assignment varies considerably according to their individual viewpoints and the state of knowledge in the particular subject.

The introductory chapter, "The Agile Role of Food: Some Historical Reflections" by James Harvey Young, was included to provide historical and sociological setting and perspective for the extremely variable role of food in human existence and endeavor. In addition to nourishment, the various roles cited include uses of food and drink as drugs or as sources of drugs, as well as fanciful uses for numerous purposes.

No effort was made to cover the diverse field of drugs which occur naturally in foods. Knowledge of this subject is not changing very rapidly and good reviews have been published elsewhere.

It is hoped that this mongraph, which is based on papers presented at the International Symposium on Nutrition and Drug Interrelations held at Iowa State University, August 4–6, 1976, will become a much needed benchmark publication in the subject. No previous symposium or publication has incorporated such a wide range of topics in this subject with this intensity. We hope that this publication will prove useful to nutritionists, pharmacologists, dietitians, and physicians, and also stimulate further research.

We wish to express our thanks to the Iowa State University Nutritional Sciences Council, especially M. Allison, W. Brewer, R. Ewan, N. Jacobson, W. Runyan, A. Trenkle, and J. Young, for help in planning, organizing, and hosting the symposium. Also, we gladly acknowledge the financial and organization support from the Nutrition Foundation, and the advice and encouragement given by Dr. William J. Darby, without which the symposium and this monograph would not have been possible.

John N. Hathcock
Julius Coon

NUTRITION AND
DRUG INTERRELATIONS

1

The Agile Role of Food: Some Historical Reflections

JAMES HARVEY YOUNG

I. FOOD AS PATRIOTISM

> Father and I went down to camp,
> Along with Captain Gooding,
> And there we see the men and boys
> As thick as hasty pudding.*
> (Sonneck, 1972; Evans, 1903–1959)

In these bicentennial days it seems appropriate to begin some reflections on the agile role of food in history by pointing to a vivid food simile appearing in "Yankee Doodle," a popular song of the American Revolution. Food and the Revolution, moreover, are bound together by ties more substantial than similes. "I know not why," John Adams wrote after the new nation had become established, "we should blush to confess that molasses was an essential ingredient in American independence"

---

*Sonneck dates a broadside containing this verse to 1775 or 1776, although other authorities believe the first published version appeared as late as 1793.

(Schlesinger, 1949, p. 239). British tax measures involving molasses, sugar, and tea had much to do with provoking the expanding discontent that eventually led to war.

Indeed, the psychohistorian Lloyd DeMause has recently termed the Boston Tea Party the "real turning point" in a "group fantasy" (Seabrook, 1976). Puritan mothers, according to his interpretation, gave their children the harsh discipline traditional in England, but moderated it with a much greater measure of love, thus rearing children who possessed the psychic strength to be rebellious enough to challenge the mother country's rule. "England was jamming food down America's throat," DeMause asserts, "just as mothers used to jam pap down their babies' throats until they threw up." In the Boston Tea Party, "the colonists didn't take it lying down."

An historian of an earlier generation, Arthur M. Schlesinger, Sr., saw economic rather than child-rearing reasons underlying American confidence in challenging Great Britain, but these reasons also related to food. The colonies possessed a food supply that was not only self-sufficient, encouraging self-reliance, but that was also ample enough for export. In his famous pamphlet *Common Sense,* Thomas Paine wryly noted that a free American nation would "always have a market while eating is the custom of Europe" (Schlesinger, 1949, pp. 238–240).

Despite America's potential food abundance, the turmoil of the Revolutionary War led to shortages and drab diets, even in the armies. John Adams complained that "Our frying-pans and gridirons slay more than the sword" (Greene, 1943). At Valley Forge the troops came close to mutiny because of poor rations. George Washington besought his chief cook to devise a meal that might enhance morale. Combining tripe, vegetables, and peppercorns, the cook invented Philadelphia Pepper Pot, which boosted the spirit of the troops considerably (Hoag, 1976).

A broader and more significant impact came from the French alliance. French military chefs began to introduce new vegetables, the practice of serving vegetables in separate dishes, and new modes of cooking food. Moments of contretemps did occur. In Cambridge, Massachusetts, Nathaniel Tracy, revealing that a little knowledge of another country's cuisine can be a dangerous thing, entertained the admiral and officers of the French fleet for dinner and served them a soup containing whole frogs (Cummings, 1941, pp. 30–31).

Food and Uncle Sam, the major figure symbolizing the nation, bear a relationship. In 1774 when Paul Revere copied for an American magazine a British cartoon showing the British prime minister forcing a draught of tea down the throat of a reluctant America, the symbol for

America was a half-naked Indian maiden.† After independence, a descendant of Yankee Doodle named Brother Jonathan supplanted the maiden. In turn Brother Jonathan was pushed aside in the 1850's by Uncle Sam, who had first made his appearance in the War of 1812, patterned after a real man who supplied meat to the armies (Murrell, 1933). When Uncle Sam took over as a symbol, he looked just like the typical American male described by a procession of European aristocrats who wrote travel books about the United States. Americans ate heavy, starchy, salty, fat-fried food and suffered from a lack of milk, fresh fruits, and leafy vegetables. They also bolted their meals; the national motto, one traveler said, should be "gobble, gulp, and go." The result, in the words of another traveler, was "a nation of moody dyspeptics" (Cummings, 1941, pp. 4 and 23–24; Schlesinger, 1949, pp. 240–242). An American observer, writing for *Harper's* in 1856, concurred in the grim judgments of the travelers from abroad (Anonymous, 1856). "We are fast becoming . . . a nation of invalids," he charged. "Foreigners already effect to see in us a degenerate offspring of a nobler race, and with them a skeleton frame, a yellow-died bilious face, an uncomfortable dyspeptic expression, an uneasy spasmodic motion, and a general ghost-like charnel-house aspect, serve to make up a type of the species Yankee." This description would serve for countless cartoon renderings of Uncle Sam (Schlesinger, 1949, pp. 241–242).

Thus food and patriotism endlessly interact and intertwine. Nor should this be at all surprising. For, like the air we breathe, but in a more complex and varied way, food is an indispensable ingredient of life. Playing for us so crucial a role, food inevitably mingles with other important ingredients in life's vast pot. Schlesinger argued that, of countless clues to the past, food is "the most basic of all" (Schlesinger, 1949, p. 234). "Men must have food if they are to think and act. Here is a want which precedes and conditions other hopes, aims and achievements." If monistic interpretations of history would serve, a dietary interpretation of history would make the most persuasive sense.

II. THE VAST VARIETY OF FOOD IMAGE AND ROLE

On the individual level, the Gestalt psychologist Fritz Perls has suggested the act of eating as a revelation of the entire personality.

---

†The cartoon, in the American Antiquarian Society, was entitled "The Able Doctor, or America Swallowing the British Draught," and appeared in the June 1774 issue of the *Royal American Magazine*.

"How . . . do you eat?" queries a popularizer of this point of view. "How do you take the world into yourself? Do you choose food carefully for its aesthetic and nutritional value? Do you pay attention to taste and texture? Chew carefully? Read when eating? As you incorporate nourishment, so you will take in and digest the world which surrounds you" (Keen, 1970).

"If you doubt this," suggests the popularizer, "give full attention to your style of eating for one week and try drawing parallels to the way in which you read, listen, think, understand, and relate to persons."

Through the ages the central importance of food to man has led him to use food as a mirror held up to reveal nature—and indeed the cosmic realms beyond. A recent issue of *Speculum* contains an article by Patrick Gallacher entitled "Food, Laxatives, and Catharsis in Chaucer's Nun's Priest's Tale" (Gallacher, 1976). Gallacher makes manifest how, not only for Chaucer, but for numerous important theorists from Plato on into the fourteenth century, eating and elimination, and efforts to accomplish both so as to keep the humors balanced and thus retain or regain health, form a fundamental analogy for the most sweeping "metaphorical, moral, and theological meanings." Man's knottiest problems are confronted, such as the relation between "free will and divine foreknowledge." Starting with food, these august thinkers construct "a model of total continuous intelligibility in the universe."

The relation of food to the mind of God transcends the relation of food to patriotism, the theme with which I began. Countless other lesser linkages have existed between food and the diverse concerns of humankind. The way in which man perceived food until less than a century ago has tended to foster such linkages.

From the earliest times man has employed the same botanicals as both food and drugs. This was certainly true at both ends of the Fertile Crescent, in ancient Egypt and in Mesopotamia. "The borderline between dietetic and pharmacological treatment," Henry Sigerist wrote, "was by no means sharp" (Sigerist, 1951, p. 486). In the Western tradition, this fusion became especially strong because of the key role given by the Hippocratic corpus to diet in the physician's effort to help his patient (Sigerist, 1951, pp. 335–336; 1961, pp. 240–241). During the medieval and Renaissance periods, spices doubled as food condiments and as drugs. One scholar points out that "the terms spices, drugs, and aromatics were generic and interchangeable through all these years" (Guerra, 1966). The late sixteenth century English herbalist, John Gerard, summed up the double role: "In the first ages of the world, . . . [plants] were the ordinary meate of men, and have continued ever since of necessary use both for meates to maintaine life, and for medicine to recover health." (Gerard, 1636).*

The striking historical circumstance, in the consideration of the same products of nature in their dual role as both food and drugs, is that, when regarded as a drug, each product might fulfill a multitude of therapeutic functions, whereas when used as food, all products were believed to serve the same single purpose. Within a decade after the appearance of Gerard's herbal, Francis Bacon wrote: "In the body there are three degrees of that we receive into it, aliment, medicine and poison."† His use of the word "aliment" revealed the continuing potency of the Hippocratic assumption that all foods contained a single principle made available to the body by digestion to repair its tissues and provide it with energy. Nor did this received doctrine suffer major challenge and revision until the nineteenth century. In 1837 Ralph Waldo Emerson could still express the general view: "The human body can be nourished on any food" (Emerson, 1903).

The perspective that nutritionally, so to speak, all foods served the same purpose had important intellectual consequences.** First, it put a damper on the development of healthy suspicion that some disease conditions might be related to the *absence* from the diet of some type of food. To be sure, here and there some people acted empirically as if vaguely harboring such a suspicion, as in the eating of fish livers by the early fishing folk of northern Europe. The single aliment notion had a second important result: if all foods were equally valuable for nourishment, then a whole host of secondary and sometimes specious reasons could develop for choosing and for rejecting individual foods. Food has served also, among other roles, as taboo, as poison, as potent marvel, as status symbol, and as handmaiden to beauty.

All major religions have had to concern themselves with something as important as food, and many ancient taboos still exercise powerful influence. The Mosaic injunction to the Jews against pork is an example. The explanation that this taboo rested on an empirical base, a sensing that eating pork might harm the health, does not seem persuasive, because the link between infected pork and trichinosis is too remote for such observational detection. A more likely reason for the taboo, Magnus Pyke argues, lies in the circumstance that the Jews were a nomadic people and pigs did not herd easily over long distances (Pyke, 1968, p.

*First edition appeared in 1597.
†Bacon is cited under "Aliment" in the "Oxford English Dictionary."
**I first explored this effort to pattern ideas in food history in Blix (1970).

12). Jealous of more settled groups who could raise pigs and eat pork, the Jews put that meat beyond the pale. The power of religious food beliefs may be suggested by another example, a quotation from a Western physician who recently practiced in India among the vegetarian Hindus (Simeons, 1968). "I know from personal experience," he writes, "that it is not uncommon for an orthodox Hindu to prefer dying of pernicious anemia to taking liver extract."

Foods have been deemed poisonous in settings solely secular. In his herbal Gerard mentioned that recent import, the potato, brought from America by Sir Walter Raleigh, and cited a Burgundian belief that its tubers caused leprosy (Gerard, 1636). European farmers generally came to share this fear. The flesh-colored nodules extending their finger-like growths made men think of the deformed hands and pale skin of leprosy. Despite many efforts to dispel this groundless suspicion, nearly 2 centuries elapsed before the potato became an accepted English field crop (Pyke, 1968, pp. 25-27). And British America from whence the potato had gone to England, brought back from the mother country traces of the fear which the potato had generated. Even after eating potatoes became acceptable, a popular American superstition held that if one ate them every day he could not live out 7 years (Weigley, 1967). In Europe, turnips, beets, and tomatoes in their day, all faced initial hostility (Renner, 1944, pp. 166-70, and 204). Only after livestock had devoured them safely for a long time did people generally take them up.

Contrariwise, other novel and exotic foods and drinks grabbed the imagination of regions into which they were newly introduced as marvelous wonders, panaceas, foods for or from the gods. So it was with maple sugar and pineapple, asparagus and celery (Young, 1961). And so it was with coffee. The Arabs drank coffee as early as the year 1000, according to one chronicler, perhaps more as a medicine than as a drink (Renner, 1944, p. 215). When coffee first appeared in Western Europe, a somewhat therapeutic mantle garbed it. "It is said to be healthy when drunk hot . . . ," wrote Sir T. H. Herbert in 1626. "It destroys melancholy, dries the tears, softens anger and produces joyful feelings. Nevertheless, the Persians would not estimate it so highly, if there were not the tradition: Invented and produced by Gabriel for restoring the sinking Mohammed." In England and on the continent coffee drinking became a sudden vogue (Renner, 1944).

Tea, the drink destined to oust coffee as England's national drink, illustrates food as status symbol. In the early eighteenth century, the urban wealthy considered tea an occasional luxury. As the years passed, each lower economic level began to desire what those above in the hierarchy increasingly drank, and by 1850 tea had become the national beverage. During the same period a similar trend occurred with respect to bread. For centuries the higher the social ranking, the whiter the bread. In the early nineteenth century, urban workers aspired to the whiter bread of their betters and, as with tea, increasingly bought it. White bread and tea entered the diets of the poor not without great social cost. "What had been mere adjuncts at the tables of the wealthy," a recent scholar states, "now constituted virtually the total diet of those who could afford no more" (Burnett, 1966, pp. 2–3).

Standards of beauty also influenced attitudes toward food. In the romantic age of the nineteenth century, a particular vision of beauty prevailed. For both men and women, paleness, frailness, slenderness became the vogue. One might achieve such an appearance by falling victim to tuberculosis and gradually waning away, becoming more ethereal the closer death approached.* Remember the heroines of all those romantic operas. If a person were not destined to contract consumption, the same ideal of beauty could be achieved by dieting. In 1824 a British magazine published advice on "Beauty Training for Ladies" which forbade them to consume milk, cream, butter, cheese, fish, or any vegetable except potatoes (Burnett, 1966, pp. 56–57). Similar dietary counsel for the same esthetic purposes enjoyed a vogue in the United States (Cummings, 1941, p. 34).

These examples illustrate the numerous secondary roles which food could play in the minds of men when food as nourishment was restricted to the single alimental role. Nor would such a vast and complex body of food folklore wither away when, during the second half of the nineteenth century, food scientists split that one universal aliment into a nutritional trinity of protein, carbohydrates, and fats.

Food in its role as medicine also contributed mightily to the massive folk tradition. Indeed, therapeutic uses for foods treasured and employed in ancient Egypt and Mesopotamia persist into our own day (Sigerist, 1951, p. 248; 1961, p. 244). Garlic, for example, served as both food and medicine for the Egyptians, the Greeks, the Romans, for medieval man, and for man ever since (Raspadori, 1966). One of Dioscorides' (1959) "herbs with a sharpe qualitie," garlic cleared out the arteries, the Greek medical writer asserted. In the 1950's garlic could still perform this indispensable healing function, if one believed the spiel of a taxi driver turned food lecturer who traveled widely in these United States (Young, 1967, pp. 333–357). Within the last year or so, an airline magazine has run an article hailing garlic's mystic healing potency.

---

*Perceptive attention to the social image of tuberculosis is paid in Dubos (1952).

III. THE AMERICAN VERSION OF FOOD FOLKLORE

Before the day of scientific nutrition, the American version of food folklore acquired its own special hue of a coloration tinting food folklore throughout the Western world. "The atmosphere of the [Romantic] age," Grete de Francesco has written, "was favourable to all sorts of nature cures, and to the development of a new kind of imposture: a falsification of Nature through overemphasis on the natural" (Francesco, 1939). All over Europe and America, lay healers in rustic settings employed all sort of "natural" remedies, water being especially prominent. Among those bemoaning the increasing artificiality of life, there began a great preoccupation with the "natural" diet.

American cultural soil permitted such ideas to grow with unusual vigor. The romantic movement furnished one impetus, and there were many others, for a major multifaceted reform movement flourished in the United States during the second quarter of the nineteenth century. Freedom's ferment expanded political democracy during the age of Andrew Jackson and addressed the rights of women and of slaves (Tyler, 1944). Health practices, from the heroic bleeding and purging prescribed by orthodox practitioners to the tightly laced corsets decreed by fashion, met challenge from reformers (Walker, 1955).

Nor were the nation's eating habits exempt from criticism. That "back to nature" should constitute the major message in appeals for food reform conformed with the basic way by which citizens of the United States sought to explain themselves. The central developing myth envisioned the nation as a garden, indeed a new opportunity for mankind almost as significant as the original Garden of Eden (Smith, 1950; Lewis, 1955; Marx, 1964). The new Adam was the American yeoman farmer. In time, the historian Frederick Jackson Turner, a native of Wisconsin, converted the garden myth into respectable historiography. His frontier hypothesis, enunciated at the Chicago Columbian Exposition in 1893 (Turner, 1920), remained the virtually unchallenged explanation of American uniqueness for 40 years. The hypothesis attributed everything good about the nation to the frontier. The converse of this idealization of nature was suspicion of too much civilization, especially that site of noisy machinery, epidemic ailments, and processed foods, the city. Intellectuals and common citizens alike shared this distrust of urban life (White and White, 1962).

In the first great urbanizing–industrializing period, coinciding with those years of freedom's ferment, Sylvester Graham became the nation's first great champion of natural foods (Shryock, 1966). A clergyman, Graham found his ideal standard of diet in the Garden of Eden. "Fruits, nuts, farinaceous seeds, and roots," he wrote in 1839, "with perhaps some milk, and it may be honey... constituted the food of the first family and the first generation of mankind" (Graham, 1883, p. 316).* During this Golden Age, Graham said, no "artificial preparation" was necessary except for shelling the nuts.

The way Americans ate in Graham's day deserved rebuke, as I have already suggested. So Graham made much sense. But some of his ideas went far astray. He made a panacea of bread baked from a kind of flour that still bears his name. He termed all meat taboo. And he came close to suggesting that his dietary regimen might bring back the Garden of Eden. "The simpler, plainer, and more natural the food of man is," Graham wrote, "... the more healthy, vigorous, and long-lived will be the body, the more perfect will be all the senses, and the more active and powerful may the intellectual and moral faculties be rendered by suitable cultivation" (Graham, 1883, p. 309).

Graham's doctrines had much influence on the dietary practice of new religious sects arising in the nation and shortly upon commerce as well. Ronald Numbers has recently published a biography of Ellen G. White, the founder of one of those new sects, the Seventh Day Adventists (Numbers, 1976). The dry cereal industry that arose in Battle Creek, Michigan, a center of Adventist strength, initially promoted itself with food reform ideas. That form of corn flakes later known as Post Toasties first bore the name of Elijah's Manna (Carson, 1957).

Packaged cereals formed one sector of an increasingly important processed food industry, made possible by advances in science and technology and made necessary by burgeoning urban population, remote from the gardens and orchards of rural America. The technology often revealed inadequacies, and the processors sometimes exhibited ethical shortcomings which they shared with other types of entrepreneurs during the Gilded Age. A vigorous critique arose, attacking food adulteration that might go so far as to fabricate so-called "strawberry jam" from apple scraps and hayseeds, and condemning the use of a host of new and perhaps dangerous preservatives. Food, in this extreme of agility, could equal fraud (Cummings, 1941, pp. 96–103; Keuchel, 1972, 1973; Anderson, 1958).

Some critics, recognizing the necessity for processed foods in an increasingly urbanized society, sought to restrain abuses through the enactment of pure food and drug laws. A small but vocal minority, however, echoed Sylvester Graham's plea of half a century earlier to return to nature.

*Graham's lectures were originally published in 1839.

Prime prophet of this doctrine during the early twentieth century was a Missouri farm boy who preached how to go back to nature in the city (Macfadden and Gauvreau, 1953; Young, 1977). Bernarr Macfadden learned better than had Graham the technique of self-promotion. He set up a magazine called *Physical Culture* to propagandize his version of nature's way, and on the streets of New York City he exhibited his own muscled body as his most potent advertisement. His regimen, long on exercise, short on clothing, condemned "the baneful habit of over-eating" (Macfadden, 1903). Like Graham, Macfadden thought ill of meat and well of raw vegetables. The carrot became for him a sort of trademark.

IV. THE NEWER NUTRITION AND ITS MANIPULATION

Macfadden, who had attended grade school only briefly, drew his ideas about food from the vast body of popular lore that had developed through the centuries when nutritional concepts were simple. He propagated his gospel during the very years that nutrition was becoming established as a true science. "In 1900," Elmer McCollum has said, "we were [still] almost blind to the relation of food to health" (McCollum, 1957). The single universal aliment had become a trinity, but as of 1900 observations and research were just building toward an awareness of the infinitely greater complexity that existed in the nexus between food and health. Charles Rosenberg (1976) has recently helped clarify how difficult a research frontier the nutritional borderlands were to enter upon. Professional specialization had already reached the point at which the clinical physician and the organic chemist did not know enough about what the other was doing, about what techniques the other was using. America's initial contributions to the newer nutrition, the discovery of vitamin A, for example, came not from medical men concerned about deficiency diseases, but from organic chemists at agricultural experiment stations concerned about the feeding of cattle. Even after early successes by the organic chemists, physicians assimilated only slowly the concept of dietary deficiency diseases. The germ theory attributed illness to the presence of unwanted invaders from outside the body, and research concentrated on tracking down all such intruders. To think of diseases as caused by an absence in the body of elusive substances that should be there required a contrasting mind-set only gradually acquired. Before this audience there is no need to trace the nutritional revolution to its major plateau about 1940, by which time more than forty vitamins and other nutrients had been proved necessary for an adequate diet in man. For the nutritional scientist, food had assumed the role of multiple nutrient.

What of the layman, be he ordinary mortal, cultist, or wily entrepreneur? For him also the nutrition revolution ushered in the dawn of a new day. To the great mythic storehouse deriving from ancient alimental days, a second vast vision relating food to health became added, bearing the imprimatur of science. Too complex for easy grasping, the new doctrine, like the older simpler one, could be easily twisted and distorted. Its basic premise readily provoked alarm. Even while eating enough of what you usually ate, you might get sick. To stay healthy some mysterious extras might be needed. You couldn't see them and you couldn't taste them, but without them you might acquire horrendous symptoms or else just wither away.

Grant that Graham and Macfadden believed fervently in their own food gospels, both the old lore and the new science offered boundless opportunities for shady commercial exploitation. Before the first World War, a form of dried cottage cheese, parading under the name of Sanatogen, was marketed claiming to be "The Re-Creator of Lost Health," "a nerve and tissue food for which the brain, spinal cord and the nerves have a special predilection" (American Medical Association, 1912). During the 1920's the word vitamin appeared with increasing frequency in food advertising, even for chocolate bars (Young, 1967, p. 335). Multivitamin panaceas began to receive widespread promotion, one of them called Catalyn, made of wheat bran, milk sugar, and epinephrine, its label boasting potency in all vitamins from A through G and claiming to cure high and low blood pressure, Bright's disease, dropsy, and goiter (U.S. v. Lee, 1939).

After World War II a new wave of questionable promotions got under way. The wartime enrichment program decreed by the Food and Nutrition Board of the National Academy of Sciences had further publicized vitamins, expanding public interest. The Food and Drug Administration, using new powers acquired in the New Deal revision of its basic law, began a vigorous campaign against traditional forms of quackery. Some hard-pressed promoters moved into the greener pastures of "nutrition."

To succeed most effectively, these vitamin vendors needed to undermine faith in the regular food supply. They sought to do this through books, pamphlets, mail-order catalogs, radio and television broadcasts, lectures, door-to-door pitches, and conversations in health food stores (Young, 1967, pp. 333–359). An integrated myth emerged of considerable persuasiveness: improper diet caused all disease; food wasn't what it used to be because of worn-out soil; chemical fertilizers poisoned the land and hence the food grown on it; pesticides heaped on more poison;

food processing destroyed nutrients; you might not realize you were sick, but you really were, suffering from subclinical deficiencies (Bell, 1958). But a way lay open to counter all these hazards: take wonder mixes of ingredients and stay out of "the marble orchard." These mixtures often wedded the ancient lore and the new science. Garlic continued to possess its marvelous curative properties known to the Egyptians. Vitamins soared beyond the value attributed to them by nutritional scientists and offered laymen a magical route to super-health and super-happiness. Promoters were clever too at turning an occasional true problem of the regular food supply to their account: an instance of excessive pesticide residue, some problems with a food additive, the discovery of mercury in fish.

Events of the 1960's expanded the nation's receptivity to food faddism and charlatanism. For then we saw, especially among the young, an upsurge of neoromanticism, a wave of disillusion with civilization and its discontents, a skepticism of big government, big business, big science, and, indeed, of the intellectual approach underlying science, rational thought. This temper drew strength from the fact that big science had invented the atomic bomb and environment-threatening chemicals, although the mood had been coming on for a long time. When reason is distrusted, unreason becomes glamorized. Romantics, depending on intuitions, always worry about their health, and are ready to intuit a variety of unorthodox cures. Romanticism, as we have seen from earlier eras, leads back to nature—in our day, sometimes all the way back to a remote rural commune, sometimes only so far as so-called organic foods for sale at a health food store. In such a climate, billions have been made by promoters preying on the susceptible.

On a case-by-case basis, the Food and Drug Administration attacked the largest and most outrageous pseudonutritional promotions right from the start (Young, 1967, pp. 206–208 and 338–359). Since World War II the regulatory task has proved especially difficult, because such a high proportion of the exaggeration has consisted of the spoken word. A printed label, primly circumspect, acquires overtones of magic when interpreted by a spieler or a clerk in a health food store. I have a bottle of multivitamin tablets given me by a student to whose uncle it was sold. Recovering from a broken leg, the uncle had hobbled to his front door to confront an itinerant salesman who took one look and then insisted that the vitamins he vended would speed the mending of the fracture. For a time after tape recorders came on the market, the courts permitted the FDA to present as evidence recordings of false and misleading claims made orally by promoters and recorded without their knowledge. In due course such recordings came to be considered unwarranted invasions of privacy. Thus enormous difficulties continue to plague regulators.

V. THE VITAMIN AMENDMENTS OF 1976

Indeed, the most recent chapter of the story seems to me to possess elements of tragedy. Powerful popular currents, shrewdly exploited by special interest groups, have led to a significant weakening of protection against promoters of nutritional nonsense. The neoromantic tide with its back-to-nature currents has been mentioned. Suspicion of bureaucracy has also mounted mightily in the last few years, certainly for some legitimate reasons, with the impact of suspicion, however, falling on the heads of both the unjust and the just. The ecological movement, while sorely needed, at times has magnified individual incidents and produced exaggerated alarm. In such an atmosphere purveyors of the food myth have found an increasing number of common citizens ready to be persuaded that our ordinary food supply is dangerously tainted and that only magical mixtures of twentieth century vitamins and dawn-age botanicals can save the nation (National Analysts, Inc., 1972).* Thus food with agility assumes a Janus-image as poison and perfector.

Striving to combat the growing market which depends on deceptions and distortions relating to food, the Food and Drug Administration has itself fallen victim to the power of the health food industry and the vast number of American citizens who have been persuaded to swallow whole the nutrition myth. In 1962 the FDA sought to bolster the case-by-case method by revising its regulations, 2 decades old and seriously outmoded, so as to introduce scientific rationality into the marketing of vitamins, minerals, and other dietary supplements. Some 54,000 pieces of mail flooded the FDA opposing its proposals, including 40,000 protesting postcards generated by the major trade association in the health food industry, the National Heath Federation (Public Health and Environment Subcommittee, 1973, pp. 1–5). A new version of the proposed regulations issued in 1966 was the subject of marathon hearings between 1968 and 1970, amassing 32,000 pages of testimony. In 1973 the FDA published final regulations, and elements of the health food industry took the FDA to court. In due course a Circuit Court of Appeals re-

---

*According to a survey sponsored by federal agencies, three out of four adult Americans were persuaded that, no matter how nutritionally adequate their diets, extra vitamins would provide them with increased energy.

quired some modification of the regulations and ruled that one issue be given renewed hearings, held this year (National Nutritional Foods Association *v.* Food and Drug Administration, 1974; Davidson, 1976). But in the main the court supported both the FDA's authority and its approach to regulating special dietary supplements. Indeed, the Court asserted that some of the most effective evidence showing the need for new regulations came from the 50,000 letters the FDA had received protesting the regulations.

The battle, however, had shifted to another front. No doubt anticipating that the courts might let the FDA set standards which, if not met, automatically brought products into violation of the law, the health food industry turned its attention to the Congress. A new law was needed, the industry asserted, because bureaucrats intended to trample the consumer's freedom of choice, depriving him of the right to buy vitamins without a prescription from a doctor (Public Health and Environment Subcommittee, 1973, pp. 5–7). Such charges were untrue, except for potentially toxic levels of vitamins A and D. Under the new regulations, consumers would retain freedom to buy individual vitamins other than A and D and to purchase other single food supplements at any level of strength (Public Health and Environment Subcommittee, 1973, pp. 11–18; Anonymous, 1974). For multi-ingredient products, to be sure, standards of identity would provide for more rational combinations than those on the market, the yardstick of rationality derived from the Recommended Daily Allowances as determined by the Food and Nutrition Board of the National Academy of Sciences. The regulations also would decree more informative labeling to help consumers buy more wisely.

Why did the Congress respond so favorably to the health food industry's attack upon the FDA? For one thing, Congressmen were buried under an avalance of mail. The industry generated over two million letters—the issue was said to have spurred more mail than Watergate—protesting the FDA regulations and demanding a law to stay the agency's hand (Kline and Davis, 1975; Anonymous, 1973). Moreover, we may assume, like some of their constituents, key members of the Congress had been beguiled into putting personal trust in facets of the nutrition myth. Also, skepticism of bureaucratic agencies was rising in the legislative branch. So during 1973 various bills were introduced, one of them co-sponsored by over 150 members of the House of Representatives (Congressional Record, 1973; Young, 1974). The bill would not only negate the FDA's proposed regulations, but would also curtail seriously the agency's legislative authority to regulate food supplements, given it by the Congress in the law of 1938. One such bill received Senate approval during the 93rd Congress (Congressional Record, 1974). The size of the vote indicated the way the wind was blowing: the bill passed 81 to 10.

In the 94th Congress, a somewhat revised Senate version of the vitamin bill was attached as a rider to a "must" bill which had almost no opposition, the National Heart and Lung Act. The House heart and lung bill passed without the vitamin rider, but the conference committee accepted it, as did, in April 1976, both Houses of the Congress. The President quickly signed the measure into law (U.S. Senate, 1975; Congressional Record, 1975, 1976).*

The Congress can not be said to have given the issue the consideration it deserved. The devious parliamentary strategy indicates this. Moreover, the 94th Congress did not even hold public hearings on the bill, despite opposition to the food supplement measure from such a wide spectrum of groups as the American Society of Clinical Nutrition, the Committee on Nutrition of the American Academy of Pediatrics, the American Association of Retired Persons, Consumers Union, and Ralph Nader's associates (Public Health and Environment Subcommittee 1973, pp. 52–56; Health Subcommittee, 1974; Holliday, 1975; Butterworth, 1975). A trade newsletter deemed the course of events "one of the 'legislative miracles' in a lifetime" (F-D-C Reports, 1975).

The 1976 amendments to the 1938 act represent the first retrogressive step in federal legislation respecting self-treatment wares since the initial Pure Food and Drugs Act became law in 1906. The amendments will prevent the Food and Drug Administration from: "Limiting the potency of vitamins and minerals in dietary supplements to nutritionally useful levels; classifying a vitamin or mineral preparation as a "drug" because it exceeds a nutritionally rational or useful potency; requiring the presence in dietary supplements of nutritionally essential vitamins and minerals; [and] prohibiting the inclusion in dietary supplements of useless ingredients with no nutritional value" (Food and Drug Administration, 1976; Hopkins, 1976).

During the course of this legislative adventure, Food and Drug Commissioner Alexander M. Schmidt spoke of the then pending bill as "a charlatan's dream" (Food and Drug Administration, 1976).

The biochemical interrelations in the human body of what we term foods and what we deem drugs, the theme of our symposium, constitutes one front of the ongoing, complex, careful, scientific inquiry regarding nutrition. That inquiry, it has been the burden of my remarks to illustrate, takes place in a bigger real world, one in which food has been and

*The enacted bill became Public Law 94-278.

will be a kaleidoscopic concept, the facets of which possess great power to spur the actions of men, often in bizarre ways inharmonious with the tenets prevailing in a nutrition laboratory.

REFERENCES

American Medical Association. (1912). "Nostrums and Quackery," pp. 470–478. Am. Med. Assoc., Chicago, Illinois.

Anderson, O. E. (1958). "The Health of a Nation: Harvey W. Wiley and the Fight for Pure Food." Univ. of Chicago Press, Chicago, Illinois.

Anonymous. (1856). Why we get sick. *Harper's Mon.* **13,** 643.

Anonymous. (1973). Vitamin buffs, FDA may clash. *Atlanta Constitution* (June 25), p. 9-A.

Anonymous. (1974). Vitamins, minerals, and FDA. *FDA Consum.* **7** (Sep.), 18–19.

Bell, J. N. (1958). Let 'em eat hay. *Today's Health* **36** (Sep.), 22–25 and 66–68.

Blix, G., ed. (1970). "Food Cultism and Nutrition Quackery," Symp. Swed. Nutr. Found., Vol. 8, pp. 9–21. Almqvist & Wiksell, Stockholm.

Burnett, J. (1966). "Plenty and Want." Nelson, London.

Butterworth, C. E. (1975). Letter from American Society for Clinical Nutrition to members of Congress. (July 8).

Carson, G. (1957). "Cornflake Crusade," pp. 145 and 196–197. Rinehart, New York.

Congressional Record. (1973). (93rd Congress, 1st Session) **119,** 53, 40936.

Congressional Record. (1974). (93rd Congress, 2d Session) **120,** 32376.

Congressional Record. (1975). (94th Congress, 1st Session) **121,** H10074, S21866.

Congressional Record. (1976). (94th Congress, 2d Session) **122,** H2796, S5154, S3244, S5507, H3381.

Cummings, R. O. (1941). "The American and His Food." Univ. of Chicago Press, Chicago, Illinois.

Davidson, D. J. (1976). "Food for Special Dietary Uses." Food and Drug Administration, Rockville, Maryland.

Dioscorides (1959). "The Greek Herbal of Dioscorides" (R. T. Gunther, ed.), pp. 187–191. Hafner, New York.

Dubos, R. J. (1952). "The White Plague." Little, Brown, Boston, Massachusetts.

Emerson, R. W. (1903). The American scholar. *In* Emerson, "Nature, Addresses and Lectures," p. 92. Houghton, Boston, Massachusetts.

Evans, C. (1903–1959). "American Bibliography," Vol. 11, p. 11. Columbia Press, Chicago, Illinois.

Food and Drug Administration. (1976). "FDA Talk Paper." FDA, Rockville, Maryland.

F-D-C Reports. (1975). **37** (Sep. 1), p. 5.

Francesco, G. (1939). "The Power of the Charlatan." Yale Univ. Press, New Haven, Connecticut.

Gallacher, P. (1976). Food, laxatives, and catharsis in Chaucer's Nun's Priest's Tale. *Speculum* **51,** 49–68.

Gerard, J. (1636). "The Herball or Generall Historie of Plantes." A. Islip, J. Norton and R. Whitakers, London.

Graham, S. (1883). "Lectures on the Science of Human Life," p. 316. Fowler & Wells, New York.

Greene, E. B. (1943). "The Revolutionary Generation," p. 253. Macmillan, New York.

Guerra, F. (1966). Drugs from the Indies and the political economy of the sixteenth century. *In* International Academy of the History of Medicine, "Materia Medica in the XVIth Century." (M. Florkin, ed.), pp. 29–30. Pergamon, Oxford.

Health Subcommittee. (1974). "Food Supplement Legislation, 1974" (Hearings on S. 2801 and S. 3867). Committee on Labor and Public Welfare, U.S. Senate, 93rd Congress, 2nd session.

Hoag, D. R. (1976). The random time machine. *Atlanta Journal and Constitution* (June 20), p. 15-B.

Holliday, M. A. (1975). Letter from Committee on Nutrition, American Academy of Pediatrics, to members of Congress (June 19).

Hopkins, H. (1976). Regulating vitamins and minerals. *FDA Consum.* **10** (July–Aug), pp. 10–11.

Keen, S. (1970). "To a Dancing God," p. 50. Harper, New York.

Keuchel, E. F. (1972). Master of the art of canning: Baltimore, 1860–1900. Md. Hist. Mag. **67,** 351–362.

Keuchel, E. F. (1973). Science, technology, and food preservation. *In* "Essays in American History in Honor of James C. Malin" (B. J. Williams, ed.), pp. 163–178. Coronado Press, Lawrence, Kansas.

Kline, O. L., and Davis, G. K. (1975). Letter to members of the American Institute of Nutrition (Sept. 2).

Lewis, R. W. B. (1955). "The American Adam." Univ. of Chicago Press, Chicago, Illinois.

McCollum, E. V. (1957). "A History of Nutrition," p. 421. Houghton, Boston, Massachusetts.

Macfadden, B. (1903). Health made and preserved by daily exercise. *Cosmopolitan* **34,** 705–712.

Macfadden, M., and Gauvreau, E. (1953). "Dumbbells and Carrot Strips." Holt, New York.

Marx, L. (1964). "The Machine in the Garden." Oxford Univ. Press, London and New York.

Murrell, W. (1933). "A History of American Graphic Humor," Vol. 1, pp. 132–133. Whitney Museum of American Art, New York.

National Analysts, Inc. (1972). "A Study of Health Practices and Opinions," pp. 11–12. Natl. Tech. Inf. Serv., Springfield, Virginia.

National Nutritional Foods Association *v.* Food and Drug Administration. (1974). 504 Fed. (2d) 761.

Numbers, R. L. (1976). "Prophetess of Health." Harper, New York.

Public Health and Environment Subcommittee. (1973). "Vitamin, Mineral, and Diet Supplements." (Committee print No. 11). Committee on Interstate and Foreign Commerce, U.S. House of Representatives, 93d Congress, 1st Session.

Pyke, M. (1968). "Food and Society." John Murray, London.

Raspadori, F. (1966). Un medicamento sempre usato: l'aglio. *Medicina nei Secoli* **3,** 8–23.

Renner, H. D. (1944). "The Origin of Food Habits." Faber & Faber, London.

Rosenberg, C. E. (1976). "No Other Gods: On Science and American Social Thought," pp. 185–195. Johns Hopkins Univ. Press, Baltimore, Maryland.

Schlesinger, A. M. (1949). "Paths to the Present," Macmillan, New York.

Seabrook, C. (1976). Psycho-historian says colonial mothers caused war. *Atlanta Journal and Constitution* (Feb. 29), p. 3-G.

Shryock, R. H. (1966). Sylvester Graham and the popular health movement, 1830–1870. *In* Shyrock, "Medicine in America," pp. 111–125. Johns Hopkins Press, Baltimore, Maryland.

Sigerist, H. E. (1951). "A History of Medicine," Vol. 1. Oxford Univ. Press, London and New York.

Sigerist, H. E. (1961). "A History of Medicine," Vol. 2. Oxford Univ. Press, London and New York.

Simeons, A. T. W. (1968). "Food: Facts, Foibles, and Fancy," p. 56. Funk & Wagnalls, New York.

Smith, H. N. (1950). "Virgin Land." Harvard Univ. Press, Cambridge, Massachusetts.

Sonneck, O. G. T. (1972). "Report on 'The Star-Spangled Banner' 'Hail Columbia' 'America' 'Yankee Doodle'," pp. 142 and 195. Dover, New York.

Turner, F. J. (1920). The significance of the frontier in American history. *In* Turner, "The Frontier in American History," pp. 1–38. Holt, New York.

Tyler, A. F. (1944). "Freedom's Ferment." Univ. of Minnesota Press, Minneapolis.

U.S. Senate. (1975). "National Biomedical Heart, Blood Vessel, Lung, Blood and Research Training Act of 1975." Senate Report 94-509, 94th Congress, 1st session.

U.S. *v.* Lee. (1939). 107 Fed. (2d) 522.

Walker, W. B. (1955). "The Health Reform Movement in the United States, 1830–1870." Johns Hopkins University, Baltimore, Maryland (unpublished doctoral dissertation).

Weigley, E. S. (1967). Food in the days of the Declaration of Independence. *In* "Essays on History of Nutrition and Dietetics," (A. M. Beeuwkes, E. N. Todhunter, and E. S. Weigley, compilers), p. 152. Am. Diet. Assoc., Chicago, Illinois.

White, M., and White, L. (1962). "The Intellectual versus the City." Harvard Univ. Press, Cambridge, Massachusetts.

Young, J. H. (1961). "The Toadstool Millionaires," p. 171. Princeton Univ. Press, Princeton, New Jersey.

Young, J. H. (1967). "The Medical Messiahs." Princeton Univ. Press, Princeton, New Jersey.

Young, J. H. (1974). "American Self-Dosage Medicines," pp. 46–50. Coronado Press, Lawrence, Kansas.

Young, J. H. (1977). Macfadden, Bernarr. *In* "Dictionary of American Biography, Supplement Five" (J. A. Garraty, ed.), pp. 452–454. Charles Scribner's Sons, New York.

Section I

DRUG EFFECTS ON NUTRIENT INTAKE, FUNCTION, AND REQUIREMENT

2

Appetite Regulation and Its Modulation by Drugs

ANN C. SULLIVAN and LORRAINE CHENG

I. INTRODUCTION

Feeding is so crucial to the survival of the species that we should not be surprised at the multitude of regulatory tactics involved in the control of appetite. Feeding behavior certainly reflects a multiplicity of inputs and the control of appetite is undoubtedly regulated by a succession of oral, gastric, intestinal, parenteral, and ultimately central processes. Peripheral (outside the brain) factors influence feeding and include taste, smell, stomach distention, osmoreception, gastrointestinal and

21

hepatic chemoreception, metabolites, ions, hormones, and temperature. Metabolic processes influence, coordinate, and integrate peripheral factors with neural elements and the animal starts, continues, or stops eating. Regulation of food intake is believed to encompass both a short-term and a long-term component. The former consists of "factors" which influence and modify individual meals, i.e., short-term satiety, and the latter includes "factors" which reflect the state of body nutrient stores and are concerned with the long-term regulation of feeding. Normal feeding behavior is intimately linked to energy balance, and animals maintain an optimal level of body weight through appropriate alterations in caloric intake. Hyperphagic obesity and anorexia nervosa represent the two major types of feeding disorders, involving significant overeating and undereating in relation to energy requirements, respectively. Anorectic agents decrease food intake and are employed in the treatment of hyperphagic obesity; orectic agents stimulate appetite and are frequently used in a therapeutic regimen for anorexia nervosa. The majority of drugs that have been demonstrated to influence food intake apparently act centrally by influencing various components involved in the neural regulation of appetite. However, other agents might reduce appetite by acting predominantly at peripheral sites believed to be involved in feeding control.

The following review presents current concepts of the neural and peripheral components of appetite regulation as well as metabolic elements which might integrate and influence these areas. Disorders of appetite regulation will be discussed, and anorectic and orectic drugs affecting appetite will be described with emphasis on their mechanism(s) and site(s) of action.

II. REGULATION OF FOOD INTAKE

A. Neural Regulation of Food Intake

The vast majority of investigations on the regulation of food intake have centered around two major syndromes of abnormal feeding: ventromedial hypothalamic hyperphagia (Brobeck et al., 1943) and lateral hypothalamic aphagia (Anand and Brobeck, 1951). From these studies the concept of a bilateral "satiety center" localized in the ventromedial hypothalamus, and a bilateral "feeding center" located in the lateral hypothalamus emerged (Stellar, 1954). This model proposed that the motivation to eat was proportional to the activity of the "feeding center" in the lateral hypothalamus, and that the "satiety center" in the ventromedial hypothalamus influenced feeding by exerting inhibitory effects on the "feeding center". These centers are believed to collect neural and chemical information regarding the nutritional state of the animal, and to receive input from peripheral sources as well as other regions of the brain (Grossman, 1975).

The involvement of neurotransmitters in these two abnormal syndromes, and in normal appetite regulation in general, has emerged from the development of several important techniques: (1) application of neurotransmitters directly into specific sites in the brain, thus extending the classical work of Grossman (1960, 1962a,b); (2) anatomic visualization and identification of monoamine systems in the brain (Anden *et al.*, 1966); and (3) selective destruction of catecholamine systems in the brain (Ungerstedt, 1971). Through the applications of these techniques, spe-

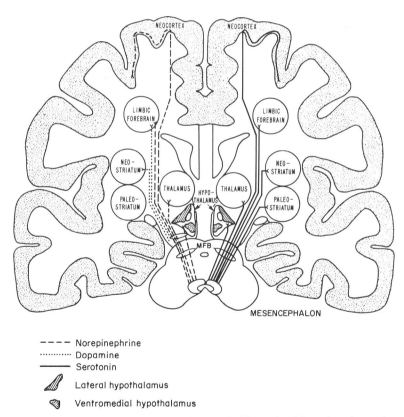

Fig. 1. Diagrammatic representation of the brain, illustrating biogenic amine pathways of three major neurotransmitters (norepinephrine, dopamine, serotonin) and two important anatomical locations (lateral hypothalamus and ventromedial hypothalamus) involved in appetite regulation.

cific transmitter systems in the brain are believed to be critical links in the transmission of various types of information to the aforementioned appetite centers, and a more integrated view of the neural regulation of food intake has emerged. The anatomical location of the important brain centers involved in appetite regulation (ventromedial and lateral hypothalamic areas) and the neurotransmitter nerve fiber systems (norepinephrine, dopamine, and serotonin) are illustrated in Fig. 1. The following discussion will describe these brain centers and the neurotransmitters believed to be involved in appetite control. Several excellent reviews (Epstein, 1971; Hoebel, 1971; Rabin, 1972; Baile, 1974; Panksepp, 1974; Grossman, 1975; Teitelbaum and Wolgin, 1975) should be consulted for further details.

1. *Brain Sites*

a. Ventromedial Hypothalamus. As first reported by Hetherington and Ranson (1940), small bilateral lesions in the ventromedial hypothalamus of rats produced overeating which led to obesity. The marked increase in body weight produced by ventromedial hypothalamic lesions is illustrated in Fig. 2. Several well-documented cases of patients with hypothalamic tumors in this same area, who developed hyperphagia and obesity were reported (Reeves and Plum, 1969; Heldenberg *et al.*, 1972). The ventromedial hypothalamus is considered an inhibitory "satiety center" since stimulation of this site resulted in cessation of feeding, while its destruction produced overeating (Table I). Hyperphagia ceased when the lateral hypothalamus was subsequently destroyed bilaterally, suggesting that the ventromedial hypothalamic region inhibited activity in the lateral hypothalamus (Anand and Brobeck, 1951).

Many investigators have analyzed the behavioral and biochemical results of ventromedial hypothalamic lesions in animals, partly because remarkable similarities existed between the behavior of obese humans and the behavior of animals that became obese after lesions of the ventromedial hypothalamus (Nisbett, 1968, 1972a; Schacter, 1971). Rats with ventromedial lesions eventually reached a "static" phase and no longer continually increased their food intake; body weight was maintained at a high but stable value. When starved back to normal body weight, however, rats returned to a "dynamic state" (similar to that observed after lesioning) and became hyperphagic (Brobeck, 1946). If prior to lesioning, an animal was made obese either by insulin administration or force-feeding, the subsequent destruction of the ventromedial hypothalamus caused little overeating and weight gain (Hoebel and

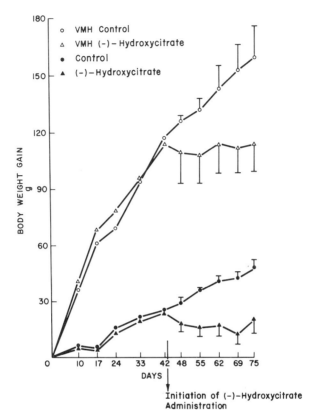

Fig. 2. Comparison of the effect of (—)-hydroxycitrate on cumulative body weight gain in ventromedial hypothalamic-lesioned and nonlesioned rats. The ventromedial hypothalamic region of 10 rats was destroyed bilaterally by electrocauterization with radiofrequency current. Ten lesioned rats and 15 nonlesioned rats were fed ad libitum a 70% glucose diet for 42 days, and on day 43 one-half of each group was given (—)-hydroxycitrate, trisodium salt (52.6 mmoles/kg diet) as a dietary admixture for 33 days. Vertical bar indicates the SE of the mean. (Sullivan and Triscari, 1977).

TABLE I
Food Intake Following Experimental Manipulation[a]

Brain region	Surgical or chemical lesion	Electrical or chemical stimulation
Ventromedial hypothalamus	↑	↓
Lateral hypothalamus	↓	↑

[a] Adapted from Epstein (1960).

Teitelbaum, 1966). These studies supported a theory first proposed by Kennedy (1950) which stated that the primary regulation performed by the ventromedial nucleus was stabilization of body fat stores. Thus, the major effect of ventromedial hypothalamic lesions was to elevate a control level for body weight or adiposity, i.e., the hyperphagia resulting from these lesions represented an adaptive response to a lesion-induced elevation in a body weight "set point" (see Section II, C, 2). The long-term regulation of feeding might reside within the ventromedial hypothalamus, and perhaps be organized around an anabolic intermediate of glucose (Panksepp, 1972, 1973, 1974). It was postulated that when body nutrient stores were low, neurons within the ventromedial hypothalamus stimulated appetite, and these neurons reduced appetite when nutrient stores were high. Hypothalamic mechanisms involved in the regulation of body weight were discussed recently (Keesey and Powley, 1975).

Current investigations suggest that some or perhaps all of the effects of the lesions in the ventromedial hypothalamus may be due to an interruption of noradrenergic fibers. Selective destruction of the ventral noradrenergic bundle which supplies the hypothalamus with most of its noradrenergic terminals, either electrolytically or with 6-hydroxydopamine (a neurotoxin that selectively destroys catecholaminergic neurons), produced overeating leading to obesity (Ahlskog and Hoebel, 1973), although the obesity was not as extensive as that observed after lesioning the ventromedial hypothalamus (Ahlskog, 1973). Additionally, some interesting behavioral differences existed between the ventromedial hypothalamic-lesioned and ventral noradrenergic bundle-lesioned rats (Teitelbaum and Wolgin, 1975).

b. Lateral Hypothalamus. As first demonstrated by Anand and Brobeck (1951), destruction of the lateral hypothalamus in rats produced aphagia (Table I) and adipsia, which might be fatal unless the animals were properly nursed through these early periods. Chemical or electrical stimulation of the lateral hypothalamus produced eating (Table I). Lateral hypothalamic-lesioned rats recovered feeding and drinking in an apparently invariable sequence of stages (stage 1, aphagia and adipsia; stage II, anorexia and adipsia; stage III, adipsia with dehydration aphagia; stage IV, partial recovery) (Teitelbaum and Epstein, 1962). These successive stages through which the lateral hypothalamic-lesioned animal passed prior to establishing free feeding and weight maintenance are believed to constitute a process of neural recovery, involving either the participation of surrounding lateral hypothalamic tissue (Teitelbaum and Epstein, 1962) or a reencephalization process which closely paralleled the development of feeding in infancy (Teitelbaum *et al.*, 1969). Sensory and motor dysfunctions as a result of lateral hypothalamic lesions were suggested to contribute significantly to the impaired feeding and drinking behavior (Baillie and Morrison, 1963; Balagura *et al.*, 1969; Marshall *et al.*, 1971). The recovered lateral hypothalamic-lesioned animals appeared to have adjusted to a new body weight "set point" (Fig. 3). These rats maintained their body weight at a reduced level, and successfully defended this new level against various dietary challenges (Powley and Keesey, 1970; Keesey and Boyle, 1973). Several clinical cases involving hypothalamic damage [e.g., tumors (Lewin *et al.*, 1972; Heron and Johnston, 1976), lesions (White and Hain, 1959), and demyelination of the lateral hypothalamus (Kamalian *et al.*, 1975)] were reported to be associated with anorexia.

The possibility that the lateral hypothalamic syndrome might be due to interruption of fiber systems rather than destruction of cellular components in the area was emphasized in several studies (Morgane, 1961; Gold, 1967). Lesions of the substantia nigra induced electrolytically or by injections of 6-hydroxydopamine produced aphagia and adipsia, thus implicating the nigrostriatal pathway which ascends through the lateral hypothalamus (Ungerstadt, 1971).

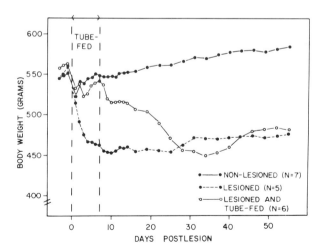

Fig. 3. The effect of force-feeding on the duration of anorexia in lateral hypothalamic-lesioned rats. Force-feeding was used to maintain the weight of the lesioned and tube-fed group at a control level for the first week following surgery. This group was then permitted to feed ad libitum. The nonlesioned and lesioned groups were permitted to feed ad libitum throughout the experiment (Keesey *et al.*, 1976).

c. **Extrahypothalamic Sites.** Possible involvement of several extrahypothalamic structures in the regulation of food intake was reviewed extensively (Grossman, 1972, 1975) and is briefly summarized below. Hyperphagia was reported after lesions in the frontal lobe (Richter and Hawkes, 1939), thalamus (Schreiner *et al.*, 1953), mammillary region (Graff and Stellar, 1962), periaqueductal gray of the brainstem (Skultety and Gary, 1962), amygdala (Grossman and Grossman, 1963), after surgical transection of the anterior, lateral, and posterior connections of the medial hypothalamus (Grossman and Grossman, 1970), and following surgical or chemical lesion in the ventral noradrenergic bundle (Ahlskog and Hoebel, 1973). Aphagia and adipsia were observed after lesions in the globus pallidus (Morgane, 1961), midbrain tegmentum (Gold, 1967), substantia nigra (Ungerstedt, 1971), amygdala (Pubols, 1966), and after lesions in the lower brainstem or basal thalamus which interrupt projections of the trigeminal nerve (Zeigler and Karten, 1974).

2. *Neurotransmitters*

a. **Adrenergic Systems.** Feeding can be elicited in satiated rats by norepinephrine administration to the lateral hypothalamus (Grossman, 1960, 1962a,b) and other hypothalamic areas (Booth, 1967, 1968a). The physiological importance of norepinephrine in the regulation of appetite is further supported by studies with drugs (administered hypothalamically) that increased the endogenously produced norepinephrine and stimulated feeding in rats (Slangen and Miller, 1969). Strong evidence that noradrenergic components of the hypothalamus were intimately involved in the regulation of food intake was derived from studies demonstrating that perfusates, collected by a push-pull technique from the hypothalamus of donor hungry monkeys, could elicit feeding in satiated recipient monkeys (Yaksh and Myers, 1972); perfusates from satiated monkey hypothalamus inhibited feeding when injected into the hypothalamus of hungry monkeys. Hypothalamic perfusates from hungry monkeys contained an increased quantity of a noradrenergic-like substance compared to perfusates from satiated monkeys. The existence of two central catecholaminergic mechanisms for the control of feeding was postulated (Leibowitz, 1970, 1976). α-Adrenergic receptors appeared to control feeding in the medial hypothalamic region and their activation stimulated feeding; β-adrenergic and dopaminergic receptors are believed to be located in the lateral hypothalamus and their activation suppressed feeding behavior (Leibowitz, 1970, 1976).

Dopaminergic neural systems also appeared to be involved in the regulation of appetite, since destruction of the ascending nigrostriatal pathway by applying 6-hydroxydopamine to the substantia nigra (the cells of origin of the dopamine system in the brain) produced marked anorexia and aphagia (Ungerstedt, 1971). No aphagia was evident when only norepinephrine depletion in this bundle was produced. Food deprivation increased hypothalamic dopamine concentrations in rats (Friedman *et al.*, 1973). Considerable support for the role of dopamine in the nigrostriatal pathway involved in feeding has appeared recently (Stricker and Zigmond, 1974, 1976).

b. Serotonergic Systems. A serotonergic mechanism might participate in the control of feeding behavior. Selective depletion of brain serotonin in rats by the intraventricular administration of *p*-chlorophenylalanine (Breisch *et al.*, 1976) or of 5,7-dihydroxytryptamine (after pretreatment with desmethylimipramine to protect the noradrenergic neurons) (Saller and Stricker, 1976) resulted in hyperphagia and weight gain. On the other hand, injections of 5-hydroxytryptophan, the precursor of serotonin, elicited a significant decrease in food intake in deprived rats with or without bilateral lesions of the lateral hypothalamus (Blundell and Leshem, 1975a). However, conflicting data on the role of serotonin in appetite regulation exist. Inhibition of serotonin synthesis with *p*-chlorophenylalanine administration reduced body weight to a stable 75% of control (Panksepp and Nance, 1974), suggesting that this neurotransmitter might be involved in the "set point" by which body weight was regulated. This weight reduction was similar to that observed after later hypothalamic lesions placed in the trajectory of ascending serotonergic fiber systems (Powley and Keesey, 1970). Further research should clarify these apparent discrepancies.

c. Cholinergic Systems. Cholinergic regulation of hypothalamically elicited eating and satiety was proposed (Stark *et al.*, 1971). Injections of acetylcholine and related synthetic cholinomimetics into the hypothalamus produced vigorous drinking but inhibited feeding (Grossman, 1962a,b). However, later studies demonstrated that atropine, a cholinergic blocking agent, failed to disinhibit feeding responses suppressed by satiation (Margules and Stein, 1969). This finding suggested that the systems which suppressed feeding either formed noncholinergic synapses in the hypothalamus or did not synapse at this level. Thus, the role of cholinergic mechanisms in feeding regulation remains to be clarified.

B. Peripheral Regulation of Food Intake

Despite the importance of hypothalamic mechanisms in the regulation of food consumption, the operation of these central neural processes requires the input of sensory, mechanical, and metabolic information from the peripheral sites. Recent investigations stressed the role(s) played by several peripheral sites in influencing particularly the short-term regulation of feeding behavior. The importance of such organs as the duodenum and liver and their neural innervations in the control of hunger and satiety has been summarized recently (Novin, 1976).

1. *Orosensory Factors*

Sensory factors are important in the control of eating (Kawamura, 1975). The initiation of feeding depends to a certain extent on olfactory and gustatory stimuli, which determine the palatability of a food. A number of studies demonstrated the interaction of hunger and palatability of food (for review, see Le Magnen, 1972); it appeared that hunger potentiated palatability and, conversely, that palatability potentiated hunger. Motivational factors were also important in the maintenance of eating behavior. Epstein and Teitelbaum (1962) suggested that cues supplied by taste and smell of food were not essential for the control of food intake. However, Snowdon (1969) noted that the motivation to eat was impaired greatly in rats trained to feed themselves in the absence of oropharyngeal stimuli by bar-pressing for food delivered intragastrically, thus demonstrating the motivational role of oropharyngeal sensations. However, orpharyngeal stimuli alone were not sufficient to elicit satiety, as shown by the hyperphagia which occurred in rats with opened gastric fistulae (Young *et al.*, 1974).

2. *Gastrointestinal Factors*

Gastric distention produced cessation of eating (Smith *et al.*, 1962), possibly due to a selective stimulation of the neural activity of the "satiety center" in the ventromedial hypothalamus (Sharma *et al.*, 1961; Anand and Pillai, 1967) through vagal afferents arising from the stomach (Anand and Pillai, 1967). The concept of tension receptors in the walls of the gastrointestinal tract which control meal size has been proposed (Davis and Campbell, 1973; Davis *et al.*, 1976). These receptors presumably could be activated in response to gastric distension and serve as a signal for the control of food intake by the hypothalamus. Removal of gastric contents served as a signal for feeding (Snowdon, 1970).

Vagal afferent and efferent information appeared important in the regulation of food intake. Subdiaphragmatic vagotomy reversed the obesity in rats made hyperphagic by bilateral lesions in the ventromedial hypothalamus (Powley and Opsahl, 1974), inhibited the feeding response induced by lateral hypothalamic stimulation in rats (Ball, 1974), and altered the meal pattern and appetite of rabbits in a manner similar to the lateral hypothalamic syndrome (Rezek *et al.*, 1975a).

A duodenal satiety mechanism appears to be involved in the short-term regulation of food intake. A chemoreceptor mechanism operating at the gastrointestinal level which might serve as a signal for appetite control was postulated by Sharma and Nasset (1962), and the results of several subsequent studies (Novin *et al.*, 1974; VanderWeele *et al.*, 1974; Rezek *et al.*, 1975b; VanderWeele and Sanderson, 1976; Rezek and Novin, 1976) were consistent with the concept of gastrointestinal glucoreceptors. These studies showed that perfusion of glucose into the duodemum of free-feeding rabbits reduced food intake; this effect was not observed in the food-deprived rabbit. The duodenally based satiety was dependent upon the feeding condition (i.e., free-feeding versus food deprivation) and was completely eliminated in vagotomized rabbits. Small intraduodenal infusions of nutrients also produced satiety in rats (Snowdon, 1975). VanderWeele *et al.* (1974) proposed as a tentative hypothesis that the vagus innervates receptors that are activated by nutrients in the gastrointestinal tract. See the discussion under "Gastrointestinal Hormones" (Section II, C, 6, g) for a further evaluation of the role of the gastrointestinal tract in the regulation of food intake.

3. *Hepatic Factors*

The concept that hepatic glucoreceptors constitute an important control mechanism for food intake was first proposed by Russek (1963, 1971) and subsequent studies from Russek's laboratory (Rodriguez-Zendejas *et al.*, 1968; Russek *et al.*, 1968; Russek, 1970b; Russek and Stevenson, 1972) support this hypothesis. These studies in cats and dogs indicated that anorexia was dependent upon liver glucose utilization and glucose concentrations; the satiating effect of glucose was observed only when it was channeled directly into the liver, since intraportal but not intrajugular injection of glucose produced anorexia. The rate of glucose turnover rather than the actual glucose concentration in the liver could also possibly serve as the stimulus for hepatic glucoreceptors (Russek and Stevenson, 1972; Sullivan and Triscari, 1976). Hepatic receptors specific for amino acids were also postulated to participate in the regulation of appetite (Russek, 1970a, 1971).

The neural pathway responsible for transmitting metabolic information from the hepatic glucoreceptors to the hypothalamic "feeding" center was thought to be the vagus nerve, since its blockade produced immediate anorexia in cats (Penaloza-Rojas and Russek, 1963). The existence of vagally innervated hepatic glucoreceptors was strongly supported by other studies. Glucose perfusion of the isolated guinea pig liver with the hepatic branch of the vagus attached, produced a dose-dependent depression of vagal afferent discharges (Niijima, 1969). *In vivo* injection of glucose produced the same results. The injection of 2-deoxyglucose (a glucose analogue which blocks glucose utilization) into the hepatic-portal circulation of rabbits stimulated food intake (Novin *et al.*, 1973). Comparable injections into the jugular vein or into the hepatic-portal circulation of vagotomized rabbits resulted in a lesser increase of food intake. Similar results were obtained by Booth (1972b). Thus, the operation of hepatic glucoreceptors appeared to require the mediation of the vagus nerve. However, there is also evidence that other neural pathways (i.e., splanchnic nerve) may also be involved in the regulation of food intake by hepatic receptors (Schmitt, 1973).

Recent data have appeared which contradict the role of hepatic receptors in the control of food intake. Neither intrajugular or intraportal injections of glucose or saline, nor the intraportal injection of amino acids significantly reduced the food-seeking response or the total food consumption in the pig (Stephens and Baldwin, 1974). Intraportal infusions of glucose resulted in no anorexia in dogs despite increased blood glucose and insulin concentrations (Bellinger *et al.*, 1976). Future research should clarify the role of hepatic chemoreceptors in feeding behavior.

C. Metabolic Regulation of Food Intake

The regulation of food intake represents a complex physiological process involving the recognition and integration of many different types of signals. Estimations of the importance and extent of the contribution of metabolic factors to this regulatory system were attempted by many investigators and are summarized below.

1. *Carbohydrates: "Glucostatic" Theory*

The "glucostatic" theory postulated by Mayer (1955) stated that insulin-dependent glucoreceptors, probably located in the ventromedial hypothalamus, mediated the short-term control of food intake. Arteriovenous glucose differences, an indicator of peripheral glucose utilization, were suggested as a possible index of activity within these receptors. Satiety and hunger would be indicated by high and low glucose utilization rates, respectively. The rate of glucose utilization rather than the absolute blood sugar levels appeared to be the critical factor monitored by glucoreceptors (Finger and Mook, 1971).

The search for glucoreceptors has suggested the existence of central and peripheral receptor mechanisms. A number of studies utilizing glucose antimetabolites supported the role of glucose-sensitive mechanisms, operating perhaps via hypothalamic glucorecptors in the regulation of appetite. Gold thioglucose produced lesions in the ventromedial hypothalamus with subsequent hyperphagia and obesity; other gold analogues produced none of these effects (Mayer and Marshall, 1956; Debons *et al.*, 1962; Liebelt and Perry, 1967; Baile *et al.*, 1970). It was postulated that gold thioglucose produced degeneration of axons leading from the ventromedial nucleus to the lateral area of the hypothalamus, consequently, hyperphagia resulted from the loss of inhibitory action of the ventromedial nucleus on the lateral hypothalamus. Insulin appeared to be required for the gold thioglucose effect, since diabetic animals were not susceptible to this compound unless treated with insulin (Debons *et al.*, 1968). However, other hormones (thyroxine, cholecystokinin, epinephrine, and hydrocortisone) were also reported to restore the sensitivity of diabetic animals to gold thioglucose (Baile *et al.*, 1971).

2-Deoxyglucose, which blocks glucose utilization, increased food intake when administered systemically to monkeys and rats (Smith and Epstein, 1969). Enhanced feeding was also observed after direct administration of 2-deoxyglucose into the lateral hypothalamus; lesions in the lateral hypothalamus and the preoptic area abolished feeding usually elicited by intraperitoneal administration of 2-deoxyglucose (Epstein and Teitelbaum, 1967). Thus, glucoreceptors appeared to be present in both the ventromedial and lateral area of the hypothalamus (Smith, 1972). Electrophysiological studies demonstrated the existence of glucoreceptor cells in both of these hypothalamic areas (Oomura *et al.*, 1969). Glucose tended to increase the frequency of discharge of ventromedial hypothalamic neurons and to decrease the discharge frequency of glucose-sensitive neurons in the lateral hypothalamus (Fig. 4) (Oomura, 1976). Note also the expected opposite effects of insulin and 3-O-methylglucose compared to glucose on rat neuronal discharge frequency.

The possible existence of gastrointestinal and hepatic glucoreceptors and their role in the regulation of appetite were discussed above (see Sections II, B, 2 and 3). Thus, the metabolism of glucose in a specialized area of the central and/or peripheral nervous system produced short-term effects on appetite regulation. Long-term precision of energy regu-

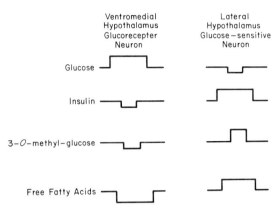

Fig. 4. Schematic representation of the effects of glucose, insulin, 3-*O*-methylglucose and free fatty acids on rat neuronal discharge frequency (Adapted from Oomura, 1976).

lation is postulated to be due to some signal, reflecting adipose tri-glyceride stores, producing appropriate adjustments in food intake.

2. Lipids: "Lipostatic" Theory

The "lipostatic" theory of appetite first proposed by Kennedy (1950, 1966) suggested that feeding was regulated to maintain a constant pro-portion of adipose tissue to body weight, and that a primary function of the ventromedial hypothalamus was to regulate body fat stores, (see Sec-tion II, A, I, a). Kennedy theorized that metabolites or signals from the adipose depots relating to their storage or utilization, transmitted infor-mation to the ventromedial hypothalamus, which subsequently modulated food intake. As discussed above, the primary effect of ven-tromedial hypothalamic lesions was to elevate the set point of the hypothalamic "lipostat".

The nature of these metabolites whose levels reflect adipose tissue status and metabolism is unknown. Certain steroid hormones were suggested to reflect adipose mass through a "tracer" dilution method (Hervey, 1969). Prostaglandins were suggested as components of a sig-nal relating fat depots and energy balance regulation (Baile *et al.*, 1973; Martin and Baile, 1973). Free fatty acids were suggested also as monitor-ing metabolites. Van Itallie and Hashim (1960) postulated that de-creased free fatty acid levels were correlated with satiety and increased levels with hunger. Free fatty acids applied electroosmotically to glucose-sensitive neurons in the rat lateral hypothalamus and to glucoreceptor neurons in the ventromedial hypothalamus, facilitated the former and inhibited the latter (Fig. 4) (Oomura, 1976). Elevated free fatty acid levels characterize the fasting state and it is interesting that obese subjects have significantly increased free fatty acid levels (Bjorntörp *et al.*, 1969). The obese individual and the hungry individual were similar in a variety of behavioral characteristics (Nisbett, 1972b).

3. *Amino Acids: "Aminostatic" Theory*

Food intake is influenced by both the proportion of amino acids in the diet and the dietary content of amino acids and protein (Harper, 1976). An inverse relationship between appetite and serum amino acid levels was postulated in man (Mellinkoff *et al.*, 1956). The amino acid pattern rather than total levels was probably more significant. High systemic levels of amino acids depressed feeding in rats more than comparable levels of the other major nutrients (Adair *et al.*, 1968). Intrahypothalamic injections of amino acids reduced feeding, suggesting that circulating amino acids could depress appetite by a relatively direct action on hypothalamic neurons (Panksepp and Booth, 1971). Further evidence implicating amino acids in neural regulation of appetite originated from observations that rats decreased consumption of diets having imbalanced amino acid contents (Rozin, 1968); appetite was restored to normal by intracarotid, but not intrajugular, infusion of the limiting amino acid (Leung and Rogers, 1969). If the prepyriform cortex of rats was bilaterally destroyed, then imbalanced amino acid diets were readily consumed (Leung and Rogers, 1971).

4. *Energy Flow: "Energostatic" Theory*

The "energostatic" theory hypothesized that feeding was regulated by the metabolic energy status of the animal, and that the type of nutrient (i.e., fat, carbohydrate, or protein) producing the metabolic energy was unimportant (Booth, 1972c). In other words, convergent intracellular metabolic events ultimately control feeding behavior. Rats compensated for the increase in caloric intake derived from an intragastric glucose load by decreasing food consumption; the caloric value of food consumption decreased was approximately equal to the caloric value of the gastric load (Booth, 1972a). Equicaloric amounts of casein, corn oil, and glucose, when administered intragastrically to ad libitum fed rats, reduced food intake in proportion to the number of administered calories (Fig. 5) (Panksepp, 1974). No differences in satiating capacity of the nutrients were detected. This accurate compensatory mechanism for adjustment of caloric intake was subsequently substantiated by other investigators (Liu and Yin, 1974; McHugh *et al.*, 1975).

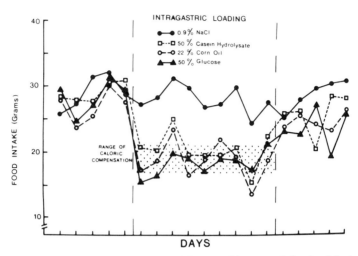

Fig. 5. Daily food intakes of animals receiving 10 ml intragastric loads of the indicated solutions each day for 9 successive days. The rats (3 males per group) had free access to food (Panksepp, 1974).

5. *Temperature: "Thermostatic" Theory*

Appetite is known to be affected by ambient temperature in man and animals, being decreased when the environmental temperature is high and increased when low (Johnson and Kark, 1947; Durrer and Hannon, 1962). Thermoreceptors were postulated to exist in the hypothalamus (Brobeck, 1948) which regulated food intake as follows: feeding was inhibited at this hypothalamic level by the heat generated during the assimilation of food, and was stimulated by a decline in central temperature. Satiety resulted from an inhibition of feeding reflexes. Temperature changes in the hypothalamus were reported to occur as a result of eating (Hamilton, 1963; Rampone and Shirasu, 1964), although the relationship between intracranial temperature changes and general feeding behavior was questioned (Rampone and Shirasu, 1964).

6. *Hormones*

An excellent review on the hormonal control of feeding behavior and energy balance has appeared recently (Panksepp, 1975), which expands a previous presentation (Bray, 1974). The following summarizes briefly the major findings on endocrine factors involved in appetite regulation.

a. Insulin. Insulin administration (Booth and Brookover, 1968; Booth and Pitt, 1968) stimulated hyperphagia. If glucose was given with the insulin the feeding effect was eliminated; nonmetabolizable 3-methylglucose was not effective in blocking enhanced eating response (Booth and Pitt, 1968). Insulin-induced hyperphagia might reflect an indirect action through influencing the peripheral utilization of glucose, or it might act directly on the hypothalamus (Fig. 4).

b. Glucagon. Glucagon administration decreased gastric hunger contractions (Stunkard *et al.*, 1955), body weight and food intake (Schulman *et al.*, 1957) in man. Gastric hunger contractions appeared to be, at least in part, under hypothalamic control (Mayer, 1960).

c. Growth Hormone. Growth hormone stimulated food intake in hypophysectomized rats which normally demonstrated hypophagia (Goldman *et al.*, 1970). Hyperphagia and weight gain in ventromedial hypothalamic lesioned-hypophysectomized rats were reduced by growth hormone treatment (York and Bray, 1972). Since growth hormone stimulated lipolysis, a hunger signal associated with lipolysis (perhaps free fatty acids) was postulated to be mediated through this hormone and act directly on the ventromedial hypothalamus (Kennedy, 1966).

d. Glucocorticoids. Glucocorticoids were apparently related to food intake and body weight, since adrenalectomy in animals (Grossie and Turner, 1965) and hypoadrenal function in man (Williams, 1968) were associated with anorexia. Glucocorticoid therapy was associated with hyperphagia and increased body weight in man (Hollifield, 1968). Normal daily release of glucocorticoids might facilitate feeding (Panksepp, 1975), since in meal-fed rats the maximal secretion of corticosterone was shifted so as to just precede the feeding period (Johnson and Levine, 1973).

Epinephrine administered parenterally significantly reduced feeding behavior in several species; norepinephrine had no effect (Russek *et al.*, 1967). As discussed above (see Section II, A, 2) feeding was stimulated in satiated rats when norepinephrine was injected into the hypothalamus.

e. Thyroxine. Thyroxine given chronically depressed body weight gain and increased food intake in rats (Grossie and Turner, 1961). The hyperphagia was probably a compensatory effort to balance the increased energy metabolism of the hyperthyroid animal.

f. Gonadal Hormones. Gonadal hormones modified feeding behavior and energy balance although, as is the case with other hormones discussed here, their mechanism of action was unknown. In the female rat food intake decreased and physical activity increased on the evening of proestrus (Tarttelin and Gorski, 1971; Wade, 1972). Recent studies suggested that estrogen but not progesterone was the ovarian hormone active in the regulation of food intake in the female rat. Neonatal castration decreased body weight in males; females increased body weight when testosterone was administered soon after birth (Bell and Zucker, 1971). In adult rats ovariectomy increased and castration decreased food intake and body weight (Kakalewski et al., 1968).

g. Gastrointestinal Hormones. Several gastrointestinal hormones may function as short-term satiety signals. An enterogastrone preparation purified from hog duodenum, but not glucagon or secretin, reduced food intake in hungry mice (Schally et al., 1967). Cholecystokinin, another polypeptide gut hormone, could function as a satiety signal (Smith and Gibbs, 1975), since, when injected intraperitoneally, it decreased food intake but not water consumption in fasted rats (Gibbs et al., 1973a) and in rats subjected to sham feeding (Gibbs et al., 1973b). Sham feeding was produced in rats equipped with chronic gastric fistulae; food stimuli were eliminated from the surface of the intestines, cholecystokinin was not released and the rats never became satiated. Gastric preloads of L-phenylalanine, a potent releaser of endogenous cholecystokinin, also decreased food intake in monkeys (Gibbs et al., 1976). Cholecystokinin elicited the complete behavioral sequence of satiety in rats following sham feeding (Antin et al., 1975; Liebling et al., 1975). Recent electrophysiological experiments suggested that cholecystokinin could modulate central neuronal activity, particularly in areas of the hypothalamus which regulate the control of appetite (Dafny et al., 1975). However, a preliminary report stated that cholecystokinin infused intravenously did not produce satiety in man (Goetz and Sturdevant, 1975).

A structural specificity was required for the satiety effect of cholecystokinin. Whereas the synthetic C-terminal octapeptide of cholecystokinin (SQ 19844), a compound with the full biological activity of cholecystokinin, was able to suppress sham feeding, the desulfated synthetic C-terminal octapeptide of cholecystokinin (SQ 19265), which is devoid of the sulfate group on the tyrosyl residue in the seventh position from the C-terminal, and which has little cholecystokinin activity, abolished the satiety effect (Gibbs et al., 1973b). Other peptides which share a portion of the octapeptide sequence, such as caerulein (Gibbs et al., 1973a; Stern et al., 1976), pentagastrin (Smith et al., 1974), gastrin I and II (Smith and Gibbs, 1976), also inhibited feeding but to a significantly

weaker extent. Intraventricular caerulein was more effective·than systemic caerulein in decreasing food intake in rats and microinjections of
caerulein into the ventromedial hypothalamus, but not into the lateral
hypothalamus, resulted in reduced eating (Stern *et al.*, 1976). Secretin
(Gibbs *et al.*, 1973a; Smith *et al.*, 1974) and pancreatic glucagon (Smith
and Gibbs, 1976), peptides which are structurally similar to cholecystokinin but lack the octapeptide sequence, did not inhibit feeding. Further work is required to determine whether cholecystokinin or its
analogues will be useful in producing short-term satiety in hyperphagic
obese subjects.

III. DISORDERS OF APPETITE REGULATION

A. Hyperphagic Obesity

Obesity results when the caloric intake which exceeds the requirement
for energy expenditure is stored as body fat. Van Itallie and Campbell
(1972) have attempted to classify obesity into three categories according
to causative mechanisms: (1) "metabolic obesity" is the result of enzymatic, endocrine, or neurologic disorders; (2) "constitutional obesity" is
caused by hyperplasia of adipocytes; and (3) "regulatory obesity" occurs
without any primary metabolic abnormality and is produced by hyperphagia. Any or all of these causative mechanisms might be involved in
the expression of obesity in a particular individual.

Hyperphagic obesity occurs twice as frequently in females and might
result from psychological and/or physiological factors. The evidence for
psychological factors in obesity, the psychiatric classification of obesity,
and the behavioral disturbances associated with obesity and weight reduction have been reviewed (Glucksman, 1972). Many studies suggested
that obese individuals differed from normal persons in their eating behavior (for review, see Nisbett, 1972b). Reports of hunger and gastric
motility were directly correlated in the nonobese, but not in the obese
(Stunkard and Koch, 1964). The lack of responsiveness of obese subjects
to internal physiological cues was suggested, and the occurrence of eating
behavior in the obese seemed to be dependent upon external stimuli
such as smell, sight, taste, and time (Schacter, 1968). Obese subjects
appeared to be less able than normal-weight or thin individuals to
achieve the point of satiety (Linton *et al.*, 1972). However, evidence that
obese subjects might not differ significantly from other weight groups in

their response to physiological hunger cues was also reported (Parham *et al.*, 1975; Warner and Balagura, 1975).

Hyperphagic obesity might also be produced by physiological factors such as increased energy intake (e.g., damage to hypothalamic areas involved in appetite regulation; see Section II, A, 1 and a recent review by Bray and Gallagher, 1975) or decreased energy output (e.g., sedentary existence). Many metabolic and endocrine aberrations characterize obesity (for review, see Sullivan *et al.*, 1976). Studies in normal volunteers made moderately obese by forced hyperphagia demonstrated that many of these metabolic aberrations are, in part, a consequence of corpulence; these alterations could be reversed by weight loss and induced by overeating (Sims *et al.*, 1973). However, two important differences existed between subjects who accumulated fat late in life or by experimentally-induced hyperphagia and those with spontaneous hyperplastic "constitutional" obesity (Bray, 1975). First, the body weight "set point" in these two groups might be different, since normal subjects who gained weight by forced overeating returned to their initial lean body weight. On the contrary, obese individuals encountered great difficulties in maintaining a lower body weight after weight reduction, and in most cases returned to their original obese weight. Second, the adipose tissue hypercellularity in the obese group could not be reversed by weight reduction.

B. Anorexia Nervosa

Anorexia nervosa predominantly afflicts female patients during adolescence (incidence is twelve times greater in females than males), although extremes in age ranging from 11 to 35 years have been reported (Seaver and Binder, 1972). The disease is rarely observed in children (Blitzer *et al.*, 1961) and in males (Crisp and Toms, 1972). Anorexia nervosa is characterized by three distinct clinical abnormalities which form the criteria for differential diagnosis (Russell, 1970): (1) behavioral disorders characterized by a consistent and abnormal avoidance of eating, particularly carbohydrates which are regarded as "fattening". Starvation may alternate with bouts of overeating, and some patients have been known to eliminate food intake by means of self-induced vomiting or purgation. (2) Psychopathology manifested by an unjustified phobia of obesity in which judgment and perception appeared to be distorted, since the patient is unable to make a correct estimate of the amount of food required or the ideal body weight. (3) Endocrine disturbance characterized by persistent amenorrhea sometimes preceding the onset of weight loss, and at other times, continuing even after weight loss has been restored, thus suggesting that it is not totally secondary to malnutrition. In male patients, the clinical manifestation of endocrine disturbance was a loss of libido and potency.

Experiments conducted during the past decade have aimed at the elucidation of the hormonal derangements underlying these clinical symptoms of endocrine disturbance. The urinary output of estrogens and human pituitary gonadotropins in patients with anorexia nervosa was measured before and after feeding in an attempt to ascertain whether malnutrition was a causative factor for endocrine dysfunction in this disease (Russell *et al.*, 1965; Bell *et al.*, 1966). "Total" estrogen output (estradiol, estrone, and estriol) and the relative proportions of these estrogens were abnormally low in the female patients studied, approaching values encountered generally in postmenopausal women. The urinary excretion of pituitary gonadotropins was likewise depressed. Refeeding with concomitant weight gain resulted in an increase in total estrogen excretion, a normalization of the excretion pattern of the estrogens, little change in pituitary gonadotropins, and a persistent absence of ovulatory activity. It appeared that the principle endocrine defect in patients with anorexia nervosa was the diminished secretion of pituitary gonadotropins, since despite refeeding, these levels remained low in a significant proportion of the patients. The observation that plasma luteinizing hormone and follicle stimulating hormone levels were low in patients with anorexia nervosa (Crisp, *et al.*, 1973) prompted a recent clinical study in which long-term treatment with luteinizing hormone-releasing hormone in patients with anorexia nervosa led to follicular maturation and ovulation with resumption of menstruation (Nillius and Wide, 1975).

The functional integrity of the pituitary gland and the hypothalamus was determined by means of a variety of endocrine evaluations in patients with anorexia nervosa (Mecklenburg *et al.*, 1974). There was no evidence of pituitary dysfunction on the basis of several criteria, but hypothalamic function appeared to be impaired. Many of the other myriad symptoms and complications of anorexia nervosa might be directly related to the condition of malnutrition (for review, see Russell, 1970; Mawson, 1974).

C. Eating Disorders Associated with Organic and Psychiatric Diseases

Anorexia is a prominent clinical feature in many organic diseases (Hall, 1975; Seaver and Binder, 1972). Diseases of the gastrointestinal tract, such as sprue, Crohn's disease, and ulcerative colitis are understandably associated with anorexia, but other diseases such as cancer and viral hepatitis are also known to cause appetite depression. The etiology of the anorexia and cachexia in patients with cancer is not known. A variety of metabolic derangements has been known to occur in patients with cancer (Theologides, 1972), but none of the observed metabolic abnormalities can offer an adequate explanation of the decreased food intake (Theologides, 1974), with the possible exception of the hypothesis of appetite regulation by circulating amino acid levels. Since patients with cancer have been shown to have abnormal amino acid concentrations and patterns in their blood, and since tumor tissue can produce and release peptides, it was suggested that these changes might provide the signal for anorexia (Theologides, 1976).

Anorexia as well as hyperphagia accompany many psychiatric disorders (Kay and Schapira, 1972; Robinson *et al.*, 1975a). Children with emotional maladjustment are more apt to have a poor appetite. Anorexia is a prominent feature in some forms of neurosis, psychosis, schizophrenia, and chronic brain syndromes. Feeding disorders associated with hypothalamic tumors and lesions were discussed previously (see Sections II, A, 1, a and b).

IV.   DRUGS AFFECTING FOOD INTAKE

A.   Anorectic Agents

1.   *Phenethylamines*

The chemical structures of phenethylamine anorectic agents are provided in Fig. 6. Several recent reviews present certain aspects of the clinical efficacy of anorectic drugs (Silverstone, 1975; Sullivan *et al.*, 1976; Craddock, 1976). Selected studies on the clinical efficacy of these drugs in promoting weight loss are summarized in Table II. Drug dose, duration of treatment, number of obese patients, dietary advice, and average weight loss on treatment are reported. The following discussion presents mechanism(s) and site(s) of action of these drugs when these data are available and highlights certain features of their clinical efficacy in the treatment of obesity.

   a.   Amphetamine.   With the advent of the newer anorectic agents, the use of amphetamine for the control of food intake is no longer justified. Whereas it effectively suppresses appetite and decreases body weight in obese patients upon short-term administration (Kornhaber,

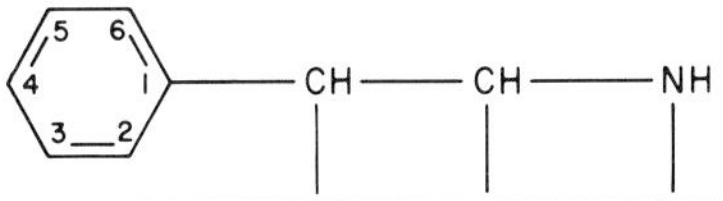

Ring structure: positions 5, 6, 4, 1, 3, 2 —CH——CH——NH

	Ring	CH	CH	NH
Phenethylamine		H	H	H
Amphetamine		H	CH_3	H
Phenylpropanolamine		OH	CH_3	H
Phentermine		H	2*	H
Clortermine	2–Cl	H	2*	H
Chlorphentermine	4–Cl	H	2*	H
Diethylpropion		3*	CH_3	4*
Phenmetrazine		1*		
Fenfluramine	3–CF_3	H	CH_3	C_2H_5
780 SE	3–CF_3	H	CH_3	$(CH_2)_2O\overset{O}{\overset{\|}{C}}C_6H_5$
Flutiorex	3–SCF_3	H	CH_3	C_2H_5
Flucetorex	3–CF_3	H	CH_3	$\overset{O}{\overset{\|}{C}}CH_2OC_6H_4NH\overset{O}{\overset{\|}{C}}CH_3$
Fenfluramine glycinate	3–CF_3	H	CH_3	CH_2COOH

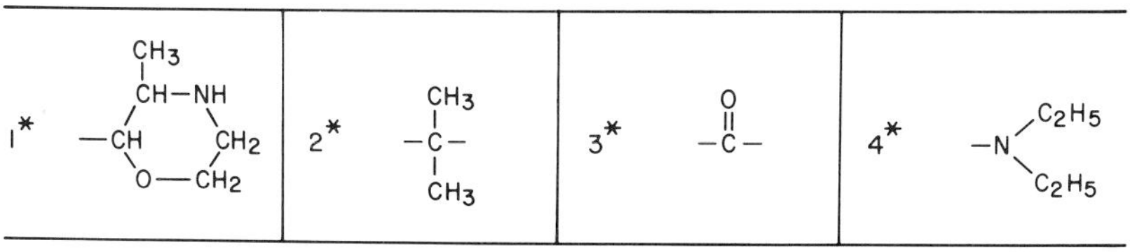

Footnotes:

1* $-CH \begin{smallmatrix} \overset{CH_3}{CH-NH} \\ CH_2 \\ O-CH_2 \end{smallmatrix}$ 2* $-\overset{CH_3}{\underset{CH_3}{C}}-$ 3* $-\overset{O}{\overset{\|}{C}}-$ 4* $-N \begin{smallmatrix} C_2H_5 \\ C_2H_5 \end{smallmatrix}$

Fig. 6. Chemical structures of phenethylamine anorectic agents.

1973; Defelice *et al.*, 1973), its long-term efficacy is not assured and chronic treatment not only leads to tolerance of the drug with a decrease in anorectic response, but also results in dependence and withdrawal reactions. The central nervous system stimulatory effects and the tendency to be abused add to the undesirability of amphetamine as an anorectic agent. However, amphetamine remains a prototype drug with powerful appetite suppressant activity, against which other compounds

TABLE II

Clinical Efficacy of Phenethylamine Anorectic Drugs

Drug	Dose	Duration (weeks)	Number of obese patients	Average weight loss Drug (kg)	Average weight loss Placebo (kg)	Diet restriction (calories)	References
Amphetamine	5 mg × 3	12	14	4.5	2.4	1000	Kornhaber, 1973
	5 mg × 3	6	20	1.5	0.5	1200	Defelice et al., 1973
Phenylpropanolamine	25 mg × 3	4	29	2.5	1.8	1000	Griboff et al., 1975
Phentermine	30 mg	14	30	7.3	1.8	1000	Langlois et al., 1974
Clortermine	50 mg	4	(7 Double-blind studies)	0.8–2.2	0.1–1.1	None	Mizrahi, 1974
	50 mg	4	(18 Double-blind studies)	2.2–5.1	1–3.7	1000	Mizrahi, 1974
Chlorphentermine	65 mg	12	29	2.7		None	Hadler, 1967b
Diethylpropion	25 mg × 3	12	41	9.1	4.5	1000	Allen, 1975
	75 mg	25	10	11.7	1.6	Strict	McKay, 1975
	25 mg × 3	12	22	4.4	1.6	1000	McQuarrie, 1975
	25 mg × 3	12	20	6.8	4.4	1000	Nolan, 1975
Phenmetrazine	75 mg	6	53	1.8	+0.6	None	Hadler, 1967a
	75 mg	12	24	2.8		None	Hadler, 1967b
	25 mg × 2	6	27	2.6		None	Hadler, 1968a
	50 mg	6	28	2.0		None	Hadler, 1968a
Phendimetrazine	105 mg	12	36	3.4	0.5	None	Hadler, 1968b
Fenfluramine	20 mg × 2	6	44	2.4	0.3	None	Dent and Preston, 1975
	40 mg	6	23	1.7	0.3	None	Dent and Preston, 1975
	60 mg	12	56	4.7	2.5	None	Tisdale and Ervin, 1976
	20 mg × 3	12	60	6.6	2.5	None	Tisdale and Ervin, 1976
	60 mg	6	16	2.4		1000	Hooper, 1975
	20 mg × 3	6	11	2.3		1000	Hooper, 1975
780 SE	720 mg[a]	6	6	2.8	+0.7		Miller et al., 1975
Flutiorex	20 mg		6	350g[b]	500g[b]		J. F. Giudicelli et al., 1976

[a] Maximum dose during third and fourth week.

[b] Food intake.

under development are compared. Studies on its mechanism of action have yielded important information on the physiology of appetite regulation and have offered scientific investigators of different disciplines a challenge to develop anorectic agents which are more potent, less toxic, and longer-acting than amphetamine.

Several studies suggested that amphetamine anorexia was mediated by the ventromedial hypothalamus, based on electrical activity in this area after amphetamine administration (Brobeck *et al.*, 1956, Krebs *et al.*, 1969) and lesion studies (Sharp *et al.*, 1962). However, recent evidence indicated that amphetamine anorexia did not require the functional integrity of the ventromedial hypothalamus (Wishart and Walls, 1973).

Numerous studies provided evidence that the lateral hypothalamus must remain intact in order for amphetamine to exert its anorectic effect. Bilateral lesions in the lateral hypothalamus attenuated the effect of amphetamine on food intake in rats (Carlisle, 1964; Russek *et al.*, 1973; Blundell and Leshem, 1974). Unilateral lesions in the lateral hypothalamus which destroyed the nigrostriatal bundle also reduced sensitivity to the appetite suppressant effect of amphetamine (Carey and Goodall, 1975). Additional evidence of lateral hypothalamic involvement was provided by studies in which an interaction was shown between amphetamine administered systemically and the electrical activity of this area, which was consistent with an inhibitory effect of amphetamine on the lateral hypothalamus (Stark and Totty, 1967; Thode and Carlisle, 1968; Reiter, 1970). A close link between amphetamine and feeding was demonstrated after administration of the drug into the lateral hypothalamus (Booth, 1968b; Leibowitz, 1975a). Amphetamine delayed the onset of eating in food-deprived rats, and increased the latency of feeding response in rats under ad libitum feeding conditions, suggesting an effect of amphetamine on the hunger mechanism (as opposed to satiety, which is correlated with early termination of a meal and a decrease in meal size) involving the lateral hypothalamus (Blundell *et al.*, 1976). Other areas of the brain were implicated in amphetamine action and include: (1) the substantia nigra, since unilateral lesions in this area attenuated amphetamine anorexia (Carey and Goodall, 1975), and (2) the ventral noradrenergic bundle, since its destruction antagonized the amphetamine-induced reduction of food consumption (Ahlskog, 1974).

The nature of the neurotransmitter(s) responsible for mediating the anorectic action of amphetamine has been investigated. α-Methyltyrosine, an inhibitor of catecholamine synthesis, antagonized the depressing effect of amphetamine on food intake in rats (Weissman *et al.*, 1966), thus providing a basis for the hypothesis of catecholaminergic mechanism of amphetamine anorexia substantiated by several investigators (Holtzman and Jewett, 1971; Frey and Schulz, 1973; Baez, 1974). Midbrain injection of 6-hydroxydopamine near the ventral noradrenergic bundle resulted in almost complete loss of forebrain norepinephrine content and abolished amphetamine anorexia in rats (Ahlskog, 1974). Norpinephrine elicited eating in rats when injected into the lateral hypothalamus, and amphetamine injected into the same site depressed appetite, offering further evidence that anorexia was probably attributed to an interaction of amphetamine with the adrenergic activity in the lateral hypothalamus (Booth, 1968a,b). Consistent with this view was the finding that L-propranolol (a β-adrenergic receptor antagonist) injected into the lateral hypothalamus abolished the anorectic effect of amphetamine (Leibowitz, 1975a). Whereas haloperidol, a dopaminergic receptor blocker, also antagonized amphetamine, the α-adrenergic receptor antagonist phentolamine did not. These data suggested that amphetamine, in suppressing feeding behavior, acted through the lateral hypothalamus, causing a release of dopamine and norepinephrine from lateral hypothalamic nerve endings, and a subsequent stimulation of dopaminergic and β-adrenergic receptors located in that region (Leibowitz, 1975b).

A dopaminergic mechanism in the mediation of amphetamine anorexia finds support in several other studies involving dopamine blockers (Kruk, 1973; Baez, 1974) and depletion of brain dopamine (Fibiger et al., 1973; Heffner et al., 1975; Carey and Goodall, 1975), since the anorectic activity of amphetamine was attenuated or abolished by these manipulations. Additionally, it was demonstrated that dopamine-β-hydroxylase inhibitors potentiated the anorectic effect of amphetamine in mice (Dobrzanski and Doggett, 1975).

The interaction of amphetamine with brain monoamines and food intake is illustrated in Table III. Amphetamine administration decreased brain norepinephrine but had no effect on serotonin levels. The anorexia produced by amphetamine was dependent upon an intact catecholaminergic system; lesions of the serotonergic system did not affect amphetamine anorexia (Garattini et al., 1975b).

Table II presents the clinical efficacy of amphetamine compared to other phenethylamine anorectic drugs.

b. Amphetamine Derivatives. i. *Phenylpropanolamine.* A recent double-blind study revealed that a formulation containing phenylpropanolamine (Propadrine), caffeine, and vitamins produced anorexia and weight loss in obese subjects with a minimum of side effects (Griboff et al., 1975) (Table II). In rats, feeding, but not drinking behavior, elicited by electrical stimulation of the lateral hypothalamus was inhibited by phenylpropanolamine when it was injected intraperitoneally or through

TABLE III
Interaction of Anorectic Agents with Brain Monoamines and Food Intake[a]

Treatment[b]	Brain norepinephrine ($\mu g/gm \pm$ SE)	Brain serotonin ($\mu g/gm \pm$ SE)	Food intake			
			Vehicle (gm/2 hours $\pm$ SE)	After lesions of catecholaminergic system (gm/2 hours $\pm$ SE)	After lesions of serotonergic system (gm/2 hours $\pm$ SE)	
Saline	0.40 ± 0.01	0.43 ± 0.01	7.8 ± 0.4	8.9 ± 0.5	8.7 ± 0.6	
Amphetamine	0.24 ± 0.02^c	0.40 ± 0.01	1.8 ± 0.5^c	7.1 ± 0.6	2.4 ± 0.8^c	
Fenfluramine	0.38 ± 0.01	0.16 ± 0.01^c	1.7 ± 0.4^c	1.0 ± 0.3^c	7.2 ± 0.8	
Mazindol	0.32 ± 0.3^c	0.50 ± 0.08	4.4 ± 0.3^c	9.7 ± 0.4^c	5.0 ± 1.4^c	

[a] Adapted from Garattini et al. (1975b).

[b] Drugs were administered ip at 15 mg/kg (brain moncamine study) and 1.3–5 mg/kg (food intake study). Each group contained 6 rats.

[c] $p < 0.05$.

lateral hypothalamic cannulae. No effects were observed if the drug was administered into medial hypothalamic cannulae (Hoebel *et al.*, 1975).

ii. *Phentermine and chlorphentermine.* A double-blind clinical study under controlled conditions established that phentermine at 15 mg or 30 mg produced a significant reduction in caloric intake as well as on hunger ratings (Silverstone, 1972). Effective weight loss was obtained at 30 mg (Langlois *et al.*, 1974) (Table II). Intermittent phentermine therapy was more effective than intermittent fenfluramine and was comparable to continuous fenfluramine in effecting weight loss, without appreciable central nervous system stimulation (Steel *et al.*, 1973). Tolerance to or dependence on phentermine did not appear to be a problem (Langlois *et al.*, 1974).

Chlorphentermine at doses ranging from 50 mg to 200 mg produced a significant and dose-related inhibition of appetite and food intake, an effect also observed for amphetamine. The two drugs differed in subjective and physiological responses, since those produced by chlorphentermine were characterized by sedation with little or no change in blood pressure, temperature, and sleep time, whereas those produced by amphetamine were mainly euphoria, hyperpyrexia, hypertension, and insomnia (Griffith *et al.*, 1976). Weight reduction was observed at a dose of 65 mg (Hadler, 1967b) (Table II).

iii. *Clortermine.* Clortermine at 50 mg once daily produced significantly greater weight loss than placebo in double-blind studies, with 76% of the patients reporting no adverse reactions; the most frequent side effects were overstimulation, insomnia, headache, and dry mouth (Mizrahi, 1974) (Table II).

iv. *Diethylpropion.* Double-blind clinical studies established that diethylpropion at a dose of 25 mg three times a day or 75 mg once a day produced weight loss without any deleterious effects on electrocardiograms, chest X-rays, blood pressure, or pulse rate (Allen, 1975; McKay, 1975; McQuarrie, 1975; Nolan, 1975) (Table II). Diethylpropion administered continuously was more efficacious than intermittent treatment (Silverstone, 1974), and no significant interacting side effects were observed when the drug was used concurrently with hypotensive agents (Seedat and Reddy, 1974).

v. *Phenmetrazine and phendimetrazine.* Double-blind studies demonstrated the effectiveness of phenmetrazine as an appetite suppressant with mild and transient side effects when administered as a single dose ranging from 50 mg to 105 mg (Hadler, 1967a,b, 1968a,b) (Table II). Phendimetrazine at 105 mg once a day also resulted in weight loss with minimal side effects (Hadler, 1968b) (Table II).

  c. Fenfluramine. A comprehensive review (Pinder *et al.*, 1975) has appeared recently, covering the many aspects of the pharmacology and therapeutic efficacy of fenfluramine. Specific reviews should be referred to for more detailed discussions on the mechanism of action (Garattini *et al.*, 1975a,b), peripheral and metabolic effects (Macrae, 1975), metabolism (Beckett, 1975), and central nervous system effects (Reuter, 1975). Valuable information on several levels of drug action may be obtained from the proceedings (Fenfluramine and Derivatives, 1975) of a symposium on fenfluramine and derivatives held in 1974.

  The site of action of amphetamine appears to reside in the lateral hypothalamus, whereas that of fenfluramine is less well defined, and perhaps involves extrahypothalamic zones. Amphetamine and fenfluramine injected into the ventromedial nucleus of the rat produced no significant change in feeding behavior, while bilateral injections into the lateral hypothalamus resulted in suppression of food intake (Blundell and Leshem, 1973). There was a difference in the time course of anorexigenic action; the effect of amphetamine was immediate following injection, that of fenfluramine was delayed. These and subsequent findings supported the hypothesis that amphetamine acted on a hypothalamic hunger system and fenfluramine acted by means of a postulated serotonergic satiety system (Blundell *et al.*, 1976). Lesion studies further demonstrated differences between amphetamine and fenfluramine. Bilateral lesions of the lateral hypothalamus produced an enhancement of fenfluramine anorexia and an attenuation of amphetamine anorexia (Blundell and Leshem, 1974, 1975b); the effect on fenfluramine action was sustained over a period of months (Blundell and Leshem, 1974). Lesions in the anterior hypothalamic area or the preoptic area enhanced the suppression of feeding behavior induced by amphetamine, but had no effect on that of fenfluramine (Blundell and Leshem, 1975b).

  Fenfluramine and amphetamine also differ in their mechanism of action. Whereas amphetamine anorexia is believed to be mediated by the release of brain norepinephrine, fenfluramine anorexia depends upon the release of endogenous serotonin from central neurons. In rats, the injection of fenfluramine resulted in a decrease in brain serotonin levels (Duhault *et al.*, 1975a,b; Fuxe *et al.*, 1975). Marked depletion of serotonin was found in the diencephalon (Ghezzi *et al.*, 1973), telencephalon (Ghezzi *et al.*, 1973; Harvey and McMaster, 1975), the amygdala (Harvey and McMaster, 1975), and the remaining brainstem (Ghezzi *et al.*, 1973). Irreversible damage in the serotonergic cell bodies of the ventromedial midbrain tegmentum was demonstrated in rats following an injection of fenfluramine (100 μmoles/kg) (Harvey and McMaster, 1975). The decrease in brain serotonin was correlated with the metabolism of fenfluramine to norfenfluramine, and was probably mediated by the presence of this metabolite in the brain (Duhault et al., 1975a,b). Since platelets are considered to be a simple model of tryptaminergic nerve endings, they were employed to study the effect of fenfluramine on the release and blockaade of ^{14}C-serotonin (Buczko et al., 1975). The results confirmed that fenfluramine enhanced the release and blocked the uptake of serotonin.

Fenfluramine reduced brain serotonin levels and its anorectic activity was dependent upon an intact serotonergic but not catecholaminergic system (Table III). Drugs or surgical lesions which modified brain serotonin metabolism also antagonized the anorexigenic action of fenfluramine. Thus, pretreatment of rats with chlorimipramine, an inhibitor of neuronal serotonin uptake (Ghezzi et al., 1973; Jespersen and Scheel-Krüger, 1973; Duhault et al., 1975b), as well as the indoleamine antagonists methergoline (Funderburk et al., 1971; Jespersen and Scheel-Krüger, 1973; Clineschmidt et al., 1974), cyproheptadine (Clineschmidt et al., 1974), and cinanserin (Clineschmidt et al., 1974) had the same effect as intraventricular injection of 5,6-dihydroxytryptamine (which caused a selective degeneration of serotonin neurons) (Clineschmidt, 1973) and electrolytic lesions of the midbrain raphe (an area rich in serotonin neurons) (Samanin et al., 1975) in antagonizing the appetite suppressant action of fenfluramine. However, in other studies, p-chlorophenylalanine (an inhibitor of tryptophan hydroxylase) (Duhault et al., 1975b), methysergide (a serotonin antagonist) (Jespersen and Scheel-Krüger, 1973) or destruction of serotonergic neurons (Sugrue et al., 1975) had no significant effect on the anorexigenic action of fenfluramine.

Evidence supporting a serotonin mechanism for fenfluramine anorexia has also been demonstrated in man. In nonobese patients with neurological disorders, fenfluramine reduced caloric intake and body weight declined, concomitant with a 66% reduction in the accumulation of 5-hydroxyindoleacetic acid, a serotonin metabolite, in the cerebrospinal fluid, but there was no change in the accumulation of homovanillic acid, a major product of dopamine metabolism (Chase and Shoulson, 1975; Shoulson and Chase, 1975).

Differences in the mechanism of action of amphetamine and fenfluramine were also suggested by the lack of development of cross-tolerance between these two drugs (Kandel et al., 1975). Rats developed tolerance to the suppression of milk consumption induced by d-amphetamine, d-methamphetamine and d,l-fenfluramine. There was cross-tolerance between the effects of *d*-amphetamine and *d*-methamphetamine, but not between those of *d*-amphetamine and *d,l*-fenfluramine.

A double-blind clinical trial established that fenfluramine at a dosage of 20 mg twice a day produced greater weight loss in obese subjects than did the same total dose given once daily or in increasingly larger doses (Dent and Preston, 1975) (Table II). The use of fenfluramine offered no significant advantage over caloric restriction alone (Rayner and Court, 1975; Wells, 1975). A long-acting formulation (60 mg) of fenfluramine appeared to be better than placebo (Owen, 1975a,b) or 20 mg three times daily (Tisdale and Ervin, 1976) in producing weight loss. Comparative studies showed the 60 mg once a day dosage to be equally as effective as (Hooper, 1975), better than (Maneksha, 1975), or less effective than (Innes *et al.*, 1975) the standard 20 mg three times daily dosage. Evidence was presented to show that norfenfluramine played an important role as a mediator of fenfluramine anorexia (Goudie *et al.*, 1974; Blundell and Campbell, 1975).

Side effects of fenfluramine are generally mild: lowered blood pressure and heart rate (Griffith *et al.*, 1975), mydriasis (Griffith *et al.*, 1975) probably mediated by norfenfluramine (Kramer *et al.*, 1973), mood depression 3–6 days following the end of treatment (Holstrand and Jonsson, 1975), olfactory and visual hallucinations accompanied by changes in mood and ideation following high doses (240 mg) (Griffith *et al.*, 1974, 1975), and fenfluramine abuse (Levin, 1975; Rosenvinge, 1975) have been reported. Fenfluramine in addition to its anorectic activity possesses effects on energy metabolism which were reviewed recently (Sullivan *et al.*, 1976).

d. Fenfluramine Derivatives. i. *780 SE.* 780 SE was a potent anorexigenic agent and produced a mild behavioral effect in rats (Taylor and Goudie, 1975). This compound reduced food intake and body weight in obese and nonobese subjects (Miller *et al.*, 1975) (Table II). In patients with maturity-onset diabetes, the drug administered in conjunction with diet restriction resulted in loss of body weight with a significant improvement in glucose tolerance (Asmal and Leary, 1975).

ii. *Flutiorex (SL 72340).* Flutiorex, SL 72340, a new anorectic agent structurally related to fenfluramine was more active than fenfluramine in suppressing food consumption in rats (R. Giudicelli *et al.*, 1976). A double-blind clinical trial has confirmed its anorectic potency (J. F. Giudicelli *et al.*, 1976) (Table II).

iii. *Flucetorex.* Studies on the structure–activity relationship of a series of phenoxyacetamide derivatives of fenfluramine showed that anorexigenic activity was associated with amine substitution in the para position on the phenoxyacetic moiety. The p-amido compounds, although less active than the p-amino compounds, were devoid of stimulating effects, and the most promising compound was the p-acetamido derivative (flucetorex) (Bourillet and Buzas, 1976).

iv. *Fenfluramine glycinates.* A number of fenfluramine glycinates and their optical isomers were submitted to pharmacological evaluation (Duhault *et al.*, 1975c). Although less potent than the parent compound in anorectic activity, these new derivatives were also less toxic, being almost devoid of sedative properties, and not inhibiting apomorphine-induced stereotypy.

v. *Lilly 110140.* A newly developed inhibitor of the uptake pump in serotonin neurons, Lilly 110140 [3-(p-trifluoromethyl-phenoxy)-N-methyl-3-phenylpropylamine hydrochloride] was reported to have a potent anorectic effect of short duration in rats (Goudie *et al.*, 1976). This compound also potentiated the anorectic effect of 5-hydroxytryptophan, the precursor of serotonin, thus supporting the concept of a serotonergic system which inhibited food intake.

2. *Nonphenethylamine Anorectic Agents*

The chemical structures of several novel nonphenethylamine anorectic agents are presented in Fig. 7. Only mazindol and 11698 JL have been studied in humans and the anorectic activity demonstrated by these drugs in several selected clinical trials is summarized in Table IV.

a. Mazindol. Double-blind studies confirmed the efficacy and safety of mazindol as an anorectic agent in obese patients (Haugen, 1975; Heber, 1975; Schwartz, 1975; Sedgwick, 1975; Smith *et al.*, 1975; Thorpe *et al.*, 1975; Wallace, 1975; Woodhouse *et al.*, 1975) (Table IV). Mazindol (3 mg/day) was equivalent to phenmetrazine (75 mg/day) (Kornhaber, 1973), equal to (Kornhaber, 1973) or superior to (Defelice *et al.*, 1973) amphetamine (15 mg/day), equal to fenfluramine (up to 160 mg/day) (Goldrick *et al.*, 1974), and superior to diethylpropion (75 mg/day) (Murphy *et al.*, 1975) in achieving weight reduction.

The mechanism of action of mazindol in producing anorexia remains unclear. Pharmacological responses of mazindol suggested that this drug modulated brain norepinephrine metabolism (Gogerty *et al.*, 1975), but unlike amphetamine, which caused norepinephrine release from neuronal stores and inhibited norepinephrine synthesis, mazindol acted primarily through inhibition of neuronal uptake mechanism (Engstrom *et al.*, 1975). Mazindol reduced mildly brain norepinephrine levels but

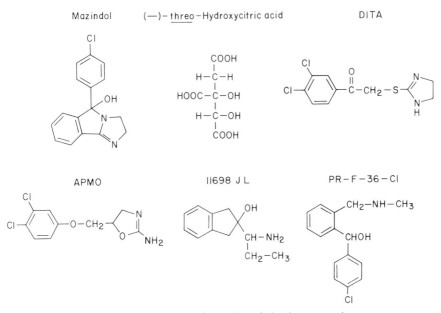

Fig. 7. Chemical structures of nonphenethylamine anorectic agents.

had no effect on serotonin levels (Table III). It was also suggested that the anorectic effect of mazindol was mediated through dopamine (Garattini *et al.*, 1975b; Kruk, 1976) or serotonin (Barrett and McSharry, 1975). The anorectic activity of mazindol was abolished by lesioning the catecholaminergic system; anorexia was independent of lesions in the serotonergic system. Structural modification of mazindol resulted in a decrease or loss in anorectic activity (Aeberli *et al.*, 1975).

b. 11698 JL.   A novel aminopropylindanol analogue, 11698 JL was an effective appetite suppressant in normal and hyperphagic rats (Dorf *et al.*, 1975). A double-blind clinical study in obese subjects demonstrated a significant loss of weight when the drug was given at a dose of 120 mg three times a day in conjunction with calorie restriction (Table IV).

c.   (—)-Hydroxycitrate.   (—)-Hydroxycitrate decreased food intake and weight gain in the normal mature rat (Fig. 8), the ventromedial hypothalamic-lesioned obese rat (Fig. 2) and the gold thioglucose-induced obese mouse (Sullivan and Triscari, 1977). The loss in body weight was

TABLE IV
Clinical Efficacy of Nonphenethylamine Anorectic Drugs

Drug	Dose	Duration (weeks)	Number of obese patients	Average weight loss		Diet restriction (calories)	References
				Drug (kg)	Placebo (kg)		
Mazindol	1 mg × 3	6	30	4.6	1.7	None	Haugen, 1975
	2 mg	12	15	6.9	1.6	1200	Heber, 1975
	2 mg	12	40	8.4	1.1	1000	Schwartz, 1975
	2 mg	12	27	8.5	6.6	1000	Sedgwick, 1975
	2 mg	12	19	1.4	0.3	Restricted	Smith et al., 1975
	1 mg × 3	8	14	5.2	3.8	1200	Thorpe et al., 1975
	2 mg	12	23	5.5	2.3	50 gm carbohydrate	Wallace, 1975
	1 mg × 3	12	12	5.2	0.6	None	Woodhouse et al., 1975
11698 JL	120 mg × 3	2	30	> Placebo		1200	Dorf et al., 1975

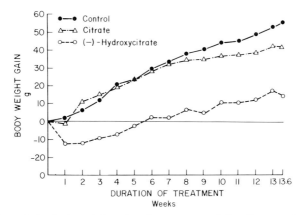

Fig. 8. Cumulative body weight gain of mature rats fed a diet containing citrate or (—)-hydroxycitrate. Mature rats were adapted to the 70% glucose diet for 30 days, then separated into 3 groups of 12–29 rats per group (control, citrate and (—)-hydroxycitrate groups contained 29, 14 and 12 rats, respectively) with equivalent age distribution (58% of each group were 10–14 months old and 42% of each group were 6 months old) and mean body weight distribution. They were fed ad libitum either the diet alone, diet containing citrate, trisodium salt (52.6 mmoles/kg diet), or diet containing (—)-hydroxycitrate, trisodium salt (52.6 mmoles/kg diet) for 13.6 weeks. Cumulative body weight gain of the (—)-hydroxycitrate treated group was significantly reduced compared to controls at each interval ($p < 0.05$). There were no significant differences in the weight gained by the citrate treatment compared to controls (Sullivan and Triscari, 1977).

due to a significant depression of body lipid levels; protein content was unaffected (Sullivan *et al.*, 1974b). Citrate administration produced no significant effects on appetite or weight gain. (—)-Hydroxycitrate decreased fatty acid (Fig. 9) and cholesterol synthesis *in vivo* in the tissues which serve as sources of newly synthesized lipid (adipose tissue, liver, small intestine) (Sullivan *et al.*, 1972, 1974a; Sullivan, 1975). This reduction of the conversion of carbohydrate and its metabolites into lipid was due to (—)-hydroxycitrate's activity as a potent competitive inhibitor of ATP citrate lyase, the enzyme which supplies acetyl CoA (the precursor of fatty acids and cholesterol) (Watson *et al.*, 1969). The anorexia produced by (—)-hydroxycitrate was due possibly to the alteration of metabolite flux resulting from this diversion of carbohydrate from lipid synthesis. In the liver some of the diverted carbohydrates were apparently channeled into glycogen as shown by the significant increases in glycogen synthesis (Fig. 10) and content (Fig. 11) (Sullivan and Triscari, 1976). As discussed above (Section II, B, 3), information regarding hepatic glycogen and/or glucose levels or the rate of change in concen-

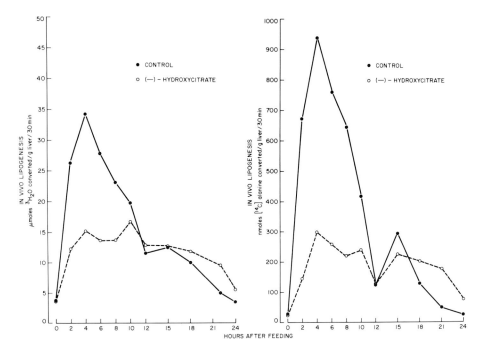

Fig. 9. Effect of oral administration of (—)-hydroxycitrate on the *in vivo* rate of hepatic lipogenesis determined over a 24-hour period. Rats were prefasted 48 hours, then meal-fed a 70% glucose diet for 6 days. On day 7, rats were given either saline or (—)-hydroxy-citrate (2.63 mmoles/kg) by gastric intubation immediately before receiving 8.7 g of food. The *in vivo* rate of lipogenesis was determined using the ^3H_2O and ^{14}C-alanine pulse at the indicated times (8–10 rats per point). The animals were killed 30 minutes after pulse administration. The μmoles ^3H_2O and nmoles ^{14}C-alanine converted into fatty acids in the (—)-hydroxycitrate-treated rats were significantly less than controls at 2, 4, 6, and 8 hours ($p < 0.05$) (Sullivan and Triscari, 1976).

tration of these metabolites may be an important factor in appetite regulation. (—)-Hydroxycitrate might exert its anorectic effect by influencing hepatic glucoreceptors.

d. DITA. DITA [3′,4′-dichloro-2-(2-imidazolin 2-ylthio)aceto-phenone] is an experimental anorectic agent which was active in several animal species and produced an increase in spontaneous locomotor activity (Abdallah and White, 1974). Its potential for abuse, as evaluated in the Rhesus monkey, was found to be one-third as potent as amphetamine (Downs and Woods, 1975).

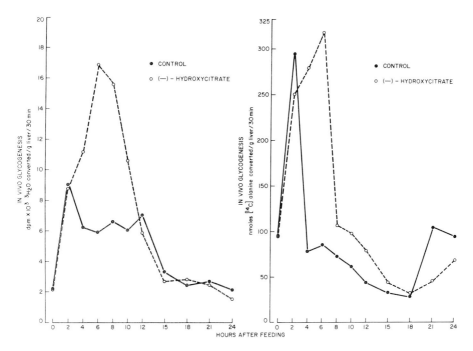

Fig. 10. Effect of the oral administration of (—)-hydroxycitrate on the *in vivo* rate of hepatic glycogenesis determined over a 24-hour period. (See Fig. 9 legend for experimental details). The dpm ^3H_2O and nmoles ^{14}C-alanine converted into glycogen in the (—)-hydroxycitrate-treated rats (5 rats per point) were significantly greater than controls at 6 and 8 hours (^3H_2O), and 6 hours (^{14}C-alanine) ($p < 0.01$) (Sullivan and Triscari, 1976).

e. APMO. APMO [2 - amino - 5 - (3,4 - dichlorophenoxymethyl) - 2 - oxazoline] produced anorexia in several animal species, and was both less active and less toxic than amphetamine (Abdallah, 1973). In equipotent anorectic doses its stimulant effects on both the central nervous and cardiovascular systems were less than those produced by amphetamine. Several analogues of APMO were synthesized which demonstrated significant anorectic activity, particularly 2-amino-5-(phenylthiomethyl)-2-oxazolone (Freiter *et al.*, 1973).

f. PR-F-36-Cl. PR-F-36-Cl [4-chloro-2′-(methylamino)methylbenzhydrol] significantly reduced food intake in rats (Freter *et al.*, 1970). Subsequent studies indicated that although the drug was one-sixth as potent as amphetamine in anorectic activity, it possessed little central nervous

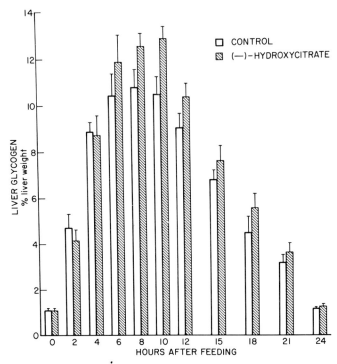

Fig. 11. Effect of the oral administration of (—)-hydroxycitrate on hepatic glycogen content determined over a 24-hour period. (See Fig. 9 legend for experimental details). Hepatic glycogen was isolated at the indicated times (10 rats per group). The amount of glycogen in (—)-hydroxycitrate-treated rats from 6 to 10 hours was significantly greater than controls ($p < 0.05$) (Sullivan and Triscari, 1976).

system or cardiovascular activities (Oliver, 1974). Turnover studies indicated that PR-F-36-Cl did not release catecholamine from storage sites as did amphetamine, but rather prevented the re-uptake of norepinephrine by adrenergic nerve fibers.

B.   Orectic Agents

1.   *Cyproheptadine*

Cyproheptadine (Fig. 12) is an antihistamine and a serotonin antagonist. Studies in the 1960's established the efficacy of cyproheptadine in stimulating appetite and increasing body weight in children and adults. This drug also proved successful in inducing weight gain in patients with anorexia nervosa (Benady, 1970). Continuous therapy with

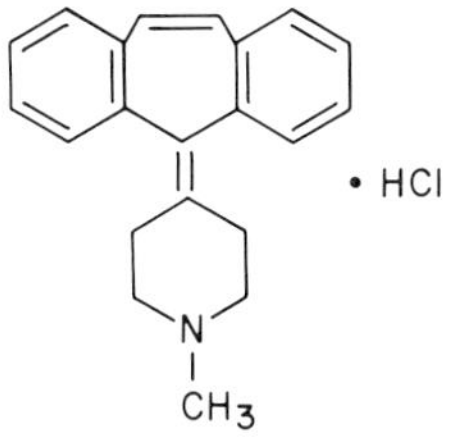

Fig. 12. Chemical structure of cyproheptadine.

cyproheptadine at a daily dose of 12 mg resulted in significantly greater increase in appetite and weight gain as compared to placebo (Mainguet, 1972; Silverstone and Schuyler, 1975; Pawlowski, 1975). According to these studies, cyproheptadine induced weight gains of 2–3.5 kg compared to 0.2–1.3 kg for placebo during a treatment regimen of 4–20 weeks.

Attempts were made to elucidate the mechanism of action of cyproheptadine in promoting weight gain and appetite. Cyproheptadine administered intravenously elicited an increase in the frequency and amplitude of firing in the lateral hypothalamus, but produced no change in the electrical activity of the ventromedial hypothalamus in cats (Chakrabarty *et al.*, 1967). Arteriovenous differences, used as an index of glucose utilization, were decreased following the administration of cyproheptadine (a possible demonstration of the glucostatic theory), and these changes were accompanied by increased food intake, weight gain, and drowsiness. By applying cyproheptadine directly to single neurons in the lateral hypothalamus and the ventromedial hypothalamus of rats, Oomura *et al.*, (1973) found that neuronal firing frequency was reduced in about 60% of the ventromedial hypothalamic neurons, and increased in about 70% of the lateral hypothalamic neurons. Most of the cyproheptadine-sensitive neurons were also glucose-sensitive, in that the firing frequency of the lateral hypothalamic and ventromedial hypothalamic neurons were decreased and increased, respectively, by the local application of glucose.

2. Psychotropic Agents

The chemical structures of a variety of psychotropic drugs which have been reported to stimulate food intake are presented in Figure 13.

a. Benzodiazepines. In the course of evaluating the pharmacology of chlordiazepoxide, it was noted that the drug stimulated the appetite of

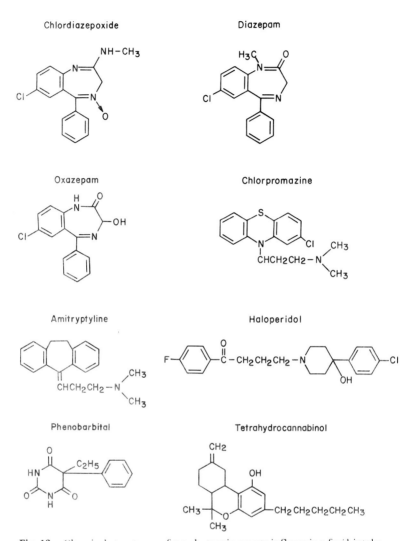

Fig. 13. Chemical structures of psychotropic agents influencing food intake.

experimental animals at doses far below the ataxic dose (Randall, 1960).
This orectic activity of chlordiazepoxide was confirmed by other workers
in experimental animals (Niki, 1965; Matsuda, 1966; Opitz and Akinlaja,
1966; Wedeking, 1974; Poschel, 1971; Stephens, 1973; Soubrié et al.,
1975; Tye et al., 1975; Boissier et al., 1976; Fratta et al., 1976; Mereu et
al., 1976) and in the clinic (McGovern et al., 1960; Feldman, 1962; Ban et
al., 1965; Jenner and Kerry, 1967). The appetite-stimulating effect of

chlordiazepoxide is not unique among the benzodiazepines. Sternbach *et al.*, (1964) presented data on the effects of a large series of benzodiazepines on food intake in starved rats. Subsequent studies have confirmed the appetite-stimulating effect of diazepam and other benzodiazepines including oxazepam, lorazepam, *N*-methyllorazepam, medazepam, nitrazepam, pinazepam, prazepam, and elfazepam (Optiz and Akinlaja, 1966; Margules and Stein, 1967; Poschel, 1971; Soper and Wise, 1971, Stephens, 1973; Wise and Dawson, 1974; Soubrié *et al.*, 1975; Boissier *et al.*, 1976; Fratta *et al.*, 1976; McLaughlin *et al.*, 1976; Mereu *et al.*, 1976).

Attempts were made to determine whether the appetite-stimulating activity of the benzodiazepines was due to disinhibition of a previously suppressed feeding response by means of their antianxiety effect, or due to specific actions on the mechanisms regulating hunger and satiety. There is evidence in the literature showing that both types of actions could account for the appetite-stimulating effect of benzodiazepines. The following observations are consistent with the antianxiety action of benzodiazepines on food intake: (1) Oxazepam increased lever pressing for a sweetened milk reward which had been suppressed in the dark by nonreinforcement of the reward (Margules and Stein, 1967), and increased the drinking behavior suppressed by bitter taste as a result of adulterating sweet milk with quinine. (2) Chlordiazepoxide caused an increase in food seeking behavior inhibited by electric shock in rats (Bainbridge, 1968). (3) In those rats which failed to eat after electrical stimulation of the lateral hypothalamus, the injection of diazepam was able to elicit a stimulation-induced eating response (Soper and Wise, 1971). (4) Benzodiazepines were shown to release the ingestive behavior of rats which had been suppressed by an aversion to a novel situation, such as an unfamiliar food substance in the case of chlordiazepoxide, diazepam, oxazepam, medazepam, and nitrazepam (Poschel, 1971), food from a novel container in the case of chlordiazepoxide (Tye *et al.*, 1975), an unknown eating environment in the case of chlordiazepoxide, diazepam, and nitrazepam (Stephens, 1973), or an unknown eating environment in addition to unfamiliar food in the case of diazepam, chlordiazepoxide, lorazepam, nitrazepam, oxazepam, and prazepam (Boissier *et al.*, 1976; Soubrié *et al.*, 1975). These results are consistent with the view that the release of eating by diazepam is mediated by its action on emotional systems involved in suppression of behavior (Soper and Wise, 1971).

Experimental data also exist which indicate that benzodiazepines may decrease satiety and increase hunger drive: (1) Oxazepam, in addition to releasing suppressed feeding behavior, also increased milk intake of satiated rats (Margules and Stein, 1967). These workers proposed that tranquilizers such as oxazepam release suppressed consummatory behavior through disinhibition, at least in part, by blocking the outflow of the ventromedial nucleus of the hypothalamus. (2) Diazepam increased intake of familiar food but not drinking in satiated rats in both novel and familiar test environments (Wise and Dawson, 1974). (3) Benzodiazepines also increased food intake in animals habituated to a test situation (Boissier *et al.*, 1976; Fratta *et al.*, 1976). (4) Chlordiazepoxide, diazepam, *N*-methyl-lorazepam, and oxazepam could increase food intake in satiated cats (Mereu *et al.*, 1976). The fact that oxazepam abolished the amphetamine-induced anorexia in rats, but had no effect on hyperactivity and sterotypy in amphetamine-treated animals led to the suggestion that the appetite-stimulating effect of benzodiazepines may be attributed to an interference with the release of catecholamines in specific neuronal circuits (Fratta *et al.*, 1976).

b. Chlorpromazine. Chlorpromazine treatment was associated with increased appetite and food intake in schizophrenic patients (Robinson *et al.*, 1975b) and at doses up to 1600 mg/day had been used satisfactorily when combined with insulin in restoring weight gain in patients with anorexia nervosa (Dally, 1967; Dally and Sargant, 1966). Patients were reported to gain between 0.2 and 0.5 kg of body weight/ day. It is possible that endogenous norepinephrine mediated eating elicited by hypothalamically injected chlorpromazine (Leibowitz and Miller, 1969). A recent study showed that chlorpromazine induced a hyperphagic response in rats during the first day of treatment, but suppressed food intake with continued treatment (Robinson *et al.*, 1975b).

c. Amitriptyline.   In a study evaluating the efficacy of amitriptyline maintenance therapy in recovered female depressive patients, it was found unexpectedly that amitriptyline produced excessive weight gain and a craving for carbohydrates (Paykel *et al.*, 1973). Patients on maintenance therapy for 6 months gained an average of 2.5 kg, whereas patients not maintained on amitriptyline gained an average of 0.2 kg during the same period. For those patients who had gained weight during maintenance therapy, withdrawal of the drug was followed by weight loss. A correlation was demonstrated between growth hormone response and the degree of carbohydrate craving; patients with a greater craving for carbohydrates showed a higher growth hormone response to insulin. The authors suggest that amitriptyline may influence the ability of the hypothalamus to recognize cues signaled by changing levels of plasma glucose.

d. Haloperidol. Haloperidol, though having no significant effect on the feeding behavior of deprived animals (Zis and Fibiger, 1975), abolished the feeding response induced by stimulation of the lateral hypothalamus, whether the response was measured by the eating incidence, total duration of eating, or the amount of food consumed (Phillips and Nikaido, 1975).

e. Marijuana and Tetrahydrocannabinol. Marijuana smoking was observed to increase the consumption of marshmallows by human subjects (Abel, 1971). Marijuana administered orally as an extract at doses equivalent to 27–39 mg (mean dose 32 mg) of tetrahydrocannabinol increased appetite and food consumption in slightly more than half of the subjects studied (Hollister, 1971).

In contrast to the paucity of reports on the effect on food intake of marijuana in man, several studies have indicated an appetite depressant effect of tetrahydrocannabinol in rats. Δ^9-Tetrahydrocannabinol, the major active component of marijuana, decreased food intake and body weight of male rats after intraperitoneal administration at doses ranging from 1.25 to 10 mg/kg (Manning *et al.*, 1971; Corcoran and Amit, 1974; Sofia and Barry, 1974; Johansson *et al.*, 1975), but administration of 1.0 mg/kg Δ^9-tetrahydrocannabinol by intubation to deprivation-experienced rats significantly increased food and water intake (Gluck and Ferraro, 1974). However, in female rats, Δ^9-tetrahydrocannabinol either did not significantly affect food intake after intraperitoneal administration (Sjödén *et al.*, 1973), or increased food consumption at a low dose but decreased it at a high dose (Glick and Milloy, 1972). When administered either orally or intraperitoneally Δ^9-tetrahydrocannabinol was found to induce in rats a dose-related aversion to the normally preferred saccharine solution (Elsmore and Fletcher, 1972). The intraperitoneal administration of Δ^8-tetrahydrocannabinol also resulted in decreased food intake and body weight in male rats (Fernandes *et al.*, 1971; Järbe and Henriksson, 1973), but a lack of effect on food intake was observed in a study employing female rats (Sjödén *et al.*, 1973). In dogs smoking marijuana daily for prolonged periods, there was an increase in food consumption at 3 months, a slowing of weight gain during 9 months, and no significant change in food intake or body weight at 27 months (Huy and Roy, 1976). Pyrahexyl, a homologue of marijuana, was found to decrease food intake in rats at a dose of 15 mg/kg (Abel and Schiff, 1969).

f. Barbiturates. Jacobs and Farel (1971) noted that pentobarbital injected intraperitoneally into satiated rats elicited an increase in the amount of wet mash consumed. They attributed this action of pentobarbital to a nonspecific increase in arousal in the presence of a goal object, and not to a specific effect on consummatory behavior. Injection of pentobarbital into the lateral ventricle of rats (Kulkosky *et al.*, 1975), into the third ventricle or lateral ventricle of sheep (Baile and Martin, 1974; Seoane and Baile, 1973, 1975), and into the lateral ventricle of pigs (Baldwin *et al.*, 1975) and cats (Kuhn, 1973) resulted in hyperphagia, possibly by depressing the inhibitory effect of the medial hypothalamus on the lateral hypothalamic feeding center and thus releasing an eating response. Other barbiturates found to stimulate food consumption included phenobarbital (Seoane and Baile, 1973; Wedeking, 1974), amobarbital (Seoane and Baile, 1973; Soubrié *et al.*, 1975) and barbital (Seoane and Baile, 1973), whereas secobarbital and thiamylal (Seoane and Baile, 1973) had no effect. It is interesting to note that pentobarbital produced an elevation in plasma insulin levels in rats prior to the observed increase in food intake (Kulkosky *et al.*, 1975), thus implicating a role of insulin in the mediation of feeding response elicited by barbiturates. Pentobarbital had been shown to antagonize amphetamine anorexia in mice (Abdallah *et al.*, 1974), and amobarbital was found to enhance the anorectic effect of amphetamine in rats (Iorio *et al.*, 1976).

V. SUMMARY AND RESEARCH NEEDS

This review presents current concepts of normal and abnormal appetite regulation and its modulation by drugs. The regulation of food intake involves a complex, multifactorial array of central and peripheral factors which are integrated by metabolic processes. Normal feeding behavior is intimately linked to energy balance, and an optimal level of body weight is maintained through appropriate alterations in caloric intake. Disorders of appetite regulation which are manifested in abnormal body weights include hyperphagic obesity, anorexia nervosa, and conditions accompanying certain organic and psychiatric diseases. Anorectic agents decrease food intake, and demonstrate clinical utility particularly as short-term adjunctive therapy to a dietary restriction program in the treatment of hyperphagic obesity. Orectic agents stimulate appetite, and are employed frequently in the therapeutic regimen for anorexia nervosa.

The field of appetite regulation is receiving increasing attention from physiological psychologists, pharmacologists, and biochemists, and enhancement of such a multidisciplinary approach is needed. The productive interrelationship between basic research and drug development is demonstrated effectively in this field, since an understanding of the mechanism(s) and site(s) of action of several anorectic agents provides insight into central processes involved in appetite regulation. Future research should be directed at the elucidation of the peripheral and metabolic components involved in appetite control. An understanding of the roles these factors play in the modulation of feeding behavior will facilitate the design and development of new drugs with greater specificity, less toxicity, and longer duration of action to treat appetite disorders. Agents could also be employed to modify feeding behavior for economic purposes, e.g., enhancing food intake and weight gain in cattle. The challenge to understand appetite regulation in both normal and abnormal states, and to utilize this information to develop pharmacological agents to treat appetite disorders is most exciting.

REFERENCES

Abdallah, A. H. (1973). Comparative study of the anorexigenic activity of 5-(3,4-Dichlorophenoxymethyl)-2-amino-2-oxazoline.HCl and d-amphetamine in different species. *Toxicol. Appl. Pharmacol.* **25**, 344–353.

Abdallah, A. H., and White, H. D. (1974). Pharmacological evaluation of 3',4'-dichloro-2-(2-imidazolin-2-yl-thio)-, acetophenone hydrobromide (DITA). A new anorexigenic compound. *Fed. Proc., Fed. Am. Soc. Exp. Biol.* **33**, 564.

Abdallah, A. H., White, H. D., and Kulkarni, A. S. (1974). Interaction of d-amphetamine with central nervous system depressants on food intake and spontaneous motor activity of mice. *Eur. J. Pharmacol.* **26**, 119–121.

Abel, E. L. (1971). Effects of marijuana on the solution of anagrams, memory and appetite. *Nature (London)* **231**, 260–261.

Abel, E. L., and Schiff, B. B. (1969). Effects of the marihuana homologue, pyrahexyl, on food and water intake and curiosity in the rat. *Psychonom. Sci.* **16**, 38.

Adair, E. R., Miller, N. E., and Booth, D. A. (1968). Effects of continuous intravenous infusion of nutritive substances on consummatory behavior in rats. *Commun. Behav. Biol., Part A* **2**, 25–37.

Aerberli, P., Eden, P., Gogerty, J. H., Houlihan, W. J., and Penberthy, C. (1975). Anorectic agents. 2. Structural analogs of 5-(p-chlorophenyl-2,3-dihydro-5H-imidazo[2,1-a]isoindol-5-ol. *J. Med. Chem.* **18**, 182–185.

Ahlskog, J. E. (1973). Brain norepinephrine and its involvement in the regulation of food consumption. Ph.D. Thesis, Princeton University, Princeton, New Jersey [Univ. Microfilms, Ann Arbor, Michigan, Order No. 74-9662. *Diss. Abstr. Int. B* **34**, 5700 (1974).]

Ahlskog, J. E. (1974). Food intake and amphetamine anorexia after selective forebrain norepinephrine loss. *Brain Res.* **82**, 211–240.

Ahlskog, J. E., and Hoebel, B. G. (1973). Overeating and obesity from damage to a noradrenergic system in the brain. *Science* **182**, 166–169.

Allen, G. S. (1975). A practical regimen for weight reduction in family practice. *J. Int. Med. Res.* **3**, 40–44.

Anand, B. K., and Brobeck, J. R. (1951). Hypothalamic control of food intake in rats and cats. *Yale J. Biol. Med.* **24**, 123–140.

Anand, B. K., and Pillai, R. V. (1967). Activity of single neurones in the hypothalamic feeding centres: Effect of gastric distension. *J. Physiol. (London)* **192**, 63–77.

Anden, N.-E., Dahlström, A., Fuxe, K., Larsson, K., Olson, L., and Ungerstedt, U. (1966). Ascending monoamine neurons to the telencephalon and diencephalon. *Acta Physiol. Scand.* **67**, 313–326.

Antin, J., Gibbs, J., Hold, J., Young, R. C., and Smith, G. P. (1975). Cholecystokinin elicits the complete behavioral sequence of satiety in rats. *J. Comp. Physiol. Psychol.* **89**, 784–790.

Asmal, A. C., and Leary, W. P. (1975). A study of the effects of 780SE on carbohydrate tolerance and plasma hormone and lipid profile in maturity-onset diabetes. *Postgrad. Med. J.* **51**, Suppl. 1, 144–148.

Baez, L. A. (1974). Role of catecholamines in the anorectic effects of amphetamine in rats. *Psychopharmacologia* **35**, 91–98.

Baile, C. A. (1974). Putative neurotransmitters in the hypothalamus and feeding. *Fed. Proc., Fed. Am. Soc. Exp. Biol.*, **33**, 1166–1175.

Baile, C. A., and Martin, F. H. (1974). Parotid secretion and feeding in sheep following intraventricular injections of 1-norepinephrine, *d*1-isoproterenol, pentobarbital, and carbachol. *J. Dairy Sci.* **57**, 308–313.

Baile, C. A., Mayer, J., Baumgardt, B. R., and Peterson, A. (1970). Comparative gold thioglucose effects on goats, sheep, dogs, rats, and mice. *J. Dairy Sci.* **53**, 801–807.

Baile, C. A., McLaughlin, C. L., Zinn, W., and Mayer, J. (1971). Exercise, lactate, hormones, and gold thioglucose lesions of the hypothalamus of diabetic mice. *Am. J. Physiol.* **221**, 150–155.

Baile, C. A., Simpson, C. W., Bean, S. M., McLaughlin, C. L., and Jacobs, H. L. (1973). Prostaglandings and food intake of rats: A component of energy balance regulator? *Physiol. Behav.* **10**, 1077–1085.

Baillie, P., and Morrison, S. D. (1963). The nature of the suppression of food intake by lateral hypothalamic lesions in rats. *J. Physiol. (London)* **165**, 227–245.

Bainbridge, J. G. (1968). The effect of psychotropic drugs on food reinforced behavior and on food consumption. *Psychopharmacologia* **12**, 204–213.

Balagura, S., Wilcox, R. H., and Coscina, D. V. (1969). The effect of diencephalic lesions on food intake and motor activity. *Physiol. Behav.* **4**, 629–633.

Baldwin, B. A., Grovum, W. L., Baile, C. A., and Brobeck, J. R. (1975). Feeding following intraventricular injection of Ca^{++}, Mg^{++} or pentobarbital in pigs. *Pharmacol., Biochem. Behav.* **3**, 915–918.

Ball, G. G. (1974). Vagotomy: Effect on electrically elicited eating and self-stimulation in the lateral hypothalamus. *Science* **184**, 484–485.

Ban, T. A., Lehmann, H. E. Matthews, V., and Donald, M. (1965). Comparative study of chlorpromazine and chlordiazepoxide in the prevention and treatment of alcohol withdrawal symptoms. *Clin. Med.* **72**, 59–64 and 66–67.

Barrett, A. M., and McSharry, L. (1975). Inhibition of drug-induced anorexia in rats by methysergide. *J. Pharm. Pharmacol.* **27**, 889–895.

Beckett, A. H. (1975). Recent research on the basic factors involved in studies on the metabolism and distribution of anorectic drugs. *Postgrad. Med. J.* **51**, Suppl. 1, 9–12.

Bell, D. D., and Zucker, I. (1971). Sex differences in body weight and eating: Organization and activation by gonadal hormones in the rat. *Physiol. Behav.* **7**, 27–34.

Bell, E. T., Harkness, R. A., Loraine, J. A., and Russell, G. F. M. (1966). Hormone assay studies in patients with anorexia nervosa. *Acta Endocrinol. (Copenhagen)* **51**, 140–148.

Bellinger, L. L., Trietley, G. J., and Bernardis, L. L. (1976). Failure of portal glucose and adrenaline infusions or liver denervation to affect food intake in dogs. *Physiol. Behav.* **16**, 299–304.

Benady, D. R. (1970). Cyproheptadine hydrochloride (Periactin) and anorexia nervosa: A case report. *Br. J. Psychiatry* **117**, 681–682.

Bjorntörp, P., Bergman, H., and Varnauskas, E. (1969). Plasma free fatty acid turnover rate in obesity. *Acta Med. Scand.* **185**, 351–356.

Blitzer, J. R., Rollins, N., and Blackwell, A. (1961). Children who starve themselves: Anorexia nervosa. *Psychosom. Med.* **23**, 369–383.

Blundell, J. E., and Campbell, D. B. (1975). The relationship between fenfluramine and norfenfluramine blood levels and anorectic activity in the rat. *Br. J. Pharmacol.* **55**, 261P.

Blundell, J. E., and Leshem, M. B. (1973). Dissociation of the anorexic effects of fenfluramine and amphetamine following intrahypothalamic injection. *Br. J. Pharmacol.* **47**, 183–185.

Blundell, J. E., and Leshem, M. B. (1974). Central action of anorexic agents: Effects of amphetamine and fenfluramine in rats with lateral hypothalamic lesions. *Eur. J. Pharmacol.* **28**, 81–88.

Blundell, J. E., and Leshem, M. B. (1975a). The effect of 5-hydroxytryptophan on food intake and on the anorexic action of amphetamine and fenfluramine. *J. Pharm. Pharmacol.* **27**, 31–37.

Blundell, J. E., and Leshem, M. B. (1975b). Hypothalamic lesions and drug-induced anorexia. *Postgrad. Med. J.* **51**, Suppl. 1, 45–54.

Blundell, J. E., Latham, C. J., and Leshem, M. B. (1976). Differences between the anorexic actions of amphetamine and fenfluramine—possible effects on hunger and satiety. *J. Pharm. Pharmacol.* **28**, 471–477.

Boissier, J. R., Simon, P., and Soubrié, P. (1976). New approaches to the study of anxiety and anxiolytic drugs in animal. *Proc. Int. Congr. Pharmacol., 6th, 1975* Vol. 3, pp. 213–222.

Booth, D. A. (1967). Localization of the adrenergic feeding system in the rat diencephalon. *Science* **158**, 515–517.

Booth, D. A. (1968a). Mechanism of action of norepinephrine in eliciting an eating response on injection into the rat hypothalamus. *J. Pharmacol. Exp. Ther.* **160**, 336–348.

Booth, D. A. (1968b). Amphetamine anorexia by direct action on the adrenergic feeding system of rat hypothalamus. *Nature (London)* **217**, 869–870.

Booth, D. A. (1972a). Satiety and behavioral caloric compensation following intragastric glucose loads in the rat. *J. Comp. Physiol. Psychol.* **78**, 412–432.

Booth, D. A. (1972b). Modulation of the feeding response to peripheral insulin, 2-deoxyglucose or 3-O-methyl glucose injection. *Physiol. Behav.* **8**, 1069–1076.

Booth, D. A. (1972c). Postabsorptively induced suppression of appetite and the energostatic control of feeding. *Physiol. Behav.* **9**, 199–202.

Booth, D. A., and Brookover, T. (1968). Hunger elicited in the rat by a single injection of bovine crystalline insulin. *Physiol. Behav.* **3**, 439–446.

Booth, D. A., and Pitt, M. E. (1968). The role of glucose in insulin-induced feeding and drinking. *Physiol. Behav.* **3**, 447–453.

Bourillet, F., and Buzas, A. (1976). Anorectic phenoxyacetamide derivatives of *m*-trifluoromethyl-phenyl-isopropylamine. *Proc. Int. Congr. Pharmacol., 6th, 1975* p. 357.

Bray, G. A. (1974). Endocrine factors in the control of food intake. *Fed. Proc., Fed. Am. Soc. Exp. Biol.,* **33**, 1140–1145.

Bray, G. A. (1975). Metablic effects of corpulence. In "Recent Advances in Obesity Research" (A. Howard, ed.), Vol. 1, pp. 56–65. Newman Publ. Ltd., London.

Bray, G. A., and Gallagher, T. F., Jr. (1975). Manifestations of hypothalamic obesity in man: A comprehensive investigation of eight patients and a review of the literature. Medicine (Baltimore) 54, 301–330.

Breisch, S. T., Zemlan, F. P., and Hoebel, B. G. (1976). Hyperphagia and obesity following serotonin depletion by intraventricular p-chlorophenylalanine. Science 192, 382–385.

Brobeck, J. R. (1946). Mechanism of the development of obesity in animals with hypothalamic lesions. Physiol. Rev. 26, 541–559.

Brobeck, J. R. (1948). Food intake as a mechanism of temperature regulation. Yale J. Biol. Med. 20, 545–552.

Brobeck, J. R., Tepperman, J., and Long, C. N. H. (1943). Experimental hypothalamic hyperphagia in the albino rat. Yale J. Biol. Med. 15, 831–853.

Brobeck, J. R., Larsson, S., and Reyes, E. (1956). A study of the electrical activity of the hypothalamic feeding mechanism. J. Physiol. (London) 132, 358–364.

Buczko, W., De Gaetano, G., and Garattini, S. (1975). Effect of fenfluramine on 5-hydroxytryptamine uptake and release by rat blood platelets. Br. J. Pharmacol. 53, 563–568.

Carey, R. J., and Goodall, E. B. (1975). Attentuation of amphetamine anorexia by unilateral nigral striatal lesions. Neuropharmacology 14, 827–834.

Carlisle, H. J. (1964). Differential effects of amphetamine on food and water intake in rats with lateral hypothalamic lesions. J. Comp. Physiol. Psychol. 58, 47–54.

Chakrabarty, A. S., Pillai, R. V., Anand, B. K., and Singh, B. (1967). Effect of cyproheptadine on the electrical activity of the hypothalamic feeding centres. Brain Res. 6, 561–569.

Chase, T. N., and Shoulson, I. (1975). Behavioural and biochemical effects of fenfluramine in patients with neurologic disease. Postgrad. Med. J. 51, Suppl. 1, 105–109.

Clineschmidt, B. V. (1973). 5,6-dihydroxytryptamine: Suppression of the anorexigenic action of fenfluramine. Eur. J. Pharmacol. 24, 405–409.

Clineschmidt, B. V., McGuffin, J. C., and Werner, A. B. (1974). Role of monoamines in the anorexigenic actions of fenfluramine, amphetamine and p-chloromethamphetamine. Eur. J. Pharmacol. 27, 313–323.

Corcoran, M. E., and Amit, Z. (1974). The effects of hashish injections on feeding and drinking in rats. Res. Commun. Chem. Pathol. Pharmacol. 9, 193–196.

Craddock, D. (1976). Anorectic drugs: Use in general practice. Drugs 11, 378–393.

Crisp, A. H., and Toms, D. A. (1972). Primary anorexia nervosa or weight phobia in the male: Report on 13 cases. Br. Med. J. 1, 334–338.

Crisp, A. H., MacKinnon, P. C. B., Chen, C., and Corker, C. S. (1973). Observations of gonadotrophic and ovarian hormone activity during recovery from anorexia nervosa. Postgrad, Med. J. 49, 584–590.

Dafny, N., Jacob, R. H., and Jacobson, E. D. (1975). Gastrointestinal hormones and neural interaction within the central nervous system. Experientia 31, 658–660.

Dally, P., and Sargant, W. (1966). Treatment and outcome of anorexia nervosa. Br. Med. J. 2, 793–795.

Dally, P. J. (1967). Anorexia nervosa—long-term follow up and effects of treatment. J. Psychosom. Res. 11, 151–155.

Davis, J. D., and Campbell, C. S. (1973). Peripheral control of meal size in the rat: Effect of sham feeding on meal size and drinking rate. J. Comp. Physiol. Psychol. 83, 379–387.

Davis, J. D., Collins, B. J., and Levine, M. W. (1976). Peripheral control of meal size: Interaction of gustatory stimulation and postingestional feedback. In "Hunger: Basic

Mechanisms and Clinical Implications" (D. Novin, W. Wyrwicka, and G. Bray, eds.), pp. 395–408. Raven, New York.

Debons, A. F., Silver, L., Cronkite, E. P., Johnson, H. A., Brecher, G., Tenzer, D., and Schwartz, I. L. (1962). Localization of gold in mouse brain in relation to gold thioglucose obesity, *Am. J. Physiol.* **202**, 743–750.

Debons, A. F., Krimsky, I., Likuski, H. J., From, A., and Cloutier, R. J. (1968). Gold thioglucose damage to the satiety center: Inhibition in diabetes. *Am. J. Physiol.* **214**, 652–658.

Defelice, E. A., Chaykin, L. B., and Cohen, A. (1973). Double-blind clinical evaluation of mazindol, dextroamphetamine, and placebo in treatment of exogenous obesity. *Curr. Ther. Res. Clin. Exp.* **15**, 358–366.

Dent, R. W., Jr., and Preston, L. W., Jr. (1975). Anorectic effectiveness of various dosages of fenfluramine and placebo: A cooperative double-blind study. *Curr. Ther. Res. Clin. Exp.* **18**, 132–143.

Dobrzanski, S., and Doggett, N. S. (1975). Effect of dopamine-β-hydroxylase inhibitors and centrally administered noradrenaline on (+)-amphetamine anorexia in mice. *Br. J. Pharmacol.* **54**, 245P–246P.

Dorf, G., Louis, A., and Benedetti, M. S. (1975). Clinical and pharmacokinetic studies of a new anorectic drug: 11698 J.L. *In* "Recent Advances in Obesity Research" (A. Howard, ed.), Vol. 1, pp. 404–406. Newman Publ. Ltd., London.

Downs, D. A., and Woods, J. H. (1975). Food- and drug-reinforced responding: Effects of DITA and *d*-amphetamine. *Psychopharmacologia* **43**, 13–17.

Duhault, J., Malen, C., Boulanger, M., Voisin, C., Beregi, L., and Schmitt, H. (1975a). Fenfluramine and 5-hydroxytryptamine. Part 1: Is fenfluramine or norfenfluramine involved in the decrease of brain 5-hydroxytryptamine? *Arzneim.-Forsch.* **25**, 1755–1758.

Duhault, J., Boulanger, M., Voisin, C., Malen, C., and Schmitt, H. (1975b). Fenfluramine and 5-hydroxytryptamine. Part 2: Involvement of brain 5-hydroxytryptamine in the anorectic activity of fenfluramine. *Arzneim.-Forsch.* **25**, 1758–1762.

Duhault, J., Beregi, L., Boulanger, M., and Hugon, P. (1975c). New glycinates with high anorectic activity. *In* "Recent Advances in Obesity Research" (A. Howard, ed.), Vol. 1, pp. 409–411. Newman Publ. Ltd., London.

Durrer, J. L., and Hannon, J. P. (1962). Seasonal variations in caloric intake of dogs living in an arctic environment. *Am. J. Physiol.* **202**, 375–378.

Elsmore, T. F., and Fletcher, G. V. (1972). Δ^9-tetrahydrocannabinol: Aversive effects in rat at high doses. *Science* **175**, 911–912.

Engstrom, R. G., Kelly, L. A., and Gogerty, J. H. (1975). The effects 5-hydroxy-5-(4′-chlorophenyl)-2,3-dihydro-5H-imidazo (2,1-a) isoindole (mazindol, SaH 42-548) on the metabolism of brain norepinephrine. *Arch. Int. Pharmacodyn. Ther.* **214**, 308–321.

Epstein, A. N. (1971). The lateral hypothalamic syndrome: Its implications for the physiological psychology of hunger and thirst. *Prog. Physiol. Psychol.* **4**, 263–317.

Epstein, A. N. (1960). Reciprocal changes in feeding behavior produced by intrahypothalamic chemical injections. *Am. J. Physiol.* **199**, 969–974.

Epstein, A. N., and Teitelbaum, P. (1962). Regulation of food intake in the absence of taste, smell, and other oropharyngeal sensations. *J. Comp. Physiol. Psychol.* **55**, 753–759.

Epstein, A. N., and Teitelbaum, P. (1967). Specific loss of the hypoglycemic control of feeding in recovered lateral rats. *Am. J. Physiol.* **213**, 1159–1167.

Feldman, P. E. (1962). An analysis of the efficacy of diazepam. *J. Neuropsychiatry* **3**, S62–S67.

Fenfluramine and Derivatives. (1975). Proceedings of a symposium held in Marbella, Spain, Mar. 11–16, 1974, organized by the Servier Research Institute. *Postgrad. Med. J.* **51**, Suppl. 1, 1–189.

Fernandes, M., Rating, D., and Kluwe, S. (1971). The influence of subchronic tetrahy-drocannabinole- and cannabis treatment on food- and water-intake, body weight and body temperature of rats. *Acta Pharmacol. Toxicol.* **29**, Suppl. 4, 89.

Fibiger, H. C., Zis, A. P., and McGeer, E. G. (1973). Feeding and drinking deficits after 6-hydroxydopamine administration in the rat: Similarities to the lateral hypothalamic syndrome. *Brain Res.* **55**, 135–148.

Finger, F. W., and Mook, D. G. (1971). Basic drives. *Annu. Rev. Psychol.* **22**, 1–38.

Fratta, W., Mereu, G., Chessa, P., Paglietti, E., and Gessa, G. (1976). Benzodiazepine-induced voraciousness in cats and inhibitions of amphetamine-anorexia. *Life Sci.* **18**, 1157–1166.

Freiter, E. R., Abdallah, A. H., and Strycker, S. J. (1973). Some 2-amino-5-substituted oxazolines and intermediates as potential anorectants. *J. Med. Chem.* **16**, 510–512.

Freter, K. R., Gotz, N., and Oliver, J. T. (1970). A new group of anorexigenic compounds. *J. Med. Chem.* **13**, 1228–1230.

Frey, H.-H., and Schulz, R. (1973). On the central mediation of anorexigenic drug effects. *Biochem. Pharmacol.* **22**, 3041–3049.

Friedman, E., Starr, N., and Gershon, S. (1973). Catecholamine synthesis and the regulation of food intake in the rat. *Life Sci.* **12**, Part 1, 317–326.

Funderburk, W. H., Hazelwood, J. C., Ruckart, R. T., and Ward, J. W. (1971). Is 5-hydroxytryptamine involved in the mechanism of action of fenfluramine? *J. Pharm. Pharmacol.* **23**, 468–470.

Fuxe, K., Hamberger, B., Farnebo, L.-O., and Örgen, S.-O. (1975). On the *in vivo* and *in vitro* actions of fenfluramine and its derivatives on central monoamine neurons, especially 5-hydroxytryptamine neurons, and their relation to the anorectic activity of fenfluramine. *Postgrad. Med. J.* **51**, Suppl. 1, 35–45.

Garattini, S., Jori, A., Buczko, W., and Samanin, R. (1975a). The mechanism of action of fenfluramine. *Postgrad. Med. J.* **51**, Suppl. 1, 27–35.

Garattini, S., Bizzi, A., deGaetano, G., Jori, A., and Samanin, R. (1975b). Recent advances in the pharmacology of anorectic agents. *In* "Recent Advances in Obesity Research" (A. Howard, ed.), Vol. 1, pp. 354–367. Newman Publ. Ltd., London.

Ghezzi, D., Samanin, R., Bernasconi, S., Tognoni, G., Gerna, M., and Garattini, S. (1973). Effect of thymoleptics on fenfluramine-induced depletion of brain serotonin in rats. *Eur. J. Pharmacol.* **24**, 205–210.

Gibbs, J., Young, R. C., and Smith, G. P. (1973a). Cholecystokinin decreases food intake in rats. *J. Comp. Physiol. Psychol.* **84**, 488–495.

Gibbs, J., Young, R. C., and Smith, G. P. (1973b). Cholecystokinin elicits satiety in rats with open gastric fistulas. *Nature (London)* **245**, 323–325.

Gibbs, J., Falasco, J. D., and McHugh, P. R. (1976). Cholecystokinin-decreased food intake in rhesus monkeys. *Am. J. Physiol.* **230**, 15–18.

Giudicelli, J. F., Richer, C., and Berdeaux, A. (1976). Preliminary assessment of flutiorex, a new anorectic drug, in man. *Br. J. Clin. Pharmacol.* **3**, 113–121.

Giudicelli, R., Lefevre, F., Jalfre, M., Branceni, D., and Najer, H. (1976). Pharmacological studies on *d*-1-(3'-trifluoromethylthio-phenyl)-2-ethylamino-propane (SL 72.340-d), a new anorexigenic agent. *Proc. Int. Congr. Pharmacol., 6th, 1975*, p. 356.

Glick, S. D., and Milloy, S. (1972). Increased and decreased eating following THC administration. *Psychonom. Sci.* **29**, 6.

Gluck, J. P., and Ferraro, D. P. (1974). Effects of Δ^9-THC on food and water intake of deprivation experienced rats. *Behav. Biol.* **11,** 395–401.

Glucksman, M. L. (1972). Psychiatric observations on obesity. *Adv. Psychosom. Med.* **7,** 194–216.

Goetz, H., and Sturdevant, R. (1975). Effect of cholecystokinin on food intake in man. *Clin. Res.* **23,** 98A.

Gogerty, J. H., Penberthy, C., Iorio, L. C., and Trapold, J. H. (1975). Pharmacological analysis of a new anorexic substance: 5-hydroxy-5-(4'-chlorophenyl)-2,3-dihydro-5H-imadazo-(2,1-a) isoindole (mazindol). *Arch. Int. Pharmacodyn. Ther.* **214,** 285–307.

Gold, R. M. (1967). Aphagia and adipsia following unilateral and bilaterally asymmetrical lesions in rats. *Physiol. Behav.* **2,** 211–220.

Goldman, J. K., Schnatz, J. D., Bernardis, L. L., and Frohman, L. A. (1970). Adipose tissue metabolism of weanling rats after destruction of ventromedial hypothalamic nuclei: Effect of hypophysectomy and growth hormone. *Metab. Clin. Exp.* **19,** 995–1005.

Goldrick, R. B., Nestel, P. J., and Havenstein, N. (1974). Comparison of a new anorectic agent AN 448 with fenfluramine in the treatment of refractory obesity. *Med. J. Aust.* **1,** 882–885.

Goudie, A. J., Taylor, M., and Wheeler, T. J. (1974). Chronic anorexic and behavioural effects of the fenfluramine metabolite, norfenfluramine: An evaluation of its role in the actions of fenfluramine. *Psychopharmacologia* **38,** 67–74.

Goudie, A. J., Thornton, E. W., and Wheeler, T. J. (1976). Effects of Lilly 110140, a specific inhibitor of 5-hydroxytryptamine uptake, on food intake and on 5-hydroxy-tryptophan-induced anorexia. Evidence for serotoninergic inhibition of feeding. *J. Pharm. Pharmacol.* **28,** 318–320.

Graff, H., and Stellar, E. (1962). Hyperphagia, obesity, and finickiness. *J. Comp. Physiol. Psychol.* **55,** 418–424.

Griboff, S. I., Berman, R., and Silverman, H. I. (1975). A double-blind clinical evaluation of a phenylpropanolamine–caffeine–vitamin combination and a placebo in the treatment of exogenous obesity. *Curr. Ther. Res. Clin. Exp.* **17,** 535–543.

Griffith, J. D., Witt, J. G., and Jasinski, D. R. (1974). A comparison of fenfluramine and *d*-amphetamine in man. *Clin. Pharmacol. Ther.* **15,** 207.

Griffith, J. D., Nutt, J. G., and Jasinski, D. R. (1975). A comparison of fenfluramine and amphetamine in man. *Clin. Pharmacol. Ther.* **18,** 563–570.

Griffith, J. D., Jasinski, D. R., and Pevnick, J. S. (1976). Chlorphentermine: Absence of amphetamine-like profile in man. *Clin. Pharmacol. Ther.* **19,** 107.

Grossie, J., and Turner, C. W. (1961). Effect of hyperthyroidism on body weight gain and feed consumption in male and female rats. *Proc. Soc. Exp. Biol. Med.* **107,** 520–523.

Grossie, J., and Turner, C. W. (1965). Effect of thyroparathyroidectomy and adrenalectomy on food intake in rats. *Proc. Soc. Exp. Biol. Med.* **118,** 25–27.

Grossman, S. P. (1960). Eating or drinking elicited by direct adrenergic or cholinergic stimulation of hypothalamus. *Science* **132,** 301–302.

Grossman, S. P. (1962a). Direct adrenergic and cholinergic stimulation of hypothalamic mechanisms. *Am. J. Physiol.* **202,** 872–882.

Grossman, S. P. (1962b). Effects of adrenergic and cholinergic blocking agents on hypothalamic mechanism. *Am. J. Physiol.* **202,** 1230–1236.

Grossman, S. P. (1972). Neurophysiologic aspects: Extrahypothalamic factors in the regulation of food intake. *Adv. Psychosom. Med.* **7,** 49–72.

Grossman, S. P. (1975). Role of the hypothalamus in the regulation of food and water intake. *Psychol. Rev.* **82,** 200–224.

Grossman, S. P., and Grossman, L. (1963). Food and water intake following lesions or electrical stimulation of the amygdala. *Am. J. Physiol.* **205,** 761–765.

Grossman, S. P., and Grossman, L. (1970). Surgical interruption of the anterior or posterior connections of the hypothalamus: Effects on aggressive and avoidance behavior. *Physiol. Behav.* **5,** 1313–1317.

Hadler, A. J. (1967a). Weight reduction with phenmetrazine: A double-blind study. *Curr. Ther. Res. Clin. Exp.* **9,** 462–467.

Hadler, A. J. (1967b). Weight reduction with phenmetrazine and chlorphentermine. A double-blind study. *Curr. Ther. Res. Clin. Exp.* **9,** 563–569.

Hadler, A. J. (1968a). Reduced-dosage sustained-action phenmetrazine in obesity. *Curr. Ther. Res. Clin. Exp.* **10,** 255–259.

Hadler, A. J. (1968b). Sustained-action phendimetrazine in obesity. *J. Clin. Pharmacol.* **8,** 113–117.

Hall, R. J. C. (1975). Progress report: Normal and abnormal food intake. *Gut* **16,** 744–752.

Hamilton, C. L. (1963). Hypothalamic temperature records of a monkey. *Proc. Soc. Exp. Biol. Med.* **112,** 55–57.

Harper, A. E. (1976). Protein and amino acids in the regulation of food intake. *In* "Hunger: Basic Mechanisms and Clinical Implications" (D. Novin, W. Wyrwicka, and G. Bray, eds.), pp. 103–113. Raven, New York.

Harvey, J. A., and McMaster, S. E. (1975). Fenfluramine: Evidence for a neurotoxic action on midbrain and a long-term depletion of serotonin. *Psychopharmacol. Commun.* **1,** 217–228.

Haugen, H. N. (1975). Double blind cross-over study of a new appetite suppressant. *Eur. J. Clin. Pharmacol.* **8,** 71–74.

Heber, K. R. (1975). Double-blind trial of mazindol in overweight patients. *Med. J. Aust.* **2,** 566–567.

Heffner, T. G., Zigmond, M. J., and Stricker, E. M. (1975). Brain dopamine involvement in amphetamine-induced anorexia. *Fed. Proc., Fed. Am. Soc. Exp. Biol.* **34,** 348.

Heldenberg, D., Tamir, I., Ashner, M., and Werben, B. (1972). Hyperphagia, obesity and diabetes insipidus due to hypothalamic lesion in a girl. *Helv. Paediatr. Acta* **27,** 489–494.

Heron, G. B., and Johnston, D. A. (1976). Hypothalamic tumor presenting as anorexia nervosa. *Am. J. Psychiatry* **133,** 580–582.

Hervey, G. R. (1969). Regulation of energy balance. *Nature (London)* **222,** 629–631.

Hetherington, A. W., and Ranson, S. W. (1940). Hypothalamic lesions and adiposity in the rat. *Anat. Rec.* **78,** 149–172.

Hoebel, B. G. (1971). Feeding: Neural control of intake. *Annu. Rev. Physiol.* **33,** 533–568.

Hoebel, B. G., and Teitelbaum, P. (1966). Weight regulation in normal and hypothalamic hyperphagic rats. *J. Comp. Physiol. Psychol.* **61,** 189–193.

Hoebel, B. G., Hernandez, L., and Thompson, R. D. (1975). Phenylpropanolamine inhibits feeding, but not drinking, induced by hypothalamic stimulation. *J. Comp. Physiol. Psychol.* **89,** 1046–1052.

Hollifield, G. (1968). Glucocorticoid-induced obesity—a model and a challenge. *Am. J. Clin. Nutr.* **21,** 1471–1474.

Hollister, L. E. (1971). Hunger and appetite after single doses of marihuana, alcohol, and dextroamphetamine. *Clin. Pharmacol. Ther.* **12,** 44–49.

Holstrand, J., and Jonsson, J. (1975). Subjective effects of two anorexigenic agents—fenfluramine and AN 488 in normal subjects. *Postgrad. Med. J.* **51,** Suppl. 1, 183–186.

Holtzman, S. G., and Jewett, R. E. (1971). The role of brain norepinephrine in the anorexic effects of dextroamphetamine and monoamine oxidase inhibitors in the rat. *Psychopharmacologia* **22**, 151–161.

Hooper, A. C. (1975). A clinical trial of a new fenfluramine preparation (Ponderax PA). *Postgrad. Med. J.* **51**, Suppl. 1, 159–160.

Huy, N. D., and Roy, P. E. (1976). Inhalation of tobacco and marijuana in dog over a period of 30 months: Effect on body weight, food intake and organ weight. *Res. Commun. Chem. Pathol. Pharmacol.* **13**, 465–472.

Innes, J. A., Millar, J., Campbell, I. W., and Munro, J. F. (1975). A comparison of the efficacy and acceptability of fenfluramine tablets (BP) and prolonged action capsules. *Postgrad. Med. J.* **51**, Suppl. 1, 160–162.

Iorio, L. C., Ryan, E. A., and Gogerty, J. H. (1976). Combinations of selected CNS depressants with *d*-amphetamine or mazindol on food intake and motor activity of rats. *Eur. J. Pharmacol.* **36**, 89–94.

Jacobs, B. L., and Farel, P. B. (1971). Motivated behaviors produced by increased arousal in the presence of goal objects. *Physiol. Behav.* **6**, 473–476.

Järbe, T. U. C., and Henriksson, B. G. (1973). Acute effects of two tetrahydrocannabinols (Δ^9-THC and Δ^8-THC) on water intake in water deprived rats: Implications for behavioral studies on marijuana compounds. *Psychopharmacologia* **30**, 315–322.

Jenner, F. A., and Kerry, R. J. (1967). Comparison of diazepam, chlordiazepoxide and amylobarbitone. (A multidose double blind crossover study.) *Dis. Nerv. Syst.* **28**, 245–249.

Jespersen, S., and Scheel-Krüger, J. (1973). Evidence for a difference in mechanism of action between fenfluramine- and amphetamine-induced anorexia. *J. Pharm. Pharmacol.* **25**, 49–54.

Johansson, J. O., Järbe, T. U. C., and Henrikkson, B. G. (1975). Acute and subchronic influences of tetrahydrocannabinols on water and food intake, body weight, and temperature in rats. *TIT J. Life Sci.* **5**, 17–27.

Johnson, J. T., and Levine, S. (1973). Influence of water deprivation on adrenocortical rhythms. *Neuroendocrinology* **11**, 268–273.

Johnson, R. E., and Kark, R. M. (1947). Environment and food intake in man. *Science* **105**, 378–379.

Kakalewski, J. W., Cox, V. C., and Valenstein, E. S. (1968). Sex differences in body weight change following gonadectomy of rats. *Psychol. Rep.* **22**, 547–554.

Kamalian, N., Keesey, R. E., and Zu Rhein, G. M. (1975). Lateral hypothalamic demyelination and cachexia in a case of "malignant" multiple sclerosis. *Neurology* **25**, 25–30.

Kandel, D., Doyle, D., and Fischman, M. W. (1975). Tolerance and cross-tolerance to the effects of amphetamine, methamphetamine and fenfluramine on milk consumption in the rat. *Pharmacol., Biochem. Behav.* **3**, 705–707.

Kawamura, Y. (1975). Role of sensory factors in chewing and feeding behavior. *Pharmacol., Biochem. Behav.* **3**, Suppl. 1, 163–173.

Kay, D. W. K., and Schapira, K. (1972). Psychiatric observations on anorexia. *Adv. Psychosom. Med.* **7**, 277–299.

Keesey, R. E., and Boyle, P. C. (1973). Effects of quinine adulteration upon body weight of LH-lesioned and intact male rats. *J. Comp. Physiol. Psychol.* **84**, 38–46.

Keesey, R. E., and Powley, T. L. (1975). Hypothalamic regulation of body weight. *Am. Sci.* **63**, 558–565.

Keesey, R. E., Boyle, P. C., Kemnitz, J. W., and Mitchel, J. S. (1976). The role of the lateral hypothalamus in determining the body weight set point. *In* "Hunger: Basic Mechanisms and Clinical Implications" (D. Novin, W. Wyrwicka, and G. Bray, eds.), pp. 243–255. Raven, New York.

Kennedy, G. C. (1950). The hypothalamic control of food intake in rats. *Proc. R. Soc. London, Ser. B* **137**, 535–549.

Kennedy, G. C. (1966). Food intake, energy balance and growth. *Br. Med. Bull.* **22**, 216–220.

Kornhaber, A. (1973). Obesity-depression: Clinical evaluation with a new anorexigenic agent. *Psychosomatics* **14**, 162–167.

Kramer, R., Rubicek, M., and Turner, P. (1973). The role of norfenfluramine in fenfluramine-induced mydriasis. *J. Pharm. Pharmacol.* **25**, 575–576.

Krebs, H., Bindra, D., and Campbell, J. F. (1969). Effects of amphetamine on neuronal activity in the hypothalamus. *Physiol. Behav.* **4**, 685–691.

Kruk, Z. L. (1973). Dopamine and 5-hydroxytryptamine inhibit feeding in rats. *Nature (London), New Biol.* **246**, 52–53.

Kruk, Z. L. (1976). Mazindol anorexia is mediated by stimulation of central dopamine receptors. *Proc. Int. Congr. Pharmacol., 6th, 1975* Abstract No. 832.

Kuhn, F. J. (1973). Hyperphagia in cats induced by injection of sodium pentobarbital into cerebral ventricles as a method for testing anorectics. *Arzneim.-Forsch.* **23**, 100–102.

Kulkosky, P. J., Porte, D., Jr., and Woods, S. C. (1975). Elevation of rat plasma insulin by intrathecal pentobarbital. *Experientia* **31**, 123–124.

Langlois, K. J., Forbes, J. A., Bell, G. W., and Grant, G. F., Jr. (1974). A double-blind clinical evaluation of the safety and efficacy of phentermine hydrochloride (Fastin) in the treatment of exogenous obesity. *Curr. Ther. Res. Clin. Exp.* **16**, 289–296.

Leibowitz, S. F. (1970). Reciprocal hunger-regulating circuits involving alpha- and beta-adrenergic receptors located, respectively, in the ventromedial and lateral hypothalamus. *Proc. Natl. Acad. Sci. U.S.A.* **67**, 1063–1070.

Leibowitz, S. F. (1975a). Amphetamine: Possible site and mode of action for producing anorexia in the rat. *Brain Res.* **84**, 160–167.

Leibowitz, S. F. (1975b). Catecholaminergic mechanisms of the lateral hypothalamus: Their role in the mediation of amphetamine anorexia. *Brain Res.* **98**, 529–545

Leibowitz, S. F. (1976). Brain catecholaminergic mechanisms for control of hunger. *In* "Hunger: Basic Mechanisms and Clinical Implications" (D. Novin, W. Wyrwicka, and G. Bray, eds.), pp. 1–18. Raven, New York.

Leibowitz, S. F., and Miller, N. E. (1969). Unexpected adrenergic effect of chlorpromazine: Eating elicited by injection into rat hypothalamus. *Science* **165**, 609–611.

Le Magnen, J. (1972). Regulation of food intake. Physiologic-biochemical aspects (peripheral regulatory factors). *Adv. Psychosom. Med.* **7**, 73–90.

Leung, P. M. B., and Rogers, Q. R. (1969). Food intake: Regulation by plasma amino acid pattern. *Life Sci.* **8**, Part 2, 1–9.

Leung, P. M. B., and Rogers, Q. R. (1971). Importance of prepyriform cortex in food-intake response of rats to amino acids. *Am. J. Physiol.* **221**, 929–935.

Levin, A. (1975). The non-medical misuse of fenfluramine by drug-dependent young South Africans. *Postgrad. Med. J.* **51**, Suppl. 1, 186–188.

Lewin, K., Mattingly, D., and Millis, R. R. (1972). Anorexia nervosa associated with hypothalamic tumour. *Br. Med. J.* **2**, 629–630.

Liebelt, R. A., and Perry, J. H. (1967). Action of gold thioglucose on the central nervous system. *Handb. Physiol., Sect. 6: Aliment. Canal.* Vol. I, pp. 271–285.

Liebling, D. S., Eisner, J. D., Gibbs, J., and Smith, G. P. (1975). Intestinal satiety in rats. *J. Comp. Physiol. Psychol.* **89**, 955–965.

Linton, P. H., Conley, M., Kuechenmeister, C., and McClusky, H. (1972). Satiety and obesity. *Am. J. Clin. Nutr.* **25**, 368–370.

Liu, C. M., and Yin, T. H. (1974). Caloric compensation to gastric loads in rats with hypothalamic hyperphagia. *Physiol. Behav.* **13**, 231–238.

McGovern, J. P., Ozkaragoz, K., Barkin, G., Haywood, T., McElhenney, T., and Hensen, A. E., Jr. (1960). Studies of chlordiazepoxide in various allergic diseases. *Ann. Allergy* **18,** 1193–1199.

McHugh, P. R., Moran, T. H., and Barton, G. N. (1975). Satiety: A graded behavioral phenomenon regulating caloric intake. *Science* **190,** 167–168.

McKay, R. H. G. (1975). Long-term use of diethylpropion in obesity. *In* "Recent Advances in Obesity Research" (A. Howard, ed.), Vol. 1, pp. 388–390. Newman Publ. Ltd., London.

McLaughlin, C. L., Krabill, L. F., Scott, G. C., and Baile, C. A. (1976). Chemical stimulants of feeding animals. *Fed. Proc., Fed. Am. Sco. Exp. Biol.* **35,** 579.

McQuarrie, H. G. (1975). Clinical assessment of the use of an anorectic drug in a total weight reduction program. *Curr. Ther. Res. Clin. Exp.* **17,** 437–443.

Macrae, S. M. (1975). Peripheral and metabolic effects of fenfluramine, 780SE, nor-fenfluramine and hydroxyethylnorfenfluramine—a review. *Postgrad. Med. J.* **51,** Suppl. 1, 13–17.

Mainguet, P. (1972). Effect of cyproheptadine on anorexia and loss of weight in adults. *Practitioner* **208,** 797–800.

Maneksha, S. (1975). Prolonged action fenfluramine capsules versus fenfluramine tablets in general practice. *Br. J. Clin. Pract.* **29,** 12–13.

Manning, F. J., McDonough, J. H., Jr., Elsmore, T. F., Saller, C., and Sodetz, F. J. (1971). Inhibition of normal growth by chronic administration of Δ^9-tetrahydrocannabinol. *Science* **174,** 424–426.

Margules, D. L., and Stein, L. (1967). Neuroleptics vs. tranquilizers: Evidence from animal behavior studies of mode and site of action. *Neuro-Psycho-Pharmacol., Proc. Int. Congr. Coll. Int. Nurop-Psycho-Pharmacol, 5th, 1966* Excerpta Med. Found. Int. Congr. Ser. No. 129, pp. 108–120.

Margules, D. L., and Stein, L. (1969). Cholinergic synapses in the ventromedial hypothalamus for the suppression of operant behavior by punishment and satiety. *J. Comp. Physiol. Psychol.* **67,** 327–335.

Marshall, J. F., Turner, G. H., and Teitelbaum, P. (1971). Sensory neglect produced by lateral hypothalamic damage. *Science* **174,** 523–525.

Martin, F. H., and Baile, C. A. (1973). Feeding elicited in sheep by intrahypothalamic injections of PGE_1. *Experientia* **29,** 306–307.

Matsuda, Y. (1966). Effects of some centrally acting drugs on food intake of normal and hypothalamus-lesioned rats. *Jpn. J. Pharmacol.* **16,** 276–286.

Mawson, A. R. (1974). Anorexia nervosa and the regulation of intake: A review. *Psychol. Med.* **4,** 289–308.

Mayer, J. (1955). Regulation of energy intake and the body weight: The glucostatic theory and the lipostatic hypothesis. *Ann. N. Y. Acad. Sci.* **63,** 15–43.

Mayer, J. (1960). The hypothalamic control of gastric hunger contractions as a component of the mechanism of regulation of food intake. *Am. J. Clin. Nutr.* **8,** 547–561.

Mayer, J., and Marshall, N. B. (1956). Specificity of gold thioglucose for ventromedial hypothalamic lesions and hyperphagia. *Nature (London)* **178,** 1399–1400.

Mecklenburg, R. S., Loriaux, D. L., Thompson, R. H., Andersen, A. E., and Lipsett, M. B. (1974). Hypothalamic dysfunction in patients with anorexia nervosa. *Medicine (Baltimore)* **53,** 147–159.

Mellinkoff, S. M., Frankland, M., Boyle, D., and Greipel, M. (1956). Relationship between serum amino acid concentration and fluctuations in appetite. *J. Appl. Physiol.* **8,** 535–538.

Mereu, G. P., Fratta, W., Chessa, P., and Gessa, G. L. (1976). Voraciousness induced in cats by benzodiazepines. *Psychopharmacology* **47,** 101–103.

Miller, D. S., Evans, E., Samuel, P., and Burland, W. L. (1975). A study of the energy and biochemical status of obese and non-obese students treated with 780SE. *Postgrad. Med. J.* **51,** Suppl. 1, 117–120.

Mizrahi, A. (1974). Drug profile: Voranil (clortermine). *J. Int. Med. Res.* **2,** 317–320.

Morgane, P. J. (1961). Alterations in feeding and drinking behavior of rats with lesions in globi pallidi. *Am. J. Physiol.* **201,** 420–428.

Murphy, J. E., Donald, J. F., Molla, A. L., and Crowder, D. (1975). A comparison of mazindol (teronac) with diethylpropion in the treatment of exogenous obesity. *J. Int. Med. Res.* **3,** 202–206.

Niijima, A. (1969). Afferent impulse discharges from glucoreceptors in the liver of the guinea pig. *Ann. N. Y. Acad. Sci.* **157,** 690–700.

Niki, H. (1965). Chlordiazepoxide and food intake in the rat. *Jpn. Psychol. Res.* **7,** 80–85.

Nillius, S. J., and Wide, L. (1975). Gonadotrophin-releasing hormone treatment for induction of follicular maturation and ovulation in amenorrhoeic women with anorexia nervosa. *Br. Med. J.* **3,** 405–408.

Nisbett, R. E. (1968). Determinants of food intake in obesity. *Science* **159,** 1254–1255.

Nisbett, R. E. (1972a). Hunger, obesity, and the ventromedial hypothalamus. *Psychol. Rev.* **79,** 433–453.

Nisbett, R. E. (1972b). Eating behavior and obesity in men and animals. *Adv. Psychosom. Med.* **7,** 173–193.

Nolan, G. R. (1975). Use of an anorexic drug in a total weight reduction program in private practice. *Curr. Ther. Res. Clin. Exp.* **18,** 332–337.

Novin, D. (1976). Visceral mechanisms in the control of food intake. *In* "Hunger: Basic Mechanisms and Clinical Implications" (D. Novin, W. Wyrwicka, and G. Bray, eds.), pp. 357–367. Raven, New York.

Novin, D., VanderWeele, D. A., and Rezek, M. (1973). Infusion of 2-deoxy-D-glucose into the hepatic-portal system causes eating: Evidence for peripheral glucoreceptors. *Science* **181,** 858–860.

Novin, D., Sanderson, J. D., and VanderWeele, D. A. (1974). The effect of isotonic glucose on eating as a function of feeding condition and infusion site. *Physiol. Behav.* **13,** 3–7.

Oliver, J. T. (1974). Anorectic activity of 4-chloro-2'-((methylamino)methyl)benzhydrol HCl, (PR-F-36-Cl). *Arch. Int. Pharmacodyn. Ther.* **211,** 253–268.

Oomura, Y. (1976). Significance of glucose, insulin and free fatty acid on the hypothalamic feeding and satiety neurons. *In* "Hunger: Basic Mechanisms and Clinical Implications" (D. Novin, W. Wyrwicka, and G. Bray, eds.), pp. 145–157. Raven, New York.

Oomura, Y., Ono, T., Ooyama, H., and Wayner, M. J. (1969). Glucose and osmosensitive neurones of the rat hypothalamus. *Nature (London)* **222,** 282–284.

Oomura, Y., Ono, T., Sugimori, M., and Nakamura, T. (1973). Effects of cyproheptadine on the feeding and satiety centers in the rat. *Pharmacol., Biochem. Behav.* **1,** 449–459.

Opitz, K., and Akinlaja, A. (1966). Zur Beeinflussung der Nahrungsaufnahme durch Psychopharmaka. *Psychopharmacologia* **9,** 307–319.

Owen, J. H. (1975a). Prolonged action fenfluramine in general practice. *Br. J. Clin. Pract.* **29,** 13–14.

Owen, J. H. (1975b). Acceptability of prolonged release fenfluramine capsules in obese patients in general practice. *Postgrad. Med. J.* **51,** Suppl. 1, 176–177.

Panksepp, J. (1972). Hypothalamic radioactivity after intragastric glucose-^{14}C in rats. *Am. J. Physiol.* **223,** 396–401.

Panksepp. J. (1973). The ventromedial hypothalamus and metabolic adjustments of feeding behavior. *Behav. Biol.* **9,** 65–75.

Panksepp, J. (1974). Hypothalamic regulation of energy balance and feeding behavior. *Fed. Proc. Fed. Am. Soc. Exp. Biol.* **33,** 1146–1149.

Panksepp, J. (1975). Hormonal control of feeding behavior and energy balance. *In* "Hormonal Correlates of Behavior" (B. E. Elefthériou and R. L. Sprott, eds.), Vol. 2, pp. 657–695. Plenum, New York.

Panksepp, J., and Booth, D. A. (1971). Decreased feeding after injections of amino-acids into the hypothalamus. *Nature (London)* **233,** 341–342.

Panksepp, J., and Nance, D. M. (1974). Effects of para-chlorophenylalanine on food intake in rats. *Physiol. Psychol.* **2,** 360–364.

Parham, E. S., Keng, H. C., and Mohiuddin, I. (1975). Sensitivity to physiological hunger cues: Are the obese really different? *Nutr. Rep. Int.* **12,** 383–386.

Pawlowski, G. J. (1975). Cyproheptadine: Weight-gain and appetite stimulation in essential anorexic adults. *Curr. Ther. Res. Clin. Exp.* **18,** 673–678.

Paykel, E. S., Mueller, P. S., and De La Vergne, P. M. (1973). Amitriptyline, weight gain and carbohydrate craving: A side effect. *Br. J. Psychiatry* **123,** 501–507.

Penaloza-Rojas, J. H., and Russek, M. (1963). Anorexia produced by direct-current blockade of the vagus nerve. *Nature (London)* **200,** 176.

Phillips, A. G., and Nikaido, R. S. (1975). Disruption of brain stimulation-induced feeding by dopamine receptor blockade. *Nature (London)* **258,** 750–751.

Pinder, R. M., Brogden, R. N., Sawyer, P. R., Speight, T. M., and Avery, G. S. (1975). Fenfluramine: A review of its pharmacological properties and therapeutic efficacy in obesity. *Drugs* **10,** 241–323.

Poschel, B. P. H. (1971). A simple and specific screen for benzodiazepine-like drugs. *Psychopharmacologia* **19,** 193–198.

Powley, T. L., and Keesey, R. E. (1970). Relationship of body weight to the lateral hypothalamic feeding syndrome. *J. Comp. Physiol. Psychol.* **70,** 25–36.

Powley, T. L., and Opsahl, C. A. (1974). Ventromedial hypothalamic obesity abolished by subdiaphragmatic vagotomy. *Am. J. Physiol.* **226,** 25–33.

Pubols, L. M. (1966). Changes in food-motivated behavior of rats as a function of septal and amygdaloid lesions. *Exp. Neurol.* **15,** 240–254.

Rabin, B. M. (1972). Ventromedial hypothalamic control of food intake and satiety: A reappraisal. *Brain Res.* **43,** 317–342.

Rampone, A. J., and Shirasu, M. E. (1964). Temperature changes in the rat in response to feeding. *Science* **144,** 317–319.

Randall, L. O. (1960). Pharmacology of methaminodiazepoxide. *Dis. Nerv. Syst.* **21,** Suppl., 7–10.

Rayner, P. H. W., and Court, J. M. (1975). The effect of dietary restriction and anorectic drugs on linear growth velocity in childhood obesity. *Postgrad. Med. J.* **51,** Suppl. 1, 120–125.

Reeves, A. G., and Plum, F. (1969). Hyperphagia, rage, and dementia accompanying a ventromedial hypothalamic neoplasm. *Arch. Neurol. (Chicago)* **20,** 616–624.

Reiter, L. (1970). Effects of amphetamine on lateral hypothalamic activity in response to amygdaloid stimulation. *Fed. Proc., Fed. Am. Soc. Exp. Biol.* **29,** 383.

Reuter, C. J. (1975). A review of the CNS effects of fenfluramine, 780SE and norfenfluramine on animals and man. *Postgrad. Med. J.* **51,** Suppl. 1, 18–27.

Rezek, M., and Novin, D. (1976). Duodenal nutrient infusion: Effects on feeding in intact and vagotomized rabbits. *J. Nutr.* **106,** 812–820.

Rezek, M., Vanderweele, D. A., and Novin, D. (1975a). Stages in the recovery of feeding following vagotomy in rabbits. *Behav. Biol.* **14,** 75–84.

Rezek, M., Havlicek, V., and Novin, D. (1975b). Satiety and hunger induced by small and large duodenal loads of isotonic glucose. *Am. J. Physiol.* **229,** 545–548.

Richter, C. P., and Hawkes, C. D. (1939). Increased spontaneous activity and food intake produced in rats by removal of the frontal poles of the brain. *J. Neurol. Psychiatry* **2**, 231–242.

Robinson, R. G., McHugh, P. R., and Folstein, M. F. (1975a). Measurement of appetite disturbances in psychiatric disorders. *J. Psychiatr. Res.* **12**, 59–68.

Robinson, R. G., McHugh, P. R., and Bloom, F. E. (1975b). Chlorpromazine induced hyperphagia in the rat. *Psychopharmacol. Commun.* **1**, 37–50.

Rodriguez-Zendejas, A. M., Vega, C., Soto-Mora, L. M., and Russek, M. (1968). Some effects of intraperitoneal glucose and of intraportal glucose and adrenaline. *Physiol. Behav.* **3**, 259–264.

Rosenvinge, H. P. (1975). Abuse of fenfluramine. *Br. Med. J.* **1**, 735.

Rozin, P. (1968). Are carbohydrate and protein intakes separately regulated? *J. Comp. Physiol. Psychol.* **65**, 23–29.

Russek, M. (1963). Participation of hepatic glucoreceptors in the control of intake of food. *Nature (London)* **197**, 79–80.

Russek, M. (1970a). Gluco-ammonia receptors in liver. *Fed. Proc., Fed. Am. Soc. Exp. Biol.* **29**, 658.

Russek, M. (1970b). Demonstration of the influence of an hepatic glucosensitive mechanism on food-intake. *Physiol. Behav.* **5**, 1207–1209.

Russek, M. (1971). Hepatic receptors and the neurophysiological mechanisms controlling feeding behavior. *Neurosci. Res.* **4**, 213–282.

Russek, M., and Stevenson, J. A. F. (1972). Correlation between the effects of several substances on food intake and on the hepatic concentration of reducing sugars. *Physiol. Behav.* **8**, 245–249.

Russek, M., Mogenson, G. J., and Stevenson, J. A. F. (1967). Calorigenic, hyperglycemic and anorexigenic effects of adrenaline and noradrenaline. *Physiol. Behav.* **2**, 429–433.

Russek, M., Rodriguez-Zendejas, A. M., and Pina, S. (1968). Hypothetical liver receptors and the anorexia caused by adrenaline and glucose. *Physiol. Behav.* **3**, 249–257.

Russek, M., Rodriguez-Zendejas, A. M., and Teitelbaum, P. (1973). The action of adrenergic anorexigenic substances on rats recovered from lateral hypothalamic lesions. *Physiol Behav.* **10**, 329–333.

Russell, G. F. M. (1970). Anorexia nervosa: Its identity as an illness and its treatment. *In* "Modern Trends in Psychological Medicine" (J. H. Price, ed.), pp. 131–164. Butterworth, London.

Russell, G. F. M., Loraine, J. A., Bell, E. T., and Harkness, R. A. (1965). Gonadotrophin and oestrogen excretion in patients with anorexia nervosa. *J. Psychosom. Res.* **9**, 79–85.

Saller, C. F., and Stricker, E. M. (1976). Hyperphagia and increased growth in rats after intraventricular injection of 5,7-dihydroxytryptamine. *Science* **192**, 385–387.

Samanin, R., Bernasconi, S., and Garattini, S. (1975). The effect of a selective lesioning of brain catecholamine-containing neurons on the activity of various anorectics in the rat. *Eur. J. Pharmacol.* **34**, 373–375.

Schacter, S. (1968). Obesity and eating. *Science* **161**, 751–756.

Schacter, S. (1971). Some extraordinary facts about obese humans and rats. *Am. Psychol.* **26**, 129–144.

Schally, A. V., Redding, T. W., and Lucien, H. W. (1967). Enterogastrone inhibits eating by fasted mice. *Science* **159**, 210–211.

Schmitt, M. (1973). Influences of hepatic portal receptors on hypothalamic feeding and satiety centers. *Am. J. Physiol.* **225**, 1089–1095.

Schreiner, L., Rioch, D. McK., Pechtel, C., and Masserman, J. H. (1953). Behavioral changes following thalamic injury in cat. *J. Neurophysiol.* **16**, 234–246.

Schulman, J. L., Carleton, J. L., Whitney, G., and Whitehorn, J. C. (1957). Effect of glucagon on food intake and body weight in man. *J. Appl. Physiol.* **11**, 419–421.

Schwartz, L. N. (1975). A non-amphetamine anorectic agent: Preclinical background and a double-blind clinical trial. *J. Int. Med. Res.* **3**, 328–332.

Seaver, R. L., and Binder, H. J. (1972). Anorexia nervosa and other anorectic states in man. General clinical considerations. *Adv. Psychosom. Med.* **7**, 257–276.

Sedgwick, J. P. (1975). Mazindol in the treatment of obesity. *Practitioner* **214**, 418–420.

Seedat, Y. K., and Reddy, J. (1974). Diethylpropion hydrochloride (tenuate dospan) in combination with hypotensive agents in the treatment of obesity associated with hypertension. *Curr. Ther. Res. Clin. Exp.* **16**, 398–413.

Seoane, J. R., and Baile, C. A. (1973). Feeding behavior in sheep as related to the hypnotic activities of barbiturates injected into the third ventricle. *Pharmacol. Biochem. Behav.* **1**, 47–53.

Seoane, J. R., and Baile, C. A. (1975). Feeding and temperature changes in sheep following injections of barbiturates, Ca^{++}, or Mg^{++} into the lateral, third, or fourth ventricle or cerebral aqueduct. *J. Dairy Sci.* **58**, 515–520.

Sharma, K. N., and Nasset, E. S. (1962). Electrical activity in mesenteric nerves after perfusion of gut lumen. *Am. J. Physiol.* **202**, 725–730.

Sharma, K. N., Anand, B. K., Dua, S., and Singh, B. (1961). Role of stomach in regulation of activities of hypothalamic feeding centers. *Am. J. Physiol.* **201**, 593–598.

Sharp, J. C., Nielson, H. C., and Porter, P. B. (1962). The effect of amphetamine upon cats with lesions in the ventromedial hypothalamus. *J. Comp. Physiol. Psychol.* **55**, 198–200.

Shoulson, I., and Chase, T. N. (1975). Fenfluramine in man: Hypophagia associated with diminished serotonin turnover. *Clin. Pharmacol. Ther.* **17**, 616–621.

Silverstone, T. (1972). The anorectic effect of a long-acting preparation of phentermine (duromine). *Psychopharmacologia* **25**, 315–320.

Silverstone, T. (1974). Intermittent treatment with anorectic drugs. *Practitioner* **213**, 245–252.

Silverstone, T. (1975). "Anorectic Drugs in Obesity," pp. 194–227. Pathogenesis and Management Publishing Science Group, Inc., Acton, Massachusetts.

Silverstone, T., and Schuyler, D. (1975). The effect of cyproheptadine on hunger, calorie intake and body weight in man. *Psychopharmacologia* **40**, 335–340.

Sims, E. A. H., Danforth, E., Horton, E. S., Bray, G. A., Glennon, J. H., and Salans, L. B. (1973). Endocrine and metabolic effects of experimental obesity in man. *Recent Prog. Horm. Res.* **29**, 457–496.

Sjödén, P.-O., Järbe, T. U. C., and Henrikkson, B. G. (1973). Influence of tetrahydrocannabinols (Δ^8-THC and Δ^9-THC) on body weight, food, and water intake in rats. *Pharmacol., Biochem. Behav.* **1**, 395–399.

Skultety, F. M., and Gary, T. M. (1962). Experimental hyperphagia in cats following destructive mid-brain lesions. *Neurology* **12**, 394–401.

Slangen, J. L., and Miller, N. E. (1969). Pharmacological tests for the function of hypothalamic norepinephrine in eating behavior. *Physiol. Behav.* **4**, 543–552.

Smith, C. J. V. (1972). Hypothalamic glucoreceptors—the influence of gold thioglucose implants in the ventromedial and lateral hypothalamic areas of normal and diabetic rats. *Physiol. Behav.* **9**, 391–396.

Smith, G. P., and Epstein, A. N. (1969). Increased feeding in response to decreased glucose utilization in the rat and monkey. *Am. J. Physiol.* **217**, 1083–1087.

Smith, G. P., and Gibbs, J. (1975). Cholecystokinin: A putative satiety signal. *Pharmacol., Biochem. Behav.* **3**, Suppl. 1, 135–138.

Smith, G. P., and Gibbs, J. (1976). Cholecystokinin and satiety: Theoretic and therapeutic implications. *In* "Hunger: Basic Mechanisms and Clinical Implications" (D. Novin, W. Wyrwicka, and G. A. Bray, eds.), pp. 349–355. Raven, New York.

Smith, G. P., Gibbs, J., and Young, R. C. (1974). Cholecystokinin and intestinal satiety in the rat. *Fed. Proc., Fed. Am. Soc. Exp. Biol.* **33,** 1146–1149.

Smith, M., Pool, R., and Weinberg, H. (1962). The role of bulk in the control of eating. *J. Comp. Physiol. Psychol.* **55,** 115–120.

Smith, R. G., Innes, J. A., and Munro, J. F. (1975). Double-blind evaluation of mazindol in refractory obesity. *Br. Med. J.* **3,** 284.

Snowdon, C. T. (1969). Motivation, regulation, and the control of meal parameters with oral and intragastric feeding. *J. Comp. Physiol. Psychol.* **69,** 91–100.

Snowdon, C. T. (1970). Gastrointestinal sensory and motor control of food intake. *J. Comp. Physiol. Psychol.* **71,** 68–76.

Snowdon, C. T. (1975). Production of satiety with small intraduodenal infusions in the rat. *J. Comp. Physiol. Psychol.* **88,** 231–238.

Sofia, R. D., and Barry, H., III. (1974). Acute and chronic effects of Δ^9-tetrahydrocannabinol on food intake by rats. *Psychopharmacologia* **39,** 213–222.

Soper, W. Y., and Wise, R. A. (1971). Hypothalamically induced eating: Eating from 'non-eaters' with diazepam. *TIT J. Life Sci.* **1,** 79–84.

Soubrié, P., Kulkarni, S., Simon, P., and Boissier, J. R. (1975). Effets des anxiolytiques sur la prise de nourriture de rats et de souris places en situation nouvelle ou familière. *Psychopharmacologia* **45,** 203–210.

Stark, P., and Totty, C. W. (1967). Effects of amphetamines on eating elicited by hypothalamic stimulation. *J. Pharmacol. Exp. Ther.* **158,** 272–278.

Stark, P., Turk, J. A., and Totty, C. W. (1971). Reciprocal adrenergic and cholinergic control of hypothalamic elicited eating and satiety. *Am. J. Physiol.* **220,** 1516–1521.

Steel, J. M., Munro, J. F., and Duncan, L. J. P. (1973). A comparative trial of different regimens of fenfluramine and phentermine in obesity. *Practitioner* **211,** 232–236.

Stellar, E. (1954). The physiology of motivation. *Psychol. Rev.* **61,** 5–22.

Stephens, D. B., and Baldwin, B. A. (1974). The lack of effect of intrajugular or intraportal injections of glucose or amino acids on food intake in pigs. *Physiol. Behav.* **12,** 923–929.

Stephens, R. J. (1973). The influence of mild stress on food consumption in untrained mice and the effect of drugs. *Br. J. Pharmacol.* **49,** 146P.

Stern, J. J., Cudillo, C. A., and Kruper, J. (1976). Ventromedial hypothalamus and short-term feeding suppression by caerulein in male rats. *J. Comp. Physiol. Psychol.* **90,** 484–490.

Sternbach, L. H., Randall, L. O., and Gustafson, S. R. (1964). 1,4-benzodiazepines (chlordiazepoxide and related compounds). *In* "Psychopharmacological Agents" (M. Gordon, ed.), pp. 137–224. Academic Press, New York.

Stricker, E. M., and Zigmond, M. J. (1974). Effects of homeostasis of intraventricular injections of 6-hydroxydopamine in rats. *J. Comp. Physiol. Psychol.* **86,** 973–994.

Stricker, E. M., and Zigmond, M. J. (1976). Brain catecholamines and the lateral hypothalamic syndrome. *In* "Hunger: Basic Mechanisms and Clinical Implications" (D. Novin, W. Wyrwicka, and G. Bray, eds.), pp. 19–32. Raven, New York.

Stunkard, A. J., Van Itallie, T. B., and Reis, B. B. (1955). The mechanism of satiety: Effect of glucagon on gastric hunger contractions in man. *Proc. Soc. Exp. Biol. Med.* **89,** 258–261.

Stunkard, A., and Koch, C. (1964). The interpretation of gastric motility. I. Apparent bias in the reports of hunger by obese persons. *Arch. Gen. Psychiatry* **11,** 74–82.

Sugrue, M. F., Goodlet, I., and McIndewar, I. (1975). Failure of depletion of rat brain 5-hydroxytryptamine to alter fenfluramine-induced anorexia. *J. Pharm. Pharmacol.* **27,** 950–953.

Sullivan, A. C. (1975). Effect of (—)-hydroxycitrate on lipid metabolism. "Modification of Lipid Metabolism" pp. 143–174. Academic Press, New York.

Sullivan, A. C., and Triscari, J. (1976). Possible interrelationship between metabolite flux and appetite. *In* "Hunger: Basic Mechanisms and Clinical Implications" (D. Novin, W. Wyrwicka, and G. Bray, eds.), pp. 115–125. Raven, New York.

Sullivan, A. C., and Triscari, J. (1977). Metabolic regulation as a control for lipid disorders. I. Influence of (—)-hydroxycitrate on experimentally induced obesity in the rodent. *Am. J. Clin. Nutr.* **30,** 767–776.

Sullivan, A. C., Hamilton, J. G., Miller, O. N., and Wheatley, V. R. (1972). Inhibition of lipogenesis in rat liver by (—)-hydroxycitrate. *Arch Biochem. Biophys.* **150,** 183–190.

Sullivan, A. C., Triscari, J., Hamilton, J. G., Miller, O. N., and Wheatley, V. R. (1974a). Effect of (—)-hydroxycitrate upon the accumulation of lipid in the rat. I. Lipogenesis. *Lipids* **9,** 121–128.

Sullivan, A. C., Triscari, J., Hamilton, J. G., and Miller, O. N. (1974b). Effect of (—)-hydroxycitrate upon the accumulation of lipid in the rat. II. Appetite. *Lipids* **9,** 129–134.

Sullivan, A. C., Cheng, L., and Hamilton, J. G. (1976). Agents for the treatment of obesity. *Annu. Rep. Med. Chem.* **11,** 200–207.

Tarttelin, M. F., and Gorski, R. A. (1971). Variations in food and water intake in the normal and acyclic female rat. *Physiol. Behav.* **7,** 847–852.

Taylor, M., and Goudie, A. J. (1975). Comparisons between the behavioural and anorexic effects of 780SE and other phenylethylamines in the rat. *Postgrad. Med. J.* **51,** Suppl. 1, 56–65.

Teitelbaum, P., and Epstein, A. N. (1962). The lateral hypothalamic syndrome: Recovery of feeding and drinking after lateral hypothalamic lesions. *Psychol. Rev.* **69,** 74–90.

Teitelbaum, P., and Wolgin, D. L. (1975). Neurotransmitters and the regulation of food intake. *Prog. Brain Res.* **42,** 235–249.

Teitelbaum, P., Cheng, M.-F., and Rozin, P. (1969). Development of feeding parallels—its recovery after hypothalamic damage. *J. Comp. Physiol. Psychol.* **67,** 430–441.

Theologides, A. (1972). Pathogenesis of cachexia in cancer. A review and a hypothesis. *Cancer* **29,** 484–488.

Theologides, A. (1974). The anorexia–cachexia syndrome: A new hypothesis. *Ann. N. Y. Acad. Sci.* **230,** 14–22.

Theologides, A. (1976). Anorexia-producing intermediary metabolites. *Am. J. Clin. Nutr.* **29,** 552–558.

Thode, W. F., and Carlisle, H. J. (1968). Effect of lateral hypothalamic stimulation on amphetamine-induced anorexia. *J. Comp. Physiol. Psychol.* **66,** 547–548.

Thorpe, P. C., Isaac, P. F., and Rodgers, J. (1975). A controlled trial of mazindol (sanjorex teronac) in the management of the obese rheumatic patients. *Curr. Ther. Res. Clin. Exp.* **17,** 149–155.

Tisdale, S. A., Jr., and Ervin, D. K. (1976). Anorectic effectiveness of differing dosage forms of fenfluramine. *Curr. Ther. Res. Clin. Exp.* **19,** 589–594.

Tye, N. C., Nicholas, D. J., and Morgan, M. J. (1975). Chlordiazepoxide and preference for free food in rats. *Pharmacol., Biochem, Behav.* **3,** 1149–1151.

Ungerstedt, U. (1971). Adipsia and aphagia after 6-hydroxydopamine induced degeneration of the nigrostriatal dopamine system. *Acta Physiol. Scand.* **81,** Suppl. 367, 95–122.

VanderWeele, D. A., and Sanderson, J. D. (1976). Peripheral glucosensitive satiety in the rabbit and the rat. *In* "Hunger: Basic Mechanisms and Clinical Implications" (D. Novin, W. Wyrwicka, and G. Bray, eds.), pp. 383–393. Raven, New York.

VanderWeele, D. A., Novin, D., Rezek, M., and Sanderson, J. D. (1974). Duodenal or hepatic-portal glucose perfusion: Evidence for duodenally-based satiety. *Physiol. Behav.* **12,** 467–473.

Van Itallie, T. B., and Campbell, R. G. (1972). Multidisciplinary approach to the problem of obesity. *J. Am. Diet. Assoc.* **61,** 385–390.

Van Itallie, T. B., and Hashim, S. A. (1960). Biochemical concomitants of hunger and satiety in man. *Am. J. Clin. Nutr.* **8,** 587–594.

Wade, G. N. (1972). Gonadal hormones and behavioral regulation of body weight. *Physiol. Behav.* **8,** 523–534.

Wallace, A. G. (1975). AN 448 Sandoz (mazindol) in the treatment of obesity. *In* "Recent Advances in Obesity Research" (A. Howard, ed.), Vol. 1, p. 415. Newman Publ. Ltd., London.

Warner, K. E., and Balagura, S. (1975). Intrameal eating patterns of obese and nonobese humans, *J. Comp. Physiol. Psychol.* **89,** 778–783.

Watson, J. A., Fang, M., and Lowenstein, J. M. (1969). Tricarballylate and hydroxycitrate: Substrate and inhibitor of ATP: Citrate oxaloacetate lyase. *Arch. Biochem. Biophys.* **135,** 209–217.

Wedeking, P. W. (1974). Schedule-dependent differences among anti-anxiety drugs. *Pharmacol., Biochem. Behav.* **2,** 465–472.

Weissman, A., Koe, B. K., and Tenen, S. S. (1966). Anti-amphetamine effects following inhibition of tyrosine hydroxylase. *J. Pharmacol. Exp. Ther.* **151,** 339–353.

Wells, H. M. (1975). A trial of fenfluramine (PACaps) and diet in overweight diabetic patients. *Postgrad. Med. J.* **51,** Suppl. 1, 137.

White, L. E., and Hain, R. F. (1959). Anorexia in association with a destructive lesion of the hypothalamus. *Arch. Pathol.* **68,** 275–281.

Williams, R. H., ed. (1968). "Textbook of Endocrinology." Saunders, Philadelphia, Pennsylvania.

Wise, R. A., and Dawson, V. (1974). Diazepam-induced eating and lever pressing for food in sated rats. *J. Comp. Physiol. Psychol.* **86,** 930–941.

Wishart, T. B., and Walls, E. K. (1973). The effects of anorexic doses of dextro-amphetamine on the ventromedial–hypothalamic hyperphagic rat. *Can. J. Physiol. Pharmacol.* **51,** 354–359.

Woodhouse, S. P., Nye, E. R., Anderson, K., and Rawlings, J. (1975). Report on a double-blind trial with mazindol. *In* "Recent Advances in Obesity Research" (A. Howard, ed.), Vol. 1, pp. 396–398. Newman Publ. Ltd., London.

Yaksh, T. L., and Myers, R. D. (1972). Neurohumoral substances released from hypothalamus of the monkey during hunger and satiety. *Am. J. Physiol.* **222,** 503–515.

York, D. A., and Bray, G. A. (1972). Dependence of hypothalamic obesity on insulin, the pituitary and the adrenal gland. *Endocrinology* **90,** 885–894.

Young, R. C., Gibbs, J., Antin, J., Hold, J., and Smith, G. P. (1974). Absence of satiety during sham feeding in the rat. *J. Comp. Physiol. Psychol.* **87,** 795–800.

Zeigler, H. P., and Karten, H. J. (1974). Central trigeminal structures and the lateral hypothalamic syndrome in the rat. *Science* **186,** 636–637.

Zis, A. P., and Fibiger, H. C. (1975). Neuroleptic-induced deficits in food and water regulations: Similarities to the lateral hypothalamic syndrome. *Psychopharmacologia* **43,** 63–68.

3

Drugs and Water-Soluble Vitamin Absorption

CHARLES H. HALSTED

I. INTRODUCTION: PRINCIPLES OF INTESTINAL ABSORPTION

Since most drugs are available for oral use, or reach the gastrointestinal tract from either the blood or bile, the gastrointestinal epithelium across which all nutrients must pass is frequently exposed to these substances. In order to understand the ways in which a drug could influence nutrient absorption it is first necessary to have some understanding of the functioning of the small intestine. In this discussion, consideration will be made of some principles underlying intestinal absorption, the specific mechanisms, where known, for the absorption of several vitamins, and finally of the effects of several frequently administered drugs on water-soluble vitamin absorption.

The small intestine, the organ of nutrient absorption, is constructed in such a way as to maximize its surface area. The luminal surface of this cylinder is thrown into folds of Kerkring (valvulae conniventes) on which lie the intestinal villi, fingerlike structures of 0.5–1.5 mm length. The surface of each villus is lined by absorptive epithelial cells, each one of which is lined by microvilli. The estimated absorptive surface area is thus magnified approximately 600 times over that of a simple cylinder to about 2 million cm^2 (Wilson, 1962). Intestinal absorption is effected through the villus epithelial cell which presents an apical brush border

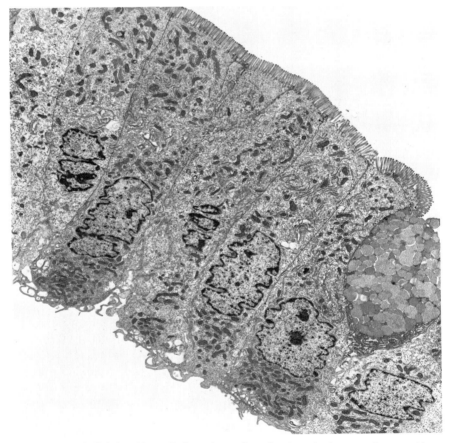

Fig. 1. Epithelial absorbing cells from the surface of rat intestinal mucosa, harvested by a vibration technique. The microvillus membrane is at the top of the picture and basement and lateral membranes at the bottom. Large structures at the base of each cell are nuclei (× 3400). Reprinted by permission of *Journal of Nutrition* (Halsted *et al.*, 1976).

membrane (containing microvilli) to the lumen and basement and lateral membranes to the capillary and lacteal circulation. Thus, to reach the circulation, a nutrient must traverse two membranes and the cell cytoplasm between them (Fig. 1). Most nutrients are effectively absorbed in the upper small intestine. However, vitamin B_{12} and bile salts share the distal ileum as an obligatory site of absorption.

Like other lipoprotein membranes, the microvillus surface of the gut poses special problems for the transport of polar, water-soluble substances. The concept of "effective pore size" has been developed to partially explain movement of solutes through the membrane (Fordtran, 1967). Pores may be located within the microvillus membrane or within the "tight junction" between two adjacent cells. Intestinal perfusion studies have demonstrated an effective pore radius of about 6.5 Å in the jejunum, large enough to accommodate substances with molecular weight less than 180, while in the ileum the pore size is about one-half that in the ileum. Several mechanisms exist to account for the movement of molecules through the gut membrane.

A. Simple Passive Diffusion and Solvent Drag

Electrochemical and osmotic concentration gradients cause the passive movement of solutes through the pores of the gut membrane. Lipid-soluble substances diffuse more freely than water-soluble substances through the lipoprotein membrane. Certain water-soluble substances may be absorbed by solvent drag, a term describing the passive movement of a substance in response to the flow of solvent (i.e., water) across a membrane. The solubility of a substance may be regulated in part by its pK, or the relative proportion of the substance in its nonpolar form at luminal pH. As will be discussed, this concept may have particular relevance to the absorption of folate, a weak acid. Drugs may potentially affect the absorption of vitamins such as folic acid by changing the pH of the luminal contents and, hence, the proportion of that vitamin in its more freely diffusible nonpolar state.

B. Active Transport and Facilitated Diffusion

"Carrier" systems are proposed, though not specifically defined, to explain the active transport of a substance against an osmotic or electrochemical gradient. As an example, glucose and galactose share (i.e., can compete for) a carrier in the brush border which transports these substances into the cell. Sodium transport is "coupled" to that of glucose, in that glucose absorption is enhanced by the presence of sodium. On the other hand, sodium transport is regulated by the presence of a pump mechanism on the lateral cell membrane which pulls sodium out of the cell, creating an osmotic gradient between the cell interior and the luminal contents. This process is inhibited by substances which poison Na^+, K^+-dependent ATPase. Thus, active transport systems require metabolic energy and can be poisoned by metabolic inhibitors. As will be discussed, the transport of vitamin B_{12} by the ileal epithelial cell requires a series of metabolic processes including binding to a receptor, transport through the cytoplasm, and release to the portal blood system. These active mechanisms may be particularly subject to drug-induced inhibition. Facilitated diffusion refers to a carrier-mediated process which does not require metabolic work and cannot transport against a concentration gradient. Examples of substances transported by facilitated diffusion include fructose, d-xylose, and possibly folic acid. Substances absorbed by either active transport or facilitated diffusion display saturation kinetics, i.e., limits on the concentration that can be transported over a given time.

II.   WATER-SOLUBLE VITAMIN ABSORPTION AND DRUG INHIBITION

With the exception of vitamin B_{12} absorption, the processes of intestinal transport of water-soluble vitamins are incompletely understood. This chapter will deal with the absorption of three vitamins, folic acid, vitamin B_{12}, and thiamine. These vitamins are chosen for discussion because of their clear role in clinical medicine, and because of the greater extent of present knowledge of their mechanisms of absorption and the effects of certain drugs on these mechanisms.

A.   Folate

1. *Mechanisms of Absorption*

Folates are a heterogeneous group of pteroylglutamates, and thus there may be no single process of folate absorption. Folates are found in highest concentration in liver and green vegetables (foliage). More than 85% of folate exists as pteroylpolyglutamate—principally pteroylheptaglutamate (Butterworth *et al.*, 1963). Pteroylmonoglutamates are largely reduced and in the form of methyl, or formyl derivatives. In the present discussion, PG-1 will be used to designate pteroylmonoglutamate or folic acid, and PG-7 will be used to designate pteroylheptaglutamate. While the daily diet may contain up to 2 mg of folates, the daily requirement is on the order of 100–300 μg. The availability of folate to the human subject may be limited by food substances. Tamura and Stokstad (1973) used urinary excretion of folate as an index of folate availability in subjects whose tissues were saturated by large doses of folic acid and who received physiologic amounts of various folates alone, or together with a variety of foods. By this method, tetrahydro-PG-1, methyletrahydro-PG-1, formyltetrahydro-PG-1, and PG-7 were found equally available, while it was shown that liver, yeast, and lima beans had more available folate than lettuce, orange juice, and egg yolk. Subsequently, they have shown that orange juice inhibits the absorption, or availability, of PG-7 but not PG-1 (Tamura et al., 1976). These studies suggested that pure folates are absorbed about equally, but that studies of natural folate absorption must take into account other factors which may selectively inhibit enzymatic reactions required for absorption. As will be shown, similar effects may occur selectively, or generally, in response to drugs.

Since folates are primarily pteroylpolyglutamates, and since PG-1 is the primary form of folate in the portal blood (Baugh et al., 1971), deconjugation must be the first step in the process of folate absorption. Folate conjugase, a γ-carboxypeptidase, is found in high concentration in the intestinal mucosa in comparison with the intraluminal contents (Hoffbrand and Peters, 1970). Mucosal deconjugation is an integral part of folate absorption. Using the technique of jejunal perfusion of separately labeled ^{3}H-pteroylmonoglutamate (PG-1) and ^{14}C-pteroylhepta-glutamate (PG-7) in normal controls (Halsted, 1975), and in patients with tropical sprue (Corcino et al., 1976) and celiac sprue (Halsted et al., 1977), we have shown (a) that the jejunal uptake of PG-1 is consistently greater than that of PG-7 in health and disease; (b) that tropical and celiac sprue severely suppress the uptake of each folate; and (c) in both health and mucosal disease, the perfusion of PG-7 is followed by the appearance within the lumen of a spectrum of its degradation products. The activity of mucosal folate conjugase, measured in vitro in mucosal biopsies, was not limited by either mucosal disease, whereas brush border disaccharidases were markedly decreased in activity. These findings suggested that mucosal folate conjugase is probably not a brush border enzyme, and are consistent with other in vitro studies suggesting an intracellular location of this enzyme (Hoffbrand and Peters, 1969; Rosenberg and Godwin, 1971; Halsted et al., 1976). Thus, present data suggest that in the sequence of folate absorption, PG-7 (molecular weight 1215) crosses the brush border to be hydrolyzed intracellularly. Hydrolytic products then efflux to the lumen to be reabsorbed, with eventual transport of pteroylmonoglutamate to the portal blood. A more plausible sequence would be brush border hydrolysis followed by transport of the smaller pteroylmonoglutamate (molecular weight 440). A recent study from our laboratory has described the presence of folate conjugase in the brush border with distinctly different characteristics than the intracellular folate conjugase activity. (Reisenauer *et al.*, 1977). Studies which have thus far failed to show a drug effect on mucosal folate conjugase have only dealt with whole homogenates of the mucosal tissue, and hence may not have dealt with the lesser, but perhaps more physiologically important brush border activity.

Delineation of the mechanism of absorption of pteroylmonoglutamate (PG-1) and its reduced and substituted derivatives has been approached by a number of methods. Studies using the method of jejunal perfusion in man have demonstrated that the absorption of PG-1 is maximal in the upper jejunum, and nonexistent in the distal ileum (Hepner *et al.*, 1968; Halsted *et al.*, 1971), is enhanced by glucose (Gerson *et al.*, 1971), and obeys saturation kinetics in the jejunum when accompanied by glucose in the perfusate (Hepner *et al.*, 1968). Thus, PG-1 may be absorbed by active transport or by facilitated diffusion. It is important to point out that perfusion studies measure disappearance from the lumen and not actual transport through the mucosa. Thus, "uptake" could reflect adherence to a mucosal binder. Leslie and Rowe (1972) have isolated a protein binder from the brush border which can be saturated by folic acid. Using a rat model and the method of *in vivo* perfusion or the *in vitro* gut sac, several groups have demonstrated a saturable transport mechanism when PG-1 is present in micromolar concentrations (Hepner, 1967; Smith *et al.*, 1970; Blair *et al.*, 1974; Burgen and Goldberg, 1962; Halsted *et al.*, 1974; Bhanthumnavin *et al.*, 1974). Blair and his colleagues have advanced the hypothesis that the rate of absorption of PG-1 is dependent on its solubility in the "acid microclimate" proposed to exist at the surface of the mucosa (Blair and Matty, 1974). The authors indicate that folic acid is entirely polar and water-soluble at pH 6.5, while 5% is nonpolar and presumably transportable by the lipoprotein membrane at pH 3.5, the pH presumed to exist at the mucosal surface. According to this scheme, absorption of PG-1 is regulated by differences in solubility and dissociation as the molecule passes to a more acid environment prior to membrane transport. However, to date no acid microclimate below pH 5.5 has been directly demonstrated, though a surface pH between 3 and 4 has been estimated (Lucas *et al.*, 1975). As will be discussed, elevation of luminal pH has been proposed as a mechanism for the inhibitory effect of dilantin on folic acid absorption.

Several studies have demonstrated that intestinal metabolism of folic acid and of its derivatives occurs during the intestinal transport process. When pharmacologic (0.5–3 mg) doses of folic acid are administered orally to man, the compound appears unchanged in the portal blood (Whitehead and Cooper, 1967; Melikian *et al.*, 1971). Using *in vitro* techniques, Olinger *et al.*, (1973) demonstrated that folic acid, present in nanomolar concentrations, is significantly reduced and methylated during transport to the serosal bathing fluid. Perry and Chanarin (1973) used everted gut sacs to show formylation and methylation during transport of PG-1. Nixon and Bertino (1972) have demonstrated rapid absorption of formyltetrahydro-PG-1 by a process involving intestinal conversion of the compound to methyltetrahydro-PG-1.

In summary, folate absorption requires a complex series of steps at the level of the intestinal mucosa: (a) a deconjugation of pteroylpolyglutamate to PG-1; (b) uptake of PG-1 by the mucosal cell by a process that may be saturable, may be pH dependent, and may involve a mucosal binding protein; and (c) at very low concentrations, probable reduction and conversion to methyltetrahydro-PG-1.

2. *Drug Inhibition of Folate Absorption*

Drugs could effect folate absorption by (a) inhibiting intestinal folate conjugase; (b) altering luminal pH and folate solubility; (c) competing for a binder or transport process; and (d) inhibiting intestinal reduction and methylation. To date, with few exceptions, there is little clear-cut proof that any drug diminishes folate absorption and, when drug-induced folate malabsorption has been shown, the mechanism remains speculative. Drugs which have been described to affect folate absorption include ethanol, Dilantin (diphenylhydantoin), oral contraceptives, and azulfidine.

a. Ethanol. The use of ethanol is ubiquitous in our society. A study of a "skid-row" hospital population of alcoholics demonstrated 44% incidence of severe folate deficiency (Herbert *et al.*, 1963). Possible mechanisms of folate deficiency anemia in alcoholics include inadequate diet, intestinal malabsorption, decreased hepatic retention (Cherrick *et al.*, 1965), altered folate utilization by the bone marrow (Sullivan *et al.*, 1964), and altered serum binding of folate (Hines, 1975). We used two approaches to demonstrate the existence of folate malabsorption in alcoholics. In the first study (Halsted *et al.*, 1967), plasma levels of tritium (^{3}H) were measured after the oral administration of ^{3}H-PG-1, 15 μg/kg body weight, to twenty-three recently drinking derelict alcoholics and twenty-three control subjects, each having been given a parenteral tissue-saturating dose of PG-1. Significantly lower plasma levels of ^{3}H were found in the alcoholic group. These findings could not be duplicated by the acute administration of an intoxicating dose of alcohol to normal subjects. However, this method of studying intestinal absorption has several drawbacks, since results could be influenced by delayed gastric emptying, altered hepatic metabolism, or increased excretion of the administered test substance. A more precise method, jejunal perfusion, was utilized subsequently (Halsted *et al.*, 1971). This technique measures the disappearance of a labeled substance from the perfused intestinal substance; results are not influenced by later hepatic metabolism or urinary excretion. Eleven recently drinking derelict alcoholics with no complicating gastrointestinal illness volunteered for the study. Eight of the eleven had eaten a poor diet (less than one meal per day) with weight loss over a 3-week period while the other three lived at home and were in a good state of nutrition. The percent jejunal uptake of tritiated folic acid (^{3}H-PG-1), administered at a concentration of 25 μg/liter in an isotonic glucose–saline solution, was lower in the eight malnourished alcoholics than the well-fed patients. Two weeks of abstinence and a nutritious diet improved folate absorption in the eight patients. However, the administration of ethanol, 192 gm/day, for 2 weeks with a nutritious diet to nine well-nourished patients, failed to suppress the jejunal uptake of ^{3}H-PG-1 (Fig. 2). These studies indicated that the jejunal uptake of PG-1 is impaired in chronic alcoholics in a poor state of nutrition, but not in well-nourished alcoholics. In a subsequent study, it was shown that the absorption of PG-1 from the perfused jejunum of rats was not impaired by a 3-week period of feeding a diet in which ethanol was isocalorically substituted for 35% of calories (Halsted *et al.*, 1974).

The most likely nutritional deficiencies which could affect intestinal malabsorption in alcoholics include deficiencies of protein and of folate. Steatorrhea (malabsorption of dietary fat) has been found in up to one-third of alcoholics in association with transient pancreatic insufficiency which can be corrected by administration of high protein diet (Mezey *et al.*, 1970). However, folate malabsorption could not be induced by feeding zero protein diets with or without alcohol to 36% of calories to rats (Halsted *et al.*, 1974). On the other hand, alcoholics with severe folate deficiency and megaloblastic anemia may exhibit morphologic changes in the intestinal mucosa, including "macrocytosis" or enlargement of the epithelial absorbing cells similar to morphologic alterations seen in the bone marrow (Bianchi *et al.*, 1970; Hermos *et al.*, 1972). Review of our series of eleven alcoholic patients indicated a significant difference in the

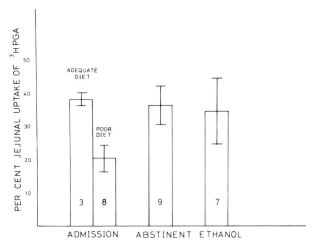

Fig. 2. The jejunal uptake of PG-1 (^{3}H-PG-A) in eleven alcoholics studied on admission, nine studied after 2 weeks of abstinence and nutritious diet, and seven studied after 2 weeks of regular hospital diet supplemented with ethanol, 192 gm/day. Decreased uptake was found on admission in eight poorly nourished alcoholics. Chronic alcohol ingestion for 2 weeks did not suppress uptake. Reprinted by permission of *New England Journal of Medicine* (Halsted *et al.*, 1971).

jejunal uptake of PG-1 between those whose serum folate levels were greater than 5 ng/ml (normal) and those who were folate-deficient. Accordingly, a prospective study was performed on four subjects, one of whom ingested ethanol, 300 gm/day on a regular diet, one of whom was made folate-deficient by diet (Herbert, 1963) and two of whom were made folate-deficient by diet supplemented with ethanol, 200 gm/day. (Halsted *et al.*, 1973a) Megaloblastosis of the bone marrow with folate deficiency was induced by diet and ethanol after 6 weeks and after 9 weeks when the diet was administered without ethanol. Sequential jejunal perfusion studies showed suppression of jejunal uptake of ^{3}H-PG-1, glucose, sodium, and water at the end point of megaloblastosis in the two subjects who ingested ethanol with the folate-deficient diet. These abnormalities were corrected by administration of folic acid, 5 mg daily, for 2 weeks in spite of continued ethanol ingestion (Fig. 3). By contrast, the jejunal uptake of 3H-PG-1 was not changed by 3 weeks of ethanol ingestion with a regular diet or by induction of folate deficiency in the absence of ethanol ingestion. Jejunal morphology was unchanged on serial intestinal biopsy in each patient. Thus, this prospective study demonstrated that the combination of dietary folate deficiency and chronic ethanol ingestion impairs the jejunal transport of PG-1, glucose, water

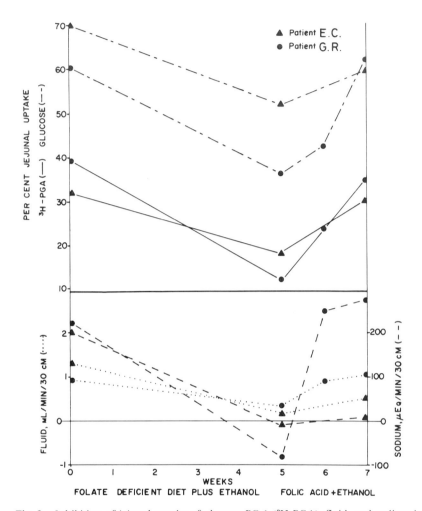

Fig. 3. Inhibition of jejunal uptake of glucose, PG-1 (^{3}H-PGA), fluid, and sodium in two alcoholic patients who were fed a folate-deficient diet supplemented with ethanol, 200 gm/day. Recovery of these functions was shown after 2 weeks of regular diet supplemented by folic acid, 5 mg/day, in spite of continued ethanol ingestion. Reprinted from *Gastroenterology* (Halsted *et al.*, 1973a).

and sodium, whereas either factor alone has no significant effect. The jejunal functional abnormalities were induced without changes in the histology of the small intestine. The effect of chronic alcoholism on decreasing fluid and electrolyte absorption has recently been confirmed in perfusion studies of ten predominantly folate-deficient alcoholics who also had normal jejunal mucosal biopsies (Krasner *et al.*, 1976a).

Ethanol could have specific or general effects on intestinal function. In evaluating studies of ethanol on the gut, it is important to distinguish between the effects on the absorbing cell of an acute rise in ethanol concentration, the effects of chronic ethanol ingestion, and the role of other nutritional factors, as described above. In experiments performed on volunteers in whom the small intestine was intubated, we showed that the acute ingestion of ethanol in an intoxicating dose of 0.8 gm/kg results in intrajejunal levels as high as 4 gm%, with levels of 500 mg% persisting for over an hour (Halsted *et al.*, 1973b) (Fig. 4). By infusing the same dose intravenously, we showed intraluminal ethanol levels similar to those in the blood, implying that ethanol freely diffuses into the gut lumen from the blood. Thus, in binge drinking, the repeated ingestion of ethanol could result in prolonged high intrajejunal levels and, after

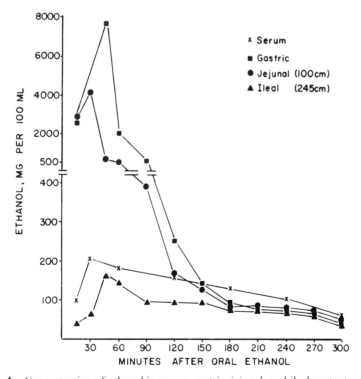

Fig. 4.   Concentration of ethanol in serum, gastric, jejunal, and ileal contents at timed intervals after the acute oral ingestion of ethanol 0.8 gm/kg body weight by a chronic alcoholic patient. Intrajejunal levels of greater than 500 mg% persist for more than 1 hour while intra-ileal levels paralleled those in the serum. Reprinted from *American Journal of Clinical Nutrition* (Halsted, 1973b).

cessation of drinking, the persistence of an intraluminal ethanol concentration throughout the small intestine similar to that in the blood.

Several studies have evaluated the acute effect of ethanol on the intestinal mucosa. Administration of ethanol to rats resulted in inflammatory changes and hemorrhagic erosions in villus tips and decreased activity of the intestinal enzymes lactase and thymidine kinase (Baraona *et al.*, 1974). These effects could be nonspecific and related to the hypertonicity of intraluminal ethanol. *In vitro* studies have demonstrated stimulation of intestinal adenyl cyclase by ethanol at a concentration of 11 gm% (Greene *et al.*, 1971). *In vitro* ethanol concentration of 0.5–3 gm% has been shown to inhibit intestinal transport of phenylalanine and methionine (Israel *et al.*, 1966), and glucose (Chang *et al.*, 1967). Ethanol could inhibit sodium and water transport, and by corollary, the absorption of water-soluble substances which are linked to sodium transport by inhibition of the "sodium pump," i.e., Na^+, K^+-dependent ATPase (Israel *et al.*, 9168). Na^+, K^+, dependent ATPase is suppressed by ethanol in other tissues (Israel and Salazar, 1967). A recent *in vitro* study demonstrated that ethanol, 2%, suppresses the concentration of guinea pig jejunal ATP but not the activity of jejunal ATPase (Krasner *et al.*, 1976b). Acute effects of ingested alcohol in man include suppressed absorption of the pentose *d*-xylose (Mezey, 1975), of methionine (Israel *et al.*, 1968) and, as will be described, thiamine (Thomson *et al.*, 1970). Following chronic alcohol ingestion by well-nourished alcoholics, folic acid absorption is probably not impaired (*vide supra*), *d*-xylose absorption is unchanged (Mezey, 1975) or increased (Lindenbaum and Lieber, 1975), and, as will be described, vitamin B_{12} absorption is decreased (Lindenbaum and Lieber, 1975). Morphologically, the chronic administration of ethanol with adequate diets to rats and man is followed by abnormalities of mitochondria and endoplasmic reticulum in the absorbing epithelial cell which are similar to those seen in the liver (Rubin *et al.*, 1972). Clearly the precise mechanism by which ethanol alters intestinal function after acute or chronic administration is not yet defined.

b. Diphenylhydantoin. The association of megaloblastic anemia and anticonvulsant therapy has been extensively reviewed by Reynolds (1968). While anemia occurs in less than 1% of treated epileptics, the incidence of subnormal serum folate levels has been reported to be between 37 and 76% in several series. Diphenylhydantoin (Dilantin) has antifolate effects on the central nervous system and administration of folic acid to Dilantin-treated patients results in increased seizure frequency (Chanarin *et al.*, 1960). On the other hand, folate-deficient anticonvulsant-treated epileptics may exhibit slowing of mentation and behavioral retardation (Reynolds, 1968).

Several studies indicate that Dilantin interferes with the absorption of folic acid, although the mechanism of the malabsorption remains controversial. In a study of fifty-nine epileptic children receiving Dilantin in doses of more than 2 mg/pound, 54% were found to have low serum folate levels which correlated with depressed whole blood folate (Dahlke *et al.*, 1967). Oral tolerance tests using a 600 μg dose of PG-1 and timed measurements of serum folate levels showed no rise in serum folate when PG-1 was administered simultaneously with the Dilantin dose, but a normal rise when Dilantin was withheld for 20 hours. The effect of oral Dilantin could not be duplicated by its intravenous administration, nor was intravenous clearance or renal excretion of folic acid affected by Dilantin. These studies indirectly indicated, therefore, that Dilantin inhibits the absorption of PG-1.

A possible inhibitory effect of Dilantin on folate conjugase was the subject of three contradictory papers. Hoffbrand and Necheles (1968) administered 200 μg oral doses of yeast-derived pteroylpolyglutamate and pure PG-1 in separate tests, both with and without 100 mg Dilantin, to epileptic patients who had been on anticonvulsant treatment for more than 1 year. Dilantin inhibited the normal rise in serum folate activity after administration of pteroylpolyglutamate but not after administration of PG-1. Using microbiologic techniques, the authors showed that Dilantin in a concentration of 25 μg/ml inhibited the activity of folate conjugase in intestinal mucosal biopsies obtained from normal volunteers, and concluded that the folate malabsorption of Dilantin treatment results from inhibition of folate deconjugation. These findings were supported by a similar study by Rosenberg *et al.* (1968), who also employed yeast-derived pteroylpolyglutamate in their oral tolerance tests and *in vitro* enzyme assays. However, other studies have contradicted these results. Using pure synthetic pteroyltriglutamate (PG-3) as substrate, Baugh and Krumdieck (1969) could find no inhibition of folate conjugase activity in human intestine, liver, or brain by Dilantin in concentrations up to 300 μg/ml. Subsequently, two groups have employed pure synthetic pteroylpolyglutamate in oral tolerance studies in patients and normal volunteers, and have failed to show a specific inhibitory effect of Dilantin on the absorption of conjugated folate (Houlihan *et al.*, 1972; Fehling *et al.*, 1973). The discrepancies between these studies is not self-evident, though the earlier studies using yeast-derived pteroylpolyglutamate did not include a pretest tissue saturating dose of folic acid in the experimental protocol. Thus, apparent pteroylpolyglutamate malabsorption may have represented more rapid disappearance of the test dose into tissue.

The technique of jejunal perfusion was used by Gerson *et al.* (1972) to measure the effect of Dilantin on the absorption of PG-1 in nine healthy adults. The perfusate contained ^{3}H-PG-1 in a concentration of 25 μg/ml and Dilantin in a concentration of 20 μg/ml, well below the maximum Dilantin concentration of 150 μg/ml which they demonstrated occurs intrajejunally after the ingestion of a 100 mg tablet. The jejunal uptake of PG-1 was reduced by a mean of 44% from the solution containing Dilantin. Since this method does not rely on hepatic or renal folate metabolism in its interpretation, these data accurately demonstrated Dilantin-induced jejunal malabsorption of PG-1.

Benn *et al.* (1971) have proposed that the inhibitory effect of Dilantin on the absorption of PG-1 is caused by a change in intraluminal pH. They reasoned that a drug which raised intraluminal pH would shift the equilibrium of the weak folic acid towards the charged ionic form of the species, thus reducing lipid solubility and membrane transport. Using a pH electrode they showed that intraduodenal pH is higher by about one unit in patients taking Dilantin. By oral tolerance tests Benn *et al.* indicated that administration of sodium bicarbonate had the same inhibitory effect as Dilantin on folic acid absorption. However, others have failed to show raised intraluminal pH after the ingestion of Dilantin (Doe *et al.*, 1971). Furthermore, in the convincing studies of Gerson *et al.* (1972), the inhibitory effect of Dilantin was observed using control and test solutions of similar pH (6.5).

In summary, present evidence indicates that Dilantin does inhibit the jejunal uptake of PG-1, but probably does not affect deconjugation of pteroylpolyglutamate. Since pteroylmonoglutamates constitute up to 20% of the normal diet, and since pteroylpolyglutamates are deconjugated to PG-1 prior to absorption, inhibition of intestinal transport of pteroylmonoglutamate could explain the folate deficiency of epileptics receiving Dilantin. However, the precise mechanism of Dilantin inhibition of folic acid absorption remains unclear.

    c. Oral Contraceptive Agents. Although much has been written on the subject, the association of folate deficiency with usage of oral contraceptive agents (OCA) is questionable and the evidence that OCA inhibit folate absorption is less tenable. In a recent literature review, Lindenbaum *et al.* (1975) point out that at least four studies have shown significantly low serum folate levels in women taking OCA but seven other studies have shown no difference in folate levels between control and OCA groups. In their experience of 120 cases of megaloblastic anemia due to folate deficiency, only two patients were taking OCA. They showed that 20% of women on OCA have megaloblastic changes in the cervicovaginal epithelial cells which did not correlate with serum folate levels. Since the morphologic changes disappeared with pharmacologic oral doses of folic acid, they suggested that OCA interfere with folate metabolism at the end organ level. Other evidence that OCA interfere with folate metabolism has been presented by LaCosta and Rothenberg (1974) who identified a binder of dihydro-PG-1 in the serum and leukocytes of women taking OCA.

The evidence for and against an effect of OCA on folate absorption can be summarized as follows. Streiff (1970) described seven women on OCA with folate deficiency anemia and normal clinical tests of intestinal absorption. The folate deficiency was responsive to oral folic acid (PG-1) at doses of 250 μg per day. Subsequently, PG-1 and yeast-derived pteroylpolyglutamate were administered in equal (200 μg) but separate doses to nine women taking OCA and nine healthy control women. Serum folate levels were normal in both groups. Following oral administration of pteroylpolyglutamate, there was a lesser rise in serum folate in the OCA group, but a similar rise in serum folate in each group following the test dose of PG-1. These studies, suggesting that OCA interfere with deconjugation of pteroylpolyglutamate, were substantiated by Necheles and Snyder (1970) using similar methodology. However, the results of both these studies may have been influenced by failure to provide for tissue folate saturation prior to the oral test doses.

Stephens *et al.* (1972) administered oral doses of folic acid and yeast-derived pteroylpolyglutamate to twenty-three control subjects and thirty-seven women taking OCA. Certain tests were preceded by tissue folate saturation by parenteral administration of PG-1 while others were not. When tissue saturation with parenteral PG-1 preceded the oral test dose there was no difference in apparent absorption of either folate between controls and OCA users, but when the saturation step was omitted, the rise in serum folate after the oral test dose of pteroylpolyglutamate was less than the rise after oral PG-1. Using biopsy-obtained intestinal mucosa, the authors could detect no *in vitro* inhibition of intestinal mucosal folate conjugase by OCA. They concluded that OCA do not inhibit folate absorption but may enhance folate clearance from the blood. Subsequently, Shojania and Hornady (1973) administered yeast-derived pteroylpolyglutamate and PG-1 to twenty-two women on OCA and to nineteen control subjects, each having received tissue saturating doses of parenteral PG-1 prior to the oral test dose. The rise in serum folate was similar in both groups after the test dose of PG-1 but less in the OCA group after the test dose of pteroylpolyglutamate. The differences were statistically related to prior evidence of folate deficiency. The rise of serum folate after the test dose of pteroylpolyglutamate was normal in a subgroup of nine of the twenty-two women on OCA with initial normal levels of serum folate, but significantly less than control in a subgroup of thirteen with initial low levels of serum folate. The absorption of pteroylpolyglutamate remained low in those women who were retested 3 months after stopping OCA. The authors suggested that folate malabsorption in women taking OCA may, in fact, be due to another condition such as occult celiac sprue. Should this be the case, these data raise an intriguing possibility that the chronic use of OCA may "uncover" latent celiac sprue.

In summary, the evidence for an effect of OCA on folate absorption is conflicting and remains unclear. Precise methodology, perhaps by use of pure synthetic substrates and direct methods of jejunal perfusion will be required to establish the presence or absence of this relationship.

d. Azulfidine. This drug is used extensively in the treatment of inflammatory bowel disease (IBD) (Crohn's disease and ulcerative colitis). Franklin and Rosenberg (1973) studied folic acid absorption in nineteen patients with IBD, both on and off azulfidine, and compared the results to a control group of healthy subjects. ^{3}H-PG-1, 200 μg, was administered by mouth and 4 hours later a 15 mg parenteral tissue saturating dose of folic acid was given. Absorption was assessed by the recovery of ^{3}H in a 48-hour urine collection. Urinary recovery of ^{3}H was significantly less in the IBD patients than the control group, and less in the IBD patients taking azulfidine than in those not receiving the drug. A significant drug-induced decrease in absorption of ^{3}H-PG-1 was noted in nine normal volunteers who were tested before and after a 1 gm oral dose of azulfidine. Azulfidine in a concentration of 1 mg% suppressed the tissue accumulation of ^{3}H-PG-1 in rings of everted rat jejunum. This effect was not noted with sulfapyridine or 5-amino-salicyclic acid, metabolites of azulfidine. The authors conclude that patients with IBD receiving azulfidine are at risk for folate deficiency secondary to drug-inhibition of folate absorption.

B. Vitamin B$_{12}$

1. *Mechanisms of Absorption*

Vitamin B$_{12}$ (molecular weight 1355), essential with folate in DNA synthesis and cell maturation, is synthesized by intestinal microorganisms and thus has an exclusive animal source. The daily requirement of vitamin B$_{12}$ is 1–2 μg per day, about 1% of that of folate. Dietary deficiency of vitamin B_{12} is found only in strict vegetarians (vegans). Therefore, when vitamin B_{12} deficiency occurs, it is almost always a result of a malabsorptive disorder. Since the process of vitamin B_{12} absorption is complex, the potential for malabsorption is varied.

In the stomach, vitamin B_{12} is transferred from its animal protein source to gastric intrinsic factor (IF). IF is a glycoprotein with a molecular weight of about 50,000, secreted by the parietal cells of the stomach. Pernicious anemia, characterized by IF deficiency, gastric achlorhydria, and ultimately the megaloblastic anemia of vitamin B_{12} lack, reflects B_{12} malabsorption at the gastric stage. In pernicious anemia, antibodies to intrinsic factor or parietal cells are frequently found. Similarly, patients who have had total gastrectomy are at absolute risk for vitamin B_{12} malabsorption and deficiency. Binding of vitamin B_{12} to IF is essential for its safe passage down the small intestine to the ileal receptor cells, the site of intestinal transport of vitamin B_{12}. Within the gastrointestinal tract, the B_{12}–IF complex is exposed to a variety of intraluminal bacteria which may compete with the human host if present in sufficient concentrations, or, in certain indigenous areas, to the fish tapeworm *Diphyllobothrium latum*. Whether bacteria utilize free B_{12} more avidly than the B_{12}–IF complex is an unsettled point (Toskes and Deren, 1973). The occurrence of subnormal vitamin B_{12} absorption was well documented in nine of twenty-two patients with pancreatic insufficiency (Toskes *et al.*, 1971), and recent studies have demonstrated neurologic and hematological changes related to vitamin B_{12} deficiency in patients with this condition (Toskes, 1976). Present evidence suggests that pancreatic trypsin is essential to prevent macromolecular complexing of B_{12}–IF (Toskes and Deren, 1973).

In the distal ileum, the B_{12}–IF complex attaches to receptor sites on the epithelial surface in a process requiring the presence of calcium and a neutral or slightly alkaline pH. The presence of IF is essential for attachment of B_{12} to the ileal receptor, though the ultimate fate of IF—whether absorbed or not—is uncertain. Subsequently, over a process of several hours, vitamin B_{12} is transported through the ileal epithelial cell and then taken up by a transport protein in the blood, termed transcobalamin II.

2. Drugs Affecting Vitamin B_{12} Absorption

Drugs affecting vitamin B_{12} absorption may act at the level of binding to IF, intraluminal precipitation of the B_{12}–IF complex, or blocking ileal uptake and/or transport. Few of the drug syndromes to be described selectively affect B_{12} absorption, but usually result in more generalized intestinal malabsorption.

a. Neomycin. This antibiotic is utilized primarily for the suppression of colonic bacteria in the treatment of hepatic encephalopathy. Early studies indicated that in addition to its antibacterial effects, the chronic administration of neomycin is followed by lowering of the serum cholesterol level in association with induction of steatorrhea (lipid malabsorption) (Jacobson et al., 1960a; Faloon et al., 1966). The administration of neomycin to volunteers is associated with decrease in intestinal disaccharidase activity (Paes et al., 1967), shortening of intestinal villi (Jacobson et al., 1960b) and enlargement of jejunal epithelial cell mitochondria (Dobbins et al., 1968). Neomycin-induced lipid malabsorption may be secondary to an effect on biliary metabolism and lipid digestion. Current evidence indicates that bile salts are precipitated in vitro and in vivo by neomycin (Faloon et al., 1966). In volunteers who received neomycin and developed steatorrhea, the total bile salt pool size decreased, in the absence of morphologic changes in the jejunal mucosa (Hardison and Rosenberg, 1969). A later study of volunteers receiving 1 gm neomycin simultaneously with a lipid test meal showed precipitation of bile and lipid in the intraluminal contents (Thompson et al., 1971). Thus, neomycin may cause lipid malabsorption by precipitating intraluminal bile. However, at least one study has also demonstrated an abnormal test of vitamin B_{12} absorption in two-thirds of patients receiving neomycin (Jacobson et al., 1960a). The effect of neomycin on vitamin B_{12} absorption could be secondary to intraluminal complexing of B_{12}–IF, or perhaps a toxic effect of the drug on the ileum, the common site of absorption of both vitamin B_{12} and bile salts.

b. Colchicine. Colchicine is a time tested anti-inflammatory agent used in the treatment of gout, with a well-recognized side effect of diarrhea. Diarrhea is sufficiently common with colchicine administration as to be used as an end point in titrating its dose. The etiology of colchicine-induced diarrhea is unknown. In a carefully controlled study, Race et al. (1970) demonstrated that colchicine administration to healthy subjects results in increased fecal excretion of sodium, potassium, lipid, and nitrogen. In addition, the authors demonstrated decreased absorption of d-xylose, shortening of jejunal villi, and decreased activity of intestinal mucosal disaccharidases. In a related study by Webb et al. (1968), the same group demonstrated that the daily administration of colchicine to normal subjects, together with labeled vitamin B_{12}, is associated with increased fecal excretion and decreased urinary excretion of the vitamin. Gastric intrinsic factor was unchanged by colchicine administration. Thus, colchicine has a nonspecific damaging effect on the intestinal mucosa. Damage to the ileal mucosa could result in both vitamin B_{12} malabsorption and diarrhea. Since both vitamin B_{12} and bile salts share the ileum as a site of absorption, colchicine-induced ileal damage could result in the colonic accumulation of bile salts, known for their cathartic properties (Mekhjian *et al.*, 1971).

c. *P*-Aminosalicyclic Acid (PAS). This anti-tuberculous agent also has a diarrhea side effect. Hypocholesterolemia and vitamin B_{12} malabsorption and deficiency were recognized as side effects of administration of this drug 10 years ago (Heinivaara and Palva, 1965). The administration of PAS to volunteers induces steatorrhea and malabsorption of d-xylose in the absence of histologic changes in the jejunal mucosa (Levine, 1968). In another report, administration of PAS, 8 gm/day, to a tuberculous patient was followed within 6 days by vitamin B_{12} deficiency and malabsorption, in the presence of normal intestinal histology and disaccharidase activity and absence of steatorrhea (Toskes and Deren, 1972). We studied the pathogenesis of intestinal malabsorption induced by PAS administration in a 78-year-old woman with tuberculosis who developed neurologic signs of vitanim B_{12} deficiency (subacute combined degeneration) 11 months after initiation of PAS, 12 gm/day (Halsted and McIntyre, 1972). Observations over a 4-year period indicated that weight loss, hypocholesterolemia, and subnormal vitamin B_{12} absorption correlated with dosage and duration of PAS administration. Normal vitamin B_{12} absorption occurred at PAS doses of 5 gm daily, while marked malabsorption of vitamin B_{12} could be demonstrated at a dose of 12 gm/day (Fig. 5). Gastric intrinsic factor was not decreased. In a prospective evaluation, 5 days of administration of PAS, 12 gm/day, was followed by steatorrhea and d-xylose malabsorption, with normal intestinal histology but subnormal mucosal disaccharidase activity. We speculated, though did not definitely prove, that PAS, like colchicine, may damage ileal transport functions, producing B_{12} malabsorption, bile acid diarrhea, and steatorrhea.

d. Ethanol. Although the megaloblastic anemia of alcoholism is almost exclusively the result of impaired folate metabolism (*vide supra*), abnormal vitamin B_{12} absorption occurs with the chronic ingestion of alcohol. Present evidence from Lindenbaum *et al.* suggests two etiologies for vitamin B_{12} malabsorption in alcoholism: folate deficiency *and* chronic ethanol ingestion. In fifteen patients with folate deficiency and megaloblastic anemia, decreased absorption of d-xylose was found in 80%, and of vitamin B_{12} in 40% (Lindenbaum and Pezzimenti, 1972). Conversely, in twenty-eight patients with vitamin B_{12} deficiency secondary to pernicious anemia, decreased vitamin B_{12} absorption (studied

Charles H. Halsted

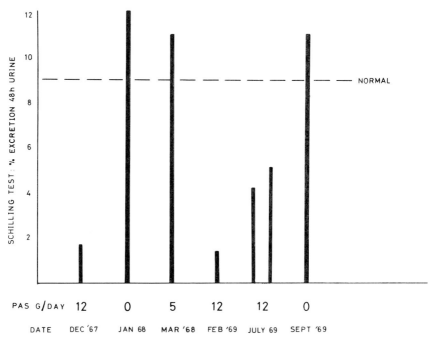

SCHILLING TEST: % EXCRETION 48h URINE

PAS G/DAY   12   0   5   12   12   0

DATE   DEC '67   JAN 68   MAR '68   FEB '69   JULY 69   SEPT '69

Fig. 5. Vitamin B_{12} absorption at intervals over a 2-year period in a 78-year-old woman being treated with PAS at varied doses. Absorption was studied by the Schilling test by measuring 48-hour urinary radioactivity after oral dose of 0.5 μg ^{57}Covitamin B_{12} and 1 mg vitamin B_{12} im Intrinsic factor was present in gastric contents. Vitamin B_{12} malabsorption correlated with dosage of PAS.

with exogenous intrinsic factor to eliminate the effect of IF deficiency on the absorption test) was found in 75% (Lindenbaum et al., 1974). These studies underscore the role of vitamin B_{12} and folate, both essential for cell maturation, on normal intestinal transport processes (Halsted, 1975). The absorption of vitamin B_{12} is also diminished by the chronic ingestion of ethanol in well-nourished alcoholics. Vitamin B_{12} absorption was measured sequentially in eight chronic alcoholics, initially after 1 month of sobriety with hospital diet and vitamin supplements, and after 1–4 weeks of ethanol ingestion in amounts of 173–253 gm/day. Following alcohol ingestion, there was decreased vitamin B_{12} absorption in six of the eight patients, while the absorption of d-xylose increased and that of dietary fat was unchanged (Lindenbaum and Lieber, 1975). In addition to the effects of folate deficiency and ethanol ingestion, vitamin B_{12} malabsorption may also result from the pancreatic insufficiency that may follow years of alcohol ingestion, as described above (Toskes *et al.*, 1971; Toskes, 1976).

   e. Biguanides. These oral hypoglycemic agents act by three possible mechanisms: enhancement of anaerobic glycolysis, decreased gluconeogenesis, and possibly by decreasing intestinal absorption of glucose. Arvanitakis *et al.* (1973) have demonstrated that the oral administration of 100 mg phenformin 45 minutes prior to testing significantly inhibits the uptake of glucose, water, and sodium from the perfused human jejunum. Jejunal biopsies obtained 75 minutes after administration of 100 mg phenformin showed mitochondrial alterations. The authors suggested that phenformin inhibits mitochondrial respiration and secondarily may limit mucosal ATP and hence the active transport of sodium and glucose. Berchtold *et al.* (1971) administered metformin, a biguanide used in Europe, to volunteers for 2–10 weeks in doses of 3 gm/day, and demonstrated drug-induced decrease in jejunal disaccharidase activity and vitamin B_{12} absorption. In another study, Tomkin *et al.* (1971) found decreased vitamin B_{12} absorption in 30% of seventy-one patients who received metformin in average doses of 1.75 gm/day for 4–6 years. Four patients in this series had low serum levels of vitamin B_{12}. Subsequently, Tomkin (1973) reported that eleven of twenty-four (46%) American patients receiving phenformin, 100 mg/day for 5 years, demonstrated low absorption of vitamin B_{12}. Thus, both biguanides impair the absorption of vitamin B_{12}, and patients receiving these drugs may be at risk for B_{12} deficiency and megaloblastic anemia. In view of the above-described effects of these biguanides on mucosal enzymes and on absorption of other substances, it is probable that biguanide has general effects on the small intestinal epithelium and inhibits vitamin B_{12} absorption at the level of ileal epithelial metabolism and transport.

C. Thiamine

   Whereas thiamine deficiency may take the form of classical beri-beri heart failure in the malnourished populations of the developing world, in clinical medicine in the United States, thiamine deficiency is almost exclusively found in the alcoholic population. In a review of 120 mostly indigent patients admitted to a large municipal hospital, thiamine deficiency was found in 31%, second in frequency to deficiency of folic acid (Leevy *et al.*, 1965). Among alcoholics, the clinical manifestations of thiamine deficiency include cardiomyopathy similar to beri-beri, and, more commonly, various neurologic manifestations. These include peripheral neuropathy, Wernicke encephalopathy, and Korsakoff psychosis. While dietary inadequacy may play the predominant role in the thiamine deficiency of alcoholism, recent evidence indicates that thiamine malabsorption may be a significant accompaniment of alcoholism.

1. Mechanism of Thiamine Absorption

Current evidence suggests that thiamine (molecular weight 337) is absorbed by a process of active transport at low concentrations and probably by passive diffusion at high concentrations. Using a method of recovery of isotope in the urine following increasing amounts of ^{35}S-thiamine administered orally to healthy volunteers, Thomson and Leevy (1972) demonstrated that the maximal absorbed dose of thiamine is about 8 mg by a rate-limited process demonstrating saturation kinetics. Recent *in vivo* and *in vitro* studies in the rat have presented convincing evidence that at thiamine concentrations of less than 1.5 μM the absorption process is saturable and can be inhibited by ouabain (an inhibitor of Na, K-dependent ATPase) and omission of sodium from the incubation media (Hoyumpa *et al.*, 1975a). A linear relationship between concentration and transport, and lack of inhibition was demonstrated at concentrations of thiamine greater than $20\mu M$. Thus a carrier-mediated process linked to sodium transport may be required for intestinal absorption of low concentrations of thiamine, while larger concentrations are absorbed passively. Of significance is the fact that the usual daily thiamine intake of 0.5–1.5 mg probably gives intraluminal thiamine concentrations of less than 2 μM, in the range for active transport.

2. Effect of Ethanol in Thiamine Absorption

Clinical evidence indicates that malabsorption contributes to the thiamine deficiency of alcoholics. Using a method of measurement of plasma levels and urinary excretion of radioactivity following oral administration of a 5 mg dose of ^{35}S-thiamine, Thomson *et al.* (1970) demonstrated (a) significant thiamine malabsorption in malnourished alcoholic patients with liver disease; (b) correction to normal of thiamine malabsorption after nutritional replenishment and abstinence from ethanol for 6 weeks; and (c) suppression of thiamine absorption in healthy volunteers who were administered ethanol, 1.5 gm/kg, prior to the dose of thiamine. Thiamine malabsorption occurred in the absence of other clinical evidence of intestinal malabsorption. These studies suggested that thiamine absorption may be limited both by nutritional deficiency and by ethanol.

Howard *et al.* (1974) demonstrated that folate deficiency limits the absorption of thiamine. Rats were pair-fed diets either folate-free or folate supplemented for periods up to 10 months, at which time markedly decreased hepatic and red cell folate levels were found in the folate-free diet group. The uptake of ^{35}S-thiamine was significantly less from *in vivo* duodenal or jejunal loops prepared in the folate-free diet group at thiamine concentrations of 0.5 μM, but not at higher concentrations of 17.5 μM. Recently, the same group demonstrated direct *in vivo* and *in vitro* effects of ethanol on thiamine absorption from rat intestine (Hoyumpa *et al.*, 1975b). Using *in vivo* intestinal loops they demonstrated that ethanol administered either intravenously or by gastric gavage significantly inhibited the duodenal absorption of a low concentration (0.5 μM) of thiamine. By *in vitro* studies of everted jejunal sacs they showed that ethanol, given intragastrically 1 hour before sacrifice, significantly limited the net transport of low concentrations of thiamine from the mucosal to serosal surface. Further analysis showed that ethanol did not impair mucosal uptake but limited the exit of thiamine from the tissue to the serosal fluid. Similar effects were shown with ouabain, an inhibitor of Na, K-dependent ATPase and sodium transport. When thiamine was present at high concentrations there was no ethanol inhibition of thiamine transport. These studies supported the previous evidence that thiamine absorption is active and linked to sodium transport when present in low concentrations but passive at high concentrations. The data suggest that ethanol inhibits thiamine transport by suppressing activity of lateral membrane Na-K-dependent ATPase (the "sodium pump").

III. DISCUSSION: RESEARCH NEEDS

The problem of drug inhibition of water-soluble vitamin absorption is extremely complex since vitamin absorption occurs through a variety of mechanisms. Drug interaction with the intestinal mucosa may be generalized or specific, and in most cases is incompletely understood. A comprehensive approach to this problem must include clear definitions of mechanisms of water-soluble vitamin absorption, precise definition of the multiple ways by which a drug may alter intestinal structure and intestinal transport processes, and a proper correlation of experimental evidence with clinical observations. The experimental approach to the study of an effect of a drug on intestinal transport should first consider the concentrations of the drug and vitamins which can be expected to be present within the intestinal lumen at the site of absorption of the vitamin in question. As examples, intraluminal drug concentrations of ethanol (Halsted *et al.*, 1973b) and Dilantin (Gerson *et al.*, 1972) have been measured, and intraluminal concentrations of thiamine have been estimated (Hoyumpa *et al.*, 1975a). On the other hand, in spite of numerous studies on possible mechanisms of folate absorption, we still have no clear understanding of the intrajejunal concentrations and biochemical species of folate that can be expected after ingestion and exposure to the intragastric environment of folate containing foods.

The methodology employed in the study of drug effects on water-soluble vitamin absorption has been extremely variable and, in many cases, imprecise. Ideally, there should be three parts involved: clinical observations, studies of absorption on human subjects, and *in vitro* studies of drug–nutrient interaction at the level of the intestinal mucosal transport site. For the most part, data are reasonably conclusive that the chronic ingestion of the drugs indicated herein is associated with the vitamin deficiencies described. (The evidence with regard to oral contraceptive use and folate deficiency remains controversial).

In many of the studies reported, the approach to human intestinal absorption has been unclear and subject to various interpretations. For example, measurement of the rise in serum folate after the oral administration of PG-1 and/or pteroylpolyglutamate to folate-deficient subjects can be interpreted as intestinal absorption or clearance from the blood to the tissues—an approach that has led to much confusion regarding possible effects of OCA on folate absorption. In this reviewer's estimation, the most accurate way to measure human intestinal absorption is by intestinal perfusion of the substance in question. By measurement of disappearance of the substance from the lumen, this method allows precise conclusions on mucosal uptake (though not on the complete intestinal transport process). Furthermore, tissue saturating doses are not required since variables of hepatic, renal or other tissue metabolism do not enter into interpretation of the results. This approach was used in the studies of the effects of Dilantin and of ethanol on PG-1 transport (Gerson *et al.*, 1972; Halsted *et al.*, 1971).

Interpretation of drug–nutrient absorption studies in human subjects is additionally complicated by questions of specificity. For example, several drugs, including neomycin, PAS, and colchicine seem to have generalized effects on mucosal enzymes and on absorption of a variety of substances. Is the effect of these drugs on vitamin B_{12} absorption related to a specific effect on the ileal absorbing cell, or generalized poorly defined effects involving the entire small intestine? If the effect is on the ileal cell, does it involve the receptor site or the transport process? Precise *in vitro* approaches will be required to answer these questions. The data on the effects of alcoholism on intestinal absorption remains confusing. One must dissect from "alcoholism" the three components of associated nutritional deficiency (e.g., folate deficiency), acute damage to the intestine from ethanol, and chronic effects on intestinal function that may arise from chronic alcohol abuse. With this in mind, the evidence suggests that folate malabsorption is the result of a combination of chronic ethanol ingestion and dietary folate deficiency, that vitamin B_{12} malabsorption requires only the chronic abuse of ethanol, and that thiamine malabsorption may result from acute ethanol ingestion or from dietary folate deficiency. A unifying mechanism whereby ethanol affects intestinal folate metabolism and/or specific vitamin transport processes has not been discovered. The experimental approaches of Howard *et al.* (1974) and Hoyumpa *et al.* (1975a,b) seem most likely to unravel these variables with regard to thiamine absorption.

In summary, research in the area of drug effects on vitamin absorption should answer the following questions, and use the following approaches:

1. Clinical observation: Is the drug effect acute, related to chronic use, or to an associated nutritional deficiency or other metabolic abnormality created by the drug?

2. Studies of human absorption: What are the ranges of levels in the intestinal lumen to be expected after ingestion of the drug and vitamin in question? Choice of the proper concentration range is essential in devising the absorption test. The method of study of intestinal absorption should be relatively free of other variables and the technique of intestinal perfusion seems most suitable.

3. Additional experimental studies should be designed to adhere closely to normal physiologic conditions and to dissect out (a) mechanisms of transport of the vitamin in question; and (b) the step or steps at which the drug (present in its physiologic concentration) interacts with these transport processes.

REFERENCES

Arvanitakis, C., Lorenzsonn, V., and Olsen, W. A. (1973). Phenformin-induced alterations of small intestinal function and mitochondrial structure in man. *J. Lab. Clin. Med.* **82,** 195–199.

Baraona, E., Pirola, R. C., and Lieber, C. S. (1974). Small intestinal damage and changes in cell population produced by ethanol ingestion in the rat. *Gastroenterology* **66,** 226–234.

Baugh, C. M. and Krumdieck, C. L. (1969). Effects of phenytoin on folic acid conjujases in Man. *Lancet* **2,** 519–521.

Baugh, C. M., Krumdieck, C. L., Baker, H. J., and Butterworth, C. E., Jr. (1971). Studies on the absorption and metabolism of folic acid. Folate absorption in the dog after exposure of isolated intestinal segments to synthetic pteroylpolyglutamates of various chain lengths. *J. Clin. Invest.* **50**, 2009-2021.

Benn, A., Swan, C. H. J., Cooke, W. T., Blair, J. A., Matty, A. J., and Smith, M. E. (1971). Effect of intraluminal pH on the absorption of pteroylmonoglutamic acid. *Br. Med. J.* **1**, 148-150.

Berchtold, P., Dahlquist, A., Gustafson, A., and Asp, N-G. (1971). Effects of a biguanide (metformin) on vitamin B_{12} and folic acid absorption and intestinal enzyme activities. *Scand. J. Gastroenterol.* **6**, 751-754.

Bhanthumnavin, K., Wright, J. R., and Halsted, C. H. (1974). Intestinal transport of tritiated folic acid (^{3}H-PGA) in the everted gut sac of different aged rats. *Johns Hopkins Med. J.* **135**, 152-160.

Bianchi, A., Chipman, D. W., Dreskin, A., and Rosensweig, N. (1970). Nutritional folic acid deficiency with megaloblastic changes in the small bowel epithelium. *N. Engl. J. Med.* **282**, 859-861.

Blair, J. A., and Matty, A. J. (1974). Acid microclimate in intestinal absorption. *Clin. Gastroenterol.* **3**, 183-197.

Blair, J. A., Johnson, I. T., and Matty, A. J. (1974). Absorption of folic acid by everted segments of rat jejunum. *J. Physiol. (London)* **236**, 653-661.

Burgen, A. S. V., and Goldberg, N. J. (1962). Absorption of folic acid from the small intestine of the rat. *Br. J. Pharmacol. Chemother.* **19**, 313-320.

Butterworth, C. E., Jr., Santini, R., and Frommeyer, W. B. (1963). The pteroylmonoglutamate components of American diets as determined by chromatographic fractionation. *J. Clin. Invest.* **42**, 1929-1939.

Chanarin, I., Laidlaw, J., Loughridge, L. W., and Mollin, D. L. (1960). Megaloblastic anemia due to phenobarbitone. The convulsant action of therapeutic doses of folic acid. *Br. Med. J.* **1**, 1099-1102.

Chang, T., Lewis, J., and Glazko, A. J. (1967). Effect of ethanol and other alcohols on the transport of amino acids and glucose by everted sacs of rat small intestine. *Biochim. Biophys. Acta* **135**, 1000-1007.

Cherrick, G. R., Baker, H., Frank, O., and Leevy, C. M. (1965). Observations on hepatic avidity for folate in Laennec's cirrbons. *J. Lab. Clin. Med.* **66**, 446-451.

Corcino, J. J., Reisenauer, A. M., and Halsted, C. H. (1976). Jejunal perfusion of simple and conjugated folate in tropical sprue. *J. Clin. Invest.* **58**, 298-305.

Dahlke, M. B., and Mertens-Roesler, E. (1967). Malabsorption of folic acid due to diphenylhydantoin. *Blood* **30**, 341-351.

Dobbins, W. O., Herrero, B. A., and Mansbach, C. M. (1968). Morphologic alterations associated with neomycin-induced malabsorption. *Am. J. Med. Sci.* **255**, 63-77.

Doe, W. F., Hoffbrand, A. V., Reed, P. I., and Scott, J. M. (1971). Jejunal pH and folic acid. *Br. Med. J.* **1**, 669-670.

Faloon, W. W., Paes, I. C., Woolfolk, D., Nankin, H., Wallace, K., and Haro, E. N. (1966). Effect of neomycin and kanamycin upon intestinal absorption. *Ann. N.Y. Acad. Sci.* **132**, 879-887.

Fehling, C., Jagerstad, M., Lindstrand, K., and Westesson, A. (1973). The effect of anticonvulsant therapy upon the absorption of folates. *Clin. Sci.* **44**, 595-600.

Fordtran, J. S. (1967). Speculations on the pathogenesis of diarrhea. *Fed. Proc., Fed. Am. Soc. Exp. Biol.* **26**, 1405-1414.

Franklin, J. L., and Rosenberg, I. H. (1973). Impaired folic acid absorption in inflammatory bowel disease: Effects of salicylazosulfapyridine (azulfidine). *Gastroenterology* **64,** 517-525.

Gerson, C. D., Cohen, N., Hepner, G. W., Brown, N., Herbert, V., and Janowitz, H. D. (1971). Folic acid absorption in man: Enhancing effects of glucose. *Gastroenterology* **61,** 224-227.

Gerson, C. D., Hepner, G. W., Brown, N., Cohen, N., Herbert, V., and Janowitz, H. D. (1972). Inhibition by diphenylhydantoin of folic acid absorption in man. *Gastroenterology* **63,** 246-251.

Greene, H. L., Herman, R. H., and Kraemer, S. (1971). Stimulation of jejunal adenyl cyclase by ethanol. *J. Lab. Clin. Med.* **78,** 336-342.

Halsted, C. H. (1975). The small intestine in vitamin B_{12} and folate deficiency. *Nutr. Rev.* **33,** 33-37.

Halsted, C. H., and McIntyre, P. A. (1972). Intestinal malabsorption caused by aminosalicyclic acid therapy. *Arch. Intern. Med.* **130,** 935-939.

Halsted, C. H., Griggs, R. C., and Harris, J. W. (1967). The effect of alcoholism on the absorption of folic acid (^{3}H-PGA) evaluated by plasma levels and urine excretion. *J. Lab. Clin. Med.* **69,** 116-131.

Halsted, C. H., Robles, E. A., and Mezey, E. (1971). Decreased jejunal uptake of labeled folic acid (^{3}H-PGA) in alcoholic patients: Roles of alcohol and nutrition. *N. Engl. J. Med.* **285,** 701-706.

Halsted, C. H., and McIntyre, P. A. (1972). Intestinal malabsorption caused by aminosalicylic acid therapy. *Arch. Intern. Med.* **130,** 935-939.

Halsted, C. H., Robles, E. A., Mezey, E. (1973a). Intestinal malabsorption in folate—deficient alcoholics. *Gastroenterology* **64,** 526-532.

Halsted, C. H., Robles, E. A., and Mezey, E. (1973b). Distribution of ethanol in the human gastrointestinal tract. *Am. J. Clin. Nutr.* **26,** 831-834.

Halsted, C. H., Bhanthumnavin, K., and Mezey, E. (1974). Jejunal uptake of tritiated folic acid in the rat studied by *in vitro* perfusion. *J. Nutr.* **104,** 1674-1680.

Halsted, C. H., Baugh, C. M., and Butterworth, C. E., Jr. (1975). Jejunal perfusion of simple and conjugated folates in man. *Gastroenterology* **68,** 261-269.

Halsted, C. H., Reisenauer, A. M., Back, C., and Gotterer, G. (1976). *In vitro* uptake and metabolism of pteroylpolyglutamate by rat small intestine. *J. Nutr.* **106,** 485-492.

Halsted, C. H., Reisenauer, A. M., Romero, J. J., Cantor, D. S., and Ruebner, B. (1977). Jejunal perfusion of simple and conjugated solates in celiac sprue. *J. Clin. Invest.* **59,** 933-940.

Hardison, W. G. M., and Rosenberg, I. H. (1969). The effect of neomycin on bile salt metabolism and fat digestion in man. *J. Lab. Clin. Med.* **74,** 564-573.

Heinivaara, O., and Palva, I. P. (1965). Malabsorption and deficiency of vitamin B_{12} caused by treatment with para-amino salicylic acid. *Acta Med. Scand.* **177,** 337-341.

Hepner, G. W. (1967). The absorption of pteroylglutamic (folic) acid in rats. *Br. J. Haematol.* **16,** 241-249.

Hepner, G. W., Booth, C. C., Cowan, J., Hoffbrand, A. V., and Mollin, D. L. (1968). Absorption of crystalline folic acid in man. *Lancet* **2,** 302-306.

Herbert, V. (1963). A palatable diet for producing experimental folate deficiency in man. *Am. J. Clin. Nutr.* **12,** 17-20.

Herbert, V., Zalusky, R., and Davidson, C. S. (1963). Correlation of folate deficiency with alcoholism and associated macroytosis, anemia, and liver disease. *Ann. Intern. Med.* **58,** 977-988.

Hermos, J. A., Adams, W. H., Lin, Y. K., and Trier, J. (1972). Mucosa of the small intestine in folate-deficient alcoholics. *Ann. Intern. Med.* **76,** 957-965.

Hines, J. D. (1975). Hemotological abnormalties involving vitamin B_6 and folate metabolism in alcoholic subjects. *Ann. N. Y. Acad. Sci.* **252**, 316-327.

Hoffbrand, A. V., and Necheles, T. F. (1968). Mechanism of folate deficiency in patients receiving phenytoin. *Lancet* **2**, 528-530.

Hoffbrand, A. V., and Peters, T. J. (1969). The subcellular localization of pteroylpolyglutamate hydrolase and folate in guinea pig intestinal mucosa. *Biochim. Biophys. Acta* **192**, 479-485.

Hoffbrand, A. V., and Peters, T. J. (1970). Recent advances in knowledge of clinical and biochemical aspects of folate. *Schweiz. Med. Wochenschr.* **100**, 1954-1970.

Houlihan, C. M., Scott, J. M., Boyle, P. H., and Weir, D. G. (1972). The effect of phenytoin on the absorption of synthetic folic acid polyglutamate. *Gut* **13**, 189-190.

Howard, L., Wagner, C., and Schenker, S. (1974). Malabsorption of thiamine in folatedeficient rats. *J. Nutr.* **104**, 1024-1032.

Hoyumpa, A. M., Middleton, H. M., Wilson, F. A., and Schenker, S. (1975a). Thiamine transport across the rat intestine. *Gastroenterology* **68**, 1218-1227.

Hoyumpa, A. M., Breen, K. J., Schenker, S., and Wilson, F. (1975b). Thiamine transport across the rat intestine. Effect of ethanol. *J. Lab. Clin. Med.* **86**, 803-816.

Israel, Y. and Salazar, I. (1967). Inhibition of brain microsomal adenosine triphosphatases by general depressants. *Arch. Biochem. Biophys.* **122**, 310-317.

Israel, Y., Salazar, I., and Rosenmann, E. (1966). Inhibitory effects of alcohol on intestinal amino acid transport *in vivo* and *in vitro*. *J. Nutr.* **96**, 499-504.

Israel, Y., Valenzuela, J. E., Salazar, I., and Ugarte, G. (1968). Alcohol and amino acid transport in the human small intestine. *J. Nutr.* **98**, 222-224.

Jacobson, E. D., Chodos, R. B., and Faloon, W. W. (1960a). An experimental malabsorption syndrome induced by neomycin. *Am. J. Med.* **28**, 524-533.

Jacobson, E. D., Prior, J. T., and Faloon, W. W. (1960b). Malabsorptive syndrome induced by neomycin: Morphologic alterations in the jejunal mucosa. *J. Lab. Clin. Med.* **56**, 245-250.

Krasner, N., Cochran, K. M., Russell, R. I., Carmichael, H. A., and Thompson, G. G. (1976a). Alcohol and absorption from the small intestine. Impairment of absorption from the small intestine in alcoholics. *Gut* **17**, 245-248.

Krasner, N., Carmichael, H. A., Russell, R. I., Thompson, G. G., and Cochran, K. M. (1976b). Alcohol and absorption from the small intestine. Effect of ethanol on ATP and ATPase activity in guinea pig jejunum. *Gut* **17**, 249-251.

LaCosta, M., and Rothenberg, S. P. (1974). Appearance of a folate binder in leukocytes and serum of women who are pregnant or taking oral contraceptives. *J. Lab. Clin. Med.* **83**, 207-214.

Leevy, C. M., Cardi, L., Frank, O., Gellene, R., and Baker, H. (1965). Incidence and significant of hypo-vitaminemia in a randomly selected municipal hospital population. *Am. J. Clin. Nutr.* **17**, 259-271.

Leslie, G. I., and Rowe, P. B. (1972). Folate binding by brush border membrane proteins of small intestinal epithelial cells. *Biochemistry* **11**, 1696-1703.

Levine, R. A. (1968). Steatorrhea induced by para-amino salicylic acid. *Ann. Intern. Med.* **68**, 1265-1270.

Lindenbaum, J., and Lieber, C. S. (1975). Effect of chronic ethanol administration on intestinal absorption in man in the absence of nutritional deficiency. *Ann. N. Y. Acad. Sci.* **252**, 228-234.

Lindenbaum, J., and Pezzimenti, J. F. (1972). Effects of B_{12} and folate deficiency on small intestinal function. *Clin. Res.* **20**, 871 (abstr.).

Lindenbaum, J., Pezzimenti, J. F., and Shea, N. (1974). Small intestine in vitamin B_{12} deficiency. *Ann. Intern. Med.* **80,** 326–331.

Lindenbaum, J., Whitehead, N., and Reyner, F. (1975). Oral contraceptive hormones, folate metabolism, and the cervical epithelium. *Am. J. Clin. Nutr.* **28,** 346–353.

Lucas, M. L., Scheider, W., Haberich, F. J., and Blair, J. A. (1975). Direct measurement by pH-microelectrode of the pH microclimate in rat proximal jejunum. *Proc. R. Soc. London* **192,** 39–48.

Mekhjian, H. S., Phillips, S. F., and Hoffman, A. F. (1971). Colonic secretion of water and electrolytes induced by bile acids. Perfusion studies in man. *J. Clin. Invest.* **50,** 1569–1577.

Melikian, V., Paton, A., Leeming, R. J., and Portman-Graham, H. (1971). Site of reduction and methylation of folic acid in man. *Lancet* **2,** 955–957.

Mezey, E. (1975). Intestinal function in chronic alcoholism. *Ann. N. Y. Acad. Sci.* **252,** 215–227.

Mezey, E., Jow, E., Slavin, R. E., and Tobon, F. (1970). Pancreatic function and intestinal absorption in chronic alcoholism. *Gastroenterology* **59,** 657–664.

Necheles, T. F., and Snyder, L. M. (1970). Malabsorption of folate polyglutamates associated with oral contraceptive therapy. *N. Engl. J. Med.* **282,** 858–859.

Nixon, P. F., and Bertino, J. R. (1972). Effective absorption and utilization of oral formyltetra-hydrofolate in man. *N. Engl. J. Med.* **286,** 175–179.

Olinger, E. J., Bertino, J., and Binder, H. J. (1973). Intestinal folate absorption. Conversion and retention of pteroylmonoglutamate by jejunum. *J. Clin. Invest.* **52,** 2138–2145.

Paes, I. C., Searl, P., Rubert, M. W., and Faloon, W. W. (1967). Intestinal lactase deficiency and saccharide malabsorption during oral neomycin distribution. *Gastroenterology* **53,** 49–58.

Perry J., and Chanarin, I. (1973). Formylation of folate as step in physiological folate absorption. *Lancet* **2,** 588 589.

Race, T. F., Paes, I. C., and Faloon, W. W. (1970). Intestinal malabsorption induced by oral colchicine. Comparison with neomycin and cathartic agents. *Am. J. Med. Sci.* **259,** 32–41.

Reisenauer, A. M., Krumdieck, C. L., and Halsted, C. H. (1977). Folate conjugase: Two separate activities in human jejunum. *Science* (in press).

Reynolds, E. H. (1968). Mental effects of anticonvulsants, and folic acid metabolism. *Brain* **91,** 197–214.

Rosenberg, I. H., and Godwin, H. A. (1971). The digestion and absorption of dietary folate. *Gastroenterology* **60,** 445–463.

Rosenberg, I. H. Godwin, H. A., Streiff, R. R., and Castle, W. B. (1968). Impairment of intestinal deconjugation of dietary folate: A possible explanation of megaloblastic anemia associated with phenytoin therapy. *Lancet* **2,** 530–532.

Rubin, E., Rybak, B. J., Lindenbaum, J., Gerson, C. D., Walker, G., and Lieber, C. S. (1972). Ultrastructural changes in the small intestine induced by ethanol. *Gastroenterology* **63,** 801–814.

Shojania A. M., and Hornady, C. J. (1973). Oral contraceptives and folate absorption. *J. Lab. Clin. Med.* **82,** 869–875.

Smith, M. E., Matty, A. J., and Blair, J. A. (1970). The transport of pteroylglutamic acid across the small intestine of the rat. *Biochim. Biophys. Acta* **219,** 37–46.

Stephens, M. E. M., Craft, I., Peters, T. J., and Hoffbrand, A. V. (1972). Oral contraceptives and folate metabolism. *Clin. Sci.* **42,** 405–414.

Streiff, R. R. (1970). Folate deficiency and oral contraceptives. *J. Am. Med. Assoc.* **214,** 105–108.

Sullivan, L. W., and Herbert, V. (1964). Suppression of hematopoiesis by ethanol. *J. Clin. Invest.* **43,** 2048–2062.

Tamura, T., and Stokstad, E. L. R.(1973). The availability of food folate in man. *Br. J. Haematol.* **25,** 513–532.

Tamura, T., Shin, Y. S., Buehring, K. V., and Stokstad, E. L. R. (1976). The availability of folates in man: Effect of orange juice supplement on intestinal conjugase. *Br. J. Haematol.* **32,** 123–133. •

Thompson, G. R., Barrowman, J., Gutierrez, L., and Dowling, R. H. (1971). Action of neomycin on the intraluminal phase of lipid absorption. *J. Clin. Invest.* **50,** 319–323.

Thomson, A. D., and Leevy, C. M. (1972). Observations on the mechanism of thiamine hydrochloride absorption in man. *Clin. Sci.* **43,** 153–163.

Thomson, A. D., Baker, H., and Leevy, C. M. (1970). Patterns of ^{35}S-thiamine hydrochloride absorption in the malnourished alcoholic patient. *J. Lab Clin. Med.* **76,** 34–45.

Tomkin, G. H. (1973). Malabsorption of vitamin B_{12} in diabetic patients treated with phenformin: A comparison with metformin. *Br. Med. J.* **3,** 673–675.

Tomkin, G. H., Hadden, D. R., Weaver, J. A., and Montgomery, D. A. D. (1971). Vitamin B_{12} status of patients on long-term metformin therapy. *Br. Med. J.* **2,** 685–687.

Toskes, P. P. (1976). Megaloblastic anemia and peripheral neuropathy secondary to vitamin B_{12} deficiency in patients with chronic pancreatitis. *Gastroenterology* **70,** A-85 (abstr.).

Toskes, P. P., and Deren, J. J. (1972). Selective inhibition of vitamin B_{12} absorption by para-amino salicylic acid. *Gastroenterology* **62,** 1232–1237.

Toskes, P. P., and Deren, J. J. (1973). Vitamin B_{12} absorption and malabsorption. *Gastroenterology* **65,** 662–683 (rev.).

Toskes, P. P., Hansell, J., Cerda, J., and Deren, J. J. (1971). Vitamin B_{12} malabsorption in chronic pancreatic insufficiency. *N. Engl. J. Med.* **284,** 627–632.

Webb, D. I., Chodos, R. B., Mahar, C. Q., and Faloon, W. W. (1968). Mechanism of vitamin B_{12} malabsorption in patients receiving colchicine. *N. Engl. J. Med.* **279,** 845–850.

Whitehead, V. M., and Cooper, B. A. (1967). Absorption of unaltered folic and from the gastrointestinal tract in man. *Br. J. Haematol.* **13,** 679–686.

Wilson, T. H. (1962). "Intestinal Absorption," 2. Saunders, Philadelphia, Pennsylvania.

4

Drug Effects on Fat-Soluble Vitamin Absorption

JAMES A. BARROWMAN

I. INTRODUCTION

Like their water-soluble counterparts the fat-soluble vitamins are only required in small amounts for health. While the absorptive capacity of the normal gastrointestinal tract for various vitamins may be quite large, dietary intake may often be close to the metabolic requirements, and derangement of digestive and absorptive function therefore may lead to

113

clinical deficiencies. It is also clear that adequate absorption does not necessarily guarantee adequate supplies of the metabolically active form of the vitamin since conversion of vitamin precursors to their active forms may occur in diverse organs such as intestinal mucosa, skin, liver, and kidney. It is important to recognize that the rate of onset of clinical deficiency of a vitamin is determined in part by the extent to which the vitamin is stored in body tissues.

Fat-soluble nutrients pose a special problem in digestion and absorption, and for optimal assimilation the function of the pancreatico–biliary system and the small intestine must be intact. The special dependence of fat-soluble vitamins on interaction with bile salts in the intestinal lumen can be regarded as the "weak point" in the sequence of their assimilation.

II. PHYSIOLOGY OF DIGESTION, ABSORPTION, AND TRANSPORT OF FAT-SOLUBLE VITAMINS

It is tempting to assume, in view of shared physical properties, that the physiological principles governing the absorption of fat-soluble vitamins apply generally to all of these substances. This may well be true in the early stages of intraluminal solubilization and intestinal mucosal uptake, though there is surprisingly little information about this. The handling of the vitamins after the uptake step however is clearly peculiar to each substance.

A. Solubilization in the Intestinal Lumen

Vitamins A, D, E, and K are relatively nonpolar lipids and the fatty acid esters of vitamins A, D, and E are even less polar. Although the distribution of fat-soluble vitamins between the emulsified oil and bile salt micellar phases in the small intestine has not been studied in detail, it is probable that they behave in a similar fashion to nonpolar solutes such as cholesterol and its esters which are able to dissolve in both phases. The distribution would be determined by such factors as esterification of vitamins A, D, and E by fatty acids, favoring their partition to the oil phase or expansion of the bile salt micellar phase by the polar products of lipolysis, namely fatty acids and monoglycerides, which are known to enhance micellar solubilization of nonpolar solutes (Borgström, 1968); the ability of fat-soluble vitamins to dissolve in mixed bile salt-fatty acid micelles is well documented by many studies *in vitro*. Although oil and bile salt micellar phases represent the major compartments of gut contents which contain the fat-soluble vitamins, it is possible that some of the vitamins may exist adsorbed to insoluble material such as dietary fiber and small amounts will be in molecular solution in the aqueous medium, these amounts being determined by the aqueous solubility of the substance.

Like other lipids, these vitamins are probably taken up by the brush border membrane of the enterocyte by a passive process. Wilson *et al.* (1971) have drawn attention to the presence of an unstirred water layer close to this membrane which offers resistance to the penetration of particles and large molecules. It is likely that highly nonpolar lipids such as hydrocarbons, sterols, and fat-soluble vitamins depend on bile salt micellar solubilization for their transport into this layer towards the surface of the cell (Borgström, 1974). In experimental animals, fat-soluble vitamins are poorly absorbed in the absence of bile (see, for example, Gagnon and Dawson, 1968). MacMahon and Thompson (1970) have shown in rats that polar lipids such as oleic acid are absorbed into mesenteric lymph almost as well from lipid emulsions as from mixed bile salt micelles, whereas α-tocopherol is poorly absorbed from an emulsion as compared with a micellar solution. The poor absorption from the emulsion is associated with low uptake into the mucosal epithelium, suggesting that it is at this stage of the absorptive process that bile salts facilitate absorption. In man the absence of bile seriously impairs the absorption of fat-soluble vitamins as judged by their appearance in lymph after feeding labeled doses of the vitamins (Forsgren, 1969).

B. Intraluminal Digestion of Esters

Bile salt micelles appear to be important as a medium in which the digestion of esters of the vitamins occurs. A substantial proportion of dietary vitamin A is in the form of retinyl esters, in particular palmitate (Olson, 1969). In certain fish liver oils, vitamin D is also esterified with long-chain fatty acids such as oleic acid. In the rat, hydrolysis in the small intestinal lumen appears to be a requisite for the absorption of the retinyl esters (Mahadevan *et al.*, 1963) and it is also likely to be so for vitamin D esters (Bell and Bryan, 1969). A parallel can be drawn between cholesterol esters and vitamin D esters which are chemically similar. It is well established that hydrolysis is necessary for cholesterol absorption from the esterified form (Vahouny and Treadwell, 1964).

Erlanson and Borgström (1968) have shown that hydrolysis of vitamin A esters by rat pancreatic juice is brought about by pancreatic carboxyl ester hydrolase acting on the bile salt micellar solubilized form of the ester and that the ester in an emulsion is split by lipase. Pancreatic juice also appears to have hydrolytic activity towards vitamin D esters (Bell and Bryan, 1969) and vitamin E esters are probably also hydrolyzed by pancreatic enzymes prior to absorption (Gallo-Torres, 1970). Pancreatic carboxyl ester hydrolase appears to be responsible for hydrolysis of esters of α-tocopherol in man (Muller *et al.*, 1975) and this enzyme provides the principal hydrolytic activity towards the fatty acid esters of the vitamin in the gut lumen. The enzyme is strongly dependent on bile salts for its activity. Thus, in addition to solubilizing the vitamin esters, bile salts function as cofactor for the enzyme which releases the free vitamins.

C. Mucosal Metabolism during Absorption

Within the mucosal epithelium some metabolism of the vitamins takes place. Beta-carotene is cleaved by 15-15′ dioxygenase yielding retinal which is readily reduced to retinol. Esterification of retinol particularly with palmitic acid is extensive both in man and animals (Olson, 1969). On the other hand, esterification of vitamin D in the mucosa appears to be only slight (Blomstrand and Forsgren, 1967). In humans and rats, α-tocopherol does not appear to be esterified to any extent in its transit through the mucosa (Johnson and Pover, 1962; Blomstrand and Forsgren, 1968b) and studies in man show that vitamin K_1 is not chemically altered during its absorption from the gut lumen into lymph (Blomstrand and Forsgren, 1968a).

D. Route and Form of Transport from the Intestine

Following absorption by the intestinal mucosa, the fat-soluble vitamins are transported from the small intestine in lymph. Experiments in both man and animals indicate that this is the principal route of transport and that the vitamins and their esters are mainly found as components of the chylomicra. Small amounts of the vitamins may be transported in the portal vein; for example MacMahon *et al.* (1971) obtained evidence suggesting that even under normal conditions a proportion of absorbed α-tocopherol may be transported in the portal vein in the rat. In the case of more polar derivatives of the vitamins, such as retinoic acid, the lymphatics play a minor part in transport and such substances are probably carried by the portal vein. While vitamin K_1 is transported in lymph in chylomicra, it is possible that the synthetic vitamin K_3 (Menadione) which has some water solubility may be partly transported by the portal vein

(Mezick *et al.*, 1968). The form of transport in lymph appears to be determined by the concurrent absorption of other lipids. Thus, when α-tocopherol is introduced into the duodenum of rats in a bile salt micellar solution together with exogenous lipids, it is transported in the lymph as a component of chylomicra. When the vitamin is given in pure bile salt micelles, however, a much smaller proportion is transported in chylomicra, the remainder probably being carried on very low-density lipoproteins (MacMahon *et al.*, 1971). In man, in the absence of bile in the gut, the absorption of all fat-soluble vitamins is greatly reduced (Forsgren, 1969); the portal vein may play some part in the transport of the vitamins when bile is absent from the gastrointestinal tract (Gagnon and Dawson, 1968).

III. DRUGS AFFECTING FAT-SOLUBLE VITAMIN ABSORPTION

A. Bile Salt Sequestrants

These drugs have been developed primarily as hypocholesterolemic agents in an attempt to reduce morbidity and mortality from arteriosclerotic disease. Several agents are now available which bind bile salts in the intestinal lumen, thus increasing their fecal excretion, and since bile salts are the major metabolic end-product of cholesterol metabolism, this results in a drain on body cholesterol and reduces serum cholesterol. Also, bile salt micellar solubilization is an important step in cholesterol absorption and this may also be impaired by bile salt sequestrants. Since hypocholesterolemic drugs must be given over a long period it is especially important to consider the possibility of a minor impairment of nutrient absorption since this could have a cumulative effect.

In addition to reducing serum cholesterol, bile salt sequestrants have proved useful in the management of diseases in which bile salts play an important part, such as the cholerrheic enteropathy of ileal resection and states of impaired bile salt secretion such as primary biliary cirrhosis and partial biliary obstruction.

These agents are nonabsorbable substances which bind bile salts and other anions either by ion exchange effect or by hydrophobic bonding. The ion exchange group includes cholestyramine, diethylaminoethyl dextran derivatives, and colestipol. Certain aminoglycoside antibiotics, notably neomycin, seem to bind and precipitate bile salts by ionic interaction. Lignins bind bile salts by an hydrophobic interaction.

1. Cholestyramine

Of the bile salt sequestrants, the most commonly used is cholestyramine. It is a strongly basic anion exchange resin containing quaternary ammonium functional groups attached to a styrene–divinyl benzene copolymer. Its bile salt binding properties could be expected to disrupt the micellar phase in the small intestine and alter sterol and fat-soluble vitamin solubilization and absorption. Johns and Bates (1970), in a study of the binding of bile salts and fatty acids to cholestyramine, have shown that its affinity for bile salts increases as the number of hydroxyl groups in the bile salt molecule falls and its affinity for fatty acids increases with increasing chain length, but decreases as the degree of unsaturation of the hydrocarbon chain rises. The binding is primarily electrostatic but a nonelectrostatic interaction related to the hydrophobicity of the molecules also operates.

In both rats (Harkins *et al.*, 1965) and man (Hashim *et al.* (1961) cholestyramine in sufficient doses causes steatorrhea. A number of animal studies indicate that cholestyramine feeding will impair fat-soluble vitamin absorption. Addition to a high fat diet, containing vitamin A in growth-limiting amounts, of 2% cholestyramine, a dose comparable to human doses, reduced body weight gain in weanling rats (Whiteside *et al.*, 1965). When larger doses of vitamin A were given, the failure of weight gain was prevented but liver storage of vitamin A was reduced. If the dietary vitamin A was in ester form, that is, vitamin A palmitate rather than the free alcohol, the effect of cholestyramine on liver storage was greater. This may reflect the importance of bile salt solubilization of esterified vitamin A for hydrolysis by pancreatic carboxylic ester hydrolase. In birds kept on marginally low vitamin K diets, 2% cholestyramine in the diet also reduced vitamin K stores in chicks and prolonged the prothrombin time, but in doses comparable with those used therapeutically no malabsorption of vitamin K_1 occurs in dogs (Robinson *et al.*, 1964). The addition of 4% cholestyramine to rat diets causes vitamin D malabsorption (Thompson and Thompson, 1969). Davies *et al.* (1972) have shown that α-tocopherol absorption in rats is more severely impaired by cholestyramine if the vitamin is fed with a long-chain rather than a medium-chain triglyceride diet. The explanation for this observation is not clear.

In human use it is commonly recommended that patients taking cholestyramine over any appreciable time should have supplements of fat-soluble vitamins. There is a little evidence that high doses of cholestyramine can cause deficiency of these vitamins but in clinical practice the problem is uncommon. While 8 gm of cholestyramine fed with a test meal containing 250,000 U.S.P. units of vitamin A acetate reduced plasma vitamin A levels, 4 gm of the drug had no significant effect (Longenecker and Basu, 1965). In fourteen healthy volunteers, the addition of 12 gm cholestyramine to a vitamin A-containing test meal reduced the expected rise in serum vitamin A by 59.5% (Barnard and Heaton, 1973).

After 4 months of 15 gm cholestyramine daily as treatment of a patient with xanthomatous biliary cirrhosis, Visintine *et al.* (1961) noted that the prothrombin time had fallen to 19% of normal, implying malabsorption of vitamin K. A similar effect was observed in treating a patient with xanthomatosis with 20 gm cholestyramine a day (Roe, 1968). Osteomalacia has been reported in a patient with terminal ileal bypass treated over 2 years with cholestyramine (Heaton *et al.*, 1972) and hypoprothrombinemia and hemorrhage occurred in a patient with postirradiation enterocolitis after 3 weeks of treatment with the drug (Gross and Brotman, 1970). These reports suggest malabsorption of vitamins D and K occasioned by cholestyramine, but it should be emphasized that in the latter two cases these deficiencies occurred in patients with impaired absorptive function particularly involving the distal ileum and both probably had compromised enterohepatic circulation of bile salts which would be aggravated by cholestyramine. Since cholestyramine is used to bind bile salts in postileectomy diarrhea, such deficiencies are always possible.

While the pruritus of primary biliary cirrhosis, considered to be due to an increased concentration of bile salts in the systemic circulation responds to cholestyramine treatment, an intraluminal deficiency of bile salts is held to be responsible for malabsorption of fat-soluble vitamins in these patients. Clearly cholestyramine could aggravate this problem.

With the exception of these isolated reports, vitamin deficiency with cholestyramine treatment is not common. In children with type II hyperlipoproteinemia treated over 10 months with 12 gm cholestyramine daily, neither vitamin A or E levels in plasma were reduced below supranormal or normal values despite reduction in serum low density lipoprotein (Glueck *et al.*, 1974), though West and Lloyd (1975) observed a significant decrease in serum concentrations of vitamins A and E over 2 years in a similar study. In adults with type II hyperlipoproteinaemia no evidence of malabsorption of vitamins A, D, E or K was obtained during an 18-week period of treatment with up to 20g cholestyramine per day. (Schade *et al.*, 1976).

2. DEAE Sephadex

Several anion exchangers, derivatives of cellulose and dextran, will bind bile salts *in vitro*. Parkinson (1967) has shown that diethylaminoethyl (DEAE)-cellulose and -Sephadex and guanidoethyl-cellulose will reduce experimental hypercholesterolemia in cockerels. DEAE–Sephadex lowers serum cholesterol in normal and hypercholesterolemic dogs and increases excretion of bile salts in the feces. When fed to pregnant rats, DEAE–Sephadex reduced the concentration of vitamin A in the liver of mothers and offspring by about 30% and had a similar effect in male weanling rats (Cecil et al., 1973).

Studies in man have suggested that DEAE–Sephadex (Secholex), that is poly(2-diethylamino)ethyl polyglycerylene dextran hydrochloride, might be a suitable agent for lowering serum cholesterol in hypercholesterolemia (Howard and Hyams, 1971; Courtenay Evans et al., 1973; Howard and Courtenay Evans, 1974; Gustafson and Lanner, 1974; Ritland et al., 1975). None of these studies indicates any interference with fat-soluble vitamin absorption, though Gustafson and Lanner (1974) did find a significant rise in the serum alkaline phosphatase in patients on the drug. Ritland et al. (1975) treating patients with hypercholesterolemia over 18 months found no change in serum vitamin A or vitamin K-dependent clotting factors. An interesting observation was that during treatment with DEAE–Sephadex, bile salt concentrations in test meals in duodenal aspirates rose. No explanation of this can be given at present but it is clear that this increase would offset the tendency of the ion exchanger to deplete bile salts in solution in the intestinal content.

As with cholestyramine, the effect of DEAE-Sephadex on lipid solubilization, digestion, and absorption is complex. Borgström (1970) has shown that DEAE–Sephadex increases the proportion of monoglyceride in a glyceride mixture formed by the action of pancreatic lipase on long-chain triglyceride in vitro in addition to binding bile salts. This is probably to be explained by a sequestration of fatty acids causing an alteration in the enzyme-catalyzed equilibrium. Thus this ion exchange resin alters the composition of the micellar phase in addition to reducing bile salt concentration.

3. Colestipol

Colestipol is a more recently introduced bile salt sequestrant. It is a high molecular weight copolymer of tetraethylene pentamine and epichlorohydrin with one of the five amine nitrogens as the chloride salt. Its affinity in vitro for bile salts is about two-thirds that of cholestyramine. Ko and Royer (1974) in an in vitro study of drug binding to colestipol have obtained results suggesting that colestipol reduces the concentration of vitamin A in a taurocholate micellar solution by binding a proportion of the bile salt and by binding some of the vitamin itself, presumably by a nonionic association. Some of the vitamin is probably also precipitated and is not associated with the polymer. There are few reports of deficiency of fat-soluble vitamins resulting from colestipol treatment. Dogs given doses equivalent to 10 times the human therapeutic dose over 1 year developed no physical signs of biochemical derangements suggesting fat-soluble vitamin deficiency (Parkinson *et al.*, 1973) nor did weanling rats fed 2000 mg colestipol per kg per day for 18 months (Webster, cited by Parkinson *et al.*, 1973). In healthy male subjects taking 12–15 gm colestipol hydrochloride daily for more than 3 years, Gundersen (cited by Parkinson *et al.*, 1973) found no prothrombin deficiency or other signs of fat-soluble vitamin deficiency; Glueck *et al.* (1972) studying twenty-five patients with familial type II hyperlipoproteinemia taking 20 gm colestipol daily over 4 months found prothrombin times were not significantly prolonged. However in eight patients with hypercholesterolemia given colestipol for 4–6 months, Miller *et al.* (1973) noted small but significant changes in serum calcium and alkaline phosphatase and, in one of the patients, a prolongation of the prothrombin time.

4. *Neomycin*

While the other drugs discussed in this section were designed as bile acid sequestrants, this property of neomycin is to be regarded as an unwanted effect of the drug. Neomycin is a polybasic nonabsorbable antibiotic of the aminoglycoside group which exerts complex effects on gastrointestinal function. In large doses (12 gm/day) in man it causes malabsorption with steatorrhea but in small doses (for example, 2 gm/day) it reduces plasma cholesterol without producing steatorrhea. Serum carotene and vitamin A levels are reduced by neomycin therapy (Levine, 1967) and prothrombin time is increased (Udall, 1965) suggesting malabsorption of vitamin K. However, in the latter instance, the role of neomycin in altering intestinal bacterial flora, thus affecting endogenous vitamin K production, may be important as well as its action on lipid solubilization in the upper small intestine.

It is postulated that some of the effects of neomycin on absorption are due to mucosal damage in the small intestine (see below). However, it is apparent that this drug is able to precipitate fatty acids and to a lesser extent bile acids from mixed bile salt–lipid micelles and thus, by disrupting the micellar phase in the small intestine, reduces the ability of nonpolar solutes such as cholesterol to stay in solution (Thompson *et al.*, 1970). When mixed sodium taurocholate–oleic acid micelles containing α-tocopherol were exposed to a variety of bile salt binding agents *in vitro* at pH 6.3 and 8.5, it was found that at concentrations of 1 mg/ml of these agents the order of efficacy in precipitating the vitamin from the micelles was neomycin, cholestyramine, lignin, and DEAE-Sephadex (P. M. Mathias, P. R. Muller, and J. A. Barrowman, unpublished results, 1976). This observation probably reflects the pronounced ability of neomycin to precipitate fatty acids, thus reducing the capacity of micelles to solubilize such nonpolar solutes. This disruption with precipitation of nonpolar solutes such as cholesterol has been proposed as the mechanism of hypocholesterolemia and steatorrhea found with neomycin treatment (Thompson *et al.*, 1971) since this drug greatly increases the percentage of bile acids and fatty acids in the precipitate in intestinal content. (Fig. 1). This explanation however has been questioned by Sedaghat *et al.* (1975) who have not been able to demonstrate increased fecal excretion of acidic steroids in patients taking 2 gm of neomycin per day. Nevertheless, the ability of neomycin to disrupt bile salt–lipid micelles in the upper small intestine remains one probable mechanism for impairment of cholesterol absorption and it may also explain impair-

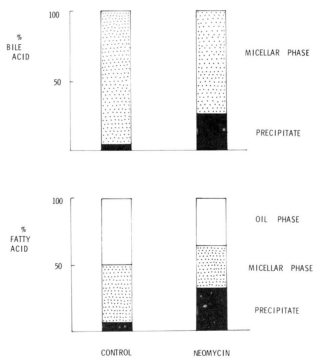

Fig. 1. Effect of neomycin on the percentage distribution of bile acid and fatty acid in ultracentrifuged intestinal contents. Results represent the means of five healthy subjects. (Courtesy of *Journal of Clinical Investigation.*)

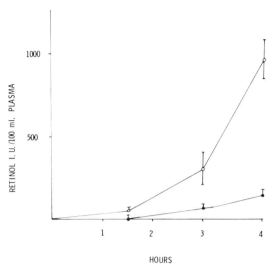

Fig. 2. Changes in plasma concentration of retinol (IU/100 ml) above fasting levels after 300,000 IU retinyl palmitate were given orally with either placebo (lactose) (-O-O-) or neomycin (-●-●-). Each point represents the mean ± SEM obtained from five subjects. (Courtesy of *European Journal of Clinical Pharmacology.*)

ment of retinol absorption (Fig. 2) (Barrowman *et al.*, 1973). The related antibiotic, kanamycin, which can cause a modest increase in fecal fat also binds bile acids *in vitro* though its affinity for bile acids is lower than neomycin (Faloon *et al.*, 1966).

5. Lignin

Lignin, an amorphous phenylpropane polymer present in many plant foods, binds bile acids probably by a hydrophobic interaction. Methylation of its phenolic hydroxyl groups enhances this binding capacity. Theoretically lignin could reduce fat-soluble vitamin absorption both by disruption of the micellar phase and by hydrophobic interaction with the vitamins themselves. There is little information on this subject but Barnard and Heaton (1973) found that large doses of lignin had no effect on the rise of serum vitamin A after an oral load.

6. Other Bile Salt Precipitants

With the explosion of information about the physiological function of bile salts in the past 10 or 15 years has come recognition that several different drugs may interact with them in the gut lumen. Old observations such as the interference with vitamin A absorption by aluminium antacids (Hoffman and Dyniewicz, 1945) may be explicable by such interactions since recent studies have indicated that aluminium hydroxide is an effective precipitant of bile salts (Clain *et al.*, 1976).

B. Mineral Oil

It has long been suggested that mineral oils, which are given as lubricants and stool softeners, impair fat-soluble vitamin absorption (Curtis and Kline, 1939; Curtis and Ballmer, 1939, Javert and Macri, 1941; Morgan, 1941). This idea has been faithfully preserved over the years but there is little proof that this is an important disadvantage of these preparations. The mechanism for such impairment of absorption is thought to be that the vitamins dissolve in an indigestible nonabsorbable lipid phase in the gut lumen and thus are excreted in this oil. For this process to be important the oil would need to be fed with the meals in quantities sufficient to dissolve the major amount of the dietary supply of the vitamins. This probably explains why 30 ml of mineral oil fed to human subjects daily at bedtime for 51 days failed to cause any abnormal decrease in plasma vitamin A levels (Mahle and Patton, 1947).

C. Drugs Affecting Small Intestinal Mucosal Morphology and Metabolism

Certain drugs, notably neomycin and colchicine, produce histological and biochemical changes in the mucosa which at least partly explain the malabsorption of fat and fat-soluble substances seen with these drugs. Triparanol, a drug once used as a hypocholesterolemic agent, but now withdrawn on account of its serious unwanted effects, also has this property (McPherson and Shorter, 1965).

In man, but not in rats, neomycin causes shortening of intestinal villi with infiltration of the lamina propria with inflammatory cells and pigment-containing macrophages (Dobbins *et al.*, 1968). Electron microscopy shows ballooning of the microvilli of the enterocytes and evidence of injury to crypt cells such as distortion of mitochondria and endoplasmic reticulum. The macrophages appear to contain material in lysosomal structures which is probably derived from cell breakdown products resulting from neomycin toxicity. These histologic changes are reversible as is a reduction of mucosal disaccharidase activity.

Steatorrhea and reduced serum carotene concentration have been found with oral colchicine treatment (Race *et al.*, 1970). Reversible depression of mucosal sucrase, lactase, and maltase activity occurs and variable mild histological abnormalities are seen, including mucosal edema and round cell infiltration of the lamina propria. At higher doses, the drug arrests division of the crypt cells which leads to villus atrophy.

D. Other Drugs Which Cause Steatorrhea

Steatorrhea and presumably some impairment of absorption of fat-soluble vitamins very occasionally follow the use of a number of unrelated drugs. These include calcium carbonate (Kramer, 1967) p-aminosalicylic acid (Levine, 1968), phenindione (Juel-Jensen, 1959), phenolphthalein (French *et al.*, 1956) and mefenamic acid (Marks and Gleeson, 1975). Among the antibiotics, a mixture of polymixin and bacitracin has been reported to increase fecal excretion of fat in man (Powell *et al.*, 1962) and in rats malabsorption of fat has been observed with tetracycline treatment; this treatment causes no morphological changes in the intestinal mucosa (Yeh and Shils, 1966). The mechanism by which most of the above drugs impair fat absorption is not clear. A moderate degree of steatorrhea is frequently found in chronic alcoholism.

IV. MISCELLANEOUS EFFECTS OF DRUGS ON FAT-SOLUBLE VITAMIN ABSORPTION

Of the fat-soluble vitamins, vitamin K is unique in that a proportion of the daily requirement is met by an endogenous supply from intestinal bacterial synthesis (Frick *et al.*, 1967). Thus chronic treatment with nonabsorbable antibiotics such as neomycin in liver disease may affect this endogenous source. It is interesting that vitamin A appears to inhibit vitamin K synthesis in the gut and this, together with an antagonism of vitamin K in prothrombin synthesis in the liver can lead to hypoprothrombinemia (Green, 1966).

In view of the importance of bile salts in the absorption of the vitamins it is not surprising that vitamin K deficiency increasing the hypoprothrombinemia produced by coumarin anticoagulants has been observed in phenothiazine-induced cholestasis (Vesell, 1972). It is important to recognize that the onset of manifestations of deficiencies of the various vitamins will reflect body stores, thus vitamin K malabsorption is most readily detected on account of the small body stores of this vitamin.

Can drugs enhance the absorption of fat-soluble vitamins? Clearly, successful drug treatment of steatorrhea, for example tetracyclines for blind-loop syndrome or quinacrine for *Giardia lamblia* infection will improve absorption of fat-soluble substances. It has been observed that

Tween 80, polyoxyethylene sorbitan mono-oleate, a nonionic surfactant, will reverse cholestyramine-induced fat malabsorption in rats (Du Bois *et al.*, 1964); in a variety of forms of human malabsorption this same compound greatly improves fat and vitamin A absorption (Jones *et al.*, 1948). It is argued that improved fat emulsification in situations of bile salt depletion is the mechanism of action of the compound, though there is little supporting evidence for this hypothesis.

V. RESEARCH NEEDS

Further clarification of the physiological processes involved in the absorption of the fat-soluble vitamins is needed. Until the behavior of the vitamins in intestinal content is fully understood, the nature of drug interaction with the process will be a matter of speculation only. The steps in transfer of the vitamins through the mucosal cell await further study particularly with reference to the influence, if any, of bile salts on mucosal metabolism and transcellular transport of the vitamins. Although existing hypocholesterolemic agents do not seem to cause deficiency of fat-soluble vitamins with any great frequency, the quest for newer and more effective agents of this type may produce drugs with this unwanted effect and such drugs need to be carefully screened to exclude this possibility. It may be that a number of other drugs are able to precipitate bile acids including certain antacids and there is need to study their effect on fat-soluble vitamin absorption. To screen drugs for such effects, practical and sensitive procedures are required to assess the fat-soluble vitamin status of patients, as many of the presently available methods are indirect or crude.

VI. CONCLUSION

Malabsorption of fat-soluble vitamins is a relatively uncommon unwanted effect of drug treatment. Bile salts play a key role in the assimilation of these vitamins and at present the only agents likely to interfere in an important way with this process are the bile salt sequestrants.

REFERENCES

Barnard, D. L., and Heaton, K. W. (1973). Bile acids and vitamin A absorption in man: The effects of two bile acid binding agents, cholestyramine and lignin. *Gut* **14,** 316–318.

Barrowman, J., D'Mello, A., and Herxheimer, A. (1973). A single dose of neomycin impairs absorption of vitamin A (retinol) in man. *Eur. J. Clin. Pharmacol.* **5**, 199–202.

Bell, N. H., and Bryan, P. (1969). Absorption of vitamin D₃ oleate in the rat. *Am. J. Clin. Nutr.* **22**, 425–430.

Blomstrand, R., and Forsgren, L. (1967). Intestinal absorption and esterification of vitamin D_3-1, 2-³H in man. *Acta Chem. Scand.* **21**, 1662–1663.

Blomstrand, R., and Forsgren, L. (1968a). Vitamin K_1 - ³H in man. Its intestinal absorption and transport in the thoracic duct lymph. *Int. Z. Vitaminforsch.* **38**, 45–64.

Blomstrand, R., and Forsgren, L. (1968b). Labelled tocopherols in man. Intestinal absorption and thoracic duct lymph transport of *dl*-alpha-tocopheryl-3,4-¹⁴C₂ acetate, *dl*-alpha-tocopheramine-3,4-¹⁴C₂, *dl*-alpha-tocopherol-(5 methyl-³H) and *N*-(methyl-³H)-*dl*-gamma tocopheramine. *Int. Z. Vitaminforsch.* **38**, 328–344.

Borgström, B. (1968). Partition of lipids between emulsified oil and micellar phases of glyceride-bile salt dispersions. *J. Lipid Res.* **8**, 598–608.

Borgström, B. (1970). Effect of ion-exchange substances on the lipolysis catalysed by pancreatic lipase. *Scand. J. Gastroenterol.* **5**, 549–553.

Borgström, B. (1974). Bile salts—their physiological functions in the gastrointestinal tract. *Acta Med. Scand.* **196**, 1–10.

Cecil, H. C., Harris, S. J., Bitman, J., and Dryden, L. P. (1973). Effect of DEAE–Sephadex on liver vitamin A of lactating rats and their offspring. *J. Nutr.* **103**, 43–48.

Clain, J., Malagelada, J. R., Chadwick, V., and Hofmann, A. F. (1976). Bile acid binding properties of antacids: An in *vitro* study. *Gastroenterology* **70**, A-13.

Courtenay Evans, R. J., Howard, A. N., and Hyams, D. E. (1973). An effective treatment of hypercholesterolaemia using a combination of Secholex and clofibrate. *Angiology* **24**, 22–28.

Curtis, A. C., and Ballmer, R. S. (1939). The prevention of carotene absorption by liquid petrolatum. *J. Am. Med. Assoc.* **113**, 1785–1788.

Curtis, A. C., and Klinc, E. M. (1939). Influence of liquid petrolatum on blood content of carotene in human beings. *Arch. Intern. Med.* **63**, 54–63.

Davies, T., Kelleher, J., Smith, C. L., Walker, B. E., and Losowsky, M. S. (1972). Effect of therapeutic measures which alter fat absorption on the absorption of alpha-tocopherol in the rat. *J. Lab. Clin. Med.* **79**, 824–831.

Dobbins, W. O., Herrero, B. A., and Mansbach, C. M. (1968). Morphologic alterations associated with neomycin-induced malabsorption. *Am. J. Med. Sci.* **255**, 63–77.

Du Bois, J. J., Holt, P. R., Kuron, G. W., Hashim, S. A., and Van Itallie, T. B. (1964). Effect of Tween 80 on cholestyramine-induced malabsorption. *Proc. Soc. Exp. Biol. Med.* **117**, 226–229.

Erlanson, C., and Borgström, B. (1968). The identity of vitamin A esterase activity of rat pancreatic juice. *Biochim. Biophys. Acta* **141**, 629–631.

Faloon, W. W., Paes, I. C., Woolfolk, D., Nankin, H., Wallace, K., and Haro, E. N. (1966). Effect of neomycin and kanamycin upon intestinal absorption. *Ann. N.Y. Acad. Sci.* **132**, 879–887.

Forsgren, L. (1969). Studies on the intestinal absorption of labelled fat-soluble vitamins (A,D,E and K) via the thoracic duct lymph in the absence of bile in man. *Acta Chir. Scand., Suppl.* **399**.

French, J. M., Gaddie, R., and Smith, N. (1956). Diarrhoea due to phenolphthalein. *Lancet* **1**, 551–553.

Frick, P. G., Riedler, G., and Brögli, H. (1967). Dose response and minimal daily requirement for vitamin K in man. *J. Appl. Physiol.* **23**, 387–389.

Gagnon, M., and Dawson, A. M. (1968). The effect of bile on vitamin A absorption in the rat. *Proc. Soc. Exp. Biol. Med.* **127**, 99–102.

Gallo-Torres, H. (1970). Obligatory role of bile for the intestinal absorption of vitamin E. *Lipids* **5**, 379–384.

Glueck, C. J., Ford, S., Scheel, D., and Steiner, P. (1972). Colestipol and cholestyramine resin. Comparative effects in familial type II hyperlipoproteinemia. *J. Am. Med. Assoc.* **222**, 676–681.

Glueck, C. J., Tsang, R. C., Fallat, R. W., and Scheel, B. A. (1974). Plasma vitamin A and E levels in children with familial type II hyperlipoproteinaemia during therapy with diet and cholestyramine resin. *Pediatrics* **54**, 51–55.

Green, J. (1966). Antagonists of vitamin K. *Vitam. Horm. (N.Y.)* **24**, 619–631.

Gross, L., and Brotman, M. (1970). Hypoprothrombinemia and hemorrhage associated with cholestyramine therapy. *Ann. Intern. Med.* **72**, 95–96.

Gustafson, A., and Lanner, A. (1974). Treatment of hyperlipoproteinaemia type II A with a new ion exchange resin Secholex. *Eur. J. Clin. Pharmacol.* **7**, 65–69.

Harkins, R. W., Hagerman, L. M., and Sarett, H. P. (1965). Absorption of dietary fats by the rat in cholestyramine-induced steatorrhea. *J. Nutr.* **87**, 85–92.

Hashim, S. A., Bergen, S. S., and Van Itallie, T. B. (1961). Experimental steatorrhea induced in man by bile acid sequestrant. *Proc. Soc. Exp. Biol. Med.* **106**, 173–175.

Heaton, K. W., Lever, J. V., and Barnard, D. (1972). Osteomalacia associated with cholestyramine therapy for postileectomy diarrhea. *Gastroenterology* **62**, 642–646.

Hoffman, W. S., and Dyniewicz, H. A. (1945). The effect of alumina gel upon the absorption of vitamin A from the intestinal tract. *Gastroenterology* **5**, 512–522.

Howard, A. N., and Courtenay Evans, R. J. (1974). Secholex [R], clofibrate and taurine in hyperlipidaemia. *Atherosclerosis* **20**, 105–116.

Howard, A. N., and Hyams, D. E. (1971). Combined use of clofibrate and cholestyramine or DEAE-Sephadex in hypercholesterolaemia. *Br. Med. J.* **3**, 25–27.

Javert, C. J., and Macri, C. (1941). Prothrombin concentration and mineral oil. *Am. J. Obstet. Gynecol.* **42**, 409–414.

Johns, W. H., and Bates, T. R. (1970). Quantification of the binding tendencies of cholestyramine. II. Mechanism of interaction with bile salt and fatty acid salt anions. *J. Pharm. Sci.* **59**, 329–333.

Johnson, P., and Pover, W. F. R. (1962). Intestinal absorption of alpha-tocopherol. *Life Sci.* **1**, 115–117.

Jones, C. M., Culver, P. J., Drummey, G. D., and Ryan, A. E. (1948). Modification of fat absorption in the digestive tract by the use of an emulsifying agent. *Ann. Intern. Med.* **29**, 1–10.

Juel-Jensen, B. E. (1959). Sensitivity to phenindione. Report of a case of severe diarrhoea. *Br. Med. J.* **2**, 173–174.

Ko, H., and Royer, M. E. (1974). *In vitro* binding of drugs to colestipol hydrochloride. *J. Pharm. Sci.* **63**, 1914–1920.

Kramer, P. (1967). The effect of antimotility and antidiarrheal drugs on the ileal excreta of human ileostomized subjects. *Gastroenterology* **52**, 1102.

Levine, R. A. (1967). Effect of dietary gluten upon neomycin-induced malabsorption. *Gastroenterology* **52**, 685–690.

Levine, R. A. (1968). Steatorrhoea induced by para-aminosalicylic acid. *Ann. Intern. Med.* **68**, 1265–1270.

Longenecker, J. B., and Basu, S. G. (1965). Effect of cholestyramine on absorption of amino acids and vitamin A in man. *Fed. Proc., Fed. Am. Soc. Exp. Biol.* **24**, 375.

MacMahon, M. T., and Thompson, G. R. (1970). Comparison of the absorption of a polar lipid, oleic acid and a nonpolar lipid, alpha-tocopherol from mixed micellar solutions and emulsions. *Eur. J. Clin. Invest.* **1**, 161–166.

MacMahon, M. T., Neale, G., and Thompson, G. R. (1971). Lymphatic and portal venous transport of alpha-tocopherol and cholesterol. *Eur. J. Clin. Invest.* **1,** 288–294.

McPherson, J. R., and Shorter, R. G. (1965). Intestinal lesions associated with triparanol. A clinical and experimental study. *Am. J. Dig. Dis.* **10,** 1024–1033.

Mahadevan, S., Seshadri Sastry, P., and Ganguly, J. (1963). Studies on metabolism of vitamin A. 3. The mode of absorption of vitamin A esters in the living rat. *Biochem. J.* **88,** 531–534.

Mahle, A. E., and Patton, H. M. (1947). Carotene and vitamin A metabolism in man: Their excretion and plasma level as influenced by orally administered mineral oil and a hydrophilic mucilloid. *Gastroenterology* **9,** 44–53.

Marks, J. S., and Gleeson, M. H. (1975). Steatorrhoea complicating therapy with mefenamic acid. *Br. Med. J.* **4,** 442.

Mezick, J. A., Tompkins, R. K., and Cornwell, D. G. (1968). Absorption and intestinal lymphatic transport of ^{14}C-menadione. *Life Sci.* **7,** 153–158.

Miller, N. E., Clifton-Bligh, P., Nestel, P. J., and Whyte, H. M. (1973). Controlled clinical trial of a new bile acid sequestering resin, colestipol, in the treatment of hypercholesterolaemia. *Med. J. Aust.* **1,** 1223–1227.

Morgan, J. W. (1941). The harmful effects of mineral oil (liquid petrolatum) purgatives. *J. Am. Med. Assoc.* **117,** 1335–1336.

Muller, D. P. R., Manning, J. A., Mathias, P. M., and Harries, J. T. (1975). The role of bile salts in the hydrolysis and absorption of vitamin E esters. *Clin. Sci. Mol. Med.* **48,** 17p.

Olson, J. A. (1969). Metabolism and function of vitamin A. *Fed. Proc., Fed. Am. Soc. Exp. Biol.* **28,** 1670–1677.

Parkinson, T. M. (1967). Hypolipidemic effects of orally administered dextran and cellulose anion exchangers in cockerels and dogs. *J. Lipid Res.* **8,** 24–29.

Parkinson, T. M., Schneider, J. C., and Phillips, W. A. (1973). Effects of colestipol hydrochloride (U-26, 597 A) on serum and fecal lipids in dogs. *Atherosclerosis* **17,** 167–179.

Powell, R. C., Nunes, W. T., Harding, R. S., and Vacca, J. B. (1962). The influence of nonabsorbable antibiotics on serum lipids and the excretion of neutral sterols and bile acids. *Am. J. Clin. Nutr.* **11,** 156–168.

Race, T. F., Paes, I. C., and Faloon, W. W. (1970). Intestinal malabsorption induced by oral colchicine. Comparison with neomycin and cathartic agents. *Am. J. Med. Sci.* **259,** 32–41.

Ritland, S., Fausa, O., Gjone, E., Blomhoff, J. P., Skrede, S., and Lanner, A. (1975). Effect of treatment with a bile-sequestering agent (Secholex[R]) on intestinal absorption, duodenal bile acids and plasma lipids. *Scand. J. Gastroenterol.* **10,** 791–800.

Robinson, M. J., Kelley, K. L., and Lehman, E. G. (1964). Effect of cholestyramine, a bile acid binding polymer on vitamin K absorption in dogs. *Proc. Soc. Exp. Biol. Med.* **115,** 112–115.

Roe, D. A. (1968). Essential hyperlipemia with xanthomatosis. *Arch. Dermatol.* **97,** 436–445.

Schade, R. W. B., van't Laar, A., Majoor, C. L. H., and Jansen, A. P. (1976). A comparative study of the effects of cholestyramine and neomycin in the treatment of type II hyperlipoproteinaemia. *Acta Med. Scand.* **199,** 175–180.

Sedaghat, A., Samuel, P., Crouse, J. R., and Ahrens, E. H. (1975). Effects of neomycin on absorption, synthesis and/or flux of cholesterol in man. *J. Clin. Invest.* **55,** 12–21.

Thompson, G. R., MacMahon, M., and Claes, P. (1970). Precipitation by neomycin compounds of fatty acid and cholesterol from mixed micellar solutions. *Eur. J. Clin. Invest.* **1,** 40–47.

Thompson, G. R., Barrowman, J., Gutierrez, L., and Dowling, R. H. (1971). Action of neomycin on the intraluminal phase of lipid absorption. *J. Clin. Invest.* **50**, 319-323.

Thompson, W. G., and Thompson, G. R. (1969). Effect of cholestyramine on the absorption of vitamin D$_3$ and calcium. *Gut* **10**, 717-722.

Udall, J. A. (1965). Human sources and absorption of vitamin K in relation to anticoagulation stability. *J. Am. Med. Assoc.* **194**, 127-129.

Vahouny, G. V., and Treadwell, C. R. (1964). Absolute requirement for free sterol for absorption by rat intestinal mucosa. *Proc. Soc. Exp. Biol. Med.* **116**, 496-498.

Vesell, E. S. (1972). Individual variations in drug response. *In* "Liver and Drugs" (F. Orlandi and A. M. Jezequel, eds.), pp. 1-40. Academic Press, New York.

Visintine, R. E., Michaels, G. D., Fukayama, G., Conklin, J., and Kinsell, L. W. (1961). Xanthomatous biliary cirrhosis treated with cholestyramine. *Lancet* **2**, 341-343.

West, R. J., and Lloyd, J. K. (1975). The effect of cholestyramine on intestinal absorption. *Gut* **16**, 93-98.

Whiteside, C. H., Harkins, R. W., Fluckiger, H. B., and Sarett, H. P. (1965). Utilization of fat-soluble vitamins by rats and chicks fed cholestyramine a bile acid sequestrant. *Am. J. Clin. Nutr.* **16**, 309-314.

Wilson, F. A., Sallee, V. L., and Dietschy, J. M. (1971). Unstirred water layers in intestine: Rate determinant of fatty acid absorption from micellar solutions. *Science* **174**, 1031-1033.

Yeh, S. D., and Shils, M. E. (1966). Effect of tetracycline on intestinal absorption of various nutrients by the rat. *Proc. Soc. Exp. Biol. Med.* **123**, 367-370.

5

Drugs and Environmental Chemicals in Relation to Vitamin Needs

MYRON BRIN

I. INTRODUCTION

If measurable effects on nutrient metabolism and/or needs can occur as a consequence of drug intake (or of environmental chemical exposure), we would expect that either clinical signs of disease or a marginal deficiency state might result. In fact, both situations occur as will be subsequently elaborated upon. Alternatively, the nutrient adequacy of a

131

person will be even more greatly stressed in individuals with marginal deficiency states than in those who are well-nourished. Accordingly, it would be well that we also recognize that condition and take corrective steps. We propose, therefore, to define the state of marginal deficiency, how extensive this condition is in the United States population, and how this relates to drug and/or chemical exposure.

II. HUMAN FINDINGS IN MARGINAL DEFICIENCY STATES

A. Methods for the Assay of Nutritional Status

The four modes for evaluating nutritional status are (1) demographic, (2) dietary history, (3) physical examination, and (4) laboratory assessment. The "demographic" mode permits presumptions about the nutritional status of a population which are based upon previous experience concerning the dietary consequences of socioeconomic status, ethnicity, and climate in a target population group. These guidelines are general and cannot usually be applied to an individual, per se, but rather to a community. Therefore, this information is often useful for public health purposes.

The second mode, "dietary history", can be applied to both the family as well as to the individual, depending upon the data collected. The "market basket surveys" (U.S. Department of Agriculture, 1965) and other government dietary history surveys (Ten State Nutrition Survey, 1970) were done essentially on a family basis, as was the 1966 survey in Puerto Rico (Fernandez et al., 1968), for instance. The two major variables and therefore, shortcomings, of this mode are the accuracy of the memory of the person being queried, and that of pride, an emotional factor which may strongly influence the results and interfere with accurate reporting. Furthermore, a record of the family food consumption does not necessarily mean that there is uniform distribution among the family members.

The third mode of "physical examination" is excellent for the diagnosis of overt clinical deficiency, such as beriberi, pellagra, pernicious anemia, and rickets. However, this mode may be nonspecific. For instance, mouth signs suggestive of ariboflavinosis may be due to other causes, such as poorly fitting dentures in the elderly. (As will be elaborated upon later, what I consider to be one of the most significant clinical signs, namely behavioral changes, are unfortunately not usually recognized by the examining physician.)

The fourth mode, "laboratory assessment", by its nature is a more objective determination of the nutritional status of an individual person. Biochemical studies may comprise the determination of nutrient levels in body fluids or perhaps a functional biochemical or physiological assay. Laboratory assessment contributes more understanding of the marginal deficiency state since it is both more objective and specific for a given nutrient than the other three modes. The four modes have been recently reviewed by an expert workshop (Anonymous, 1973a).

It should be noted that alternative methods are available for the functional assessment of nutritional status (Anonymous, 1973b). In Table I we differentiate between static methods by which nutrient levels are determined in tissues, and functional ones by which a determination is made as to the adequacy of a nutrient level to carry out a specific biochemical or physiological function. It is the latter concept which we initiated in our research some years ago with the thiamine–transketolase relationship (Brin, 1962, 1964; Brin et al., 1958, 1965) and which has now been extended to include various assays for vitamin B_2 (Sharada and Bamji, 1972; Glatzle et al., 1968) and vitamin B_6 (Brin et al., 1960b; Brin, 1964; Sauberlich et al., 1972). It is our feeling that the functional

TABLE I
Static versus Functional Assay for Evaluating Vitamin Status[a]

Vitamin	Static assay	Functional assay
A	Plasma	Night vision
D	Serum calcium	Bone X-ray
E	Plasma	Peroxidative RBC hemolysis
K	Plasma	Prothrombin time
B_1	Plasma, urine	RBC TPP-effect (TK)
B_2	Plasma, urine	RBC FAD-effect (GSH-R)
Niacin	Urine	—
B_6	Urine, Plasma PLP	Tryptophan load, RBC PLP-effect (AT's), methionine-load test
Folic acid	Plasma	Histidine-load test
B_{12}	Plasma	Schilling test, methylmalonate excretion
C	Serum, WBC	—

[a] Vitamin determinations can often be made in serum or plasma. Key to abbreviations are: RBC = red blood cell; TPP = thiamine pyrophosphate; FAD = flavine adenine dinucleotide; TK = transketolase activity; GSH-R = glutathione reductase activity; AT'S = aspartic and glutamic amino-transferases; WBC = white blood cells.

type of test is the one of choice to reveal the marginal and, therefore, the critical deficiency state, particularly in the context of drug or pollutant interreactions.

B. Nutritional Status in the United States

The USDA market basket survey for 1966 revealed inadequacies in certain portions of our population (U.S. Department of Agriculture, 1965) for iron, calcium, and vitamins A, C, B_1, B_2 and B_6. Iron deficiency anemia was revealed to be the most prevalent inadequacy in the largest portion of the population, with a large portion of this sensitive group being inadequate in more than one nutrient. The data for vitamin B_6 were derived from dietary histories according to Handbook 36 (U.S. Department of Agriculture, 1969), and it was recognized that a large proportion of our population consumes only approximately half of the United States Recommended Daily Allowance (USRDA) (Food and Nutrition Board, 1974) of 2 mg a day for this nutrient. (It should be noted that the average consumption of half an RDA means that 50% of the population consumes less than that.) These findings were essentially confirmed by the Ten State Nutrition Survey (1970) of the United States Department of Health, Education and Welfare. They have also been largely confirmed and extended by the HANES Survey (Health and Nutrition Examination Survey, 1974) in which, as of their last report, 50% of the population was less than adequate in at least two nutrients.

Furthermore, recent studies on liver vitamin A stores in human subjects have shown that 12–37% of five population groups may be markedly depleted in vitamin A despite lack of clinical signs (Raica *et al.*, 1972). Their findings agreed with other studies from Canada and New York City; comparable values have been published from other surveys also.

C. The Marginal Deficiency State

In order to understand the sequence of events in the development of a marginal deficiency state, one should refer to the outline in Table II (Brin, 1964). The first stage of deficiency is "preliminary" in that it is a period during which there is a gradual depletion of body stores due to dietary lack, some other disease condition, or malabsorption. As the depletion process continues, the state of depletion becomes "biochemical" with a reduction in coenzyme or prosthetic group formation from the essential nutrients, resulting in biochemical defects which can be measured in erythrocytes and plasma, as biopsy tissues, or by load tests

TABLE II
The Development of Vitamin Deficiency

Sequence	Deficiency stage	Demonstrable symptoms and comments
1	Preliminary	Inadequate availability of vitamin due to diet, malabsorption, and abnormal metabolism. Urinary vitamin reduced markedly
2	Biochemical	Enzyme-coenzyme activity depressed. Urinary vitamin reduced to negligible levels
3	Physiological	Loss of body weight concurrent with appetite loss, general malaise, insomnia, and increased irritability
4	Clinical	Increased malaise, loss of body weight with the appearance of deficiency syndromes
5	Anatomical	Establishment of specific deficiency disease with specific tissue pathology. Unless reversed by repletion, death results

(Luhby *et al.*, 1971). Again, a more severe depletion of a micronutrient, in this case a vitamin, results in what one might call "physiological" signs of inadequacy. These, however, do not comprise specific clinical disease, but are largely behavioral and/or anthropometric in nature, such as general malaise, insomnia, irritability, somnolence, and loss of weight and appetite. As the depletion process progresses, "clinical" deficiency signs appear. These may include nonspecific findings such as skin lesions or a more specific distribution of them such as in pellagra, or ariboflavinosis. There could also be purpura or anemia. As a consequence of a continuation of the depletion process, there develops "anatomical" tissue pathology because of severe biochemical inadequacy, and the appearance of specific syndromes. Here vital organ function is significantly impaired and death may ensue unless corrective therapy is undertaken to reverse the depletion process.

This series of stages was delineated for the purpose of demonstrating that the biochemical defects generally appear before any physiological or clinical signs are seen in the individual under study. What is noteworthy is that the "physiological" signs of loss in body weight and appetite, general malaise and irritability, are behavioral effects which would not in themselves result in a diagnosis of nutritional deficiency since they are nonspecific. Nevertheless, they have routinely been observed to occur where specific deficiencies have been studied under laboratory conditions and often during drug therapy. Accordingly, it is our belief that the behavioral aspects of nutritional inadequacy are particularly pertinent

TABLE III
Nutrient Adequacy of Type A School Lunch

Nutrient	Percent of meals less than 1/3 RDA
Calories	100
Protein	0^a
Vitamin C	56
Vitamin B_1	77
Vitamin B_2	0^a
Vitamin A	28
Iron	87
Calcium	72^a

[a] These numbers would be higher if milk were not consumed.

for study in drug-nutrient interactions because they are effectively covert and therefore might be completely overlooked by the attending physician.

The depletion process may often develop inadvertently, even as a consequency of well-meaning nutritional intervention programs. A case in point is the Type A school lunch program (Murphy *et al.*, 1969; Head *et al.*, 1973). The Type A lunch prescribes a specific distribution of food groups to be included in every federally paid lunch program and is delivered by all participating school boards. It is generally believed that the Type A lunch is both acceptable to children and is nutritionally adequate. Yet both of these assumptions have been shown to be unfulfilled. For instance, studies on school lunch programs (Murphy *et al.*, 1969) have shown that a large percentage of children do not consume all that is placed on their tray including the milk. With regard to the second assumption, a study was done in twenty-one schools in North Carolina (Head *et al.*, 1973) (when food was much cheaper than currently) in order to determine the nutritional adequacy of the Type A school lunch as served. A summary of the data is shown in Table III. In this study whole trays of food were collected as served and submitted for nutrient analyses. It was clearly evident that over 50% of lunches did not meet one-third of an RDA for iron, calcium, and vitamins B_1 and C. One must conclude that the Type A school lunch is generally nutritionally inadequate, even assuming that all children eat all of the food and milk on their trays, which clearly they may not.

III. SOME DRUG-VITAMIN INTERRELATIONS

A. Effects of Vitamin Inadequacy on Drug Utilization

The effects of nutrient adequacy on microsomal drug metabolism are shown in Table IV. It is observed that vitamin E deficiency, while resulting in no change in microsomal cytochrome P-450, shows markedly reduced hydroxylation and demethylation of drug substrates (Carpenter, 1972; Horn *et al.*, 1976; Giasuddin *et al.*, 1975). With vitamin A deficiency, there is decreased microsomal cytochrome P-450 and decreased hydroxylation and demethylation of drug substrate, with no effect on nitroreductase (Becking, 1972). Thiamine deficiency, on the other hand, results in increased metabolism of heptachlor and aniline and large doses decrease the rate of metabolism of zoxazolamine (Wade *et al.*, 1969; Grosse and Wade, 1971). In the case of riboflavin, there is decreased metabolism by azoreductase, and of benzopyrene and *p*nitrobenzene but increased oxidative metabolism of aminopyrine, hexobarbital, and aniline (Williams *et al.*, 1970; Catz *et al.*, 1970). In vitamin C deficiency, there is decreased hydroxylation and demethylation of drug substrate but no change in microsomal cytochrome P-450 (Axelrod *et al.*, 1954; Degkwitz *et al.*, 1975; Kato *et al.*, 1969; Zannoni and Sato, 1975). However, elevated dose levels result in somewhat increased

TABLE IV
Effects of Vitamin Status upon Drug Metabolism[a]

Vitamin	Status	Effects on	
		Cytochrome P-450	Microsomal metabolism
E	D	0	−
A	D	−	−
B₁	D		+
	E		−
B₂	D		−
C	D	0	−
	E	+	+

[a] Key to abbreviation: D, Deficiency; E, Level of administration in excess of ANRC recommendations; 0, No effect; +, Increased; −, Decreased. All data obtained from experimental animals.

rates of microsomal demethylation of drug substrate (Sato and Zannoni, 1974).

It is considered significant that marginal deficiencies for vitamins A, E, and C resulted in reduced drug metabolism before there were any clinical signs of vitamin deficiency. In other words, animals known to have been depleted but which appear otherwise clinically normal have reduced microsomal capacity to metabolize drugs and environmental chemicals.

Furthermore, a recent report has demonstrated that vitamin E deficiency can result in enhanced transport of passively absorbed drugs from the intestine (Meshali and Nightingale, 1976).

These two effects on drug utilization by vitamin inadequacy, namely the reduction in the rate of degradation and the increased absorption under conditions of deficiency, may individually result in an increased residence time of the drug in the body and, therefore, a possible potentiation of the drug action. This possible potentiation may not have been accorded adequate attention.

B. Effects of Drug Administration on Vitamin Needs

Some of these effects are summarized in Table V. We note that our needs for both fat- and water-soluble vitamins are increased as a conse-

TABLE V
Increased Vitamin Needs as a Consequence of Drug and/or Environmental Chemical Exposure

Nutrient	Exposures resulting in increased vitamin needs or reduced blood levels
Vitamin A	Polychlorobiphenyls, benzopyrene, spironolactone, DDT
Folacin	Oral contraceptives, anticonvulsants, methotrexate, pyrimethamine, alcohol
Vitamin B_{12}	Biguanides, anticonvulsants, oral contraceptive steroids
Vitamin B_6	Isonicotinic hydrazide, thiosemicarbazide, penicillamine, L-dopa, hydralazine, oral contraceptive steroids, alcohol
Niacin	Polychlorobiphenyls, isonicotinic hydrazide, phenylbutazone
Riboflavin	Boric acid
Vitamin D	Anticonvulsants
Vitamin K	Anticonvulsants, antibiotics
Vitamin C	Smoking, aspirin, oral contraceptive steroids, nitrosamines
Vitamin E	Oxygen, ozone

quence of drug therapy or exposure to environmental chemicals. In some cases, as in the increased vitamin D need in children given anticonvulsants, there is overt development of clinical disease, in this case rickets (Richens and Rowe, 1970). In other situations such as with oral contraceptive steroids or aspirin, only marginal deficiency states may result as reflected by reduced blood or urine levels of vitamins and/or reduced enzyme activity. In the case of oral contraceptive steroid therapy, the activity of certain enzymes may be greatly and specifically induced (Luhby *et al.*, 1971; Brin, 1971), so that vitamin B_6 requirement is increased to levels in excess of what may be possibly obtainable from diet. In the case of antituberculosis drugs and penicillamine, the therapeutic agents combine directly with the vitamin B_6 and/or compete for vitamin B_6 at the enzyme binding sites, thereby again markedly increasing the requirement. In Table V are also included the effects of certain environmental pollutants such as nitrosamines for which the adverse effects can sometimes be reversed by vitamin C (Mirvish, 1975; Kamm *et al.*, 1975); the atmospheric pollutants, ozone and NO_2, for which the adverse effects on the pulmonary tree and biochemical changes can be markedly reduced, at least in animals, by the administration of vitamin E (Kann *et al.*, 1964); and certain pesticides. In most cases an increased need has been defined on the basis of the best biochemical criteria now available for the measurement of vitamin adequacy (Anonymous, 1973a; Sauberlich *et al.*, 1974). While in most cases the taking of an additional USRDA of the nutrient per day will correct the abnormal findings, up to ten times the USRDA for vitamin B_6 may be necessary to correct the biochemical abnormalities in the case of oral contraceptive steroid therapy (Luhby *et al.*, 1971).

IV. IMPLICATIONS OF MARGINAL DEFICIENCY ON HUMAN PERFORMANCE

If one considers human performance at its ultimate, it would include maximal physical and mental performance and/or achievement in daily life. These factors are very hard to measure since they are subjective and are prone to be judged in the context of various concepts. However, one can give some consideration to biochemical as well as behavioral effects of marginal deficiency (such as might occur as a consequence of drug or environmental chemical exposure) and from these draw some conclusions and recommendations.

A. Biochemical Effects

In focusing upon human performance, there should be functional effects related to biochemical change. The body generally has a large reserve enzyme capacity to carry out biochemical work. For instance in our initial work on thiamine inadequacy (Brin, 1962), it was demonstrated that TPP-effect values of up to 15% (which means that there can be a 15% depletion of thiamine pyrophosphate of coenzyme from the erythrocyte transketolase enzyme) were associated with no clinical signs whatever, while values in excess of that were associated with some behavioral changes such as in appetite. On the other hand, Wernicke's encephalopathy was associated with a TPP-effect value of 50% or higher (Brin, 1964). Thiamine inadequacy is one of the earliest biochemical (and clinical) effects of nutrient inadequacy in chronic alcoholism, and lateral gaze paralysis (ophthalmoplegia) is a cardinal sign of alcoholic beriberi. If the alcoholic in fact consumes a poor diet, he is probably inadequate in a variety of nutrients. Why, then does thiamine deficiency assert itself earlier than other biochemical defects? To gain more information, a study was undertaken to determine the rate of depletion of vitamin B_1 in fasting human subjects. [It had already been known that the biochemical defect develops within 4 days in experimental animals (Brin et al., 1960a.)] Individuals kept on starvation diets for the reduction of obesity were studied daily during the period of two successive starvation periods. Typical data are shown in Fig. 1 (Haro et al., 1966). TPP-effect values of 15% or greater were observed within 4 days of total

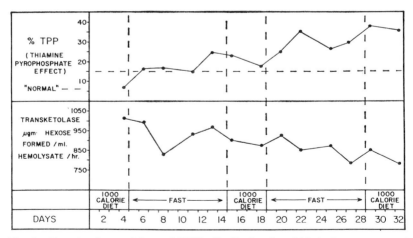

Fig. 1. Transketolase activity and "TPP-effect" of patient "A" during two successive fasts.

fasting on successive starvation periods, and exceeded 15% during the second starvation period. These data suggested that vitamin depletion can occur rapidly in humans also, even though the person is on a calorie-free, dietary regime. These data highlight the need for daily intake of vitamins whether from dietary or other sources in order to prevent vitamin insufficiency, regardless of caloric intake. The rapid rate of depletion also emphasizes the need to maintain nutritional adequacy carefully during periods of exposure to drugs or other environmental chemicals to avoid marginal deficiency.

Additional studies on alcoholics have shown that they are less able to use food as a source of folate, thiamine, and vitamin B_6 (Baker *et al.*, 1975). It is suggested that while vitamin B_6 and folate in food do not serve as readily available sources of the vitamins for alcoholics, pure vitamin B_6 and folate monoglutamate were readily absorbed. This demonstrates that the pure vitamins (in unbound form) can sometimes be better sources of nutrients than natural food, per se. These data certainly suggest the fact that a portion of our population which imbibes may have marginal vitamin insufficiency, perhaps also resulting in impaired drug metabolism.

B. Behavioral Effects of Marginal Deficiency

Detailed studies on semi-starvation included the study of biochemical, physiological, and behavioral changes in this condition (Brozek, 1953). General tiredness, muscle soreness, dizziness, apathy, irritability, and reduced self-discipline, mental alertness, and ability to concentrate were the behavioral hallmarks in this malnourished physiological condition. The psychologists on the starvation team then undertook to determine whether these findings were a consequence of deprivation of vitamins or other nutrients. One of the first studied was thiamine restriction in normal young men (Brozek, 1957). We note that large changes in the direction of deterioration were observed on the psychoneurotic scales of the Minnesota Multi-Phasic Personality Inventory. These changes were reversed by thiamine supplementation. In our studies on thiamine deficiency we undertook to study this with a self-answered questionnaire and the findings essentially confirm the prior studies (M. Brin, M. Tai, A. S. Ostashever, and H Kalinsky, unpublished results, 1962).

More recently the Medical Nutrition Laboratory of the United States Army has cooperated with other investigators to study the behavioral effects in various deficiencies including vitamins C and B_2 (Kinsman and Hood, 1971). It was found that during deprivation, changes occurred in measures of personality and psychomotor performance and in certain physical fitness tasks. Scores in the "neurotic triad" of the Minnesota Multi-Phasic Personality Inventory (the hypochondriasis, depression, and hysteria scales) became elevated as the deficiency of ascorbic acid developed. In another report from the same group, more definitive findings were given for individuals (Hodges *et al.,* 1969). Fatigability, especially of the lower limbs, and mild general malaise began insidiously before or about the time of development of objective manifestations of scurvy, suggesting that these behavioral changes were still marginal effects of vitamin C inadequacy. It is most noteworthy that the personality changes preceded decrements in psychomotor performance that were associated with the reduced arousal or motivational level such as are present during scurvy. This, in effect, confirms the sequence of events shown in Table II (Brin, 1964), in which the behavioral changes followed biochemical depletion but preceded clinical disease.

Another study by the Medical Nutrition Laboratory was designed to evaluate within-subject behavioral effects of riboflavin depletion in humans (Sterner and Price, 1973). It was shown that significant adverse changes were found in five personality subscales of the Minnesota Multi-Phasic Index (such as hypochondriasis, depression, hysteria, psychopathic-deviate, and hypomania). Reduction in hand-grip strength was also noted. The effects were noted by the thirty-ninth and fifty-second day of restriction, respectively, in the absence of any clinical symptomatology, again suggesting that the behavioral effects preceded any clinical findings of disease in the vitamin depletion sequence. What may be considered highly significant is the observation that the behavioral effects of riboflavin depletion were not reversed during a 14 day repletion period. Unfortunately, data are not available for beyond that period. However, it is noteworthy that the authors clearly suggest that select behavioral measures can afford improved means for assessing the onset and recovery of specific vitamin deficiencies. This, then, suggests that behavioral change can be an objective measure of marginal vitamin deficiency if properly managed.

Another behavioral effect, in this case as a consequence of drug administration, is the depression associated with oral contraception (Adams *et al.,* 1973). It was observed that of twenty-two depressed women whose symptoms were judged to be due to the effects of oral contraceptive steroids, eleven showed biochemical evidence of an absolute deficiency for vitamin B_6. In a doubleblind crossover trial, this deficient group of women responded clinically to the administration of pyridoxine hydrochloride while the remaining eleven showed no such response. The authors show the p value to be less than 0.005 suggesting strong statistical support for the contention that in certain susceptible women on oral contraceptive steroids, vitamin B_6 may be therapeutic for depression, again suggesting that drug administration markedly increases vitamin needs. Whether there is a similar correlation between the individuals who showed depression on oral contraceptive steroids with those who show abnormal glucose tolerance (Spellacy *et al.*, 1972; Rose *et al.*, 1975) has never been studied.

It is our feeling, therefore, that a marginal deficiency state such as may be induced by drug administration may cause behavioral effects which could seriously influence human performance. Where possible, therefore, the physician should be knowledgeable concerning the nutritional consequences of his therapy. Also, he should take steps to avoid the development of marginal (or clinical) deficiencies for a specific mode of therapy.

V. PREVENTIVE/CORRECTIVE PROPOSALS TO ATTAIN NUTRITIONAL ADEQUACY

Ideally, intervention would not be necessary to attain nutritional adequacy if suitable diets were consumed, thereby resulting in continuously maintained nutritional sufficiency in all people. As shown by the nutritional surveys described, this ideal is not universally reached, however. Intervention procedures might comprise three approaches; they are discussed below.

A. Education of Physicians and the General Population

While physicians and the laity express continuous interest in nutrition, this does not comprise thorough knowledge of the nutrient content of foods and/or appropriate food habits. Individuals are often attracted to food fads, while physicians tend to concentrate on the prescribing of therapeutic diets, often overlooking the opportunity to give their patients suitable nutritional advice to maintain health. The lack of adequate nutritional training for physicians has been amply documented (Dutra de Oliveira, 1974). Fortunately the Nutrition Foundation has undertaken to develop nutrition training programs in numerous medical schools to help rectify this problem.

Education of the general population should be in terms of nutrient delivery rather than food delivery only because the food habits of the population do not result from food choices on the basis of nutrient content. This is clearly shown by the various surveys we have mentioned previously and the fact that so many empty-calorie foods, not adequately enriched with vitamins and minerals, are consumed along with beverages which may have no nutrient value other than calories. Training of the general population, however, to change ethnic and other dietary habits is very difficult unless there is strong motivation for the individual subject to do so. Classical examples of the lack of success of educational programs have been reported (Fernandez et al., 1969; Head, 1974). Also, the nutrition education efforts associated with the general population have been highly unsuccessful. A recent USDA survey (U.S. Department of Agriculture, 1975) demonstrated that less than 50% of the people queried understood the need for a variety of food in their diets, 40% consumed diets not composed of the four food groups, and 99% did not recognize that milk intake was inadequate in their family diets. One attempt to improve nutritional status as a consequence of the White House Conference and the Federal Food Intervention Programs has been recent food labeling regulations which would help the consumer to evaluate their purchasing patterns (Federal Register, 1973). Surveys of consumers, however, have shown that they either do not understand the material on the label, or if they can understand it, they have no base-line by which they can apply the information towards improving their family's nutritional status (U.S. Department of Agriculture, 1975).

It is clear, then, that although education of physicians and the general population must continue, uppermost is the fact that food flavor and attractiveness are the cardinal factors which influence food purchasing and eating patterns. Therefore, unless the various attractive foods available in the supermarkets are properly prepared to have suitable nutrient content, nutritional status in the United States may not improve for long periods of time despite educational efforts.

B. Food Delivery of Nutrients by Appropriate Enrichment

The flour enrichment regulations of 1942 prescribed mandatory enrichment of bread with thiamine, niacin, riboflavin, and iron with the option of adding calcium (Federal Register, 1943). Over the 25 years since the promulgation of these Federal regulations, only about 37 out of 50 states have adopted them, leaving 12–13 states without mandatory enrichment. Furthermore, the flour enrichment regulations do not make it mandatory to use enriched flour in snack foods such as pretzels, which are consumed in large quantities by all portions of our population. In a study by a subcommittee of the United States Food and Nutrition Board, all of these factors were weighed and evaluated and new proposals for the broadened and improved fortification of cereal grains were proposed (Food and Nutrition Board, 1974). It was recommended that

TABLE VI
Nutrients and Levels Recommended for Inclusion in Fortification
of Cereal Grain Products[a,b]

	Amount (mg/lb)	Amount (mg/100 gm)
Vitamin A[c]	2.2	0.48
Thiamine	2.9	0.64
Riboflavin	1.8	0.40
Niacin	24.0	5.29
Vitamin B_6	2.0	0.44
Folic Acid	0.3	0.07
Iron	40.0	8.81
Calcium	900.0	198.2
Magnesium	200.0	44.1
Zinc	10.0	2.2

[a] US-NAS/NRC Food and Nutrition Board.
[b] Wheat flour, corn grits, cornmeal, rice. Other cereal grain products in proportion to their cereal grain content.
[c] Retinol equivalent.

flour enrichment be made "at the mill" rather than at the bakery, assuring that all flour used in commerce would be appropriately enriched and, therefore, would permeate the entire cereal grain food chain in the United States, including snack foods. It was recommended that enrichment be broadened to include not only the original four nutrients (thiamine, riboflavin, niacin, and iron) but to add vitamins A, B_6, and folic acid to the vitamin group, and calcium, magnesium, and zinc to the mineral group. This proposed enrichment profile is shown in Table VI. It is observed that except, perhaps, for vitamin A and iron which are added at a level of about 1.5–2 RDA per pound of flour, respectively, the other nutrients would be added at no greater level than about an RDA per pound of flour. Since a pound of flour is equivalent to approximately 1700 calories the probability of a person consuming an excessive amount of any one nutrient is avoided. Furthermore, since the flour would be enriched at the mill and enter the entire cereal grain food chain, a diverse choice of food daily would assure a person of obtaining at least a major portion of his micronutrient requirement.

In our opinion, the food industries, the United States Departments of Agriculture, and of Health, Education and Welfare, and nutrition professionals should undertake to study these proposals in depth, and to facilitate their implementation. This action would contribute significantly toward assuring that the nutritional status in the United States is in the sufficiency range.

C. Supplementation with Essential Nutrients

Where drug administration has increased the vitamin need beyond that which could be obtained through diet, however, such as in the case of vitamin B_6 and oral contraceptive steroids, it is essential for the physician to be conscious of the need for the supplementation of specific nutrients. Where generally poor dietary intake is known, a USRDA type of daily multivitamin supplement may be necessary to avoid nutritional complications of drug therapy.

Should improved and broadened fortification of cereal grains and other food products not be implemented, supplementation could restore nutritional adequacy to the population and correct the "at risk" condition as described by the various surveys.

A recent project at Tulane University which studied the effect of vitamin and mineral intervention on nutritional assessment as well as behavioral measures is noteworthy in this context (Smith *et al.,* 1975). The Nutricube supplement they used was specially designed for their purpose in the form of a beverage powder, and was given to the children on their way home for lunch. The micronutrient effects in the Nutricube group were as good as those in children participating in the school lunch program which included calories as well as the nutrients contained in the food. The Nutricube, of course, cost far less than the lunch itself. It was also noted that children who received breakfast and lunch (the Nutricube group was not given behavior testing) improved significantly in performance in disjunctive reaction time and in continued trials of associative reaction time. It was reported that: "These studies indicated a relationship between mild levels of nutrient deficiency and performance tasks demanding attentativeness and alertness." Accordingly, improved nutritional status can be associated with improved behavioral performance.

Under certain conditions, therefore, nutritional intervention by daily supplements should not be overlooked, particularly where acute situations may tend to develop, and certainly where inadequate nutritional status is suspected.

VI. SUMMARY

Nutritional status is measurable by the four modes of demographic analysis, dietary history, physical examination, and/or laboratory methods. The latter, or more specifically biochemical methods, permit one to best reveal the marginal deficiency state. Large population groups in the United States have been declared "at risk", or otherwise stated, marginally deficient, in recent authoritative government sponsored surveys.

It was emphasized that nutritional deficiencies do not just occur, but are the result of five successive stages of a continual depletion process. The marginal deficiency state is identified with behavioral and/or anthropometric change. It was shown, for example, that behavioral changes precede clinical signs in the development of deficiencies of vitamins B_1, B_2, and C.

Vitamin inadequacy often results in reduced ability to metabolize drugs, thereby possibly potentiating the effects of drugs and/or environmental chemicals. Obversely, the administration of drugs may markedly reduce body vitamin levels, or in fact cause clinical deficiency disease, sometimes associated with behavioral changes. Accordingly, the continuous maintenance of a state of nutritional adequacy is highly desirable.

Three preventive/corrective proposals were made. These included education of medical professionals and the laity, and broadened enrichment of cereal grains "at the mill" by implementing the recent Food and Nutrition Board proposals, to assure nutritional adequacy. The third proposal, appropriate where nutritional adequacy is not assured, or where specifically indicated as a consequence of a special therapeutic mode, is supplementation with a specific nutrient or multivitamin supplement.

REFERENCES

Adams, P. W., Rose, D. P., Folkard, J., Wynn, V., Seed, M., and Strong, R. (1973). Effect of pyridoxine hydrocholoride (Vitamin B_6) upon depression associated with oral contraception. *Lancet.* **1**, 897–907.
Anonymous. (1973a). Nutritional assessment in health programs. *Am. J. Public Health* **63**, Suppl.
Anonymous. (1973b). *Am. J. Public Health* **63**, 28–37.
Axelrod, J., Udenfriend, S., and Brodie, B. B. (1954). Ascorbic acid in aromatic hydroxylation III. Effect of ascorbic acid on hydroxylation of acetanilids, aniline, and antipyrine *in vivo. J. Pharacol. Exp. Ther.* **111**, 176–181.
Baker, H., Frank, O., Zetterman, R. K., Rajan, K. S., Tenhove, W., and Leevy, C. M. (1975). Inability of chronic alcoholics with liver disease to use food as a source of folates, thiamine and vitamin B_6. *Am. J. Clin. Nutr.* **28**, 1377–1380.
Becking, G. C. (1972). Vitamin A status and drug metabolism in the rat. *Can. J. Physiol. Pharmacol.* **51**, 6–11.
Brin, M. (1962). Erthrocyte transketolase in early thiamine deficiency. *Ann. N.Y. Acad. Sci.* **98**, 528–541.

Brin, M. (1964). Erythrocyte as a biopsy tissue in the functional evaluation of nutritional status. *J. Am. Med. Assoc.* **187**, 762–766.

Brin, M. (1971). Abnormal tryptophan metabolism in pregnancy and with oral contraceptive pill. I. Specific effects of an oral contraceptive steroid on the tryptophan oxygenase and two aminotransferase activities in livers of ovariectomized-adrenalectomized rats. *Am. J. Clin. Nutr.* **24**, 699–703.

Brin, M., Shohet, S. S., and Davidson, C. S. (1958). The effect of thiamine deficiency on the glucose oxidative pathway of rat erythrocytes. *J. Biol. Chem.* **230**, 319–326.

Brin, M., Tai, M., Ostashever, A. S., and Kalinsky, H. (1960a). The effect of thiamine deficiency on the activity of erythrocyte transketolase. *J. Nutr.* **71**, 273–281.

Brin, M., Tai, M. Ostashever, A. S., and Kalinsky, H. (1960b). The relative effects of pyridoxine deficiency on two plasma transaminases in the growing and in the adult rat. *J. Nutr.* **71**, 416–420.

Brin, M., Vincent, W. A., and Watson, J. Mac D. (1962). Unpublished observations.

Brin, M., Dibble, M. V., Peel, A., McMullen, E., Bourquin, A., and Chen, N. (1965). Some preliminary findings on the nutritional status of the aged in Onondaga County, New York. *Am. J. Clin. Nutr.* **17**, 240–258.

Brozek, J. (1953). Semistarvation and nutritional rehabilitation; a qualitative study with emphasis on behavior. *Am. J. Clin. Nutr.* **1**, 107–118.

Brozek, J. (1957). Psychological effects of thiamine restriction and deprivation in normal young men. *Am. J. Clin. Nutr.* **5**, 109–120.

Carpenter, M. (1972). Vitamin E and microsomal drug hydroxylation. *Ann. N.Y. Acad. Sci.* **203**, 81–92.

Catz, C. S., Juchau, M. R., and Yaffe, S. J. (1970). Effects of iron, riboflavin and iodine deficiencies on hepatic drug metabolizing systems. *J. Pharmacol. Exp. Ther.* **174**, 197–205.

Degkwitz, E., Walsch, S., Dubberstein, M., and Winter, J. (1975). Ascorbic acid and cytochromes. *Ann. N.Y. Acad. Sci.* **258**, 201–208.

Dutra de Oliveira, J. E. (1974). Teaching nutrition in medical schools: Some problems and proposed solutions. *J. Nutr. Educ.* **6**, 49–51.

Federal Register. (1943). Vol. 8, p. 10780.

Federal Register. (1973). Food Labeling 6950–6975.

Fernandez, N. A., Burgos, J. C., Roberts, L. J., and Asenjo, C. F. (1968). Nutritional status in Puerto Rican slum area. *Am. J. Clin. Nutr.* **21**, 646–656.

Fernandez, N. A., Burgos, J. C., Asenjo, C. F., and Rosa Rosa, I. (1969). Nutrition survey of two rural Puerto Rican areas before and after a community improvement program. *Am. J. Clin. Nutr.* **22**, 1639–1657.

Food and Nutrition Board. (1974). "Proposed Fortification Policy for Cereal Grain Products." Natl. Acad. Sci.—Natl. Res. Counc., Washington, D.C.

Giasuddin, A. S. M., Caygill, C. P. J., Diplock, A. T., and Jeffrey, E. (1975). The dependence on vitamin E and selenium of drug demethylation in rat liver microsomes. *Biochem. J.* **146**, 339–350.

Glatzle, D., Weber, F., and Wiss, O. (1968). Enzymatic test for the detection of a riboflavin deficiency. *Experientia* **24**, 1122.

Grosse, W., III, and Wade, A. E. (1971). The effect of thiamine consumption on liver microsomal drug metabolism. *J. Pharmacol. Exp. Ther.* **176**, 758–765.

Haro, E. N., Brin, M., and Faloon, W. W. (1966). Fasting in obesity: Thiamine depletion as measured by erythrocyte transketolase changes. *Arch. Intern. Med.* **117**, 175–181.

Head, M. K. (1974). A nutrition education program at three grade levels. *J. Nutr. Educ.* **6**, 56–59.

Head, M. K., Weaks, R. J., and Gibbs, E. (1973). Major nutrients in the Type A lunch. *J. Am. Diet. Assoc.* **63**, 620–625.

Health and Nutrition Examination Survey. (1974). Publ. No. (HRA) 74-1219-1. U.S. Dept. of Health, Education and Welfare, Rockville, Maryland.

Hodges, R. E., Baker, E. M., Hood, J., Sauberlich, H. E., and March, S. C. (1969). Experimental scurvy in man. *Am. J. Clin. Nutr.* **22**, 535–548.

Horn, L. R., Machlin, L. J., Barker, M. O., and Brin, M. (1976). Drug metabolism and hepatic heme proteins in the vitamin E deficient rat. *Arch. Biochem. Biophys.* **172**, 270–277.

Kamm, J. J., Dashman, T., Conney, A. H., and Burns, J. J. (1975). Effect of ascorbic acid on amine-nitrite toxicity. *Ann. N.Y. Acad. Sci.* **258**, 169–174.

Kann, H. E., Jr., Mengel, C. E., Smith, W., and Horton, B. (1964). Oxygen toxicity and vitamin E. *Aerosp. Med.* **35**, 840–844.

Kato, R., Takanaka, A., and Oshima, T. (1969). Effect of vitamin C deficiency on the metabolism of drugs and NADPH-linked electron transport system in liver microsomes. *Jpn. J. Pharmacol.* **19**, 25–33.

Kinsman, R. A., and Hood, J. (1971). Some behavioral effects of ascorbic acid deficiency. *Am. J. Clin. Nutr.* **24**, 455–464.

Luhby, A. L., Brin, M., Gordon, M., Davis, P., Murphy, M., and Spiegel, H. (1971). Vitamin B_6 metabolism in users of oral contraceptive agents. I. Abnormal urinary xanthurenic acid excretion and its correction by pyridoxine. *Am. J. Clin. Nutr.* **24**, 684–693.

Meshali, M. M., and Nightingale, C. H. (1976). Effect of alpha tocopherol (vitamin E) deficiency on intestinal transport of passively absorbed drugs. *J. Pharm. Sci.* **65**, 344–349.

Mirvish, S. S. (1975). Blocking the formation of N-nitroso compounds with ascorbic acid *in vitro* and *in vivo*. *Ann. N.Y. Acad. Sci.* **258**, 175–180.

Murphy, E. W., Koons, P. C., and Page, L. (1969). Vitamin content of Type A school lunches. *J. Am. Diet. Assoc.* **55**, 372–378.

Raica, N., Jr., Scott, J., Lowry, L., and Sauberlich, H. E. (1972). Vitamin A concentration in human tissues collected from five areas of the United States. *Am. J. Clin. Nutr.* **25**, 291–296.

Richens, A., and Rowe, D. J. F. (1970). Interaction between anticonvulsant drugs and vitamin D. *Br. J. Pharmacol.* **40**, 593–595.

Rose, D. P., Leklem, J. E., Brown, R. R., and Linkswiler, H. M. (1975). Effect of oral contraceptives and vitamin B_6 deficiency on carbohydrate metabolism. *Am. J. Clin. Nutr.* **28**, 872–878.

Sato, P., and Zannoni, V. G. (1974). Stimulation of drug metabolism by ascorbic acid in weanling guinea pigs. *Biochem. Pharmacol.* **23**, 3121–3128.

Sauberlich, H. E., Canham, J. E., Baker, E. M., Raica, N., and Herman, Y. F. (1972). Biochemical assessment of the nutritional status of vitamin B_6 in the human. *Am. J. Clin. Nutr.* **25**, 629–642.

Sauberlich, H. E., Skala, J. H., and Dowdy, R. P. (1974). "Laboratory Tests for the Assessment of Nutritional Status." CRC Press, Cleveland, Ohio.

Sharada, D., and Bamji, M. S. (1972). Erythrocyte glutathione reductase activity and riboflavin concentration in experimental deficiency of some water soluble vitamins. *Int. J. Vitam. Nutr. Res.* **42**, 43–49.

Smith, J. L., Sulzer, J. L., and Goldsmith, G. A. (1975). Prevention of vitamin and mineral deficiencies with protein-calorie malnutrition. *In* "Protein-Calorie Malnutrition" (R. E. Olson, ed.), pp. 415–429. Academic Press, New York.

Spellacy, W. N., Buhi, W. C., and Birk, S. A. (1972). Effects of vitamin B_6 on carbohydrate metabolism in women taking steroid contraceptives. *Contraception* **6,** 265–273.

Sterner, R. T., and Price, W. R. (1973). Restricted riboflavin: Within-subject behavioral effects in humans. *Am. J. Clin. Nutr.* **26,** 150–159.

Ten State Nutrition Survey. (1970). Publ. No. 72-8130 to 72-8134. U.S. Dept. of Health, Education and Welfare, Washington, D.C.

U.S. Department of Agriculture. (1965). "Household Food Consumption Survey." USDA/ARS, Washington, D.C.

U.S. Department of Agriculture. (1969). Pantothenic acid, vitamin B_6, and vitamin B_{12} content of foods. *U.S., Dep. Agric., Home Econ. Res. Rep.* **36.**

U.S. Department of Agriculture. (1975). Homemakers' food and nutrition knowledge, practices and opinions. *U.S. Dep. Agric., Home Econ. Res. Rep.* **39.**

Wade, A. E., Greene, F. E., Ciordia, R. H., and Caster, W. O. (1969). Effects of dietary thiamine intake on hepatic drug metabolism in the male rat. *Biochem. Pharmacol.* **18,** 2288–2292.

Williams, J. R., Jr., Grantham, P. H., Yamamoto, R. S. and Weisburger, J. H. (1970). Effect of dietary riboflavin on azo dye reductase in liver and in bacteria of cecal contents of rats. *Biochem. Pharmacol.* **19,** 2523–2525.

Zannoni, V. G., and Sato, P. (1975). Effects of ascorbic acid on microsomal drug metabolism. *Ann. N.Y. Acad. Sci.* **258,** 119–131.

6

Effects of Oral Contraceptives on Nutrient Utilization

DAVID P. ROSE

I. INTRODUCTION

It is estimated that oral contraceptives are taken by more than twenty million women, largely in North America and Western Europe, but to an increasing extent in Latin America.

The oral contraceptives are all preparations of synthetic steroids; those most commonly in use are a combination of an estrogen and a progestogen which are taken each day for 21 days, followed by a 7-day break during which menstruation occurs. The estrogenic component is either ethinylestradiol, or the 3-methyl ether (mestranol) of this steroid. Mestranol itself is an extremely weak estrogen with low affinity for

.

cytoplasmic steroid receptors, and is only effective after it has been de-methylated to yield ethinylestradiol (Eisenfeld, 1974). Consequently, on a weight for weight basis, ethinylestradiol has more estrogenic activity than mestranol when administered by mouth.

A number of different progestogens are used in combination with ethinylestradiol or mestranol. Chemically they fall into two groups, the nortestosterone derivatives and those derived from 17-hydroxypro-gesterone. Some of the progestogens, for example norethynodrel, are themselves weakly estrogenic; others, structurally more closely related to testosterone, have some androgenic activity.

When the combined oral contraceptives were first introduced, the estrogen dose was 80 or 100 μg. Recognition that smaller doses were equally effective, and that thromboembolic disease complicating oral contraception was related to the estrogen level, led to a reduction in the amount of estrogen contained in these preparations. Most of those pre-scribed currently contain 50 μg of estrogen, but products are available in which there is only 30 μg of this component. With time, the progestogen dose has also decreased; most now contain 0.5–1.0 mg.

Although the estrogen–progestogen combination is the form of oral contraception most widely prescribed in both North America and Europe, until recently, a minority of women were taking 'sequential' preparations in which a 21–23-day course of estrogen is followed by a short course of estrogen combined with progestogen. A recent report that the sequential types of oral contraceptives are associated with an increased risk of uterine cancer (Silverberg and Makowski, 1975) has resulted in the removal of these preparations from the market.

Estrogen-containing oral contraceptives act both at the neuroendo-crine level, and locally on the reproductive tract. They suppress ovulation by exerting an inhibitory effect on hypothalamic centers. In addition, they interfere with tubal transport of the ova and implantation, and the movement of spermatozoa through the cervical mucus.

The original progestogen-only oral contraceptives, chlormadinone acetate and megestrol acetate, are no longer used in the United States or Britain because toxicity trials showed that they induce mammary tumors in beagles. Before they were withdrawn, several comparative metabolic and nutritional studies of these progestogens and the estrogen-contain-ing oral contraceptives were completed.

Most of the nutritional complications of the oral contraceptives appear attributable to the estrogenic component. In many cases, estrogen induc-tion of protein, frequently enzyme, synthesis appears to be involved, and repeatedly a parallel is found between the effects of oral contraception and pregnancy.

At the outset it should be stressed that the majority of the side-effects to be described are of a minor character. Clinical manifestations of a nutritional disturbance attributable to oral contraception are few and far between. Generally, one is observing a biochemical abnormality in an apparently healthy woman. Concern arises because the long-term consequences of these steroid-induced changes are unknown, and there are no comparable clinical situations on which to base a prediction. A special case in point is the use of this form of contraception in the underdeveloped countries. Here, against a background of endemic malnutrition, the question inevitably arises as to the extent to which oral contraceptives may aggravate the preexisting deficiencies.

II. EFFECTS OF ORAL CONTRACEPTIVES ON AMINO ACID AND PROTEIN METABOLISM

A. Tryptophan Metabolism

Tryptophan is one of the essential amino acids for man. Aside from protein synthesis, several metabolic pathways exist for its utilization, the most important biologically being those which lead to the synthesis of 5-hydroxytryptamine (serotonin) and nicotinic acid (Fig. 1).

The metabolism of tryptophan to 5-hydroxytryptamine involves two enzymatic steps, the first a hydroxylation to yield 5-hydroxytryptophan, and the second a decarboxylation which requires pyridoxal phosphate as a cofactor. Although 5-hydroxytryptamine is synthesized in both liver and kidney, the amine formed at these sites cannot cross the blood–brain barrier and so that present within the brain is produced *in situ*. This has important physiological and pharmacological implications because 5-hydroxytryptamine is a key neurotransmitter.

Several of the enzymatic reactions on the tryptophan–nicotinic acid ribonucleotide metabolic pathway are also pyridoxal phosphate-dependent (Fig. 1).

In consequence, vitamin B_6 deficiency is characterized by abnormal tryptophan metabolism, the most widely described features of which are elevated excretions of kynurenine, 3-hydroxykynurenine, and xanthurenic acid in urine collected after an oral dose of the amino acid. These changes appear to arise because the kynureninase responsible for the conversion of 3-hydroxykynurenine to 3-hydroxyanthranilic acid is more sensitive to a lack of pyridoxal phosphate than are the other vitamin B_6-dependent enzymes (Ogasawara *et al.*, 1962). An apparent anomaly is that an increased urinary excretion of quinolinic acid also

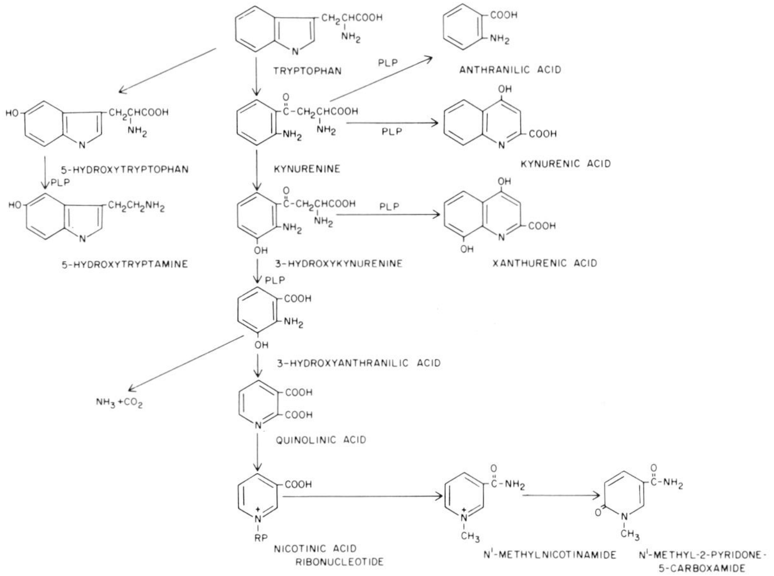

154   David P. Rose

Fig. 1. Metabolic pathways for the formation of nicotinic acid ribonucleotide and 5-hydroxytryptamine from L-tryptophan. PLP indicates the pyridoxal phosphate-dependent reactions.

occurs in experimentally induced dietary vitamin B_6 deficiency (Brown *et al.*, 1965) and after treatment with the antagonist deoxypyridoxine (Rose and Toseland, 1973). This suggests that there may be an unrecognized pyridoxal phosphate-requiring step beyond 3-hydroxyanthranilic acid.

3-Hydroxyanthranilic acid excretion is also elevated in vitamin B_6 deficiency, although to a lesser degree than are the metabolites which are proximal to it on the metabolic pathway (Rose *et al.*, 1972).

In 1966, Rose reported that women taking oral contraceptives excreted increased levels of xanthurenic acid and other tryptophan metabolites. The changes were similar to those seen in vitamin B_6 deficiency, they were reversed by large doses of pyridoxine, and an identical abnormality resulted from treatment with an estrogen alone. Later, it was shown that the urinary excretion of quinolinic acid is also elevated by estrogen-containing oral contraceptives, the levels returning to normal after pyridoxine administration (Rose and Toseland, 1973).

These findings have been confirmed and extended by other workers (Price *et al.*, 1967; Luhby *et al.*, 1971a; Aly *et al.*, 1971; Coelingh Bennink and Schrews, 1974). It appears that all of the available estrogen–progestogen combinations used for contraceptive purposes may produce abnormal tryptophan metabolism, and that an increased excretion of metabolites occurs in about 70% of users. A 2 gm L-tryptophan load test usually demonstrates an increased xanthurenic acid excretion within 21 days of starting treatment; after 3 months the urinary levels of xanthurenic acid, kynurenine, 3-hydroxykynurenine, and 3-hydroxyanthranilic acid may all be elevated. When the oral contraceptive is discontinued it may be 3 months or longer before tryptophan metabolism reverts to normal (Rose and Adams, 1972).

In addition to tryptophan metabolites, oral contraceptive-treated women excrete increased amounts of the niacin metabolite N^1-methyl-nicotinamide, but not its derivative N^1-methyl-2-pyridone-5-carboxamide, in urine collected with or without a tryptophan load (Rose et al., 1968; Leklem et al., 1975a). Stilbestrol-treated males excrete increased urinary levels of both of these compounds (Wolf et al., 1970). One interpretation of these observations is that estrogens promote the conversion of tryptophan to nicotinic acid ribonucleotide, perhaps by stimulating tryptophan oxygenase activity so that a greater proportion of the available amino acid enters this biosynthetic pathway.

There is no doubt that it is the estrogen in the combined type of oral contraceptives which is responsible for abnormalities in tryptophan metabolism. Not only are identical changes produced by estrogens alone, but progestogens reduce the effect of the estrogenic component when the two steroids are used in combination (Rose et al., 1973b). Megestrol acetate, a progestogen which has been employed as a single agent contraceptive, has no effect on tryptophan metabolism (Rose and Adams, 1972); other progestogens reduce the urinary levels of nicotinic acid derivatives (Wolf et al., 1970).

The pharmacological actions of the contraceptive steroids which are responsible for abnormalities in tryptophan metabolism have still not been established with certainty. Obviously vitamin B_6 is involved in some way because the elevated metabolite excretions are reversed by treatment with pyridoxine; in addition we must account for the increased urinary niacin metabolites.

Before the effect of oral contraceptives on tryptophan metabolism was recognized, Mason and Gullekson (1960) had shown that sulfate esters of estrogens interfere in vitro with the activity of pyridoxal phosphate-dependent enzymes by competing with the coenzyme for receptor sites on the apoenzyme molecule. There is evidence that pyridoxal phosphate is more tightly bound to mitochondrial kynurenine aminotransferase than to the supernatant kynureninase (Ogasawara et al., 1962; Ueda, 1967). Possibly this permits estrogen conjugates to inhibit hepatic kynureninase preferentially, so that 3-hydroxykynurenine accumulates and is then metabolized to xanthurenic acid. Treatment with large doses of pyridoxine could reverse this inhibition because a high concentration of pyridoxal phosphate in the liver would displace the estrogen conjugates from the apoenzyme. The presence of conjugated synthetic estrogens derived from the oral contraceptives may have a similar inhibitory effect on kynureninase.

In addition to enzyme inhibition, some women taking oral contraceptives appear to develop a true vitamin B_6 deficiency. The evidence that this does occur in a minority of oral contraceptive users is reviewed in Section III, A.

It has been suggested already in this chapter that synthetic estrogens may increase the turnover of the tryptophan–nicotinic acid ribonucleotide pathway, and that an increased yield of niacin is responsible for the elevated urinary N^1-methylnicotinamide excretion. This proposal is based on the fact that tryptophan oxygenase, the first and rate-limiting enzyme on the pathway, is inducible in rat liver by estrogen administration. Whether this occurs also in the human liver is not known, but treatment with hydrocortisone does stimulate this enzyme and cause a corresponding elevation in urinary kynurenine excretion (Altman and Greengard, 1966).

Later in this section it will be shown that estrogens may accelerate a number of pyridoxal phosphate-requiring pathways of amino acid metabolism; a redistribution of the coenzyme or an absolute increase in requirement may stem from such an effect.

B. Other Amino Acids

A reduction of α-amino nitrogen in the plasma of oral contraceptive-treated women was first recognized by Craft and co-workers (1970; Craft and Wise, 1969); it was considered to result from an increased incorporation of amino acids into protein.

Later Craft and Peters (1971) determined the concentrations of individual plasma amino acids in oral contraceptive users and controls at different times in the menstrual cycle. Significant decreases in serine, glutamate, and ornithine occurred during the second half of the controls menstrual cycles compared to the levels early in the follicular phase. Likewise, the oral contraceptive users had reductions in plasma alanine, glycine, tyrosine, proline, valine, and leucine late in their 21-day "pill cycle", when compared with the corresponding concentrations in samples obtained towards the end of their monthly break in treatment. In addition to these differences, the plasma glutamate, glycine, isoleucine, and tyrosine levels were lower in the oral contraceptive users than nonusers in the second half of the cycle. These data indicate that plasma amino acids are influenced by both cyclical changes in endogenous hormones and contraceptive steroids.

One possible mechanism is that reductions in plasma amino acids arise from a hormonally induced amino aciduria; this is at least partly responsible for the changes which occur in the third trimester of pregnancy (Zinneman *et al.*, 1967). There is a lack of information on urinary amino acid excretions by oral contraceptive-treated women, but Zinneman and his co-workers did examine the effect of progesterone given alone or in combination with stilbestrol on both plasma and urinary free amino acids in male subjects. Progesterone administration caused a significant decrease in the plasma concentrations of threonine, alanine, cystine, ornithine, and arginine, and an increase in phenylalanine. The only urinary changes were increases in taurine and phenylalanine excretions. When both progesterone and stilbestrol were given there were significant decreases in plasma serine, citrulline, glycine, alanine, valine, ornithine, lysine, and arginine, but only taurine, valine and cystathionine were increased in urine.

In summary, the work of Zinneman and his colleagues does not support a renal mechanism for the effect of oral contraceptives on plasma amino acids. Their results are, however, compatible with the conclusion reached by Craft *et al.* (1970; Craft and Peters, 1971) that the progestogenic component of the combined oral contraceptives is the steroid responsible, and that it stimulates anabolic activity with increased utilization by the liver.

But not all of the effects of oral contraceptives on plasma amino acids can be attributed to the progestogen. In another study, Zinneman *et al.* (1965) examined the effect of stilbestrol; after 5 days treatment there were significant decreases in plasma tyrosine, glutamic acid, and ornithine. Corresponding increases in urinary glutamic acid and ornithine, although small, suggest that the reduced plasma concentrations of these two amino acids were due to altered renal tubular function. On the other hand, the urinary excretion of tyrosine was decreased which, considered with the reduced plasma concentration, points to a prerenal effect of estrogens on this particular amino acid.

Rose and Cramp (1970) pursued this further and found that both estrogen-containing oral contraceptives and ethinylestradiol alone reduce the plasma tyrosine. They attributed the abnormality to an estrogen-induced elevation in hepatic tyrosine aminotransferase, with a consequent increase in the rate of degradation of the amino acid. Tyrosine aminotransferase, like tryptophan oxygenase, is a glucocorticoid-inducible enzyme, and treatment with hydrocortisone is known to reduce the plasma tyrosine concentration (Rivlin and Melmon, 1965). Both of these amino acid-catabolizing enzymes, and alanine aminotransferase, are elevated in the livers of estrogen-treated rats; effects which are largely or entirely dependent on the presence of the adrenal glands (Braidman and Rose, 1971).

The fasting plasma alanine is not reduced in oral contraceptive users (Craft and Peters, 1971; Aly et al., 1971). However, Rose et al. (1976) have recently studied the metabolism of an oral alanine load by oral contraceptive-treated women and age-matched female controls. After ingesting the amino acid, the elevation above fasting concentrations were significantly less for the oral contraceptive users (Fig. 2). The fasting blood pyruvate levels were higher in these women, and further increases occurred after alanine loading. (Fig. 3). These results are consistent with the hypothesis that the estrogenic component, by stimulating hepatic alanine aminotransferase, enhances the rate of clearance of alanine from the plasma and its transamination to pyruvate.

Aly et al. (1971) reported a study of plasma amino acid levels in oral contraceptive users which, in spite of the small number of subjects, is of special value because they regulated the diet. The total and individual plasma amino acids were determined for five women taking an estrogen-containing oral contraceptive and five controls. A diet of known composition was fed for 6 days. It provided 81 gm protein daily, and met the recommended daily allowance for all nutrients except iron and

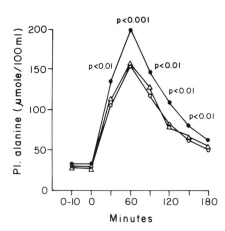

Fig. 2. Mean responses of the plasma alanine concentrations to a 200 mg/kg body weight oral dose of L-alanine for 30 oral contraceptive users (○), 11 oral contraceptive users after pyridoxine supplementation (△), and 14 controls (●). The p values refer to the significance of differences between the 30 oral contraceptive users and 14 controls (from Rose et al., 1976).

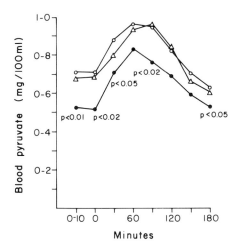

Fig. 3. Mean blood pyruvate concentrations before and after oral alanine loads for oral contraceptive users (○), oral contraceptive users after pyridoxine (△) and controls (●). The p values refer to the significance of differences between the 30 oral contraceptive users and 14 controls (from Rose *et al.*, 1976).

calories. Additional calories in the form of carbohydrates, fat, or both, were supplied in sufficient quantity to maintain body weight. Total plasma amino acid levels were significantly lower in subjects taking oral contraceptives, largely because of decreases in nonessential amino acids (Table I). Nearly all of these were low, and particularly so in the case of tyrosine, glycine, proline, and arginine. Two essential amino acids, methionine and phenylalanine, were also decreased in the oral contraceptive-treated group.

Methionine is an amino acid of special interest in the context of the present discussion because, like tryptophan, its metabolism is disturbed by vitamin B_6 deficiency.

Homocysteine, the demethylation product of methionine, is converted to cystathionine by the incorporation of serine; the reaction is catalyzed by cystathionine synthetase, a pyridoxal phosphate-requiring enzyme (Fig. 4). Cystathionase, another vitamin B_6-dependent enzyme, splits cystathionine to yield homoserine and cysteine. Homocystine and cystine are the stable oxidation products of homocysteine and cysteine respectively.

Park and Linkswiler (1970) studied methionine metabolism in normal male subjects before and after the induction of dietary vitamin B_6 deficiency. The excretions of methionine and its metabolites were determined in 24 hour collections of urine obtained before and after 3 gm oral

TABLE I

Plasma Amino Acid Levels (μmole/100 ml mean± SEM) in Five Oral Contraceptive Users and Five Controls[a]

Amino acid	Controls	OC users
Essential		
Threonine	28.2 ± 1.5	28.2 ± 1.9
Lysine	20.6 ± 1.7	20.5 ± 1.2
Leucine	13.7 ± 0.5	13.4 ± 0.8
Isoleucine	6.7 ± 0.3	6.4 ± 0.5
Phenylalanine	6.5 ± 0.4	5.3 ± 0.2[b]
Methionine	2.7 ± 0.1	1.8 ± 0.1[d]
Total	78.4 ± 3.4	75.6 ± 4.4
Nonessential		
Alanine	38.3 ± 3.1	31.7 ± 1.8
Glycine	24.6 ± 1.5	14.2 ± 1.8[c]
Proline	20.1 ± 1.3	11.7 ± 1.0[d]
Serine	13.9 ± 0.6	12.1 ± 0.8
Glutamic acid	10.3 ± 0.3	9.5 ± 1.9
Arginine	9.4 ± 0.6	7.0 ± 0.6[c]
Histidine	8.8 ± 0.4	9.6 ± 0.6
Tyrosine	6.9 ± 0.3	3.9 ± 0.2[c]
Aspartic acid	0.9 ± 0.1	0.9 ± 0.2
Total	133.2 ± 4.2	100.6 ± 6.3

[a] From Aly et al., 1971.
[b] Significantly lower than controls: $p < 0.02$.
[c] $p < 0.002$.
[d] $p < 0.001$.

L-methionine loads. When the vitamin B_6-deficient diet had been fed for 13 days there were marked increases in both the basal and post-methionine excretions of cystathionine. Homocystine was not detectable in urine collected before the deficiency period, and, even with methionine loading, only became present in measurable quantity after 21 days of vitamin B_6 depletion. At this time the pre- and post-methionine loading excretions were respectively twelve and twenty-two fold the predeficiency values. Thus, it appears that cystathionase is more sensitive to vitamin B_6 deficiency than cystathionine synthetase, presumably because the latter has a greater binding affinity for pyridoxal phosphate.

In a recent study, Leklem et al. (1975a) determined the effect of a dietary-induced vitamin B_6 deficiency on the urinary cystathionine excretion by fifteen oral contraceptive users and nine female controls. Urine collections were made after a 3 gm oral L-methionine load. Before

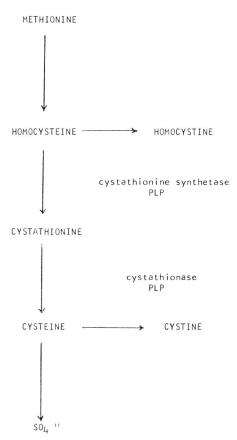

Fig. 4. Methionine metabolism. In vitamin B_6 deficiency cystathionase activity is impaired; cystathionine synthetase activity is maintained because this enzyme has a high binding affinity for the coenzyme. Hence cystathionine, rather than homocysteine, appears in the urine after a methionine load.

the depletion period the cystathionine levels were similar in both groups. This was an unexpected finding because of the gross abnormalities in tryptophan metabolite excretions which are known to occur in oral contraceptive users. The competitive inhibition of pyridoxal phosphate-dependent enzymes by steroid derivatives has been discussed earlier in this section, and it was expected that cystathionase would be affected in the same way as kynureninase.

After 2 weeks on the vitamin B_6-deficient diet, both the oral contraceptive users and controls did excrete elevated cystathionine levels, and further increases occurred during the remainder of the 4-week

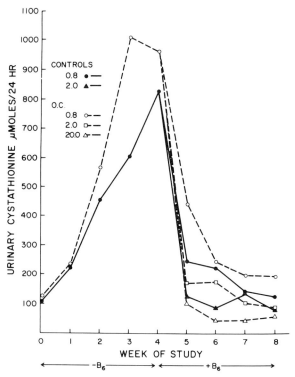

Fig. 5. Urinary cystathionine excretion after a 3.0 gm oral methionine load in oral contraceptive users and control women. During the second 4-week period the vitamin B_6-deficient diet was supplemented daily with 0.8, 2.0, or 20 mg of pyridoxine hydrochloride (from Leklem *et al.*, 1975b).

depletion period (Fig. 5). This abnormality was more marked in the oral contraceptive-treated group, suggesting that the effect of vitamin B_6 deficiency on methionine metabolism is accentuated by contraceptive steroids. Further, supplementation of the vitamin B_6-deficient diet (which provided the equivalent of 0.19 mg pyridoxine per day) with 0.8 mg pyridoxine hydrochloride per day restored the urinary cystathionine excretion to predepletion levels in the controls, but not in the oral contraceptive users.

C. Protein Metabolism

Oral contraceptive treatment is accompanied by a complexity of changes in the plasma proteins, many of which also occur in the later stages of pregnancy. Virtually all of these effects are also produced by estrogens alone.

Oral contraceptives decrease the serum albumin concentration. Robertson (1967) studied thirty-three women before and at intervals after starting their use. After 12 months treatment the serum albumin had decreased by an average of 17%. This abnormality appears to be due mainly to inhibition of albumin synthesis (Hønger and Rossing, 1969), perhaps because there is an insufficient supply of one or more of the limiting amino acids.

The reduction in serum albumin is almost certainly of no clinical significance in a well-nourished population. However, as with other nutritional side-effects of oral contraception, it might assume importance in conditions where protein-calorie malnutrition is endemic. In kwashiorkor the total serum protein concentration is reduced, and this is largely due to hypoalbuminemia (Edozien, 1960). When the dietary deficiency is corrected there is a rapid increase in serum albumin, indicating that the hypoalbuminemia is not due to impaired liver function, but rather to a lack of limiting amino acids such as tyrosine. There is an urgent need for studies of plasma protein and amino acid concentrations, and amino acid metabolism in oral contraceptive-treated women at special risk of protein deficiency.

Oral contraceptives cause a small decrease in the γ-globulins, and increases in some of the α_1, α_2 and β-globulins; the net result is that there is little, if any, change in the total plasma globulins (Robertson, 1967; Laurell et al., 1968). The most prominent abnormalities involve the hormone-binding and other transport globulins; as a secondary phenomenon there are increases in plasma hormone and metal concentrations. Examples are the marked elevations in corticosteroid-binding globulins, which are responsible for high plasma cortisol concentrations (Burke, 1970), and in the thyroxine-binding globulins which cause increases in the serum protein-bound iodine (Larsson-Cohn, 1966). Women using oral contraceptives do not develop Cushing's syndrome or hyperthyroidism, because the protein-binding prevents hormonal activity.

Several studies have demonstrated raised serum ceruloplasmin levels in oral contraceptive-treated women; these may be as much as 200–300% above control values (Carruthers et al., 1966; Laurell et al., 1968; Musa et al., 1967). Ceruloplasmin is a copper-binding α_2-globulin, and its elevation accounts for the high serum copper levels which occur in oral contraceptive users (Section IV). Similarly, the serum iron and total iron-binding capacity are increased by oral contraceptives (Burton, 1967), but in this case there is lack of agreement on the effect of these steroids on serum transferrin levels; Laurell *et al.* (1968) reported elevations in this protein, but others found it unchanged (Musa *et al.*, 1967; Mendenhall, 1970).

A large number of publications have appeared dealing with the effect of oral contraceptives on the blood clotting process. This work has been stimulated by the recognition that the estrogen-containing oral contraceptives are associated with an increased risk of thromboembolic disease (Inman *et al.*, 1970). The consensus is that these preparations do cause elevations in factors VII, VIII, X, and fibrinogen (Briggs *et al.*, 1970), but the role that these changes play in vascular complications of oral contraception remains uncertain.

Reports of effects of contraceptive steroids on other serum proteins include decreases in orosomucoid and haptoglobin, and increases in plasminogen and α_2-macroglobulins (Laurell *et al.*, 1968). These changes have not been associated with any clinical sequelae, but they must be borne in mind when assays of serum proteins are used for diagnostic purposes.

III. VITAMIN REQUIREMENTS AND UTILIZATION

A. Vitamin B_6

The reports that oral contraceptive users frequently exhibit an abnormality of tryptophan metabolism which is identical to that seen in vitamin B_6 deficiency were reviewed in the previous section. Although these studies showed that oral contraceptives interfered in some way with pyridoxal phosphate-dependent reactions on the tryptophan–nicotinic acid ribonucleotide pathway, the question remained as to whether this was due to a direct pharmacological effect of these steroids on the enzymes concerned, or was indicative of a true vitamin B_6 deficiency.

One approach to this problem was to measure alanine aminotransferase and aspartate aminotransferase levels in erythrocytes from oral contraceptive users and matched controls. Previous work had shown that decreases in the activity of the enzymes occur in dietary vitamin B_6 deficiency; an even more sensitive indicator was an increase in stimulation of activity obtained *in vitro* by the addition of pyridoxal phosphate to the assay system (Raica and Sauberlich, 1964; Cinnamon and Beaton, 1970).

The first application of this index of vitamin B_6 deficiency to the study of oral contraceptive users was made by Doberenz *et al.*, (1971). They determined erythrocyte alanine aminotransferase activity with and without stimulation *in vitro* by pyridoxal phosphate in thirteen women using oral contraceptives and eleven controls. The mean basal enzyme activity was significantly lower, and the percentage of stimulation by pyridoxal phosphate significantly greater, in the oral contraceptive-treated group. In a much larger study involving eighty oral contraceptive users and fifty untreated women, Rose *et al.* (1973a) could detect no difference in basal alanine aminotransferase activity. They did find an increased stimulation of the enzyme *in vitro* by pyridoxal phosphate in the oral contraceptive group, but this was restricted to twelve of the eighty women (15%).

Aly *et al.* (1971) assayed both erythrocyte alanine aminotransferase and aspartate aminotransferase in five oral contraceptive users and five controls when they had been consuming a standard diet, which provided 1.3 mg vitamin B_6 daily, for 6 days. The two groups had identical erythrocyte alanine aminotransferase levels; the effect of stimulation *in vitro* was not reported. Erythrocyte aspartate aminotransferase activity was significantly *higher* in the oral contraceptive users compared with the controls, but the percentage stimulation *in vitro* by pyridoxal phosphate was similar for the two groups of subjects. This effect of oral contraceptives on erythrocyte aspartate aminotransferase has been confirmed by Rose *et al.* (1972, 1973a), and in female rats treatment with ethinylestradiol causes an elevation of enzyme activity in both erythrocytes and liver (C. C. Li-Chen and D. P. Rose, unpublished).

Salkeld *et al.* (1973) employed the stimulation *in vitro* of erythrocyte aspartate aminotransferase by pyridoxal phosphate as an index of vitamin B_6 deficiency. Normal values were established by assaying samples from more than 300 blood donors. The groups for study comprised 233 oral contraceptive users and 76 age-matched nonusers who were also attending the gynecology clinic. Abnormal stimulation tests, classified as indicating vitamin B_6 deficiency, were found in 37% of the oral contraceptive-treated women, but in only 13% of the nonusers. A further 11% and 5%, respectively, were considered to have only marginally adequate vitamin B_6 nutritional status.

The results from investigations in which erythrocyte aspartate aminotransferase is employed as the indicator of vitamin B_6 deficiency are difficult to interpret because, as discussed, estrogens have a direct effect on this enzyme. An alternative approach is the direct assay of vitamin B_6 or its metabolites.

Miller *et al.* (1974) described a study in which three women taking estrogen containing oral contraceptives and two controls of similar age were fed a fixed diet, providing 1.9 mg vitamin B_6 daily, for 11 days. The oral contraceptive users excreted approximately 30% less urinary vitamin B_6 (determined by microbiological assay) than the controls. No difference in urinary 4-pyridoxic acid excretion was detected, although in a study of thirty-one oral contraceptive users consuming a self-selected diet Rose *et al.* (1972) had found that seven (22%) excreted reduced levels of this metabolite. In blood, Miller and her colleagues measured pyridoxine, pyridoxamine, and pyridoxal by selective microbiological assays. Only slight reductions, of doubtful significance, were found in the oral contraceptive users, but the mean concentration of vitamin B_6 was inversely related to the duration of steroid administration. One difficulty pointed out by the authors was that in the preliminary preparation of the blood samples trichloroacetic acid was used, which may have excluded protein-bound pyridoxal phosphate from the assay.

Plasma pyridoxal phosphate concentrations in oral contraceptive users and controls have been reported by Lumeng *et al.* (1974). Twenty percent of fifty-five women who had been taking contraceptive steroids for at least 6 months had subnormal levels. A longitudinal study of ten others showed that after an initial fall when oral contraception was commenced, there was a tendency for the plasma pyridoxal phosphate to rise again towards normal over a 6 month period. This effect may have been due to a redistribution of vitamin B_6 between tissues, or changes in dietary intake or intestinal absorption.

A series of papers from the University of Wisconsin have described a dietary study of tryptophan metabolism and vitamin B_6 nutrition in a group of oral contraceptive users and matched controls. These have been summarized in a review article (Leklem *et al.*, 1975b). The experimental design was constructed so as to compare the rate at which the two volunteer groups became depleted of vitamin B_6 while consuming an identical deficient diet, and also the rates of repletion when they were supplemented with differing doses of pyridoxine hydrochloride. The deficient diet provided 0.19 mg of pyridoxine equivalents per day.

The urinary excretion of 4-pyridoxic acid and of tryptophan metabolites after a 2 gm oral load of the amino acid, urinary cystathionine levels after a 3 gm L-methionine load, plasma pyridoxal phosphate and erythrocyte alanine aminotransferase and aspartate aminotransferase activities were used as indices of vitamin B_6 deficiency.

Before starting on the deficient diet, the oral contraceptive users excreted elevated levels of kynurenine, acetylkynurenine, 3-hydroxy-kynurenine, and xanthurenic acid compared to the controls. These differences became more marked during the period of vitamin B_6 depletion. The control subjects who were subsequently given pyridoxine hydrochloride in daily doses of 0.8 mg showed a prompt decline in tryptophan metabolite excretions, and by 3 weeks of supplementation they had reached predepletion levels. The oral contraceptive users receiving an 0.8 mg pyridoxine hydrochloride supplement also exhibited a marked reduction in excretion levels, but even after 4 weeks they were still slightly higher than the corresponding predepletion values, and significantly higher than the control subjects excretions at the same stage of study. Supplementation of the oral contraceptive users vitamin B_6 intake with 20 mg of pyridoxine hydrochloride, however, did decrease their excretions to control levels.

No difference in the rate of decline in urinary 4-pyridoxic acid excretion by the oral contraceptive users compared with the controls was apparent, during the period of vitamin B_6 depletion, nor in the rate of increase during the supplementation stage with pyridoxine hydrochloride at 0.8 mg or 2.0 mg per day. Before starting the vitamin B_6 deficient diet, the oral contraceptive-treated group had slightly lower plasma pyridoxal phosphate concentrations than the controls, and this difference was maintained, to some degree, throughout the depletion period. A supplementary dose of 0.8 mg of pyridoxine hydrochloride daily was insufficient to restore the plasma pyridoxal phosphate to predepletion levels in either group, for both the levels were higher than before the induction of deficiency when they had received 2.0 mg per day for 2–3 weeks.

The results from a study of methionine metabolism have been described earlier in this chapter (Section II, B).

Erythrocyte alanine aminotransferase was assayed throughout the study period. Initially, there was no difference between the oral contraceptive users and controls in the activity of this enzyme; the two groups showed reductions of similar degree during the vitamin B_6 depletion. Supplementation with 2.0 mg of pyridoxine hydrochloride daily, but not 0.8 mg, restored the enzyme activities of both groups to predepletion levels. As expected, addition of pyridoxal phosphate to the enzyme assay system stimulated activity to an increasing degree as the deficiency became more severe, but, again, no difference was evident between the steroid-treated group and controls. Similar changes were observed in erythrocyte aspartate aminotransferase.

This study was designed to see whether the biochemical changes induced by a dietary vitamin B_6 deficiency are accentuated by oral contraceptives. Although this appears true for tryptophan and methionine metabolism, only slight, statistically insignificant, differences were found in plasma pyridoxal phosphate, and none in urinary 4-pyridoxic acid excretion or erythrocyte aminotransferase activities. None of the oral contraceptive users had any of the reported abnormalities suggestive of vitamin B_6 deficiency before they commenced the deficient diet. But, it should be noted that, because of its complexity, only fifteen oral contraceptive users and nine controls were included in the study. Rose (1974), from a review of the literature and his own observations, concluded that biochemical evidence of vitamin B_6 deficiency can be expected in approximately 15% of women taking estrogen-containing oral contraceptives; the majority show no abnormality other than an increase in urinary tryptophan metabolites. Thus, the investigation under discussion cannot be regarded as having excluded the possibility that contraceptive steroids can cause vitamin B_6 deficiency in susceptible women.

The author's current belief is that the estrogenic component of the combination type of oral contraceptives may affect vitamin B_6 nutrition adversely by the induction of certain amino acid-metabolizing enzymes. Evidence for this effect has been discussed in Section II, B of this chapter. Increased activity of pyridoxal phosphate-dependent aminotransferases, together with an enhanced rate in the metabolic turnover of tryptophan and perhaps other amino acids, may divert the available vitamin B_6 from equally essential roles and decrease the circulating levels of the vitamin.

Two side-effects of oral contraception in which vitamin B_6 may be involved deserve special consideration: mental depression and an altered carbohydrate tolerance which is akin to that seen in adult-onset diabetes.

Several studies have indicated that mental depression occurs with increased frequency in oral contraceptive users (Larsson-Cohn, 1966; Nilsson and Almgren, 1968; Herzberg et al., 1970). Tryptophan is a precursor of the biogenic amine serotonin (5-hydroxytryptamine); low levels of 5-hydroxyindole acetic acid, the metabolite of serotonin, have been demonstrated in the cerebrospinal fluid of depressed patients (Ashcroft et al., 1966). Some depressed individuals who committed suicide had a low concentration of serotonin in the brain (Shaw et al., 1967), and tryptophan may have antidepressant activity (Coppen et al., 1967, 1972; Broadhurst, 1970).

Because of these associations, the question naturally arose of whether depression complicating oral contraception resulted from altered tryptophan metabolism. Three possible mechanisms may be postulated: divergence of tryptophan away from serotonin synthesis because of increased tryptophan oxygenase activity (Section II, A), interference with brain uptake of tryptophan by kynurenine and other metabolites of the tryptophan–niacin pathway known to be elevated in oral contraceptive users (Green and Curzon, 1970), and vitamin B_6 deficiency with resulting loss of 5-hydroxytryptophan decarboxylase activity (Winston, 1969).

Baumblatt and Winston (1970) first reported that large doses of pyridoxine had a beneficial effect on depressed oral contraceptive users, but their finding was challenged because the study was uncontrolled and of questionable validity on statistical grounds.

The matter was pursued by Adams et al. (1973) using a double-blind crossover form of clinical trial. Pyridoxine hydrochloride, 20 mg twice daily, or a placebo, was administered for 2 months to women who had developed depression for the first time while taking an estrogen-containing oral contraceptive. There was then a crossover from pyridoxine to placebo or vice versa and observation was continued for a further 2 months. Tryptophan metabolite excretion, and particularly the ratio of 3-hydroxykynurenine to 3-hydroxyanthranilic acid, urinary 4-pyridoxic acid, and erythrocyte aminotransferase levels were used as indices of vitamin B_6 deficiency. Therapeutic response was judged by a Beck self-rating depression questionnaire.

Eleven of the thirty-two patients were considered to have vitamin B_6 deficiency and these, but not the remainder, benefited from pyridoxine treatment. The placebo was without sustained effect. These data were examined statistically and the conclusion validated. A further report from this group, in which the series was enlarged to thirty-nine women, confirmed the original finding (Adams et al., 1974).

Abnormal carbohydrate metabolism brought about by the use of oral contraceptives has been investigated extensively; the characteristic change is a deterioration in glucose tolerance (Spellacy, 1969). In one longitudinal study of women before and during treatment with contraceptive steroids, 78% showed a deterioration in glucose tolerance, while in 13% the tests became frankly abnormal and were classified as indicating the presence of subclinical ("chemical") diabetes. The changes returned to normal when steroid administration was discontinued, but the duration of treatment had been relatively short (Wynn and Doar, 1970).

The significance of impaired glucose tolerance in oral contraceptive users remains to be established. Concern stems not so much from the excessive elevations in plasma glucose during tolerance testing, but from changes in the insulin response to a glucose load. In this context the report by Javier et al. (1968) is particularly significant. They found that the plasma insulin rose in the early stages of oral contraceptive use, but later, in spite of further deterioration in glucose tolerance, the insulin levels tended to be low. These observations suggest that initial peripheral insulin resistance may result, with long-term exposure to the contraceptive steroids, in exhaustion of the pancreatic islets capacity to secrete the hormone. The risk of permanent damage to pancreatic endocrine function has also been discussed by Kalkhoff *et al.* (1969) and Spellacy (1969).

Consideration of a possible association between altered carbohydrate metabolism and vitamin B_6 in oral contraceptive users arose because of some experimental studies performed by Kotake (1955). He had found that feeding rats a high tryptophan–fatty acid diet caused an elevated xanthurenic acid excretion, hyperglycemia, glycosuria, and damage to the β cells of the pancreatic islets. Similar abnormalities were produced by feeding a high tryptophan–vitamin B_6-deficient diet, and also by intraperitoneal injection of xanthurenic acid into rats receiving a normal diet. Later work showed that xanthurenic acid and insulin will form a complex *in vitro* and that this has only about half the hypoglycemic activity of an equivalent amount of free insulin when injected into a dog or rabbit (Kotake *et al.*, 1968).

Spellacy *et al.* (1972) published a preliminary report of the effect of pyridoxine treatment in twelve women whose oral glucose tolerance had deteriorated while taking contraceptive steroids. On the whole a significant improvement in glucose tolerance was achieved by giving pyridoxine 25 mg each day for 1 month, although in fact this was restricted to eight of the subjects. No attempt was made to assess vitamin B_6 nutritional status in this investigation.

Adams *et al.* (1976) studied forty-six oral contraceptive users, and classified them according to the presence or absence of biochemical evidence of vitamin B_6 deficiency. Glucose tolerance was improved by pyridoxine hydrochloride supplementation, 20 mg twice daily for 4 weeks, only in the eighteen who were considered to be deficient in the vitamin.

Recently, D. P. Rose (unpublished observations, 1976) attempted to demonstrate a deleterious effect of xanthurenic acid on carbohydrate metabolism by contraceptive steroid-treated women. Oral glucose tolerance tests were performed, and repeated after a 7-day period during which tryptophan was administered in a dose of 2 gm daily. Although increasing the dietary tryptophan intake approximately three-fold did produce a significant increase in xanthurenic acid excretion, none of the women showed any changes in their glucose tolerance or insulin responses. In the study of vitamin B_6 and carbohydrate metabolism reported by Adams *et al.* (1976), there was no significant difference in urinary xanthurenic acid excretion by those who did, and did not, respond to pyridoxine. These observations make it unlikely that the formation of an xanthurenic acid–insulin complex has a role in impaired glucose tolerance associated with oral contraception.

An alternative mechanism proposed by Adams *et al.* (1976) is based on experimental evidence that the tryptophan metabolites 3-hydroxy-anthranilic acid and quinolinic acid can inhibit gluconeogenesis by suppressing phosphoenolpyruvate carboxykinase activity. They suggested that impaired glucose tolerance in vitamin B_6-deficient oral contraceptive users arises because the levels of these metabolites are subnormal, with a consequent elevation in the activity of this enzyme. It is difficult to reconcile this hypothesis with reports that both 3-hydroxyanthranilic acid (Rose, 1966; Price *et al.*, 1972) and quinolinic acid (Rose and Toseland, 1973) are elevated in both experimental vitamin B_6 deficiency and oral contraceptive users.

Regardless of mechanism, the reports that abnormal carbohydrate metabolism by some oral contraceptive users can be reversed with pyridoxine are of considerable interest. Inevitably, together with the claims that vitamin B_6 may improve mental depression arising as a complication of contraceptive steroids, they have raised the question of whether pyridoxine supplements should be taken routinely by women employing this means of contraception.

In the author's opinion the present evidence of potential benefit is inadequate to justify such a recommendation. Further research is necessary, both to confirm the therapeutic efficacy of vitamin B_6 supplementation and to exclude the possibility that the continuous administration of pyridoxine in large doses may itself have adverse metabolic consequences.

B. Folic Acid

Shojania *et al.* (1968, 1969) were the first to report that oral contraceptive users have reduced serum and erythrocyte folic acid levels, and excrete elevated levels of formiminoglutamic acid (FIGLU) in their urine after an oral histidine load. This observation was followed by a number of case reports of women who developed megaloblastic anemia while taking contraceptive steroids. By 1970, Streiff noted that he was aware of forty-seven examples of this association, and 5 years later Lindenbaum *et al.* (1975) found twenty-nine additional cases described in the medical literature.

Clearly, in view of the population at risk any effect of oral contraceptives on folic acid nutrition is likely to be found of a minor degree for most women. Perhaps, then, it is not surprising that its very existence has become subject to controversy. Although later publications by Shojania *et al.* (1969, 1971) confirmed their original finding, at least seven other groups of workers have failed to find altered serum folate levels in oral contraceptive-treated women (Spray, 1968; McLean *et al.*, 1969; Maniego-Bautista and Bazzano, 1969; Castren and Rossi, 1970; Pritchard *et al.*, 1971; Stephens *et al.*, 1972; Paine *et al.*, 1975). On the other hand, at least six other publications had reported reduced serum and erythrocyte levels of this vitamin (Luhby *et al.*, 1971b; Wertalik *et al.*, 1972; Alperin, 1973; Roetz and Nevinny-Stickel, 1973; Gaafar *et al.*, 1973; Ahmed *et al.*, 1975). Differences in socioeconomic status, general state of nutrition, and failure to employ properly matched controls may have contributed to the discrepancy.

The duration of contraceptive use may be an important factor influencing the incidence of low serum folate levels. Thus, Shojania *et al.* (1971) studied 176 women receiving oral contraceptives and 140 untreated controls. They found that the percentage of oral contraceptive users with low serum folate levels (< 3 ng/ml.; *L. casei* assay) rose progressively with treatment duration, from 9% at less than 1 year to 21% at 2 years and 42% after 4 years. There was also a suggestion from their data that preparations containing the higher doses of contraceptive steroids had a more severe effect on the serum folate levels. None of the oral contraceptive users studied had megaloblastic anemia.

Streiff (1970) studied seven women who developed folic acid deficiency with megaloblastic anemia while taking an oral contraceptive. Their dietary intake of the vitamin appeared to be adequate. Laboratory investigation did not reveal any evidence of malabsorption, although jejunal biopsy was not performed and cases of adult celiac disease have been described in which impaired folate absorption was the only manifestation other than intestinal villous atrophy. Two of the seven patients underwent hematologic remission without folic acid therapy when oral contraceptives were discontinued.

As part of this investigation, Streiff performed an elegant absorption study to determine the mechanism whereby oral contraceptives might adversely affect folate nutritional status. Equivalent doses of pteroylpolyglutamates, which constitute most of the dietary folate, and monoglutamic folate were administered orally to nine oral contraceptive users and nine controls, and the increases in serum folate determined by serial blood sampling. All of these subjects had normal fasting serum folate concentrations. The oral contraceptive users showed a decrease in pteroylpolyglutamate absorption of approximately 50%, but normal uptakes of the monoglutamic folate; the controls absorbed both preparations to the same extent (Fig. 6). Streiff concluded from his experiment that contraceptive steroids probably inhibit jejunal pteroylglutamate hydrolase (folate conjugase). This enzyme is responsible for split-

ORAL TEST DOSE: MONOGLUTAMIC FOLATE (200 µg)

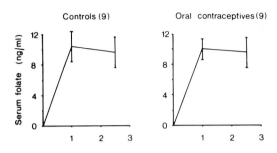

ORAL TEST DOSE: POLYGLUTAMIC FOLATE

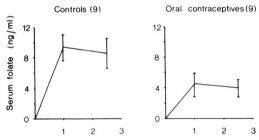

Fig. 6. Serum folate levels in 9 oral contraceptive users and 9 control women after oral administration of 200 µg of monoglutamic folate and after the molecular equivalent of polyglutamic foliate (from Streiff, 1970. *JAMA* **214,** 105, Copyright 1970, American Medical Association).

ting off the polyglutamate chain, an essential preliminary to the intestinal absorption of much of the dietary folate.

In a similar study, Necheles and Snyder (1970) observed lesser increases in serum folate after pteroylpolyglutamate ingestion by two women taking oral contraceptives than when their use had been discontinued.

The interpretation of these two investigations has not gone unquestioned. Stephens *et al.* (1972) found lesser serum folate increases in oral contraceptive users given pteroylpolyglutamate compared with controls, but this difference disappeared when they were given tissue saturating doses of folic acid prior to the test. In addition, the mean serum folate increase after pteroylmonoglutamate was also lower in the oral contraceptive-treated group when they were studied without prior folate saturation, although this difference just failed to reach statistical significance.

One interpretation of these observations is that the oral contraceptive users had a mild folic acid deficiency which was also responsible for rapid clearance of folate from the plasma. Repletion of the tissue folate stores would reverse this effect. This explanation seems unlikely, however, because there was no correlation between the fasting serum folate and the peak rise after either pteroylmonoglutamate or polyglutamate. As an alternative, the authors suggested that a direct effect of contraceptive steroids on folic acid metabolism was responsible for an increase in the plasma clearance rate of absorbed folic acid.

Shojania and Hornady (1973) also questioned the interpretation which Streiff placed on his data. They, too, performed absorption studies after their subjects had received saturating doses of folic acid and found lowered increases in serum folate after pteroylmonoglutamate or polyglutamate only in the minority of women with low fasting levels. They concluded that these women had folate malabsorption which was unrelated to oral contraceptive usage, and that in this circumstance the steroids might precipitate megaloblastic anemia by a direct effect on folic acid metabolism. Johnson et al. (1973) have described examples of this situation; two women developed megaloblastic anemia due to folic acid deficiency while taking an oral contraceptive, one of whom was found to have subclinical adult celiac disease and the other regional enteritis.

The nature of the postulated effect of oral contraceptives on folic acid metabolism remains obscure. Inhibition of jejunal folate conjugase is one possibility, and Streiff and Green (1970) have reported that this can be demonstrated in experiments in vitro. Stephens et al. (1972) stated that they failed to confirm this observation with "synthetic sex hormones", and are so quoted by Shojania and Hornady (1973). But the steroids examined in their in vitro assay system were estradiol, estrone and progesterone, and not the synthetic contraceptive steroids. The assumption that the natural estrogens and progesterone behave pharmacologically in a manner identical to contraceptive steroids is known to be erroneous in other areas, such as lipid metabolism, and may well be in the context under consideration.

Alternative mechanisms for an effect of oral contraceptives on folic acid nutrition include a redistribution of folate derivatives between the various body compartments. Da Costa and Rothenberg (1974) have described a macromolecular factor which binds folic acid in leukocyte lysates and serum from some pregnant women and oral contraceptive users. They suggest that this factor is a hormone-inducible protein, analogous to corticosteroid-binding globulin which is also elevated in pregnancy and by synthetic estrogens. Binding of folate to a plasma component such as this may render the vitamin unavailable for the performance of its coenzymic roles, and so precipitate megaloblastosis in women with a marginally adequate dietary intake or impaired intestinal absorption of folic acid.

Elsewhere in this chapter we have discussed how pyridoxal phosphate-dependent enzymes may be induced by contraceptive steroids with a possible sequestering of the vitamer. In a similar manner, sex hormones induce adaptive changes in jejunal folate-metabolizing enzymes (Stifel *et al.*, 1970). Lindenbaum *et al.* (1975), who have demonstrated abnormalities of the cervicovaginal epithelium analogous to megaloblastic dyshemopoiesis, consider that oral contraceptives cause an increased utilization of folate because they stimulate protein synthesis in estrogen target organs. In consequence, a local depletion of folate coenzymes occurs, resulting in disturbed DNA synthesis which is reflected by the abnormal cervical epithelium and, in extreme cases, megaloblastosis.

To summarize, it seems that, whatever the mechanism, the effect of oral contraceptives alone on folic acid nutrition is of minor degree. However, they may assume importance, and precipitate megaloblastic anemia, if other factors are operative. Particular consideration should be given to the possibility that this method of contraception may increase the risk of severe folic acid deficiency in malnourished populations such as those in the developing countries. One specific high-risk group may be women who become pregnant shortly after discontinuing oral contraception (Shojania *et al.*, 1971). Thus, the same factors are operative as those already discussed with regard to vitamin B_6.

C. Other Vitamins

1. *Vitamin B_{12}*

There have been a number of reports that serum vitamin B_{12} levels are reduced by oral contraceptives, but in no instance has this abnormality been associated with megaloblastic anemia. Shojania (1971) studied 106 women taking these steroids and 82 controls. Although, as a group, the oral contraceptive users had significantly lower serum vitamin B_{12} concentrations than the nonusers, in only four cases were the results classified as subnormal and they had normal hemoglobin levels.

Briggs and Briggs (1972a) determined the serum vitamin B_{12} in Africans and Europeans living in Zambia. They found that European women who were taking oral contraceptives, and African women who were not, had lower levels than European nonusers. Many of the African oral contraceptive users had extremely low vitamin B_{12} concentrations, which implies that not only may oral contraceptives reduce the circulating level of this vitamin, but that their effect summates with the consequences of poor nutrition.

Wertalik *et al.* (1972) performed serum vitamin B_{12} assays on twenty oral contraceptive users and twenty-three controls. Half of the women taking oral contraceptives had subnormal levels (less than 200 pg/ml), and 15% were considered to be unequivocally vitamin B_{12}-deficient with concentrations below 100 pg/ml. Four women were studied before commencing oral contraception and again after 2–5 months of treatment. All four showed a decrease in serum vitamin B_{12}.

The mechanism for the observed effect of oral contraceptives on serum vitamin B_{12} levels is unknown. Wertalik *et al.* (1972) were unable to confirm an earlier report by Bianchine *et al.* (1969) that these steroids increase the serum vitamin B_{12} binding capacity. However, further investigations along these lines are indicated in view of the general experience that synthetic estrogens do elevate the level of carrier proteins, such as those for iron, copper, corticosteroids, thyroxine, and, perhaps, folic acid.

In comparison with some of the other metabolic and nutritional side-effects of oral contraceptives the changes in serum vitamin B_{12} levels appear to be of minor clinical importance. An exception may be the case of African women living in areas where vitamin B_{12} deficiency occurs as a consequence of malnutrition.

2. Thiamine and Riboflavin

Erythrocyte transketolase, and more particularly the extent to which the enzyme activity is stimulated *in vitro* by the addition of thiamine pyrophosphate to the assay medium, is used as an index of thiamine nutritional status. Briggs and Briggs (1975) studied twenty professional Australian women before commencing oral contraception, and again 3 months after its use. In the pretreatment samples erythrocyte transketolase activity was stimulated by $23 \pm 7\%$ in the presence of thiamine pyrophosphate; after oral contraceptive administration the percentage stimulation was $30 \pm 11\%$. This significant increase was interpreted as indicating that contraceptive steroids will induce a mild thiamine deficiency.

A study of Indian women has been reported by Ahmed *et al.* (1975). This work is of particular value because it was concerned with a low to middle income group whose diets had been shown to be only marginally adequate for many nutrients. Oral contraception was associated with a small, but statistically significant, decrease in erythrocyte transketolase activity, but no alteration in the *in vitro* stimulation by thiamine pyrophosphate. The cause of this effect is unclear, for it is not that expected in thiamine deficiency.

Riboflavin deficiency, with angular stomatitis and glossitis, is a common nutritional problem in India and the Far Eastern countries. It is prevalent particularly in pregnant women from the poorer segments of the population (Iyengar, 1973). The vitamin may be measured directly in blood or urine, but a convenient alternative is the assay of erythrocyte glutathione reductase, and the degree of stimulation which occurs *in vitro* when FAD is added to the incubation medium.

In their nutritional survey, Ahmed *et al.* (1975) found biochemical evidence of riboflavin deficiency in many of their control women, although none had clinical manifestations. Treatment with oral contraceptives produced a marked decline in erythrocyte glutathione reductase activity, a corresponding increase in stimulation *in vitro* by FAD, and a fall in the erythrocyte riboflavin concentration. A few of these women did develop glossitis.

Similar reports on the effect of oral contraceptives on erythrocyte glutathione reductase have been published from Zambia (Briggs and Briggs, 1974) and Thailand (Sanpitak and Chayutimonkul, 1974).

3. *Ascorbic Acid*

Briggs and Briggs (1972b) measured leukocyte and platelet ascorbic acid, and found it to be reduced in oral contraceptive users. Leukocyte ascorbic acid was assayed before and after supplementation with 50–200 mg of the vitamin each day for 3 weeks by McLeroy and Schendel (1973). The mean ascorbic acid intake calculated from 3-day dietary records, was 86±45 mg for sixty-three oral contraceptive users and 84 ± 48 mg for sixty-three age-matched female controls. These intakes should have been more than sufficient to maintain high tissue vitamin C levels, but before supplementation the experimental group had low leukocyte ascorbic acid concentrations, and, unlike the controls, no change occurred as a result of supplementation.

Rivers and Devine (1972) measured plasma ascorbic acid in four women taking oral contraceptives and two controls over 2½ menstrual cycles. They were all given saturating levels of ascorbic acid. In the controls, the plasma ascorbic acid concentrations exhibited a cyclic pattern, being highest at about the time of ovulation. This cyclic pattern was not observed in the oral contraceptive users, and the plasma ascorbic acid level for all phases of the cycle was lower than in the controls. Urinary ascorbic acid excretion was determined after loading doses of the vitamin. There was no consistent relationship between ascorbic acid excretion and fasting plasma levels, nor was the urinary ascorbic acid related to the phase of the menstrual cycle in either controls or oral contraceptive users.

As is the case with many of the nutritional side-effects of the oral contraceptives, it appears that the estrogenic component is responsible for altered plasma and tissue ascorbic acid concentrations. Briggs and Briggs (1972b, 1973) reported that whereas postmenopausal women receiving estrogen replacement therapy had reduced ascorbic acid levels in plasma, leukocytes and platelets, progestogen administration was without effect. The mechanisms involved are not known. Ceruloplasmin, which is increased in the plasma of oral contraceptive users (Section II, C) has ascorbic acid oxidase activity, and several workers have suggested that this may be responsible for destruction of the vitamin (Briggs and Briggs, 1972b; McLeroy and Schendel, 1973; Kalesh et al., 1971). A review article by Rivers (1975) describes unpublished work from his laboratory which does not support this explanation. He studied the catabolism and tissue uptake of ascorbic acid in rats and guinea pigs treated with ethinylestradiol, norgestrel, a combination of these steroids, or progesterone. The preliminary data suggest that the contraceptive steroids do not affect the rate of ascorbic acid breakdown, but that they do alter tissue uptake patterns. It may be that changes in ascorbic acid distribution between the various body tissues is responsible for the reduction in blood levels.

The clinical significance of the effect of oral contraceptives on ascorbic acid levels is doubtful at the present time. Although the reported reductions in leukocytes are of the order of 30 to 40%, the absolute values are still well above those seen in scorbutic patients. Further research is clearly indicated, but current knowledge does not provide a basis on which to recommend routine supplementation with the vitamin in women using this form of contraception.

4. Vitamins A and E

Experimentally induced increases in circulating vitamin A produce congenital malformations in animals, and this effect is known to be accentuated by cortisone administration. Estrogens increase tissue storage of vitamin A when given to rats, whereas progestogens exert the reverse effect; stilbestrol, when used to suppress lactation, reduces the plasma vitamin A concentration (Gal et al., 1971). It was these considerations which led to the study of vitamin A in women using oral contraceptives.

Gal et al. (1971) found that the plasma vitamin A in oral contraceptive users was increased by 30–80%; there was no effect on β-carotene levels. This observation has been confirmed by other workers (Briggs et al.,

1972; Wild *et al.*, 1974; Yeung, 1974; Yeung and Chan, 1975). It appears that the estrogenic component is responsible for the abnormality; the progestogen norethindrone administered alone was without effect at a low dose, but at a higher concentration it did appear to enhance the effect of mestranol (Yeung and Chan, 1975). Briggs *et al.* (1972) reported that medroxyprogesterone acetate was without effect on the plasma vitamin A.

Several mechanisms have been postulated, including increased plasma-binding, altered metabolism, and a redistribution of the tissue stores. One possibility is that the estrogen induces an elevated level of plasma retinol-binding protein; this would be in keeping with the known effects of the synthetic estrogens on transport proteins. Yeung (1974) was unable to produce an increase in the plasma vitamin A levels of rats by treatment with contraceptive steroids, but there were increases in the liver depletion rate and rate of utilization of vitamin A.

The significance of these observations is unclear. Wild *et al.* (1974) could not detect an increased incidence of spontaneous abortion or congenital abnormalities in fifty-five women with plasma vitamin A levels in early pregnancy comparable to those of oral contraceptive users. Also, women who became pregnant 2–11 weeks after discontinuing oral contraception did not show plasma vitamin A levels which were significantly different from pregnant women who had not taken oral contraceptives. One possibility worthy of careful investigation is that binding of vitamin A to elevated concentrations of retinol-binding protein may aggravate a preexisting dietary deficiency. This could be of importance in those areas of the world where vitamin A deficiency is endemic.

An elevation in plasma vitamin E concentrations has been reported in oral contraceptive users (Yeung and Chan, 1975). This effect probably arises because vitamin E circulates bound to low-density lipoproteins and these are increased in oral contraceptive users. No clinical consequences have been ascribed to this alteration in vitamin E nutritional status.

IV. METALS

A number of publications have described the effect of oral contraceptives on metals, including iron, copper, zinc, and magnesium. In part, these changes appear as a consequence of increases in plasma transport globulins.

The serum iron and ironbinding capacity are elevated in oral contraceptive users. Burton (1967) considered that the change in serum iron was secondary to an estrogen-induced elevation in the iron-binding protein, transferrin. Although one study, by Mardell and Zilva (1967), showed serum iron and iron-binding capacity to vary independently in oral contraceptive-treated women, this still seems the most likely explanation. An additional factor in some women may be that the contraceptive steroids regulate previously excessive menstrual blood loss, and so permit repletion of the iron stores. Thus, Burton (1967) did find a higher packed blood cell volume in the oral contraceptive users compared with controls.

Oral contraceptives cause an increase in serum copper which is attributable to steroidal induction of ceruloplasmin, the α_2-copper-binding globulin. Carruthers *et al.* (1966) showed that there is a positive correlation between serum copper and ceruloplasmin levels in oral contraceptive users, and that despite the high levels the urinary copper excretion is normal. Although others have confirmed the effect of contraceptive steroids on serum copper, their influence on zinc levels is less clear. Halsted *et al.* (1968) determined both trace metals in oral contraceptive users and women in the last trimester of pregnancy. The two groups of subjects showed elevated serum copper, but decreased zinc concentrations, compared with control values. However, in another study (O'Leary and Spellacy, 1969), although the previously reported changes in circulating copper and zinc associated with pregnancy were confirmed, both metals were found to be increased in oral contraceptive users.

A similar conflict exists over the effect of oral contraceptives on serum magnesium levels; Goldsmith *et al.* (1970) reported reduced concentrations, whereas Dale and Simpson (1972) found no change.

A review of the literature suggests that the influence of oral contraceptives on metals is of little clinical importance, and is unlikely to result in any nutritional complications.

V. CONCLUSIONS AND FUTURE RESEARCH

This review has shown that oral contraceptives affect all of the recognized classes of nutrients; some of these effects are primarily metabolic in character, for example those involving carbohydrates, while others do appear to result in nutritional deficiencies. But, although widespread biochemical changes have been identified, in most cases their clinical significance remains in doubt.

The complexity of the problem is well illustrated by a consideration of tryptophan metabolism and vitamin B_6 nutrition. In general, published studies have reported a disturbance in the metabolism of this amino acid, with complete reversal after treatment with large doses of pyridoxine, in about three-quarters of oral contraceptive users. But, in the author's experience this situation is changing; the overall incidence of abnormal tryptophan metabolism has declined because most women are now taking the low dose estrogen oral contraceptives. Some of these preparations have little or no effect on the urinary excretion of tryptophan metabolites because not only is their estrogen content small (50 μg), but the action of these steroids is opposed by the progestogenic component. It remains to be seen whether the new generation of oral contraceptives, which contain only 30 μg of estrogen, have any adverse effect at all on tryptophan metabolism.

We have discussed at length the relationship between altered tryptophan metabolism in oral contraceptive users and vitamin B_6 nutritional status. The essential point is that, in this particular situation, the determination of urinary tryptophan metabolite excretions does not provide a reliable indication of vitamin B_6 deficiency. Only a minority of oral contraceptive-treated women with abnormal tryptophan metabolism, perhaps 15–20%, have direct evidence of vitamin B_6 deficiency, as judged by erythrocyte aminotransferase activities, plasma pyridoxal phosphate levels, and urinary 4-pyridoxic acid excretions. Nevertheless, the beneficial effects of treatment with large doses of pyridoxine on two complications of oral contraception, impaired glucose tolerance and mental depression, provide the only two examples of clinically significant abnormalities which appear to be associated with a nutritional factor. It is to be hoped that research in these two important areas will be continued and expanded.

The list of other nutritional changes in oral contraceptive users is an impressive one; hypoalbuminemia, hypoaminoacidemias, subnormal folate, vitamin B_{12}, ascorbic acid, thiamine and riboflavin levels, and increases in plasma vitamin A and E have all been discussed. But again, there is considerable uncertainty as to their practical importance.

Most of the reported studies have been concerned with well-nourished women in the United States or Western Europe. The pressing need now is for investigations located in those parts of the world where population control is mandatory, but nutrition is inadequate because of dietary deficiencies. It is in this setting that the otherwise minor effects of oral contraception may be sufficient to precipitate clinically overt disease in women whose nutritional status is already compromised.

Inevitably, the question has arisen as to whether all women taking an oral contraceptive should receive vitamin supplements to correct possible deficiencies. A multivitamin preparation designed specifically with this in mind, and advertised as such, has been marketed in the United States; in Spain an oral contraceptive preparation is available which has a

25 mg dose of pyridoxine incorporated into each tablet. It is the author's opinion that there is no justification for such routine medication. Evidence is lacking that the reported biochemical abnormalities are sufficient to cause concern, whilst the possible adverse effects of long-term treatment with large doses of vitamin B_6 are unknown. These effects may not be nutritional; the stimulation of pyridoxal phosphate-requiring enzymes has been discussed elsewhere in this chapter. But, in addition, recent work has shown that vitamin B_6 administration can influence pituitary hormones, probably by altering the concentrations of neurotransmitters, such as 5-hydroxytryptamine and dopamine in the hypothalamus.

REFERENCES

Adams, P. W., Wynn, V., Rose, D. P., Seed, M., Folkard, J., and Strong, R. (1973). Effect of pyridoxine hydrochloride (vitamin B_6) upon depression associated with oral contraception. *Lancet* **1,** 897–904.
Adams, P. W., Wynn, V., Seed, M., and Folkard, J. (1974). Vitamin B_6, depression and oral contraception. *Lancet* **2,** 516–517.
Adams, P. W., Wynn, V., Folkard, J., and Seed, M. (1976). Influence of oral contraceptives, pyridoxine (vitamin B_6), and tryptophan on carbohydrate metabolism. *Lancet* **1,** 759–764.
Ahmed, F., Bamji, M. S., and Iyengar, L. (1975). Effect of oral contraceptive agents on vitamin nutrition status. *Am. J. Clin. Nutr.* **28,** 606–615.
Alperin, J. B. (1973). Folate metabolism in women using oral contraceptive agents. *Am. J. Clin. Nutr.* **26,** XIX (abstr.).
Altman, K., and Greengard, O. (1966). Correlation of kynurenine excretion with tryptophan pyrrolase levels in disease and after hydrocortisone induction. *J. Clin. Invest.* **45,** 1527–1534.
Aly, H. E., Donald, E. A., and Simpson, M. H. W. (1971). Oral contraceptives and vitamin B_6 metabolism. *Am. J. Clin. Nutr.* **24,** 297–303.
Ashcroft, G. W., Crawford, T. B. B., Eccleston, D., Sharman, D. F., MacDougall, E. J., Stanton, J. B., and Binns, J. K. (1966). 5-Hydroxyindole compounds in the cerebrospinal fluid of patients with psychiatric or neurological diseases. *Lancet* **2,** 1049–1052.
Baumblatt, M. J., and Winston, F. (1970). Pyridoxine and the pill. *Lancet* **2,** 832–833.
Bianchine, J. R., Bonnlander, B., MaCaraeg, P. V. J., Hersey, R., Bianchine, J. W., and McIntyre, P. A. (1969). Serum vitamin B_{12} binding capacity and oral contraceptive hormones. *J. Clin. Endocrinol. Metab.* **29,** 1425–1428.
Braidman, I. P., and Rose, D. P. (1971). Effects of sex hormones on the glucocorticoid-inducible enzymes concerned with amino acid metabolism in rat liver. *Endocrinology* **89,** 1250–1255.
Briggs, M. H., and Briggs, M. (1972a). Endocrine effects on serum vitamin B_{12}. *Lancet* **2,** 1037.
Briggs, M. H., and Briggs, M. (1972b). Vitamin C requirements and oral contraceptives. *Nature (London)* **238,** 277.

Briggs, M. H., and Briggs, M. (1973). Vitamin C and colds. *Lancet* **1,** 998.

Briggs, M. H., and Briggs, M. (1974). Oral contraceptives and vitamin nutrition. *Lancet* **1,** 1234-1235.

Briggs, M. H., and Briggs, M. (1975). Thiamine status and oral contraceptives. *Contraception* **11,** 151-154.

Briggs, M. H., Pitchford, A. G., Staniford, M., Barker, H. M., and Taylor, D. (1970). Metabolic effects of steroid contraceptives. *Adv. Steroid Biochem. Pharmacol.* **2,** 111-222.

Briggs, M. H., Briggs, M., and Bennun, M. (1972). Steroid contraceptives and plasma carotenoids. *Contraception* **6,** 275-280.

Broadhurst, A. D. (1970). L-Tryptophan versus E. C. T. *Lancet* **1,** 1392-1393.

Brown, R. R., Yess, N., Price, J. M., Linkswiler, H., Swan, P., and Hankes, L. V. (1965). Vitamin B_6 depletion in man: Urinary excretion of quinolinic acid and niacin metabolites. *J. Nutr.* **87,** 419-423.

Burke, C. W. (1970). The effect of oral contraceptives on cortisol metabolism. *J. Clin. Pathol.* **23,** suppl. 3, 11-18.

Burton, J. L. (1967). Effect of oral contraceptives on hemoglobin, packed-cell volume, serum iron, and total iron-binding capacity in healthy women. *Lancet* **1,** 978-980.

Carruthers, M. E., Hobbs, C. B., and Warren, R. L. (1966). Raised serum copper and caeruloplasmin levels in subjects taking oral contraceptives. *J. Clin. Pathol.* **19,** 498-500.

Castren, O. M., and Rossi, R. R. (1970). Effect of oral contraceptives on serum folic acid content. *J. Obstet. Gynaecol. Br. Commonw.* **77,** 548-550.

Cinnamon, A. D., and Beaton, J. R. (1970). Biochemical assessment of vitamin B_6 status in man. *Am. J. Clin. Nutr.* **23,** 696-702.

Coelingh Bennink, H. J. T., and Schrews, W. H. P. (1974). Disturbance of tryptophan metabolism and its correction during hormonal contraception. *Contraception* **9,** 347-356.

Coppen, A., Shaw, D. M., Hertzberg, B., and Maggs, R. (1967). Tryptophan in the treatment of depression. *Lancet* **2,** 1178-1180.

Coppen, A., Brooksbank, B. W. L., and Peet, M. (1972). Tryptophan concentration in the cerebrospinal fluid of depressed patients. *Lancet* **1,** 1393.

Craft, I. L., and Peters, T. J. (1971). Quantiative changes in plasma amino acids induced by oral contraceptives. *Clin. Sci.* **41,** 301-307.

Craft, I. L., and Wise, I. J. (1969). Oral contraceptives and plasma amino acids. *Nature (London)* **222,** 487-488.

Craft, I. L., Wise, I. J., and Briggs, M. H. (1970). Oral contraceptives and amino acid utilization. *Am. J. Obstet. Gynecol.* **108,** 1120-1125.

Da Costa, M., and Rothenberg, S. P. (1974). Appearance of a folate binder in leukocytes and serum of women who are pregnant or taking oral contraceptives. *J. Lab. Clin. Med.* **83,** 207-214.

Dale, E., and Simpson, G. (1972). Serum magnesium levels of women taking an oral or long-term injectable progestational contraceptive. *Obstet. Gynecol.* **39,** 115-119.

Doberenz, A. R., Van Miller, J. P., Green, J. R., and Beaton, J. R. (1971). Vitamin B_6 depletion in women using oral contraceptives as determined by erythrocyte glutamic-pyruvic transaminase activities. *Proc. Soc. Exp. Biol. Med.* **137,** 1100-1103.

Edozien, J. C. (1960). The serum proteins in kwashiorkor. *J. Pediats.* **57,** 594-603.

Eisenfeld, A. (1974). Oral contraceptives: Ethinyl estradiol binds with higher affinity than mestranol to macromolecules from the sites of anti-fertility action. *Endocrinology* **97,** 803-807.

184   David P. Rose

Gaafar, A., Toppozada, H. K., and Hozayen, A. (1973). Study of folate status in long-term Egyptian users of oral contraceptive pills. *Contraception* **8**, 43-52.

Gal, I., Parkinson, C., and Craft, I. (1971). Effects of oral contraceptives on human plasma vitamin A levels. *Br. Med. J.* **2**, 436-438.

Goldsmith, N., Pace, N., Baumberger, J., and Ury, H. (1970). Magnesium and citrate during the menstrual cycle: Effect of an oral contraceptive on serum magnesium. *Fertil. Steril.* **21**, 292-300.

Green, A. R., and Curzon, G. (1970). The effect of tryptophan metabolites on brain 5-hydroxytryptamine metabolism. *Biochem. Pharmacol.* **19**, 2061-2068.

Halsted, J., Hackley, B., and Smith, J. (1968). Plasma zinc and copper in pregnancy and after oral contraceptives. *Lancet* **2**, 278-279.

Herzberg, B. N., Johnson, A. L., and Brown, S. (1970). Depressive symptoms and oral contraceptives. *Br. Med. J.* **4**, 142-145.

Hønger, P. E., and Rossing, N. (1969). Albumin metabolism and oral contraception. *Clin. Sci.* **36**, 41-45.

Inman, W. H. W., Vessey, M. P., Westerholm, B., and Engelund, A. (1970). Thromboembolic disease and the steroidal content of oral contraceptives: A report to the Committee on Safety of Drugs. *Br. Med. J.* **2**, 203-209.

Iyengar, L. (1973). Oral lesions in pregnancy. *Lancet* **1**, 680-681.

Javier, Z., Gershberg, H., and Hulse, M. (1968). Ovulatory suppressants, estrogens, and carbohydrate metabolism. *Metab. Clin. Exp.* **17**, 443-456.

Johnson, G. K., Geenen, J. E., Hensley, G. T., and Soergel, K. H. (1973). Small intestinal disease, folate deficiency anemia, and oral contraceptive agents. *Am. J. Dig. Dis.* **18**, 185-190.

Kalesh, D. G., Mallikarjuneswara, V. R., and Clemetson, C. A. B. (1971). Effect of estrogen containing oral contraceptives on platelet and plasma ascorbic acid concentrations. *Contraception* **4**, 183-192.

Kalkhoff, R. K., Kim, H. J., and Stoddard, F. J. (1969). Acquired subclinical diabetes mellitus in women receiving oral contraceptive agents. *In* "Metabolic Effects of Gonadal Hormones and Contraceptive Steroids" (H. A. Salhanick, D. M. Kipnis, and R. L. Vande Wiele, eds.), pp. 193-203. Plenum, New York.

Kotake, Y. (1955). Xanthurenic acid, an abnormal metabolite of tryptophan and the diabetic symptoms caused in albino rats by its production. *J. Biochem. (Tokyo)* **2**, 157-171.

Kotake, Y., Sotokawa, T., Murakami, E., Hisatake, A., Abe, M., and Ikeda, Y. (1968). Studies on the xanthurenic acid–insulin complex. II. Physiological activities. *J. Biochem. (Tokyo)* **63**, 578-581.

Larsson-Cohn, U. (1966). An appraisal of the clinical effect of three different oral contraceptive agents and their influence on transaminase activity. *Acta Obstet. Gynecol. Scand.* **45**, 499-514.

Laurell, C. B., Kullander, S., and Thorell, J. (1968). Effect of administration of a combined estrogen-progestin contraceptive on the level of individual plasma proteins. *Scand. J. Clin. Lab. Invest.* **21**, 337-343.

Leklem, J. E., Brown, R. R., Rose, D. P., Linkswiler, H., and Arend, R. A. (1975a). Metabolism of tryptophan and niacin in oral contraceptive users receiving controlled intakes of vitamin B₆. *Am. J. Clin. Nutr.* **28**, 146-156.

Leklem, J. E., Brown, R. R., Rose, D. P., and Linkswiler, H. M. (1975b). Vitamin B₆ requirements of women using oral contraceptives. *Am. J. Clin. Nutr.* **28**, 535-541.

Lindenbaum, J., Whitehead, N., and Rayner, F. (1975). Oral contraceptive hormones, folate metabolism, and the cervical epithelium. *Am. J. Clin. Nutr.* **28**, 346-353.

Luhby, A. L., Brin, M., Gordon, M., David, P., Murphy, M., and Spiegel, H. (1971a). Vitamin B_6 metabolism in users of oral contraceptive agents. I. Abnormal urinary xanthurenic acid excretion and its correction by pyridoxine. *Am. J. Clin. Nutr.* **24,** 684-693.

Luhby, A. L., Shimizu, N., Davis, P., and Cooperman, J. M. (1971b). Folic acid deficiency in users of oral contraceptive agents. *Fed. Proc., Fed. Am. Soc. Exp. Biol.* **30,** 239.

Lumeng, L., Cleary, R. E., and Li, T. K. (1974). Effect of oral contraceptives on the plasma concentration of pyridoxal phosphate. *Am. J. Clin. Nutr.* **27,** 326-333.

McLean, F. W., Heine, M. W., Held, B., and Streiff, R. R. (1969). Relationship between the oral contraceptive and folic acid metabolism: serum folate concentrations. *Am. J. Obstet. Gynecol.* **104,** 745-747.

McLeroy, V. J., and Schendel, H. E. (1973). Influence of oral contraceptives on ascorbic acid concentrations in healthy, sexually mature women. *Am. J. Clin. Nutr.* **26,** 191-196.

Maniego-Bautista, L. P., and Bazzano, G. (1969). Effect of oral contraceptives on serum lipid and folate levels. *J. Lab. Clin. Med.* **74,** 988.

Mardell, M., and Zilva, J. F. (1967). Effect of oral contraceptives on the variations in serum-iron during the menstrual cycle. *Lancet* **2,** 1323-1325.

Mason, M., and Gullekson, E. (1960). Estrogen-enzyme interactions: Inhibition and protection of kynurenine transaminase by the sulfate esters of diethylstilbestrol, estradiol, and estrone. *J. Biol. Chem.* **235,** 1312-1316.

Mendenhall, H. W. (1970). Effect of oral contraceptives on serum protein concentrations. *Am. J. Obstet. Gynecol.* **109,** 140-149.

Miller, L. T., Benson, E. M., Edwards, M. A., and Young, J. (1974). Vitamin B_6 metabolism in women using oral contraceptives. *Am. J. Clin. Nutr.* **27,** 797-805.

Musa, B. U., Doe, R. P., and Seal, U.S. (1967). Serum protein alterations produced in women by synthetic estrogens. *J. Clin. Endocrinol. Metab.* **27,** 1463-1469.

Necheles, T. F., and Snyder, L. M. (1970). Malabsorption of folate polyglutamates associated with oral contraceptive therapy. *N. Engl. J. Med.* **282,** 858-859.

Nilsson, A., and Almgren, P. E. (1968). Psychiatric symptoms during the postpartum period as related to use of oral contraceptives. *Br. Med. J.* **2,** 453-455.

Ogasawara, H., Hagino, Y., and Kotake, Y. (1962). Kynurenine transaminase, kynureninase and the increase of xanthurenic acid excretion. *J. Biochem. (Tokyo)* **52,** 162-166.

O'Leary, J. A., and Spellacy, W. N. (1969). Zinc and copper levels in pregnant women and those taking oral contraceptives. *Am. J. Obstet. Gynecol.* **103,** 131-132.

Paine, C. J., Grafton, W. D., Dickson, V. L., and Eichner, E. R. (1975). Oral contraceptives, serum folate, and hematologic status. *J. Am. Med. Assoc.* **231,** 731-733.

Park, Y. K., and Linkswiler, H. (1970). Effect of vitamin B_6 depletion in adult men on the excretion of cystathionine and other methionine metabolites. *J. Nutr.* **100,** 110-116.

Price, J. M., Thornton, M. J., and Mueller, L. M. (1967). Tryptophan metabolism in women using steroid hormones for ovulation control. *Am. J. Clin. Nutr.* **20,** 452-456.

Price, S. A., Rose, D. P., and Toseland, P. A. (1972). Effects of dietary vitamin B_6 deficiency and oral contraceptives on the spontaneous urinary excretion of 3-hydroxyanthranilic acid. *Am. J. Clin. Nutr.* **25,** 494-498.

Pritchard, J. A., Scott, D. E., and Whalley, P. J. (1971). Maternal folate deficiency and pregnancy wastage. IV. Effects of folic acid supplements, anticonvulsants, and oral contraceptives. *Am. J. Obstet. Gynecol.* **109,** 341-346.

Raica, N., and Sauberlich, H. E. (1964). Blood-cell transaminase activity in human vitamin B_6 deficiency. *Am. J. Clin. Nutr.* **15,** 67-72.

186   David P. Rose

Rivers, J. M. (1975). Oral contraceptives and ascorbic acid. *Am. J. Clin. Nutr.* **28,** 550–554.
Rivers, J. M., and Devine, M. M. (1972). Plasma ascorbic acid concentrations and oral contraceptives. *Am. J. Clin. Nutr.* **25,** 684–689.
Rivlin, R. S., and Melmon, K. L. (1965). Cortisone-provoked depression of plasma tyrosine concentration: Relation to enzyme induction in man. *J. Clin. Invest.* **44,** 1690–1698.
Robertson, G. S. (1967). Serum protein and cholinesterase changes in association with contraceptive pills. *Lancet* **1,** 232–233.
Roetz, R., and Nevinny-Stickel, J. (1973). Serumfolat, Serumeisen und totale Eisenbindungskapazität des Serums unter hormonaler Kontrazeption. Ergebnisse einer prospektiven Untersuchung. *Geburtshilfe Frauenheilkd.* **33,** 629–635.
Rose, D. P. (1966). The influence of oestrogens upon tryptophan metabolism in man. *Clin. Sci.* **31,** 265–272.
Rose, D. P. (1974). Assessment of tryptophan metabolism and vitamin B₆ nutrition in pregnancy and oral contraceptive users. *In* "Biochemistry of Women: Methods for Clinical Investigation" (A. S. Curry and J. V. Hewitt, eds.), pp. 317–349. CRC Press, Cleveland, Ohio.
Rose, D. P., and Adams, P. W. (1972). Oral contraceptives and tryptophan metabolism: effects of oestrogen in low dose combined with a progestagen and of a low-dose progestagen (megestrol acetate) given alone. *J. Clin. Pathol.* **25,** 252–258.
Rose, D. P., and Cramp, D. G. (1970). Reduction of plasma tyrosine by oral contraceptives and oestrogens: A possible consequence of tyrosine aminotransferase induction. *Clin. Chim. Acta* **29,** 49–53.
Rose, D. P., and Toseland, P. A. (1973). Urinary excretion of quinolinic acid and other tryptophan metabolites after deoxypyridoxine or oral contraceptive administration. *Metab., Clin. Exp.* **22,** 165–171.
Rose, D. P., Brown, R. R., and Price, J. M. (1968). Metabolism of tryptophan to nicotinic acid derivatives by women taking oestrogen-progestogen preparations. *Nature (London)* **291,** 1259–1260.
Rose, D. P., Strong, R., Adams, P. W., and Harding, P. E. (1972). Experimental vitamin B₆ deficiency and the effect of oestrogen-containing oral contraceptives on tryptophan metabolism and vitamin B₆ requirements. *Clin. Sci.* **42,** 465–477.
Rose, D. P., Strong, R., Folkard, J., and Adams, P. W. (1973a). Erythrocyte aminotransferase activities in women using oral contraceptives and the effect of vitamin B₆ supplementation. *Am. J. Clin. Nutr.* **26,** 48–52.
Rose, D. P., Adams, P. W., and Strong, R. (1973b). Influence of the progestogenic component of oral contraceptives on tryptophan metabolism. *Br. J. Obstet. Gynecol.* **80,** 82–85.
Rose, D. P., Leklem, J. E., Brown, R. R., and Potera, C. (1976). Effect of oral contraceptives and vitamin B₆ supplements on alanine and glycine metabolism. *Am. J. Clin. Nutr.* **29,** 956–960.
Salkeld, R. M., Knörr, K., and Korner, W. F. (1973). The effect of oral contraceptives on vitamin B₆ status. *Clin. Chim. Acta* **49,** 195–199.
Sanpitak, N., and Chayutimonkul, L. (1974). Oral contraceptives and riboflavin nutrition. *Lancet* **1,** 836–837.
Shaw, D. M., Camps, F. E., and Eccleston, E. G. (1967). 5-Hydroxytryptamine in the hind-brain of depressive suicides. *Br. J. Psychiatry* **113,** 1407–1411.
Shojania, A. M. (1971). Effect of oral contraceptives on vitamin B₁₂ metabolism. *Lancet* **2,** 932.
Shojania, A. M., and Hornady, G. J. (1973). Oral contraceptives and folate absorption. *J. Lab. Clin. Med.* **82,** 869–875.

Shojania, A. M., Hornady, G., and Barnes, P. H. (1968). Oral contraceptives and serum folate level. *Lancet* **1,** 1376–1377.
Shojania, A. M., Hornady, G., and Barnes, P. H. (1969). Oral contraceptives and folate metabolism. *Lancet* **1,** 886.
Shojania, A. M., Hornady, G. J., and Barnes, P. H. (1971). The effect of oral contraceptives on folate metabolism. *Am. J. Obstet. Gynecol.* **111,** 782–791.
Silverberg, S. G., and Makowski, E. L. (1975). Endometrial carcinoma in young women taking oral contraceptives. *Obstet. Gynecol.* **46,** 503–506.
Spellacy, W. N. (1969). A review of carbohydrate metabolism and the oral contraceptives. *Am. J. Obstet. Gynecol.* **104,** 448–460.
Spellacy, W. N., Buhi, W. C., and Birk, S. A. (1972). The effects of vitamin B_6 on carbohydrate metabolism in women taking steroid contraceptives: Preliminary report. *Contraception* **6,** 265–273.
Spray, G. H. (1968). Oral contraceptives and serum folate levels. *Lancet* **2,** 110–111.
Stephens, M. E. M., Craft, I., Peters, T. J., and Hoffbrand, A. V. (1972). Oral contraceptives and folate metabolism. *Clin. Sci.* **42,** 405–414.
Stifel, F. B., Herman, R. H., and Rosensweig, N. S. (1970). Dietary regulation of glycolytic enzymes X. The effect of oral, intramuscular and conjugated sex steroids on jejunal folate-metabolizing enzyme activities in normal and castrated male and female rats. *Biochim. Biophys. Acta* **222,** 71–78.
Streiff, R. R. (1970). Folate deficiency and oral contraceptives. *J. Am. Med. Assoc.* **214,** 105–108.
Streiff, R. R., and Green, B. (1970). Drug inhibition of folate conjugase. *Clin. Res.* **18,** 418.
Ueda, T. (1967). Studies on the intracellular change of vitamin B_6 content and kynurenine aminotransferase activity in the vitamin B_6 deficient rat. *Nagoya J. Med. Sci.* **30,** 259–268.
Wertalik, L. F., Metz, E. N., LoBuglio, A. F., and Balcerzak, S. P. (1972). Decreased serum B_{12} levels with oral contraceptive use. *J. Am. Med. Assoc.* **221,** 1371–1374.
Wild, J., Schorah, C. J., and Smithells, R. W. (1974). Vitamin A, pregnancy and oral contraceptives. *Br. Med. J.* **1,** 57–59.
Winston, F. (1969). Oral contraceptives and depression. *Lancet* **2,** 377.
Wolf, H., Brown, R. R., Price, J. M., and Madsen, P. O. (1970). Effect of hormones on the biosynthesis of nicotinic acid from tryptophan in man. *J. Clin. Endocrinol. Metale.* **30,** 380–385.
Wynn, V., and Doar, J. W. H. (1970). Effects of oral contraceptives on carbohydrate metabolism. *J. Clin. Pathol.* **23,** Suppl. 3, 19–36.
Yeung, D. L. (1974). Effects of oral contraceptives on vitamin A metabolism in the human and the rat. *Am. J. Clin. Nutr.* **27,** 125–129.
Yeung, D. L., and Chan, P. L. (1975). Effects of a progestogen and a sequential type oral contraceptive on plasma vitamin A, vitamin E, cholesterol and triglycerides. *Am. J. Clin. Nutr.* **28,** 686–691.
Zinneman, H. H., Musa, B. U., and Doe, R. P. (1965). Changes in plasma and urinary amino acids following estrogen administration to males. *Metab., Clin. Exp.* **14,** 1214–1219.
Zinneman, H. H., Seal, U. S., and Doe, R. P. (1967). Urinary amino acids in pregnancy, following progesterone, and estrogen-progesterone. *J. Clin. Endocrinol. Metab.* **27,** 397–405.

7

Nutritional Impact of Intestinal Drug–Microbe Interactions

R. A. PRINS

I. INTRODUCTION AND DEFINITIONS

When a drug is ingested or in some other way reaches the lumen of the gastrointestinal tract, at least some of the drug molecules will interact with the microorganisms residing there. It is now recognized that the microflora in the intestines can metabolize a large number of both exogenous and endogenous compounds and that drug metabolism in animals is influenced by the character of the flora.

A drug may affect the growth of these bacteria. It can act as a bacteriostat, a bactericide, or it may even act as a stimulator of bacterial growth. In all these cases, changes will be brought about in the number of microbial cells, and in the amounts and proportions of fermentation products turned out by these microbes, some at the benefit of their hosts.

A drug may also be profoundly altered by microbial metabolism, thereby losing old and acquiring new properties. Depending upon the action of the drug one is studying, the compound can be detoxified or activated. The microbial drug metabolites may cause several effects of toxicological or of nutritional importance.

According to the dictionary, a drug is "any substance used in the treatment of disease, healing or relieving pain". In this chapter the term drug should be read to include all other foreign compounds and anutrients present in feeds either naturally (e.g., plant secondary compounds), added intentionally (feed additives), or as contaminants, and which have a profound influence on the gastrointestinal flora or are converted to more or less toxic products by microbial metabolism in the gut.

Before discussing the possible nutritional importance of drug–microbe interactions in the alimentary tract, it is necessary first to deal with the role of the intestinal microbes in host nutrition and to review briefly the major types of biochemical reactions involved in microbial drug transformations in the gut.

II.   THE ROLE OF THE INTESTINAL MICROFLORA IN HOST NUTRITION

The nutritional importance of intestinal drug–microbe interactions depends on the role of the intestinal flora in host nutrition. The participation by intestinal microorganisms in the digestion of food components in its turn depends upon the presence of segments of the alimentary tract, where digesta can be retained for prolonged periods of time. In a large number of animal species, certain regions of the gut have become enlarged to become storage organs, permitting retention of the food; here we find massive growing populations of anaerobic microbes. These microbes ferment many food components, or use compounds present in digestive secretions and sloughed-off mucosal cells as substrates. In return, they provide the host with their metabolic waste products (mainly organic acids) and the microbial cells may be digested and become a source of amino acids, vitamins, and other nutrients to the host. However, the quantitative importance of the absorption of microbial cell components depends on the position of the "fermentation vat" in relation to the main digestive and absorptive sites: the stomach and the small intestine.

For the purpose of comparison, three main types (or models) of digestive systems can be distinguished (Hungate, 1972):

1. the simple alimentary tract of monogastric animals (omnivores and carnivores; man, laboratory rat, cats, and dogs). The stomach is simple and there is no enlarged cecum.

2. the alimentary tract of polygastric herbivores (and some omnivores). The stomach is complex and divided into several compartments, at least some of which allow storage of food separate from the acid region.

3. The alimentary tract of nonruminating herbivores. The stomach is either simple or more complex, showing some kind of a division in two or more functional regions. The forestomach(s) are lined with squamous nonsecretory epithelium. The cecum and colon are very much enlarged to allow storage of food.

A. The Monogastric Animal

In the first model, the nutritional contribution of the gut flora is bound to be small. Rapid rates of passage of digesta, the lack of a retention mechanism in the alimentary tract, the acidity of the stomach, and the large quantities of digestive enzymes turned out by the host, together with the presence of a large absorptive area in the small intestine, make it hard for the microbes to compete with their hosts for substrate.

Even when the diet contains plant polysaccharides, the contribution of volatile fatty acids (VFA) formed in the lower intestines from dietary fiber is only small in man. Fermentation products from cellulose contributed only 0.03–0.38% to the metabolizable energy and pentosans (hemicellulose) 0.6–1.2% (Southgate and Durnin, 1970). Some fermentation of sugars and starch yielding largely lactate and acetate may occur in the stomach of monogastric animals.

It is generally acknowledged that the gut flora of monogastric animals has only a marginal influence on the protein nutrition of its host when the diet contains sufficient amounts of a good quality protein (Salter, 1973). Only when this is not the case and protein intakes are restricted, or the quality is poor, it is possible that synthesis of nonessential amino acids from ammonia released in the gut from urea or from partly digested protein, or recycling of endogenous nitrogen, may be of value.

Biohydrogenation of unsaturated fatty acids and unsaturated steroids and the transformation of primary bile acids into a variety of secondary bile acids occurs in the large intestine and in the ileum (Eyssen, 1973). The unconjugated bile acids may interact with many physiological functions (Midvedt, 1974).

Some uptake of vitamins from lysed bacteria in the lower gut may occur but its significance is probably minor.

B. The Polygastric Animal

In the second model, the contribution of the intestinal microbes to the nutrition of the host is of great importance. Microbial fermentation of the food in the enormously developed forestomachs of ruminants provides the host with fermentation products (chiefly acetate, propionate, and butyrate), which serve as energy sources and as precursors for biosynthetic processes. Due to the arrangement of the forestomachs, ahead of the main digestive sites of the animal, the host is able to digest the microbes in the acid stomach and in the small intestine and to use the microorganisms from the rumen, reticulum, and omasum as a source of vitamins and protein. The fermentation in the cecum in these animals is not important on low rates of passage, but may become increasingly important with high rates of passage of digesta or with food ingredients that are digested very slowly. The nutritional and biochemical consequences of this type of association between microorganisms and animal are manifold. The ruminant animal is less dependent on the quality of its diet than other animals and is able to colonize nutritionally "difficult" areas. Many books (e.g., Hungate, 1966) and proceedings of symposia (e.g., Phillipson, 1969; McDonald and Warner, 1975) deal with the rumen fermentation. This type of alimentary tract is not only found in ruminants in the order *Artiodactyla,* but in many other forms of life (camels, peccary, hippopotamus, macropod marsupials, sloths).

C. Hindgut Fermenters

In the third type of alimentary tract we find a combination of the two models described above. First, the host digests the food in the stomach and small intestine, whereafter the undigested residues are subjected to a microbial fermentation in an enlarged portion of the lower intestinal tract, the cecum and/or the colon. The situation is found in horses, ponies, elephants, many rodents, lagomorphs, hyrax, in gallinaceous birds, and to some extent in swine. Mammals generally have a simple cecum, gallinaceous birds have two ceca, but many different forms exist (Arvy, 1972; Behmann, 1973).

The VFA absorbed from the cecum and colon may provide up to 30% of the animal's daily energy requirement (McBee, 1971). The microbial cells are not or only partially digested, and unless coprophagy takes place, are of no great importance as a source of vitamins and protein to the host, although some uptake of cell constituents from lysed microbes in the lower gut may occur. In birds, bacterial competition with the host for vitamins is not of importance, unless the diet contains limiting amounts of these vitamins. With the exception of folic acid, probably no other vitamins are absorbed from the lower gut (Hill, 1971).

Coprophagy is obligatory in the guinea pig (Sharkey, 1971). Prevention of coprophagy in rodents often leads to a decrease in the apparent digestion of proteins and carbohydrates and has a negative influence on the vitamin status of the animal. Coprophagy is not seen in the elephant, horse, or birds and these animals miss the benefit of cecal protein synthesis.

In all hindgut fermenters a rapid fermentation of starch and sugars occurs in the upper parts of the alimentary tract (crop, esophageal region of the stomach) yielding primarily lactate and acetate (see Argenzio et al., 1974; Clemens et al., 1975a,b).

III. TRANSFORMATIONS OF FOREIGN COMPOUNDS BY INTESTINAL MICROORGANISMS

Excellent reviews on the metabolism of foreign compounds by intestinal and ruminal microorganisms have been written by Scheline (1973) and by James et al. (1975) and much information can be found in the publications by Drasar et al. (1970) and Drasar and Hill (1974). It is therefore not necessary to reproduce all the information at this place, but the more important reactions have been grouped (Table I) according to Walker (1973) and some of these transformations will be briefly commented on below.

A. Hydrolysis

The hydrolysis of glucuronide detoxification products excreted with the bile is one of the most common and important reactions carried out by the microbes in the lower intestinal tract. Many intestinal anaerobes possess β-glucuronidase activity and are capable of liberating the agly-

TABLE I
Transformations of Anutrient Compounds by
Intestinal Microflora

---

1. Hydrolysis of:
   (a) Glucuronides
   (b) Glycosides
   (c) Amides
   (d) Esters
   (e) Ethereal sulfates
   (f) Sulfamates
2. Reduction of:
   (a) Carbon–carbon double bonds
   (b) Nitrogen–nitrogen double bonds
   (c) Nitro groups
   (d) N-oxides, N-hydroxy compounds
   (e) Aldehydes, ketones, alcohols
   (f) Arsonic acids
   (g) Epoxides
3. Degradation by:
   (a) Decarboxylation
   (b) Dealkylation
   (c) Dehalogenation
   (d) Dehydroxylation
   (e) Deamination
   (f) Ring fission
4. Other reactions:
   (a) Esterification
   (b) Acetylation
   (c) Nitrosamine formation
   (d) Aromatization

---

cons from the glucuronide conjugates, which are of endogenous origin
unlike many other anutrient compounds which reach the intestines.
When the aglycon is reabsorbed after intestinal hydrolysis, an enterohepatic circulation of the compound will be established. The enterohepatic circulation of stilbestrol is a famous example.

Numerous glycosidase activities are present in the mixed microbial
population of the intestines, and β-galactosidase and β-glucosidase activity are most prominent. The hydrolysis of flavonoid glycosides and
cyanogenic glycosides has received considerable attention. The toxicological consequences of the hydrolytic reactions depend primarily on
the toxicity of the aglycons and on the site of hydrolysis in the gastrointestinal tract. The toxic properties of cyanogenic glycosides and of cycasin (methylazoxymethanol-β-D-glucoside; Fig. 1), a glycoside present in
several cycad plants, are associated with the aglycons and intestinal hy-

$$CH_3-\overset{\overset{\text{O}}{\uparrow}}{N}=N-CH_2O-\beta-D-glucose$$

cycasin

chlorogenic acid   caffeic acid   quinic acid

cyclamate   cyclohexylamine

salicylazosulfa pyridine

vanillyl alcohol   4-methylguaiacol

isovanillyl alcohol   4-methylcatechol

gallic acid   pyrogallol

protocatechuic acid   catechol

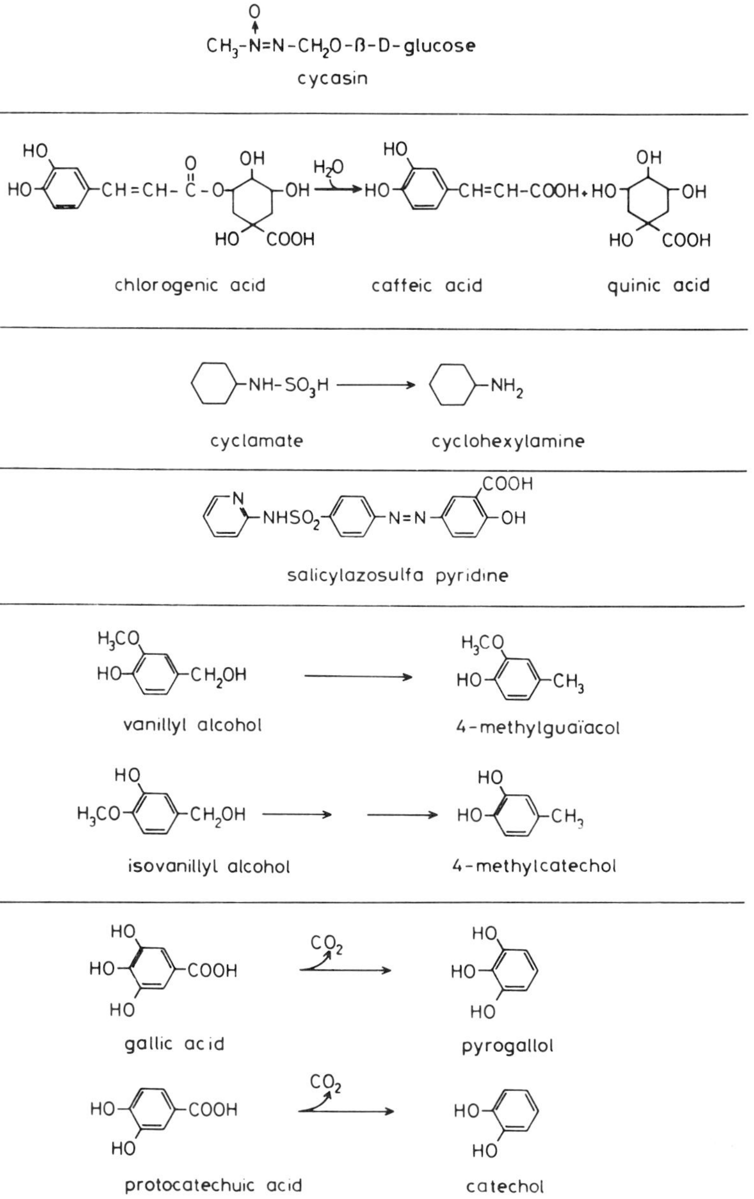

Fig. 1. Some examples of transformation of foreign compounds by intestinal microorganisms.

drolysis is required for the expression of toxicity. However, when the glycoside has more biological activity than the aglycon (e.g., with the cardiac glycosides), hydrolysis may result in a detoxification. In the latter case, ruminants have an advantage, since the glycosides are hydrolyzed in the rumen before appreciable absorption of the intact glycoside can occur.

Amidases of gut bacteria hydrolyze the amide linkage in phenacetin (Smith and Griffiths, 1974), in chloramphenicol, in penicillins, in N-acyl derivatives of sulfonamides, amines (N-acetylhistamine) and amino acids (glycocholic and taurocholic acids).

Microbial *esterases* hydrolyze many esters, as in chlorogenic acid (Fig. 1), pentacyclic triterpenoid compounds, esters of antibiotics and other therapeutic drugs. However, it should be pointed out that esterase activity in the intestines may be associated with enzymes in intestinal secretions or in the mucosa.

The hydrolysis of sulfate esters by gut microbes has mostly been studied with ethereal sulfates as substrates. The results suggest that intestinal hydrolysis of sulfate esters is a reaction of limited occurrence, which is probably related to the fact that the endogenously produced sulfate esters are primarily excreted with the urine and not via the bile.

The metabolism of the sweetening agent cyclamate (cyclohexylsulfamic acid) to cyclohexylamine (Fig. 1) by the intestinal microorganisms occurs after prolonged exposure to the drug *in vivo*. The reaction has drawn considerable attention because of its pharmacologic and toxicologic aspects (see also Bickel *et al.*, 1974). Prolonged oral feeding of cyclamate leads to an enrichment of the natural intestinal flora with anaerobic bacteria capable of using the sulfur from cyclamate for assimilation, when other sources of sulfur (sulfates, sulfur-containing amino acids, notably cysteine) are lacking. Cysteine inhibits the conversion of cyclamate to cyclohexylamine and it has been proposed that this conversion is controlled by the prevailing sulfur metabolism of the intestinal bacteria (Roxon and Tesoriero, 1974; Tesoriero and Roxon, 1975).

B. Reduction

Reduction of double bonds in various derivatives of cinnamic acid and the related ferulic acid and caffeic acid, but also of indolylacrylic acid, lead to the production of phenylpropionic acid (and derivatives) and indolylpropionic acid, respectively. The reactions resemble the well-known reduction of the double bonds of unsaturated long-chain fatty acids and of ricinoleic acid by intestinal and rumen microorganisms (see review by Prins, 1977). Reduction of the methylene group in pyrrolizidine alkaloids in the rumen is another example of this type of reaction (see Section V., B, 1, b).

The azo bonds in numerous synthetic coloring water-soluble agents (amaranth, ponceau SX, tartrazine, acid yellow, Brown FK) used in the manufacture of food and beverages are reduced in the intestines to the component amines, which are often excreted with the urine. The azo reductase activity is widespread among the members of the gut flora. Even fat-soluble dyes (e.g., butter yellow) containing azo groups are metabolized, once they have been absorbed and excreted in the bile as water-soluble conjugates.

A widely known example of the reduction of an azo group in a drug is the metabolism of salicylazosulfapyridine (Fig. 1). This compound is reduced and cleaved to sulfapyridine (an antibacterial drug) and 5-amino-salicylate (an anti-inflammatory compound) and this explains the effectiveness of the drug in the treatment of ulcerative colitis. The original design of the drug was based on the assumption that the parent drug would have the two therapeutic activities that could be attributed to its constituents (see Goldman *et al.*, 1974)! Another well-known example of bioactivation by intestinal azo group reduction is the conversion of the dyes prontosil and neoprontosil to yield sulfanilamide, which explains the therapeutic activity of these compounds *in vivo*.

Reduction of the nitro group in organic chemicals via the hydroxylamino intermediates to the amines is also one of the oldest known reactions to be carried out by the gut flora. In the rumen, the nitro groups of chloramphenicol, parathion, nitrophenols, and other nitro compounds are reduced. With parathion this results in a detoxification, while the activity of metronidazole against protozoa depends upon this reduction (see Section V, F, 1, b).

Reduction of aldehydes and alcohols in the gut has been concluded from *in vivo* and *in vitro* experiments. Even aromatic alcohols are further reduced to the corresponding toluene derivatives provided a free *p*-hydroxyl group is present, e.g., vanillyl alcohol (Fig. 1) is reduced to 4-methylguaiacol (Strand and Scheline, 1975). However, these reactions are not a major route of intestinal metabolism.

A novel biotransformation recently discovered is the reduction of epoxides to olefins (Ivie, 1976). This reduction is a significant detoxification mechanism since it is the epoxide moiety that confers biological activity to several alkylating agents, carcinogens, and pesticides. The reduction may function nutritionally in the reduction of oxidized foodstuffs (fatty acid and cutin epoxides).

C. Degradation

In the intestines not only amino acids are decarboxylated, but also phenolic acids may be converted to simple phenols, which are excreted with the urine. Phenolic, phenylacetic, and cinnamic acids are decarboxylated, but phenylpropionic acids are not, showing that there is a limit to the length of the side chain. Decarboxylation of phenolic acids occurs primarily with the p-hydroxylated compounds, but further ring substitution leads to varying degrees of inhibition of the reaction, and the rate of the reaction diminishes also when adjacent substituents are present, e.g., p-hydroxyphenylacetic acid is decarboxylated but 2-hydroxyphenylacetic acid is not. A very slow decarboxylation of benzoate was observed in pure cultures of *Methanobacterium ruminantium* (R. A. Prins, unpublished results).

Both O-dealkylation and N-dealkylation by intestinal microflora have been described. O-Dealkylation has only been reported for methoxyl compounds and dealkylation of higher homologues has not been described. Several methoxylated isoflavones are demethylated in the rumen (see Section V, B, 2, b) and isovanillyl alcohol (Fig. 1) is probably demethoxylated in the rat intestines, since 4-methylcatechol was found as an end product. When the methoxyl group is the sole ring substituent, the process may be slow, but it increases when di- and trihydric derivaties are presented. The m-methoxyl group of 3,4,5,-trimethoxycinnamic acid is more labile than the p-methoxyl group. Examples are given by Scheline (1973) which show that the intestinal demethylation is more important than the demethylation in the tissues of the body. It is not known whether the methyl group serves as a precursor for methane. N-Dealkylation is not restricted to demethylation, but dealkylation of higher homologues is possible (however, see Smith and Griffiths, 1974). Examples are the dealkylations of trifluralin (see Section V, C, 1, d) and of organometallic compounds like alkyltin chlorides.

Dehalogenation of compounds by intestinal microorganisms has only been described for organic chlorine compounds and not for bromine compounds or other halogenated derivatives. A familiar example is the conversion of DDT to DDD (see Section V, C, 2, a).

C-Dehydroxylation of bile acids and of phenolic acids occurs in the gut. Dehydroxylation at the *para* position of substituted catechols is not found with mammalian enzymes, but is seen in the intestinal metabolism of such compounds as L-dopa and caffeic acid (see Goldman *et al.*, 1974). The dehydroxylation is increased with compounds that have longer side chains, e.g., with gallic acid and protocatechuic acid (Fig. 1), decarboxylation is a more rapid process than dehydroxylation. Also, catechol is not converted to phenol. *N*-Dehydroxylating activity is not restricted to the intestines, but also resides in the tissues.

A most intriguing reaction is the fission of aromatic ring structures by anaerobic intestinal bacteria. Several heterocyclic ring systems are broken down in the gut, yielding products that are not produced elsewhere in the body. The ring systems may be chemically diverse, containing either oxygen or nitrogen. The reaction has been studied with coumarins, which are reductively cleaved to phenylpropionic acid derivatives. Another group of interest are the flavonoid compounds. The mixed rumen microbiota degrades flavonoid compounds anaerobically (Simpson *et al.*, 1969). Only a few genera of rumen bacteria were found capable of attacking flavonoids in pure culture and these could be divided in two groups: (a) those capable of hydrolyzing the glycoside and fermenting the sugar, but unable to attack the heterocyclic ring, and (b) those capable of both using the sugar and cleaving the heterocyclic ring.

A *Butyrivibrio* sp. was found to cleave the heterocyclic ring of several bioflavonoids but not of the corresponding aglycons (quercetin and naringenin, respectively, Fig. 2-I, 2-II). The utilization depended on the substrate being presented as glycoside, possibly because of the insolubility of the aglycon and its inability to enter the cell. Products from the hydrolytic cleavage of the flavonol quercetin (Fig. 2-I) were 3,4-dihydroxy benzaldehyde (III), 3,4-dihydroxyphenylacetic acid (IV), carbon dioxide and phloroglucinol (V) (Cheng *et al.*, 1969; Krishnamurty *et al.*, 1970). The glycoside naringin is hydrolyzed by the same organism to the flavanone naringenin and the sugar neohesperidose. Subsequently naringenin (Fig. 2-II) is cleaved anaerobically by reductive fission to

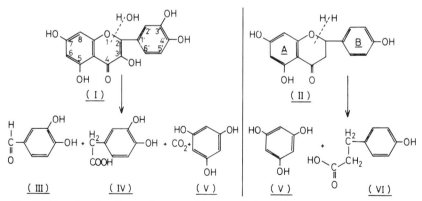

Fig. 2. Postulated pathways for anaerobic degradation of quercetin (I) and naringenin (II) by a *Butyrivibrio* sp. (after Krishnamurty *et al.*, 1970; Cheng *et al.*, 1971). For explanation see text; ———shows plane of cleavage of the heterocyclic ring.

phloroglucinol (V) and *p*-hydroxyphenylpropionic acid (VI) (Cheng *et al.*, 1971). Phloroglucinol is derived from the A ring of the flavonoids, but even phloroglucinol may be degraded to water-soluble products by *Streptococcus bovis* and *Coprococcus* sp. (Tsai and Jones, 1975), suggesting fission of the benzene nucleus. Although it is known that reductive cleavage of the aromatic ring, for example, of benzoate (See Ferry and Wolfe, 1976) occurs in anaerobic systems, this degradation is probably of minor importance in the rumen and gastrointestinal tract of animals, since the process is too slow. In ruminants both benzoic acid and phenyl-propionic acid accumulate in the rumen, phenylpropionic acid is oxidized in the liver to benzoic acid and thus benzoic acid becomes the major urinary acid (Martin, 1975).

Nitrogen-containing ring systems of azo compounds and the imidazole ring of histamine can be split anaerobically (Scheline, 1973), but no evidence was obtained that rupture of the pyrrolizidine ring of the alkaloids heliotrine and lasiocarpine occurs in the rumen (Lanigan and Smith, 1970), and no heterocyclic ring scission products were found after feeding hydroxyethylrutosides to rats (Barrow and Griffiths, 1974).

Other reactions carried out by the microorganisms in the intestines include esterification, acetylation, the formation (Mirvish, 1975) and degradation (Rowland and Grasso, 1975) of nitrosamines and the aromatization of ring structures as found in quinic acid. It is clear that the division made in Table I is not a precise one, since hydrolytic and reductive reactions often lead to degradation of a compound.

Since the intestinal microflora is chiefly composed of strict anaerobes, the types of reactions encountered are limited in one sense, i.e., the occurrence of oxygen-dependent transformations. Even in parasitic worms, which have a primarily anaerobic energy metabolism, transformations of foreign compounds take place chiefly by hydrolysis and reduction, while oxidation or the formation of conjugates does not occur (Dough and Blair, 1975).

It will be evident that microbial drug transformations themselves can be changed by drugs or by the nutritional status of the microorganisms.

IV. THE NUTRITIONAL CONSEQUENCES OF DRUG–MICROBE INTERACTIONS IN THE INTESTINES OF MONOGASTRIC ANIMALS

The demonstration that a drug is metabolized by the intestinal micro-flora *in vitro* does not imply that this process also takes place *in vivo*. There are several factors which may preclude *in vivo* metabolism of foreign compounds by gut microorganisms. The movement of foreign compounds across the gut wall is greatly facilitated when the substance is lipid-soluble, contains no polar groups and is not ionic at physiological pH. Once absorbed, the compound is converted by the microsomal system of the liver to an easily excretable form, which is water-soluble, contains polar groups and is ionic at physiological pH. Rapid uptake of a drug from the upper parts of the alimentary tract will prevent its metabolism by microorganisms in the intestines, unless the compound is excreted in the bile. In general, only those foreign compounds which are poorly absorbed, or which are excreted in the bile after hepatic metabolism (detoxification), reach the large intestines.

The following criteria are often considered proof of the occurrence of a drug-metabolizing reaction by gut microbes *in vivo:* (a) the reaction occurs more extensively after oral rather than after parenteral administration, (b) the reaction is altered (most often diminished) in animals treated with antibiotics, and (c) the reaction cannot be shown to occur in germfree animals.

Many of the pharmacological and toxicological implications of drug metabolism by gastrointestinal microorganisms have been described (Scheline, 1973) and the role of the bacterial metabolism in the formation of chemicals, possibly of importance in the etiology of cancer of the colon, breast and stomach, have been discussed (Draser and Hill, 1972, 1974; Hill, 1975).

The nutritional impact of drug–microbe interactions in monogastric animals is much less clear. Almost all the literature dealing with this topic is concerned with the influence of antibiotics, chemotherapeutics, or other antimicrobial agents on the health and growth of rats, swine, and poultry. Numerous articles have appeared on the effect of antibiotics and of antimicrobial therapy on the ecology of the intestinal flora. Again, not all antibacterial drugs reach the lower gut or affect the microbes of the intestines. Reviews have appeared which describe the activity of antimicrobial agents against gut anaerobes (Finegold, 1970; Hamilton-Miller, 1975). On the other hand, several food additives, drugs, and their intestinal metabolites may also have antimicrobial properties. Unexpectedly, the phenolic compound butylated hydroxyanisole, which is added to numerous food products to serve as an antioxidant, has antimicrobial properties, especially against gram-positive bacteria (Chang and Branen, 1975).

It is obvious that medical treatment of microbial infections of the gastrointestinal tract with antimicrobial compounds will help to restore the normal function of the gut in digestion and absorption. Malabsorption related to bacterial overgrowth in the small intestine (Neale *et al.*, 1972; Drasar and Hill, 1974) or to intestinal infection with higher parasites (Layrisse and Vargas, 1975) is based on a competition for vitamins and other nutrients between parasite and host. The value of antimicrobial therapy in these and other situations (diverticulitis, intestinal strangulation) is well established. In developing countries many children die as a consequence of malnutrition, and malabsorption of nutrients as a result of enteritis is an important factor in these cases. The question of the potential of feeding low doses of antibiotics to children in these countries where malnutrition is a problem has been asked by Rosenberg *et al.* (1974). The clinical implications in man of the presence of drug residues in foods are normally of minor importance (Hewitt, 1975).

Changes in the flora brought about by antibiotics may not only change the production of VFA, the metabolism of bile acids in the bowel, but also the activation or degradation and inactivation of drugs, including antibiotics. It has often been expected that suppression of the bacterial flora by antimicrobial drugs could interfere with the production of vitamin K in the large intestines of man, but even in cases of hypoprothrombinemia related to the usage of antibiotics, a direct effect of the antibiotic on normal regulatory genes in the hepatic cell may be the key factor (see Finegold, 1970). A review of the literature shows that: "... the fear of vitamin impoverishment of the human organism during antibiotic therapy, which alledgedly should lead to an impairment of the intestinal flora, is unfounded" (Haenel and Bendig, 1975).

There is evidence that changes in the intestinal flora by dietary administration of antibiotics may lead to a "sparing effect" on the vitamin requirements of rats. This may stimulate the growth of weanling rats fed diets deficient in these vitamins (see Boyd, 1973). The excretion of methylmalonic acid (MMA) has been considered a rather specific index of vitamin B_{12} deficiency, and excretion of this compound has been reported to be reduced in rats fed antibiotics (Armstrong and Curnow, 1967). This information should not be used as evidence that antibiotic treatment increased the intestinal synthesis of the vitamin, since the formation of propionic acid, an important precursor of MMA, can be decreased under these conditions (Anonymous, 1972).

Low-level feeding of antibiotics in animal husbandry (e.g., Menke and Krampitz, 1973) is common practice and often results in faster growth rates of the animals and greater feed efficiency (see Chapter 20). Both quantitative and qualitative changes are brought about in the bacterial flora of the gut, but these often revert to pretreatment levels (McCoy,

1957). The mechanism of action of these feed antibiotics is still not well understood, but amongst others is believed to be related to: (a) diminished utilization of nutrients and vitamins by the bacteria (especially in the small intestine), making more substrate available for direct intestinal absorption (see, e.g., Vervaeke *et al.*, 1975); (b) decreased formation of bacterial metabolites and toxins which may interfere with digestion and absorption of nutrients and water by the gut wall, or are toxic otherwise. Detoxification of such products is an energy cost to the animal; (c) direct anabolic effects on the host. The outcome of low-level feeding of antibiotics will depend on the diet, the animal species, the composition of the flora and environmental factors. Administration of antimicrobial agents to mice made pathogen-free decreased the weight gain of the animals, while in conventional animals the anaerobic flora is hardly disturbed, anerobic organisms are decreased, and weight gain increased (see Schaedler, 1973).

The significance of the cell wall damage induced in *Escherichia coli* by feed antibiotics (Walton and Bird, 1975; Walton, 1975) is not clear, since numbers of enterobacteria are often unchanged with many of these antibiotics, while numbers of gram-positive facultative anaerobes in the small intestine are decreased.

In animals with a predominantly gram-positive intestinal flora (guinea pig, hamster), administration of certain antibiotics (penicillin, lincomycin) leads to a shift in the gut flora, inflammatory response of the intestinal tract, often coliform bacteremia, and death (Small, 1968). As is clear from recent studies on the toxicity of di-*n*-octyltindichloride (DOTC) (Seinen *et al.*, 1977), the enterocolitis is not always seen upon feeding of antibacterial compounds to guinea pigs. However, a drastic reduction in the weight of the animals as well as in the VFA concentrations in the ceca occurred, when 50, 100 or 200 ppm of DOTC were present in the feed. It was discovered that DOTC produced deleterious effects on the epithelium of the stomach and small intestine, digestion and absorption being severely impaired. The cecal weights of the experimental animals became considerably increased, as often noted with antibacterial drugs that alter the cecal flora (Savage and McAllister, 1971), while the VFA concentrations in the ceca started to recover after 2–3 weeks to attain normal values after 6 weeks of DOTC feeding. This recovery is probably related to the fermentation of undigested food in the ceca by the adapted microbial flora. This would mean that under the adverse conditions of DOTC feeding, VFA produced and absorbed in the cecum can at least partially compensate for the diminished uptake of nutrients from the upper parts of the alimentary tract.

V. THE INFLUENCE OF ANUTRIENTS, FOREIGN COMPOUNDS, AND DRUGS ON THE FERMENTATION IN THE FORESTOMACHS OF POLYGASTRIC ANIMALS

A. Introduction

In the following sections some representative examples will be given of research dealing with the metabolism of anutrients, drugs and foreign compounds in the forestomachs of polygastric animals (mainly ruminants) and the influence of these compounds on fermentation.

B. Toxic Products and Plant Secondary Compounds

A wide variety of anutrient chemicals occurs in plants and each plant species has his own set of chemicals. The presence of these so-called plant secondary compounds has been explained as a means of protection from herbivores (Arnold and Hill, 1972; Freeland and Janzen, 1974). Although every textbook on toxicology (e.g., Radeleff, 1970; Hapke, 1975; Casarett and Doull, 1975) will contain at least a few examples of plants which are poisonous to ruminants especially, and of other plants which are poisonous to monogastric animals mainly, little is known about the fate of the poisonous chemicals in the rumen, even when it has been suggested that rumen metabolism could be the cause of these apparent anomalies. As has been pointed out by James *et al.* (1975), there have been surprisingly few studies on the metabolism, e.g., of plant secondary compounds in the rumen.

After a toxic plant (or potentially toxic plant) is consumed by a ruminant, it will depend on the balance of many factors whether toxicity will be expressed. Some plant poisons are rapidly inactivated in the rumen by the microbiota, while other (potentially toxic) compounds may be activated by the microbes faster than they will be detoxified in the gut. In this case the microsomal enzyme system of the animal will have to act as a safeguard. Still another category of compounds will show especially inhibitory effects on the rumen microorganisms. Some examples of these three extremes will be given, but many more can be found in the literature (see James *et al.*, 1975; Freeland and Janzen, 1974). Plant components which reduce the quantity eaten or the availability of nutrients, lower the animal's productivity from forage plants.

1. Toxic Plant Products Which Are Detoxified in the Forestomachs by Microbial Fermentation

Among the toxic compounds which may be degraded in the rumen are oxalates, pyrrolizidine alkaloids, essential oils, but also cyanides (see

Jones, 1972), seleniferous amino acids, mimosine (see Bell, 1972), cheiroline, digitalis alkaloids and caffeic acid, but in almost all cases the causative organisms have not been identified.

a. **Oxalates.** Ruminants can be adapted to consume plants containing large amounts of soluble oxalates. Following addition of such plants to the diet, increased rates of oxalate breakdown are found in the rumen and anaerobic bacteria seem to be responsible for this metabolism. The organisms could not be isolated (see James *et al.*, 1975). It could be that the anaerobic metabolism of oxalate is linked to methanogenesis, and thus occurs only in the mixed culture.

Intestinal detoxification of large amounts of oxalates occurs in rodents (pack rat, sand rat, hamster) belonging to the Cricetidae, but to a much lesser extent in the white laboratory rat which belongs to the family of the Muridae (Shirley and Schmidt-Nielsen, 1967). The stomach of the laboratory rat is simple when compared to the complex stomach of other small rodents, such as the Cricetidae. The stomach of these latter animals may be divided into two or three more or less distinct regions (Carleton, 1973). The stronger the constriction is between the forestomach (lined with squamous epithelium) and the hindstomach (with glandular epithelium), the higher the pH in the forestomach and the more active its bacterial flora (Williams-Smith, 1967). Bacterial decomposition of oxalates is the probable reason for the survival of several desert rat species on diets rich in soluble oxalate content.

b. **Pyrrolizidine Alkaloids.** The toxic agents in several species of herbaceous plants of the genera *Crotalaria, Echium, Heliotropum,* and *Senecio,* which all cause chronic liver diseases, are the pyrrolizidine alkaloids. The major alkaloids of the plant *Heliotropum europaeum* are heliotrine (Fig. 3-I) and lasiocarpine (II). These compounds are metabolized and detoxified in the rumen by reductive fission to *l*-goreensine (III) and heliotric acid (V) [reaction (a) in Fig. 3] or 7α-angeloxy-1-methylene-8α-pyrrolizidine (IV) [reaction (b)]. The intermediates III and IV are ultimately metabolized to the common end product 7α-hydroxy-1α-methyl-8α-pyrrolizidine (VI) [reactions (c) and (d); Lanigan and Smith, 1970; Lanigan, 1970)]. An organism was isolated from the rumen of sheep, which brings about reaction (a) with either H_2 or formate acting as hydrogen donor (Russell and Smith, 1968). Lanigan (1971) then studied the effect of molecular hydrogen on heliotrine metabolism in rumen fluid. A tenfold stimulation in the metabolism of heliotrine was observed upon inclusion of gaseous hydrogen in the gas phase of *in vitro* incubations, showing that hydrogen is limiting for the reductive break-

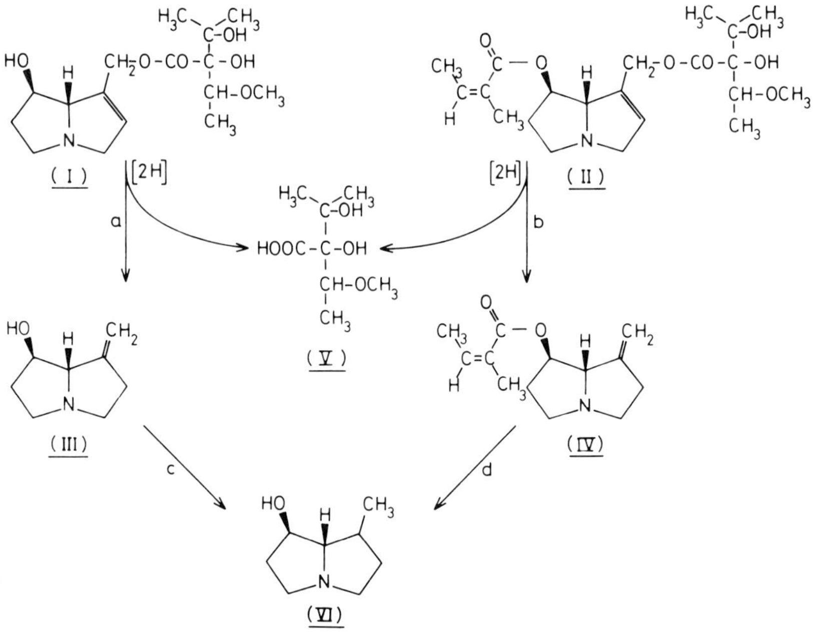

Fig. 3. Reductive degradation of the plant alkaloids heliotrine (1) and lasiocarpine (II) in the rumen. For explanation see text.

down of the alkaloid. It was then argued by Lanigan, that, since the major users of metabolic hydrogen in the rumen are the methanogenic bacteria, selective inhibition of these bacteria should permit a faster rate of heliotrine reduction. Applications of the methane inhibitors chloroform, carbon tetrachloride, and chloral hydrate, indeed, accelerated heliotrine metabolism and also shortened the lag-time which is usually observed before heliotrine breakdown starts. The results of these experiments led to the suggestion that antimethanogenic agents might have protective value for sheep ingesting *H. europaeum*. It was shown that by inhibiting rumen methanogenesis *in vivo*, the time taken for metabolism of 2 gm of *H. europaeum* alkaloids was reduced to 25–40% of that taken in control animals (Lanigan, 1972).

c. Essential Oils. The koala (*Phascolarctos cinereus*) is an arboreal marsupial, feeding predominantly on leaves of eucalyptus trees. These leaves contain large amounts of steam-volatile oils and the oils of *E. punctata* leaf, a suitable food for the koala, have been characterized in detail (Southwell, 1973). Feeding of *E. punctata* leaves to captive koalas followed by analyses of the feces and the urine showed that 7–30% of the volatile oils ingested was excreted in a steam-volatile form in the feces, 10% in the urine, while the remainder was excreted in the form of glucuronides (Eberhard *et al.*, 1975). A large portion of some of the oil constituents which are regarded most toxic (cryptone, cuminal, and *p*-cymene), was not recovered in the feces and it was suggested that these constituents were either absorbed or transformed in the gut by the cecal microorganisms to other products, since the appearance of some new products in the feces was noted. However, only the macropod marsupials have a divided stomach (Moir, 1968) and in these animals microbial detoxification of toxic plant components could even be of more importance.

2. Production of Toxic Principles from Natural Plant Ingredients in the Forestomachs by Microbial Fermentation

a. **Timber Milk Vetch Poisoning (Miserotoxin).** Miserotoxin is the β-glucoside of 3-nitro-1-propanol and the toxic principle of certain varieties of *Astragalus miser* (var. *serotina* = timber milk vetch). In the rumen the glycoside will be hydrolyzed and under the reducing conditions found in the rumen, glucose and 3-nitro-1-propanol (which is toxic) are produced. In monogastric animals miserotoxin is hydrolyzed to glucose and the less toxic 3-nitropropionic acid under the acidic conditions of the stomach (see James *et al.*, 1975).

b. **Clover Disease.** Red clover (*Trifolium pratense*) and subterranean clover (*Trifolium subterraneum*) are known to contain certain isoflavones such as formononetin, biochanin A, and genistein. Ruminants grazing these plants may show serious reproductive disorders. Pure biochanin A and genistein turned out to be estrogenic when administered parenterally in mice and sheep, but not so much in sheep when administered intraruminally. Formononetin appears inactive in mice and active in sheep only after intraruminal administration. The riddle was solved by the discovery that the highly active components biochanin A and genistein are metabolized in the rumen to the inactive compound *p*-ethylphenol, whereas the inactive formononetin was converted to the weakly estrogenic compound equol (Fig. 4). Since the daily intake of formononetin by sheep may be as high as 20 gm per day, enough equol is produced to cause the disorders (see Lindsay and Kelly, 1970). The demethylation and reduction reactions in the metabolism of formononetin may be reversed and in this case 4'-O-methyl equol is formed (Nottle and Beck, 1974), which under these conditions replaces equol as the

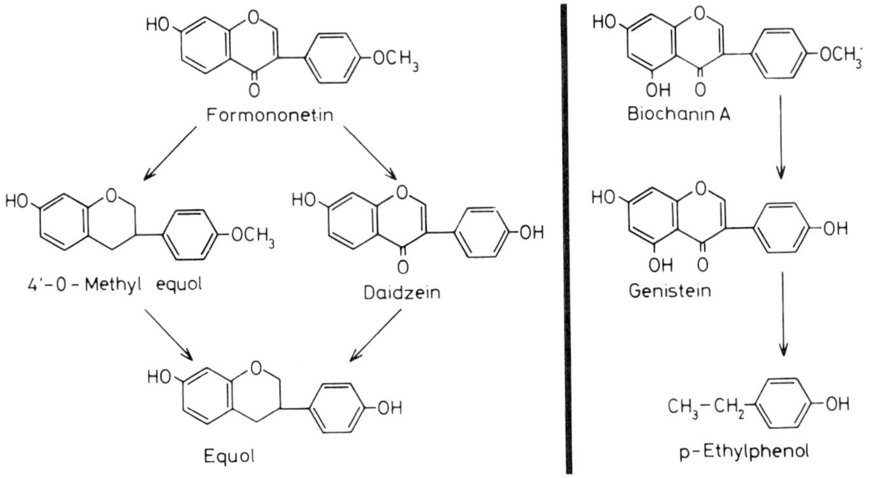

Fig. 4. The principal isoflavones of *Trifolium* sp. and their ruminal metabolites.

main (estrogenic) metabolite. Thus, the metabolism of the isoflavones in the rumen clearly shows that both activation and inactivation of plant toxins may occur in the forestomachs of animals.

c. **Kale Poisoning (S-Methylcysteine Sulfoxide).** Another striking example of the production of toxic principles is found in kale poisoning in cattle, described in an extremely interesting review by Smith (1974). When ruminants are fed exclusively on kale (*Brassica oleracea* var. *acephala*) or cabbage (*B. oleracea*) they may develop a severe hemolytic anemia. One of the first signs of the disease is the appearance of refractile, stainable granules within the red cells, the so-called Heinz-Ehrlich bodies. The disease is restricted to ruminants and is believed to be caused mainly by the production of dimethylsulfide (DMS) from the compound S-methylL-cysteine sulfoxide (SMCO) which is contained in these plants in large amounts. It is proposed (see Smith, 1974) that the microbial enzyme S-alkylL-cysteine sulfoxide-lyase will convert SMCO into methyl methanethiol sulfinate (MMS), pyruvate and ammonia [reaction (a) in Fig. 5], after which MMS is reduced in the rumen to DMS [reaction (b)] or even further to methanethiol [reaction (c)]. Strains of *Veillonella alcalescens*, *Megasphaera elsdenii*, *Anaerovibrio lipolytica* and of a *Lactobacillus* sp. were found capable of producing significant amounts of DMS and methanethiol from SMCO.

Reductive cleavage (dimethiolation) of methionine or S-methylL-cysteine also yields dimethylsulfide and methanethiol (see review by

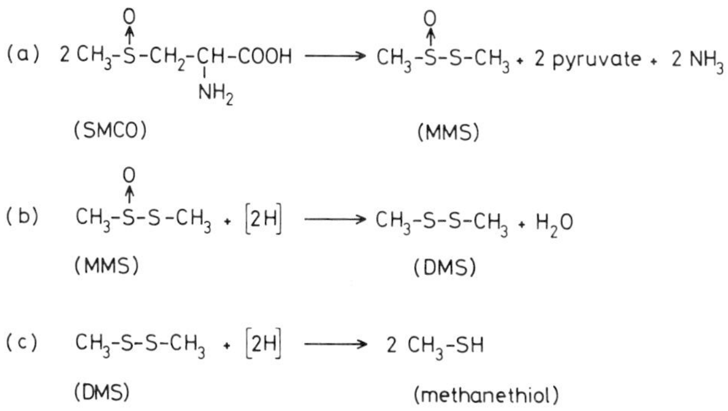

(a) $2\ CH_3\text{-}\overset{O}{\overset{\uparrow}{S}}\text{-}CH_2\text{-}\underset{NH_2}{\underset{|}{CH}}\text{-}COOH \longrightarrow CH_3\text{-}\overset{O}{\overset{\uparrow}{S}}\text{-}S\text{-}CH_3 + 2\ \text{pyruvate} + 2\ NH_3$

(SMCO)   (MMS)

(b) $CH_3\text{-}\overset{O}{\overset{\uparrow}{S}}\text{-}S\text{-}CH_3 + [2H] \longrightarrow CH_3\text{-}S\text{-}S\text{-}CH_3 + H_2O$

(MMS)   (DMS)

(c) $CH_3\text{-}S\text{-}S\text{-}CH_3 + [2H] \longrightarrow 2\ CH_3\text{-}SH$

(DMS)   (methanethiol)

Fig. 5. Microbial conversion of S-methylcysteine sulfoxide (SMCO) to methanethiol via methyl methanethiol sulfinate (MMS) and dimethyl sulfide (DMS) by rumen organisms.

Prins, 1977) and it is suggested by Smith (1974) that the hemolytic anemia observed in rats fed supplementary methionine (Mengel and Klavins, 1967) could be the result of the action of the gut flora on methionine.

d. Photosensitizing Agents (Phylloerythrin). Metabolism of chlorophyll pigments in the rumen produces pheophytins and the pheophytins of chlorophyll a and b will subsequently be metabolized to the pigment phylloerythrin by loss of the phytol side chain (Dawson and Hemington, 1974). Phylloerythrin is absorbed from the alimentary tract and is excreted in the bile. Any interference with biliary secretion causes retention of this photodynamic compound and consequently results in photosensitization of the unprotected skin when exposed to sunlight. The syndrome has experimentally been produced in horses by ligation of the bile duct. Chlorophyll is degraded in the horse cecum (Ford and Gopinath, 1974).

3. Plant Products Which Are Toxic to the Microorganisms in the Forestomachs

Unlike nutritional chemicals which are generally believed to increase palatability of plants, nonnutritional chemicals are regarded as deterrents which increase the resistance of the plant to animals. Examples of cases where these anutrients were responsible for refusal of the plant by animals are given by Radwan (1974).

a. Alkaloids. Alkaloids present in *Phalaris tuberosa* cause the disease phalaris staggers in livestock grazing this plant. The responsible agents are alkaloid derivatives of tryptamine. Unpalatable clones of reed canary-grass contained higher concentrations of indole-alkaloid derivatives than did palatable clones.

In these and other examples the alkaloids exert their toxicity on the animal. However, one of the principal alkaloids of *Lolium perenne* and the principal alkaloid of tall fescue (*Festuca arundinacea*) is perloline. This compound not only is suspected of causing ryegrass staggers, it is also toxic to the rumen microorganisms. Cellulose breakdown and VFA formation are strongly inhibited *in vitro* by concentrations of $10^{-4}M$ or higher (Bush *et al.*, 1972).

b. Essential Oils. Volatile components ("essential oils") from certain plants (*Artemisia, Eucalyptus, Pseudotsuga* and *Juniperus* sp.) are inhibitory to the growth of many aerobic bacteria and anaerobic bacteria in the rumen (Nagy *et al.*, 1964; Nagy and Tengerdy, 1967a,b; Oh *et al.*, 1968; Longhurst *et al.*, 1968; James *et al.*, 1975).

Of the essential oils isolated from Douglas fir needles (Sakai *et al.*, 1967) monoterpene hydrocarbons and sesquiterpenes had no effect on rumen microbial activity, whereas the oxygenated monoterpenes, particularly monoterpene alcohols (α-terpineol, terpinen-4-ol, citronellol, fenchyl alcohol) strongly inhibited these organisms (Oh *et al.*, 1967). More of the acyclic oxygenated monoterpenes are found in tips of Douglas fir as the plant matures (Maarse and Kepner, 1970), and oils from old needles are more inhibitory to the microorganisms than those from new growth (Oh *et al.*, 1970). Clones of Douglas fir which are resistant to deer browsing in general have lower dry matter digestibilities and essential oils with greater inhibitory action on rumen microbial activity (Radwan, 1972). No studies have been made of the fate of terpenes in the rumen.

Plants with high levels of inhibitory components cannot serve as a total diet, although there is some evidence that adaptation of the microbes will occur to a certain degree. Different ruminant species with different complements of rumen microorganisms may have different tolerance levels for the same plants.

c. Tannins. Natural tannins are complex polyphenols of high molecular weight (> 500), and can be divided in two groups the hydrolyzable tannins, which occur mainly in fruit pods and plant galls, and the condensed tannins, which are commonly found in forages. In contrast to the hydrolyzable tannins, the condensed tannins have no carbohydrate core and are not hydrolyzed in the gut by either acid in the stomach or by enzymes. The tannins bind easily to proteins; under anaerobic conditions the binding will be primarily by reversible hydrogen-binding. As a result, the activities of many enzyme systems are inhibited by these plant compounds and in general tannins are toxic. In the rumen especially the digestion of protein is reduced, but despite this action, ruminants appear to tolerate high levels of tannins in the food. Treatment of the food with tannins has been suggested, in order to obtain a more efficient use of dietary protein by ruminants. From the foregoing it is clear that only hydrolyzable tannins can be used for protein protection (see the review by McLeod, 1974).

d. Fungal Toxins and Antibiotics. Toxins produced by fungi may contaminate foods and feeding stuffs and may affect the health of man and animals. Microbial products accumulated in deteriorated feedstuffs not only are directly toxic to animals, they also disturb the natural intestinal flora and enhance the incidence of infectious diseases. The little information there is on interactions between these compounds and rumen microbes is summarized by Gedek (1973) and by James et al. (1975). Aflatoxin B_1 is not metabolized in the rumen but inhibits the growth of rumen bacteria (Mathur et al., 1976).

Much more information is available about the effects of commercial antibiotics employed as feed additives and as therapeutics (see Section V, D, 3).

C. Toxic Contaminants of Food (Pesticides)

Among the numerous possible chemicals that may be present as contaminants in animal feeds, pesticides are of interest and many studies have been devoted to the metabolism of such compounds in the rumen and of their effect on the rumen fermentation.

1. *Herbicides*

a. Phenoxyalkanoic Acids. The herbicide 4-(2,4-dichlorophenoxybutyric) acid is rapidly altered in the rumen, but 2,4-dichlorophenoxyacetic acid (2,4-D) is not among the products, as is commonly seen in plants or soil (Gutenmann et al., 1963a), and 2,4-D itself is not metabolized in the rumen (Gutenmann et al., 1963b; Clark et al., 1964). The benzoic acid derivative Dicamba, 2,4-D, and 2,4,5-T are excreted largely unchanged in the urine of cattle (see James et al., 1975).

b. Benzoic Acid Derivatives. The herbicide Disugran ($5 \times 10^{-6} M$) is rapidly degraded in rumen fluid from sheep on low- and high-energy diets (Ivie et al., 1974). The rate of breakdown was highest with rumen fluid from animals fed the low-energy diet. The suggested pathway (Fig. 6) of Disugran (I) metabolism in the rumen is through initial cleavage of the methylether, followed by hydrolysis of the methylester. Principal metabolites were 3,6-dichlorosalicylate (III) and its methylester, while only traces of Dicamba (IV) were found. Dicamba is stable in rumen fluid.

   c. **Trazines.**   Propazine and probably also Simazin and Atrazine are not degraded by rumen microbes (Williams *et al.*, 1968).

   d. **Dinitroanilines.**   A pathway has been proposed for the microbial degradation of Trifluralin, a preemergent soil-incorporated herbicide (Golab *et al.*, 1969). The pathway (Fig. 7) is very similar to that of trifluralin degradation in anaerobic soils. The major route is via reduction of the nitro groups to yield a mixture of polar products. Dealkylation is much less important. Of twelve selected strains of rumen bacteria only two metabolized Trifluralin (Williams and Feil, 1971). A strain of *Bacteroides ruminicola* subsp. *brevis* and a strain of *Lachnospira multiparus* reduced one or both of the nitro groups. In these pure cultures no loss of the trifluoromethyl group or cleavage of the Trifluralin ring was evident.

   Reduction of organic nitro groups is commonly seen and also the compounds dinitrocresol (DNOC) and dinitrobutylphenol (DNBP) are reduced in the rumen via the 6-amino derivatives to aminophenols (Froslie, 1974) and upon intraruminal administration these compounds therefore not only show their effect as uncouplers, but in addition the diamino metabolites cause methemoglobinemia and hemoconcentration. The antioxidant diphenylamine is stable in rumen fluid (Gutenmann and Lisk, 1975).

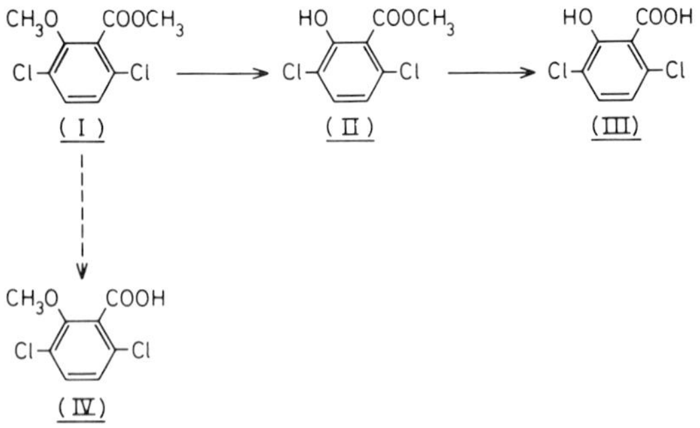

Fig. 6. Ruminal metabolism of the herbicide Disugram (I) to 3,6-dichloro-salicylic acid (III) and its methylester (II). Dicamba (IV) is a minor product.

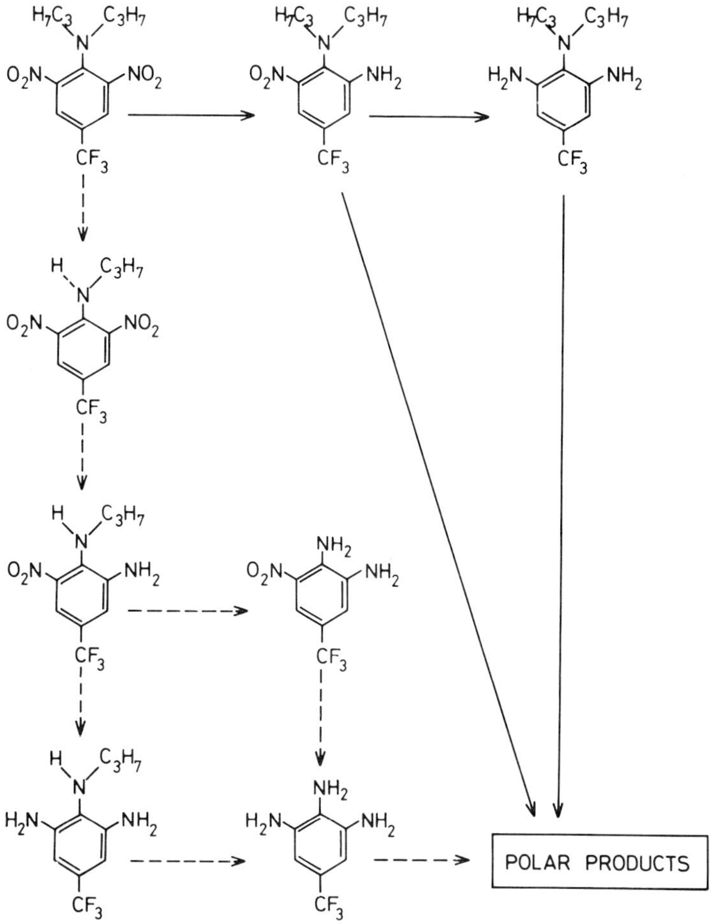

Fig. 7.   Pathway postulated for Trifluralin degradation in rumen fluid (after Golab *et al.*, 1969).

2. *Insecticides*

a.   **Chlorinated Hydrocarbons.**   Surveys of pesticide levels in wild North American ruminants have shown that stored levels of DDT in these animals are considerably higher than those of its metabolite DDE, which is the reverse of the normal situation in man (Watson *et al.*, 1975). Since the residue most commonly ingested in usually DDE rather than DDT, the authors suggested that DDE would be converted in the rumen to DDT. However, DDT is converted to DDD in the rumen by reductive dechlorination (Fries *et al.*, 1969), as has been demonstrated with microflora from the digestive tract of the rat (Braunberg and Beck, 1968; Mendel and Walton, 1966) and in rumen contents (Miskus *et al.*, 1965; Rumsey *et al.*, 1970). The rumen ciliate protozoa do not take part in this reaction (Kutches and Church, 1971). Feeding of DDT (30 mg per kg of body weight daily) to steers did reduce the concentration of VFA and the numbers of ciliate protozoa when the diet consisted of concentrates, but with a roughage diet no such changes were seen (Rumsey *et al.*, 1970).

A number of reasons for the persistence of DDT in nature have been proposed by Alexander (1973). Additional reasons may lay in the function of DDT as an inhibitor of methanogenesis (as are many other halogenated hydrocarbons) and in the fact that halogenated ring structures could interfere with the anaerobic degradation of ring structures (see Ferry and Wolfe, 1976).

Lindane was only partially (10%) metabolized by a strain of *E. coli* isolated from rat feces to a single metabolite 2,3,4,5,6-pentachlorcyclohexene (γ-PCCH) also found in aerobic degradation (Francis *et al.*, 1975). In the rumen dieldrin is reduced to aldrin (Ivie, 1976).

b. Organophosphates. Some of these inhibitors of cholinesterase are rendered less toxic by metabolism in the rumen (for references, see Williams *et al.*, 1963; James *et al.*, 1975). The aromatic nitro group of parathion is reduced in the rumen, especially by the protozoal fraction, to the less toxic aminoparathion, which is excreted. Malathion is cleaved by microbial phosphatase action in the rumen to dimethylphosphate and O,O'-dimethyl phosphorothioate.

The voluntary intake of hay by ruminating bull calves was inversely related to intake of Supracide, when this insecticide was mixed with the diet (Polan *et al.*, 1969). Three out of five animals receiving 2.0 mg of Supracide per kg body weight died within 34 days of continuous treatment. Supracide is not degraded in the rumen (St. John and Lisk, 1974).

c. Carbamates. The carbmate insecticide Mobam(benzo[*b*]thien-4-yl-methylcarbamate) is metabolized by mixtures of ruminal bacteria and esterase-processing rods (possibly *Butyrivibrio fibrisolvens?*) to 4-hydroxybenzothiophene, carbon dioxide, and several nonidentified polar products from the methylcarbamate moiety (Williams and Stolzenberg, 1972). Other carbamates (Furadan, Sevin) probably are also hydrolyzed in the rumen.

3. Effects of Pesticides on Rumen Function

Several studies have been made to test the effect of various pesticides on rumen metabolism. In general no relation is seen between the extent of metabolism of these compounds in the rumen and their toxicity for the rumen microbes. Even with pesticides that are not metabolized, there may be effects on the microbial population and hence on the fermentation in the rumen.

Results of a study to determine the effect of various concentrations of selected pesticides (aldrin, dieldrin, 2,4-D, DDT, Toxaphene, Parathion, Malathion, EPN, Sevin, Mobam, Zectran, Baygon, Black Leaf-40, Bordeaux Mixture and MemaRM) on goat or deer rumen microbial function indicated that no significant effects on *in vitro* dry matter and cell wall constituent digestion will occur at pesticide concentrations lower than 100 ppm (Schwartz *et al.*, 1973; Schwartz and Nagy, 1974), although it was reported that *in vitro* cellulose digestion may be impaired at concentrations ≤ 100 ppm of all pesticides (Barber *et al.*, 1970). Since contaminated forage usually contains low residue concentrations, it was concluded by Schwartz *et al.* (1973) and Schwartz and Nagy (1974) that pesticides will have a negligible effect on rumen microbial function. Rumen levels of several of the tested pesticides required for inhibition of dry matter digestion were so high (1000 ppm) that the amounts would be well over the calculated LD_{50} for these compounds. Another study with twelve pesticides (Bromacil, Dicamba, Diuron, DDT, Sevin, Simazine, Tordon, Toxaphene, 2,3,6-TBA, 2,4-D, and 2,4,5-T) also led to the conclusion that relatively high concentrations (up to 500 ppm) were tolerated by mixed rumen microorganisms from a fistulated sheep fed a forage diet (Kutches *et al.*, 1970).

Trifluralin did not cause changes in the fermentation by rumen bacteria or protozoa, nor influenced the formation of VFA *in vitro* (Williams and Feil, 1971). The herbicide Propazine had no influence on rumen metabolism in sheep dosed with 80 mg of the herbicide per kg of body weight (Williams *et al.*, 1968).

A stimulation of *in vitro* gas production by *Isotracha* sp. was seen with the pesticides Lindane, Thioday, Sevin, Diazinon, Dimethoate (Williams *et al.*, 1963) and 100 ppm levels of the compounds tested by Kutches *et al.* (1970) stimulated protozoal numbers *in vitro*. M15, a synthetic herbicide containing 70% of calcium trichloroacetate, and Dalapon, when added in 50 ppm levels to incubations of suspensions of mixed rumen protozoa and rice starch, stimulated VFA production rates over the controls by 37 and 55% respectively (Abou Akkada *et al.*, 1973). In general it would seem that the protozoa are less sensitive to pesticides than the rumen bacteria. No attention has been paid to the possibility that some of these pesticides in addition to DDT may act as inhibitors of methanogenesis. The carbamate fungicide Ziram (zinc N,N-dimethyldithiocarbamate) in a concentration of 5 ppm inhibits the fermentation of cellulose by bovine rumen contents *in vitro,* but much higher levels of Ziram are required for inhibition after feeding the compound with the ration, suggesting adaptation of the bacteria (Madella Amadei, 1966). As has already been pointed out, *in vitro* fermentations are more readily inhibited than the fermentation *in vivo.* Also, pure cultures of rumen bacteria, especially cellulolytic organisms are more sensitive to certain pesticides than the mixed rumen population (Barber and Nagy, 1971).

D. Drugs Administered Orally to Ruminants in Veterinary Practice

It is not unlikely that at least some of the compounds which are administered orally to ruminants (Rossoff, 1974), with the intention of curing a disease not associated with the rumen, will nevertheless influence rumen function. Yet, the fact that many compounds which are given orally to calves, swine, and horses are given parenterally to ruminants, show that practical experience in veterinary medicine has learned how to evade possible complications. The influence of several ruminal parameters on the distribution and excretion of orally ingested drugs are discussed by Jenkins *et al.* (1975).

1. *Anthelmintics*

Tetramisole (2,3,5,6-tetrahydro-6-phenylimidazo-[2,1-*b*]-thiazole) is an anthelmintic used against pulmonary and gastrointestinal nematodes and the inhibition of the fumarate reductase reaction in the parasite is one of the biochemical mechanisms of action of this drug. Since the reduction of fumarate to succinate is also an intermediate step in many rumen bacteria, which form succinate or propionate by way of the dicarboxylic acid pathway, the possibility of rumen propionate inhibition by Tetramisole was investigated (Prins *et al.,* 1972a). No consistent effect on the formation of acetate, propionate, butyrate, lactate, or methane from glucose or from a mixed sugar substrate was seen *in vitro.*

Inactivation of drugs may occur in the rumen. Anthelmintics, e.g., containing organic nitro compounds as active principle, can only be given orally to ruminants after coating the drug to prevent inactivation as a result of reduction of the nitro group.

2. Antiprotozoals

A number of antiprotozoals were tested (O'Connor *et al.*, 1970) and especially metronidazole and dimetridazole and the compounds Su-14,276 and Su-15,412 were toxic to rumen protozoa. These compounds together with niridazole (all at 10 mg per 50 ml of incubation fluid) inhibited formation of VFA *in vitro*. The Su-compounds stimulated propionate formation *in vitro,* but this could not be reproduced *in vivo* (O'Connor *et al.*, 1971).

3. Antibiotics

A large number of studies have been devoted to the effect of antibiotics on *in vitro* cellulose digestion. In general only those antibiotics active against anaerobes (Hamilton-Miller, 1975) have a pronounced inhibitory effect on this process (Prins, 1969). Fewer studies have been made of the effect on VFA production. In the study by O'Connor *et al.* (1970), zinc bacitracin, streptomycin, bacitracin, chlortetracycline, neomycin, oleandomycin, oxytetracycline, and rifocin had only small effects or even no effect on VFA formation *in vitro,* whereas penicillin and spiramycin depressed VFA most when given at the high levels of 10 mg per 50 ml incubation fluid. Tylosin, spiramycin, and penicillin especially depressed propionate formation.

The rumen protozoa are in general less susceptible than rumen bacteria to a number of antibiotics (Harmeyer, 1965). Addition of antibiotics to the rumen often results in an increase of the bacterial population (e.g., Satapathy and Purser, 1967).

4. Sulfonamides and Other Compounds

Temporary inappetence, reduction of water intake, transient depression of ruminal motility, diminished glucose fermentation rate, cessation of cellulolytic activity, and a transient reduction in the concentration of VFA in rumen fluid, were the most prominent features recorded after intraruminal administration of sulfadimidine to adult sheep (Jenkins, 1969). Much higher concentrations of sulfonamides than of antibiotics are needed to affect the digestion of cellulose by rumen contents *in vitro* (Prins, 1969).

Thiamine inhibitors, sulfonamides, nitrofurans, and antihistamines were without major effects of VFA production *in vitro* when applied in low levels (O'Connor *et al.*, 1970). Antihistamines have been used to study the rate of histamine degradation in the rumen (Dickinson and Huber, 1972).

5. Ruminal Synthesis of Antithiamine Compounds

The disease of sheep and cattle which is called cerebrocortical necrosis (CCN) is characterized by multiple foci of necrosis of the cerebral neurones. The presence of a thiaminase I activity was detected in the rumens of the affected animals and has been regarded as the cause of CCN. Where thiaminase I activity was detected in the rumen contents, it was also found to be present in intestinal contents and in unvoided feces (Edwin and Jackman, 1973). CCN has also been experimentally reproduced by oral administration of the thiamine antagonist Amprolium to calves and lambs (for references, see Edwin and Jackman, 1970, 1973). The action of thiaminase I would render the animals thiamine-deficient by cutting off their supply of this vitamin, but it is also possible that the production of antithiamine compounds by thiaminase I (Fig. 8) is the cause of the problems. Much would depend on the type of cosubstrate in the thiaminase reaction. Even a number of drugs commonly used as anthelmintics and tranquilizers can be active as second substrates (Roberts and Boyd, 1974). When nicotinic acid is the cosubstrate, depletion of both these vitamins could occur. These antithiamine compounds would be responsible for the thiamine deficiency, rather than simple destruction of thiamine. This seems likely (Zintzen, 1973) since even under conditions where a high thiaminase I activity is found in the rumen, it is conceivable that at least a sizable portion of the thiamine (present and functioning within the microbial cells) would escape destruction and be absorbed in the abomasum and small intestines.

High levels (2–4 mM) of the thiamine analogues oxythiamine and neopyrithiamine did not influence cellulose digestion of VFA production in vitro, but lower concentrations of thiopental (0.72 mM) or hexetidine (15 μM) were inhibitory (Milligan et al., 1965).

Long-term feeding of a nonprotein nitrogen diet devoid of B vitamins to sheep leads to the development of a thiamine deficiency and possibly of other B vitamins (Naga et al., 1975).

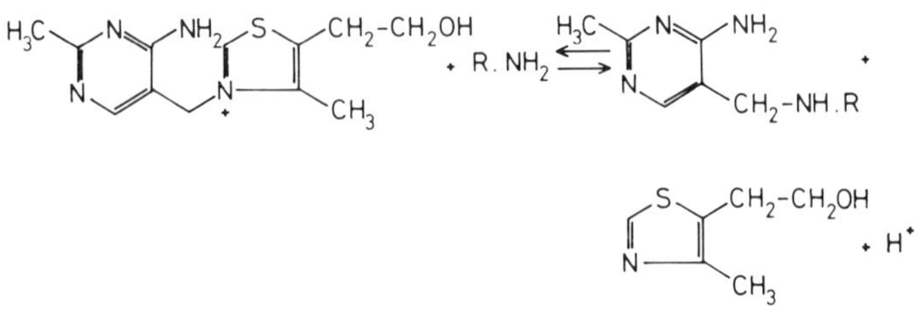

Fig. 8. The decomposition of thiamine by thiaminase I involves the transfer of the pyrimidine moiety to an amine.

E.   Prevention and Treatment of Rumen Disturbances

Toxic products can be formed from natural feed ingredients (nutrients). There are several examples of the formation of excessive amounts of normal fermentation end products or rumen intermediates, and the accumulation of such products may cause harm to the host animal. A number of these rumen abnormalities have been reviewed by James *et al.* (1975).

Some rumen bacteria are capable of using nitrate as an electron acceptor and the accumulation of the first reduction product nitrite may cause methemoglobinemia upon feeding diets rich in nitrate.

The rapid breakdown of particular nitrogenous compounds (e.g., urea) may lead to excessive ammonia levels in the rumen and in the blood, causing alkalosis and ammonia intoxication.

Bacterial decarboxylases may form toxic amines from the corresponding amino acids at the low pH values in the rumen seen in acidosis as a result of overfeeding (see review by Slyter, 1976).

In experimental studies feeding of tryptophan of indoleacetic acid caused pulmonary edema and emphysema in cattle; the microbial metabolite 3-methylindole (skatole) is thought to be responsible for the development of the symptoms (Carlson, *et al.,* 1975; Yokoyama *et al.,* 1975).

The rapid fermentation of sugars and starch in ruminants not adapted to easily digestable rations may lead to the accumulation of lactate (especially the D-isomer), causing acidosis of the rumen and blood (Dunlop and Hammond, 1965; Dunlop, 1972).

In many of such cases the oral application of antibiotics or other compounds with antimicrobial activity has been advocated in veterinary medicine or has been studied in experimental situations and examples can be found in the literature. However, emptying of the rumen, changing the diet, and appropriate medication to revert the blood changes seen are better treatments, because of the digestive upsets and the destruction of the microflora of the gut following the treatment with massive doses of antibiotics (Buck, 1969).

A drastic reduction in the incidence of experimental legume bloat was obtained by feeding alkyl aryl sulfonate, an inhibitor of the enzyme pectin methyl esterase (Nichols, 1963). Hydrolysis of pectic substances by this enzyme liberates methanol and polygalacturonic acids, and the latter were believed to form an important contributing factor to the high viscosity of ruminal contents observed in legume bloat (Gupta and Nichols, 1962). The free pectic acid binds free water, rendering the ruminal contents more viscid, so that bubbles of gas could be trapped, thus stabilizing the froth so formed.

Meyer and Bartley (1972) tested 235 drugs (synthetic detergents) for their effect on froth production, microbial activity, surface tension, and relative viscosity in order to find a promising drug for the treatment of feedlot bloat. One drug was finally selected which controlled froth formation and prevented bloat. The drug (a dimethyl dialkyl quaternary ammonium compound) did not affect the microbial fermentation, but was found to inhibit capsule and slime formation (see Bartley *et al.*, 1975).

F. Manipulation of the Normal Rumen Fermentation to Improve the Animal's Productivity

1. *Nitrogen Metabolism*

a. Inhibitors of Protein Fermentation and Urease Inhibitors. One of the drawbacks of having a forestomach fermentation is the extensive microbial degradation of food proteins in animals which cannot meet their requirements from the microbial proteins synthesized in the rumen and from the undegraded food proteins which bypass the rumen.

Rumen microbial proteases hydrolyze especially the proteins that are soluble in the rumen to peptides and amino acids. Some species of rumen bacteria use these peptides and amino acids for the synthesis of their cell proteins, but the major fraction is fermented to ammonia and other products. Since a higher rate of protein degradation is observed with proteins that are more soluble in the rumen fluid, methods have been devised to decrease protein breakdown in the rumen by lowering their solubility. These include heat treatment and chemical treatment of foods (Phillipson, 1972; Ferguson, 1975). Other methods to bypass the rumen are stimulation of esophageal groove closure, encapsulation of supplementary amino acids, or the feeding of amino acid analogues which should resist rumen degradation, be absorbable from the intestines, and have biological potency in tissue metabolism (see review by Chalupa, 1975).

There is little information on the possibility to decrease protein fermentation by feeding drugs. Experiments with antibiotics to control ruminal protein breakdown did not result in encouraging results, since these depressed feed intake and caused temporary digestive disturbances (see Chalupa, 1975). Chloral hydrate does inhibit the fermentation of casein to VFA (Prins, 1967), presumably by interfering with the fermentation of amino acids, since there is no effect of this compound on the proteolytic activity of rumen contents (Oyaert and Bouckaert, 1959). Feeding of 15 gm of chloral hydrate per day in a single dose to lactating dairy cows fed a hay and concentrate mixture, resulted in a fivefold lowering of the ruminal NH_3-N concentration (Prins, 1967). Amicloral, a hemiacetal of chloral and starch, produces a decreased ruminal deamination of amino acids *in vitro* (Chalupa, 1975) and feeding of bromochloromethane lowered ammonia levels in the rumen of lambs fed natural diets (Singh and Trei, 1971).

Hydrazine, an effective inhibitor of amino acid fermentation by rumen microbes *in vitro* (Broderick and Smith, 1974), cannot hold promises for *in vivo* application, because it is a general metabolic inhibitor. Another compound, 4,4'-dimethyldiphenyliodonium chloride, inhibits the degradation of amino acids in the rumen, increases nitrogen retention and growth rates of calves (Chalupa *et al.*, 1976). Other diaryliodonium compounds are also active inhibitors of amino acid fermentation (Chalupa and Scott, 1976).

As a normal constitutent of body water, the detoxification product urea enters the lumen of the gastrointestinal tract and is hydrolyzed by the microbial ureases. Uric acid may also contribute to the ammonia pool in the gut (see review by Prins, 1977). In man and other monogastric species the quantity of urea hydrolyzed in the gastrointestinal tract is estimated at about 20–25% of the daily excretion. Although the hydrolysis of urea by the enteric flora does not result in a net loss of urea from the body, it delays the excretion of nitrogen and represents an energy cost, since most of the intestinal ammonia is reconverted to urea by the liver. Intestinal ammonia can also be utilized in the synthesis of amino acids in the body and thus for protein synthesis, but only when adequate amounts of essential amino acids are available (for a review, see Visek, 1972).

Many approaches have been used to reduce the intestinal ammonia production from urea including feeding of antibacterial compounds and urease immunization of animals. All treatments have produced increased growth of chicks and rats on purified diets. In urease-immunized sheep showing substantial increases in growth over controls, the sites of maximum reduction in urea hydrolysis were the small and large intestines rather than the rumen. Urea was the only source of nitrogen in the purified diet of these animals (Visek, 1972). The results of these experiments are difficult to understand since the immunization of the animals was done with jack-bean urease and this enzyme differs considerably from ruminal urease (Mahadevan *et al.*, 1976).

Acetohydroxamate (AHA) is a noncompetitive inhibitor of bacterial urease of low toxicity and the application of AHA in the treatment of hyperammonemic states in man by reducing the contribution of urea to blood ammonia, as a result of intestinal microbial urease activity, has been proposed (Fishbein *et al.*, 1965). The compound could prevent urea poisoning in ruminants and improved the nitrogen retention in sheep fed a urea-containing diet (Streeter *et al.*, 1969). Although AHA is believed to be relatively nontoxic to bacteria and animals, the effect of this drug on the mixed rumen population *in vitro* is not limited to inhibition of urease (Jones, 1968). Both the total VFA production, as well as the relative proportions of acetate and propionate produced from added cellulose by the rumen microorganisms, were modified. The VFA production was lowered and the ratio of acetate/propionate was increased. Meanwhile, AHA was slowly degraded and 80% of the activity was lost within 24 hours of incubation.

Caprylohydroxamic acid (CHA) is an even stronger inhibitor of bacterial urease (Shimbayashi *et al.*, 1973a). Urease activity and ammonia concentration in the rumen of urea-fed sheep as well as urease activity in the intestines of rats and ammonia levels in portal and cardiac blood of these rats, were effectively reduced after inclusion of CHA in the diet. The total production of VFA and the pH were reported not to be affected. Only VFA concentrations and no production rates were measured (Shimbayashi *et al.*, 1973b).

The chain length of the hydroxamates of amino acids is of importance in determining the inhibitory properties on urease. Aspartic acid β-hydroxamate and L-glutamic acid γ-monohydroxamate are much less active than the hydroxamates of DL-alanine, L-arginine, and DL-threonine (Mahadevan *et al.*, 1976).

b. Defaunation Experiments. Students of rumen physiology have always been puzzled by the question about the role and the importance of the rumen ciliate protozoa in the nutrition of their hosts. The rumen protozoa are chiefly particle eaters and satisfy their nutritional needs largely by ingesting bacteria (predation) or other rumen protozoa (predation and cannibalism). The amino acids of the microbial proteins are incorporated into protozoal protein with little interconversion between the amino acids. *De novo* synthesis of amino acids by the protozoa occurs, but is of little quantitative importance and the major part of the amino acids needed is derived from the proteins of ingested microorganisms. The nitrogenous materials released by the protozoa during digestion of their prey are largely recycled back to ammonia by fermentation. Ciliates do not synthesize purine or pyrimidine bases *de novo* and have to use the so-called salvage pathways for biosynthesis. The bacterial nucleic acids are degraded by the rumen protozoa as far as the individual nucleotides or nucleosides and these are incorporated preferentially, since the ciliates also lack the ability to form ribose. It has been estimated that

30–40% of the microbial cells are degraded in the rumen each day (for a review, see Prins and Van den Vorstenbosch, 1975).

Numerous studies have been undertaken on the effect of defaunation on the ruminant animal and in order to obtain defaunated animals, as many methods have been advocated. One of the oldest used a combined starvation–copper sulfate treatment (Becker, 1929). Copper sulfate however affects the animal's health and *in vitro* studies have shown that copper ions inhibit the rumen fermentation, especially when concentrates are fermented (Slyter and Wolin, 1967). In later studies many other compounds were found to have deleterious effects on the rumen ciliates, but almost all of these compounds also have an inhibitory effect on the bacteria as well.

Dosing cattle with 30 gm of dioctyl sodium sulfosuccinate on 2 consecutive days completely eliminated both ciliate and flagellate protozoa and the animals recovered from the depression in the rumen fermentation at the fourth day (Abou Akkada *et al.,* 1968). The same detergent led to a complete suppression of the hydrogenation of linoleic acid and oleic acid by rumen contents of sheep. As the animal recovered from the effects of the detergent, the ability to hydrogenate both substrates was almost completely recovered, even though the rumen of the sheep remained devoid of ciliate protozoa (Dawson and Kemp, 1969). Anionic detergents such as long-chain sulfates and phosphates and even long-chain unsaturated fatty acids in general are toxic to the rumen protozoa, but may depress rumen microbial bacterial activity (Willard and Kodras, 1967; Meyer and Bartley, 1972). Well-known inhibitors of cell metabolism such as hydrogen peroxide, iodoacetic acid, sodium arsenate are also toxic to the enzyme systems of rumen protozoa (Willard and Kodras, 1967; Prins and Prast, 1973), but of course are unsuitable as defaunating agents.

Other compounds that have been used as defaunating agents are antiprotozoal drugs as the imidazoles and the drugs Su-14,276 and Su-15,412 (Willard and Kodras, 1967; Clarke and Reid, 1969; O'Connor *et al.,* 1970). Dimetridazol has been used in a dose of 16 gm per day on 3 consecutive days to defaunate cattle in a study on the effect of defaunation on the incidence of legume bloat in dry and lactating cows (Clarke *et al.,* 1969) and although both incidence and severity of bloat were reduced, the drug was considered to hold little practical value as a bloat prophylactic, since both food intake and milk production were reduced. The compound resulted in a marked inhibition of the rumen fermentation. Not only the protozoa were killed but a 50% reduction was seen in the formation of VFA by metronidazole and dimetridazole *in vitro* (O'Connor *et al.,* 1970). Metronidazole has been used for many years in the oral treatment of trichomoniasis, amoebiasis, giardiasis, and Vincent's stomatitis in man, and the drug displays a wide spectrum of activity against many anaerobic bacteria and protozoa. The compound acts as a preferential electron acceptor from reduced ferridoxin in *Trichomonas vaginalis* (Edwards and Mathison, 1970) and in *Clostridium acetobutylicum* (O'Brien and Morris, 1972) and thus inhibits hydrogen evolution by these organisms. *T. foetus* also possesses a mechanism for hydrogen evolution similar to that found in the saccharolytic clostridia (Bauchop, 1971). In sensitive cells of *T. vaginalis* the nitro group of metronidazole is reduced in the process and by analogy with the nitrofurans (McCalla *et al.*, 1975), the most probable pathway of metronidazole reduction in anaerobes would be via some potentially very reactive intermediates (hydroxylamines), which could react with DNA and protein (Ings *et al.*, 1974). The reduced nitrofuran derivatives also cause breakage of DNA and the potency of these compounds as mutagens and carcinogens is correlated with the amount of damage caused to DNA (McCalla *et al.*, 1975). Other organic drugs with nitro groups found to be highly toxic to the rumen ciliates are *p*-nitroaniline and nitrofurazone (Willard and Kodras, 1967).

Stimulation of the protozoa by a drug has sometimes been reported. Feeding of diethylstilbestrol (DES) increases rate of gain, feed efficiency, and nitrogen retention in ruminants. The total number of rumen ciliates of dairy cows on semi-purified or natural diets in continuous feeding experiments were significantly increased, but a decrease was seen in the relative abundancy of *Entodinium* sp. (Ibrahim *et al.*, 1970). Another reported effect of DES is that it prevents the disappearance of ciliate protozoa from the rumen of ruminants fed high concentrate pelleted diets (Christiansen *et al.*, 1964). In both cases the stimulatory action was tentatively explained on the basis of the estrogenic activity of the drug. However, in a study by Dearth *et al.* (1974) with lambs, no effect of dietary DES on either growth of the animals or on rumen protozoal numbers was seen. Implantation of DES in steers increased body weight gain, but this was not associated with increases in rumen protozoal numbers (Slyter *et al.*, 1970). It was discovered by Hino *et al.* (1973) that several neutral plant sterols as well as cholesterol are stimulatory to the growth of *Entodinium* sp. *in vitro*. It is possible that there is a relation between this observation and the alleged effect of DES. Protein synthesis in a cell-free preparation from *Entodinium* sp. was not stimulated by DES (Hoshino and Sugiyama, 1974) and no influence of DES was found on the rate of storage of amylopectin or the formation of gaseous hydrogen from glucose by *Dasytricha ruminantium* in short-term incubation studies *in vitro* (R. A. Prins and W. van Hoven, unpublished experiments).

When they are present in the rumen, the ciliate protozoa undoubtedly play an important role in the fermentation of food materials and they are of nutritional importance to their hosts. Upon defaunation, however, bacterial numbers increase in the rumen and it is likely that bacteria take over many of the protozoal functions. The results of the many studies on the effects of defaunation have not been unanimous (reviewed by Hungate, 1966; Harmeyer, 1973). In general, growth and well-being of calves reared without ciliate rumen protozoa are not greatly affected (Williams and Dinusson, 1973), but several changes in rumen and blood parameters as well as in some other physiological criteris have been reported in defaunated animals. These include lower rumen NH_3 levels, often lower levels of rumen butyrate, and a lower excretion of nitrogenous compounds in the urine. Much depends on the diet composition and level of intake. It has also been claimed that the serum and tissue linoleic acid concentrations of steers were increased in the absence of ruminal protozoa (Clemens et al., 1974; Abaza et al., 1975).

2. Carbohydrate Fermentation

Many methods have been described that alter the rumen fermentation of food by manipulating the diet. The extent of the rumen fermentation can be influenced by feeding level, choice of food, and by applying different processes in the preparation of feeding stuffs (Thomson, 1972; Singleton, 1972). Increased rates of passage of digesta allows more food to escape from the rumen fermentation. At the same time, several of these manipulations also affect the rumen fermentation pattern. Higher fermentation rates are seen with higher rates of digesta passage and the higher rates of fermentation increase the rates of formation of propionate, valerate, or butyrate. Higher fermentation rates also allow a more efficient microbial growth, since maintenance energy requirements for the microbes become relatively smaller. The high fermentation rates can be obtained, e.g., by lowering the ratio of roughage to concentrates in the diet, by diminution of the particle size, by increasing the level or frequency of feeding, by the choice and the processing of carbohydrates (for a full discussion, see Ørskov, 1975).

In the rumen fermentation, propionate is very efficiently produced since hydrogen is taken up in its formation from glucose. An increase in propionate and a decrease in acetate (or to a lesser extent in butyrate) is associated with a more efficient fermentation, since the energy loss in the production of methane is reduced. In the following we will discuss a number of chemicals and feed ingredients that stimulate the formation of propionate in the rumen. Some of these are highly inhibitory to the production of methane.

a. **Unsaturated Long-Chain Fatty Acids and Related Compounds.**
It has repeatedly been shown (see Prins *et al.*, 1972b; Demeyer and
Van Nevel, 1975) that the feeding of vegetable oils to cattle resulted in
an increase in rumen propionic acid levels. This effect is probably the
result of the antibacterial activity of unsaturated long-chain fatty acids
(Demeyer and Henderickx, 1966; Czerkawski *et al.*, 1966) which are
released in the rumen by lipases of microbial and of plant origin (Prins *et
al.*, 1975; Faruque *et al.*, 1974). The results of studies with natural rumen
contents (Demeyer and Henderickx, 1967; Van Nevel *et al.*, 1971) or
with pure cultures of *Methanobacterium* sp. (Prins *et al.*, 1972b) and other
rumen bacteria (Henderson, 1973) clearly show that unsaturated long-
chain fatty acids are toxic to methane bacteria especially. For the expression of toxicity a free carboxyl group is required, triglycerides being
ineffective. Substitution of the polar carboxyl group by less polar groups
or nonpolar groups diminishes or abolishes the inhibitory effect on
methane production. Other compounds which combine an aliphatic
chain with a polar group (sulfate alcohols, Blaxter and Czerkawski,
1966; tertiary branched-chain carboxylic acids, Clapperton and Czerkawski, 1971) also are effective as methane inhibitors (Table II). Toxicity
of the unsaturated long-chain fatty acids depends on the type of unsaturation (acetylenic > ethylenic) and is increased with the number of
nonconjugated double bonds. *Cis*-unsaturated acids are more active than
trans-isomers. Anacardic acids (8-An 15:1 and 8,11,14-An 15:3) were
extremely toxic to methanogenic bacteria in rumen contents (Van Nevel
et al., 1971). Anacardic acids are salicylic acids substituted in position 6
with saturated or unsaturated long-chain alkyl groups.

Lipophilic acids also have been used as antimicrobial food additives or
preservatives (Freese *et al.*, 1973) and antimicrobial agents for cosmetics
and pharmaceuticals (Kabara, 1975). The activity of several fatty acids
and fatty acid derivatives against aerobic gram-positive organisms also
shows that chain length and position of the unsaturated bonds are of
importance in determining antimicrobial activity. Results with straight
chain C_{18} acids demonstrate that the highest inhibitory action was obtained when unsaturation is located at the Δ^2 or Δ^8 position (Kabara,
1975).

Gram-negative bacteria (though more sensitive to inhibition by short-
chain fatty acids) are more resistant than gram-positive organisms towards the inhibitory action on growth, amino acid transport, and oxygen
consumption of long-chain fatty acids. This is related to the screening
action of the lipopolysaccharide layer, which prevents the accumulation
of the acids on the inner membrane at inhibitory concentrations (Sheu
and Freese, 1973).

TABLE II
Summary of Results of Experiments in which Aliphatic Compounds Were Given
to Sheep[a]

Compound		Depression of CH_4 production (kcal/100 kcal of compound)
Saturated acids		
Acetic	inf.[b]	4.2
n-Butyric	inf.	1.5
Caproic		16.6
Caprylic		12.3
Capric		27.4
Lauric		67.5
Myristic		48.6
Palmitic		22.8
Stearic		23.2
Unsaturated acids		
Oleic	inf.	13.8
Linoleic	inf.	14.2
Linolenic	inf.	16.4
Linolenic		28.9
Alcohols		
Oleyl alcohol	inf.	0.1
Lauryl alcohol	inf.	3.7
Sulfated alcohols		
Sulfated C_{16} and C_{18} alcohols	inf.	80.7
Sulfated lauryl alcohols	inf.	92.9
Hydrocarbons		
C_{18}	inf.	0.5

[a] From Blaxter and Czerkawski, 1966.
[b] Added to the rumen by infusion; in other cases the compounds were mixed with the diet.

The inhibitory effect of unsaturated fatty acids on methanogenic bacteria is not the result of competition for hydrogen (used in the hydrogenation of unsaturated fatty acids) but is a direct toxic effect on methane-producing bacteria (Prins et al., 1972b). Accumulation of gaseous hydrogen in vivo or in vitro, as is seen with other more selective inhibitors of methanogenesis (see below), is not always seen when long-chain fatty acids are added to the fermentation.

Not only methanogenic bacteria are affected however since other rumen anaerobic bacteria such as cellulolytic Ruminococcus and Butyrivibrio species studied by Henderson (1973) are inhibited. Rumen ciliate protozoa are killed and these observations may be related to the decreased butyrate formation in rumen contents *in vivo* observed upon infusion of linseed oil fatty acids (Demeyer *et al.*, 1969).

Feeding linseed oil hydrolysate (4%) in rations for beef production did not give the expected beneficial effect on animal performance; sulfite (0.8%), another inhibitor of rumen methanogenesis (Prins *et al.*, 1972b; see review by Weigand, 1974) also did not influence digestibility parameters, daily gain, or feed conversion (Cottyn *et al.*, 1973). This could be explained by the fact that tallow was included in the control diet to make the diets isocaloric, and the saturated long-chain fatty acids already may have depressed methane formation, since rates of methane production were low (Van Nevel *et al.*, 1973). The escape of large amounts of carbohydrate in these diets from ruminal fermentation was also postulated and this in itself would have increased the efficiency of utilization of the metabolizable energy from these rations.

When a mixed diet of hay and concentrates fed to sheep was supplemented with 20 gm of cod liver oil per day, a marked fall in the ratio of acetate to propionate was observed, but no clear differences were seen in the amount of energy fermented in the rumen (64% of the digestible energy), or in the efficiency of microbial protein synthesis, which averaged 200 gm/kg organic matter apparently digested in the rumen (Sutton *et al.*, 1975). No increase in microbial fat synthesis was found as was observed by Czerkawski (1973) and Czerkawski *et al.* (1975).

b. Halogenated Compounds. A large number of polyhalogenated compounds appear to interfere with the formation of methane. The halogenated methane analogues (alkyl halides) are very powerful inhibitors of methanogenesis. On a molar basis these compounds are a thousand times more effective in decreasing methane formation than the long-chain fatty acids (see Table III). However, since these compounds are too volatile (methyl chloride and methyl bromide are already gaseous at room temperature) to be used in diets as feed additives, a large number of halogenated compounds including various polyhalogenated alcohols, aldehydes, acids, hemiacetals of sugars and starch, and esters, have been synthesized and tested for their effects on the rumen fermentation. In Table IV the main groups of these compounds are listed with references to the pertaining literature. Most of these compounds inhibit methanogenesis, lower the acetate/propionate ratio in the rumen and sometimes an increase in the lactate concentration is seen. Hydrogen often accumulates in the gas phase and this is an important difference with the situation encountered after the addition of unsaturated long-chain fatty acids. A number of other characteristics that have been noted

TABLE III
Concentrations of Methane Inhibitors Needed for 50% or 100% Inhibition of Methane Production *in Vitro*

Compound	Rumen fluid		Pure cultures of *Methanobacterium* sp.
	50% inhibition[a]	100% inhibition[d]	50% inhibition[c]
CCl_4	$1.4 \times 10^{-6} M$	$10.0 \times 10^{-6} M$	$32.0 \times 10^{-6} M$
$CHCl_3$	$7.8 \times 10^{-6} M$	$20.0 \times 10^{-6} M$	$8.0 \times 10^{-6} M$
Chloral hydrate		$\geqslant 2.0 \times 10^{-4} M$	$1.4 \times 10^{-4} M$
Linoleate			$3.2 \times 10^{-3} M$
Linolenate	$1 \times 10^{-3} M$ [b]		$1.8 \times 10^{-3} M$
Linseed oil hydrolysate		$\geqslant 1 \times 10^{-3} M$	
Sulfite	$3.0 \times 10^{-3} M$ [c]	$10.0 \times 10^{-3} M$	$1.2 \times 10^{-3} M$

[a] Bauchop (1967)
[b] Demeyer and Henderickx (1967)
[c] Van Nevel (1972)
[d] Van Nevel *et al.* (1970)
[e] Prins *et al.* (1972b)

are the inhibition of the fermentation of pyruvate, lactate, sugars, and cellulose.

The efficacy of a number of polyhalogenated acids and derivatives in decreasing *in vitro* methane formation is shown in Table V (data taken from Trei *et al.*, 1971). The halogens on the compounds are essential for activity, e.g., while polyhalogenated aldehydes were active, their nonsubstituted counterparts were not (Quaghebeur and Oyaert, 1971b). Iodine compounds are more effective than bromine compounds and these in turn are more active than their chlorinated analogues. The more halogens on the molecule the stronger the influence.

The relative activity of various esters of polyhalogenated alcohols (shown in Table VI) is probably determined by the ease with which the compounds are absorbed by the microbes (Czerkawski and Breckenridge, 1975a). Chloral hydrate (Prins, 1965) and its sugar derivatives are partly metabolized by the rumen microbes with the release of the methane inhibitors trichloroethanol and chloroform (Prins and Seekles, 1968), though evidence was presented by Quaghebeur and Oyaert (1971b) to show that this conversion also occurs spontaneously with chloral hydrate.

TABLE IV

Halogenated Methane Inhibitors and Literature References on the Application of These Compounds *in Vitro* and *in Vivo*

Compounds	*In vitro*	*In vivo*
Polyhalogenated methane analogues		
CCl_4	Bauchop (1967); Rufener and Wolin (1968); Parish and Trei (1971); Prins et al. (1972b)	Quaghebeur and Oyaert (1971a); Clapperton (1974)
$CHCl_3$	Bauchop (1967); Prins (1967); Prins (1970); Parish and Trei (1971); Prins et al. (1972b)	
CH_2Cl_2	Bauchop (1967)	
CBr_4	Quaghebeur and Oyaert (1971a,b)	
$CHBr_3$	Quaghebeur and Oyaert (1971a,b)	
CH_2Br_2	Van Nevel et al. (1970); Parish and Trei (1971); Quaghebeur and Oyaert (1971a,b)	
$CHClBr_2$	Van Nevel et al. (1970)	Johnson et al. (1972)
CI_4	Quaghebeur and Oyaert (1971a,b)	
CHI_3	Quaghebeur and Oyaert (1971a,b)	
CH_2I_2	Quaghebeur and Oyaert (1971a,b)	
CH_3I	Quaghebeur and Oyaert (1971a,b)	
Polyhalogenated alcohols		
Trichloroethanol	Czerkawski and Breckenridge (1975a)	
4-Chloro-1-butanol	Prins (1967); Prins and Seekles (1968)	
Polyhalogenated aldehydes	Quaghebeur and Oyaert (1971a)	Quaghebeur and Oyaert (1971b)
α,α,β-Trichloro-n-butyraldehyde	Quaghebeur and Oyaert (1971a,b)	

Compound	References	
Chloroacetaldehyde	Quaghebeur and Oyaert (1971a,b)	
Bromoacetaldehyde-diethylacetal	Quaghebeur and Oyaert (1971a,b)	
Polyhalogenated acids		
2,2,2-Tribromoacetic acid	Trei et al. (1971)	Patchett et al. (1972b)
Bis (chloromethyl) sulfone		
Polyhaologenated alcoholesters	Czerkawski and Breckenridge (1975a)	Czerkawski and Breckenridge (1975b)
Polyhalogenated alkylamides		
2,2,2-Trichloroacetamide	Trei and Olson (1969); Parish and Trei (1972a; 1973b); Clapperton (1974)	Trei et al. (1971); Parish and Trei (1972a;1973b); Clapperton (1974)
N-(2-Hydroxypropyl)dichloracetamide		Patchett et al. (1972a)
Bis(polyhalomethyl)derivatives	Parish and Trei (1972b)	Parish and Trei (1972b)
Hydrates of polyhalogenated aldehydes and polyhalohemiacetals		
Chloral hydrate	Prins (1965;1967;1970); Prins and Seekles (1968) Prins et al. (1972b); Van Nevel et al. (1969)	Prins (1967); Prins and Seekles (1968); Quaghebeur and Oyaert (1971a); Czerkawski and Breckenridge (1975a)
β-Chloralose, dichloralose	Prins (1967); Prins and Seekles (1968)	
Polyhalohemiacetal derivatives of saccharides		
Bromal	Parish and Trei (1971) Quaghebeur and Oyaert (1971a,b)	Johnson (1972); Trei et al. (1972) Quaghebeur and Oyaert (1971a)

TABLE V

Percentage of Inhibition of Rumen Methanogenesis by Several
Haloaliphatic Acids and Derivatives[a]

Compound: R-CO-X		Level in ppm (volume)	
R	X	3	13
CH_2Cl	OH	60	75
CH_2Cl	NH_2	—	25
$CHCl_2$	OH	50	75
$CHCl_2$	NH_2	80	95
CCl_3	OH	10	25
CCl_3	NH_2	80	93
CCl_3	$NHCH_3$	20	93
CCl_3	NHC_2H_5	17	96
CCl_3	NHC_8H_{17}	—	85
CCl_3	$NHCH_2CH_2OH$	80	90
CCl_3	$N(CH_3)_2$	45	95
CH_2Br	OH	—	[b]
$CHBr_2$	OH	70	—
$CHBr_2$	NH_2	73	—
CBr_3	OH	93	96
CF_3	NH_2	0	0
CF_2Cl	OH	0	0
CF_2Cl	NH_2	—	9
CH_3CHBr	OH	28	64
$(CH_3)_2CBr$	OH	0	0
$CH_2ClCHCl$	NH_2	—	10
CH_2I	OH	[b]	[b]
CH_2I	NH_2	[b]	[b]

[a] After Trei et al., 1971.
[b] Overall fermentation reduced.

Methanogenesis is also inhibited by other organic compounds such as
DDT (McBride and Wolfe, 1971) and other halogenated pesticides (R.
A. Prins and A. Lankhorst, unpublished results). The inhibitory activity
of DDT is centered in the trichloroethane portion of the molecule
(McBride and Wolfe, 1971). In natural systems such as anaerobic sewage
sludge or anaerobic sediments of lakes, methane analogues also inhibit
methanogenesis (Sykes and Kirsch, 1972; Thiel, 1969; Cappenberg,
1974).

In older publications it was suggested that halogenated methane
analogues block the formation of methane by reacting with reduced
vitamin B_{12}, at that time supposed to be a cofactor in methanogenesis
(see review by Wolfe, 1971), but doubt of this explanation has arisen

TABLE VI

Relative Inhibitory Activity (RIA) of Various Compounds with Respect to Methane Production during Incubation of Sheep Rumen Contents *in Vitro*[a,b]

Compound	RIA	Compound	RIA
Halogen-substituted ethanols		Esters of trichoroacetic acid	
Monochloroethanol	1	(TCA)	
Dichloroethanol	22	TCA	4
TCE	909	TCE TCA	714
Trifluoroethanol	0	Ethyl TCA	17
Tribromoethanol (TBE)	10000	Isobutyl TCA	21
Esters of halogen-substituted		t-Butyl TCA	96
ethanols and pivalic acid		Isobutyl isobutyrate	1
Monochloroethyl pivalate	0	Isobutyraldehyde	1
Dichloroethyl pivalate	6	-Pentyl TCA	8
TCE pivalate	1000	Amyl TCA	14
Trifluroethyl pivalatz	1	Neopentyl TCA	23
TBE pivalate	2500	2,5-Hexanediol TCA	43
		1,6-Hexanediol TCA	8
Esters of TCE and fatty acids			
TCE acetate	500	Esters of sulfonic acids	
TCE butyrate	909	Methane sulfonic acid	0
TCE isobutyrate	833	TCE methane sulfonate	588
TCE valerate	1250	Trichloromethane	9
TCE isovalerate	1000	sulfonic acid	
TCE hexanoate	1250	TCE trichloromethane	93
TCE isohexanoate	625	sulfonate	
TCE palmitate	278	Ethyl trichloromethane	64
TCE versatate	217	sulfonate	
TCE linolenate	51	TCE tosylate	294
Esters of dibasic acids		Trichloro C_3 compounds	
TCE succinate	1000	Trichloroacetone	340
TCE glutarate	1667	Trichloro-2-propanol	454
TCE adipate	1428	Trichloro-2-propanol	214
TBE succinate	5000	pivalate	
TBE adipate	2500		
Isobutyl adipate	13	General	
		Chloral hydrate	526
		TCA	714
		TCE benzoate	500

[a] The concentrations of the test compounds and of the trichloroethanol (TCE) ester of pivalic acid incubated at the same time and required to give 50% inhibition of methane production were used to calculate the RIA under standard conditions; RIA is the concentration of TCE pivalate divided by the concentration of the test compound and multiplied by 1000.

[b] Taken from Czerkawski and Breckenridge (1975b).

when it was found that DDT also acts as an inhibitor, although it cannot alkylate B_{12} chemically (McBride and Wolfe, 1971). In the newly proposed metabolic scheme of the process of methanogenesis, vitamin B_{12} derivatives do not appear to play a role as cofactor (R. S. Wolfe, personal communication). In one of the two pathways for the formation of propionate in the rumen, isomerization of succinyl-CoA to methylmalonyl-CoA requires the intervention of dimethylbenzimidazole cobalamide, a vitamin B_{12} compound, yet the formation of propionate through this pathway is not decreased by chloral hydrate (Prins and van der Meer, 1976).

Inhibition of the nonoxidative decarboxylation of pyruvate and of alcohol dehydrogenase has been postulated as a mechanism of action of chloral hydrate and halogenated compounds (Quaghebeur and Oyaert, 1971c). However, these reactions are not of importance in the rumen (see Prins, 1977).

The mechanism by which the increase in the production of propionate is brought about by halogenated methane analogues, is related to the fact that hydrogen is the main precursor of rumen methane. During fermentation of carbohydrates in the rumen, pyridine nucleotide cofactors are reduced and gaseous hydrogen can be produced from the reduced cofactors, especially when the partial pressure of hydrogen in the medium is kept low (Chung, 1976; for references, also see Van Nevel *et al.*, 1974; Wolin, 1974, 1975; Prins, 1977), or the reduced cofactors are oxidized in processes such as propionate formation. Another system for the release of hydrogen gas is constituted by the combined action of pyruvate: ferredoxin oxidoreductase and ferredoxin-linked hydrogenase in the metabolism of pyruvate. In the normal rumen the concentration of dissolved hydrogen gas is kept low by methanogenesis and other hydrogen consuming reactions.

When hydrogen-oxidizing *Methanobacterium* sp. are grown together with hydrogen-producing anaerobes, removal of the hydrogen by the methanogenics results in (a) a shift in fermentation products by the hydrogen-former in the sense that more acetate (with either hydrogen and carbon dioxide or with formate) and less lactic acid, ethanol, butyric acid, succinic acid or propionic acid are formed, when compared to controls (Wolin, 1975; Prins and van den Vorstenbosch, 1975; Chung, 1976), and (b) increased growth of the hydrogen-forming strain, since more ATP becomes available to the organism in the acetigenic fermentation.

When the formation of methane in the rumen is specifically-inhibited, hydrogen accumulates. Calculation of the balance of metabolic hydrogen shows that some hydrogen is missing when methanogenesis is blocked by halogenated methane analogues, but not when unsaturated fatty acids are used (Demeyer and Van Nevel, 1975). In the former case the accumualtion of an unknown reduced precursor of methane was postulated. The accumulation of hydrogen leads to a diminished formation of hydrogen itself and of acetate by inhibition of pyruvate degradation (Chung, 1976). Electrons generated in glycolysis have to be shunted away to other reductive processes and more electron acceptors derived from pyruvate have to be used for regeneration of NAD^+. This results in a stimulation of propionate formation, or sometimes in increased formation of valerate or caproate. Whem rumen fluid or pure cultures of ruminal propionate or succinate-forming bacteria are incubated under a gas phase containing added hydrogen gas, propionate formation may be increased (Prins, 1970; Van Nevel *et al.*, 1974). The flux of carbon in the fermentation of lactate in the rumen is increased through both the acrylate and the dicarboxylic acid pathways (Prins and van der Meer, 1976).

As in the case of unsaturated fatty acids, feeding of methane analogues and other halogenated inhibitors has not always given the expected improvements in animal performance. It would seem that the following factors are of importance in determining the outcome of such studies:

1. *Composition and level of the diet.* Best results would have to be expected with roughage diets fed at 1 × maintenance. Little or no improvement might be expected from the application of inhibitors with concentrate rations fed *ad libitum,* which already in themselves result in narrow acetate/propionate ratios.

2. *Depression of feed intake.* Sometimes a lowered intake of feed is seen possibly as a result of:

3. *A depressed overall fermentation rate.* Inhibitors may cause a reduced fermentation of substrate in the rumen when the dose is too high or because the selectivity of the drug is too low.

4. *Pharmacodynamics of the drug.* A rapid wash-out of water-soluble inhibitors fed once or twice a day or the volatibility of certain compounds may render the drugs ineffective.

5. *Adaptation of the microflora.* This phenomenon poses a real threat to the usefulness of several inhibitors (see Trei *et al.,* 1971; Clapperton, 1974). Reversal to normal pretreatment rates of methane formation and VFA patterns similar to the original fermentation pattern are often seen in long-term experiments.

6. *Eructation of hydrogen gas is still an energy loss.*

7. *Toxicity of the inhibitor.* The methane inhibitor itself may have desired but as yet unknown effects on the host animal.

At least some of the above problems (3, 5, and 6) do not occur with the

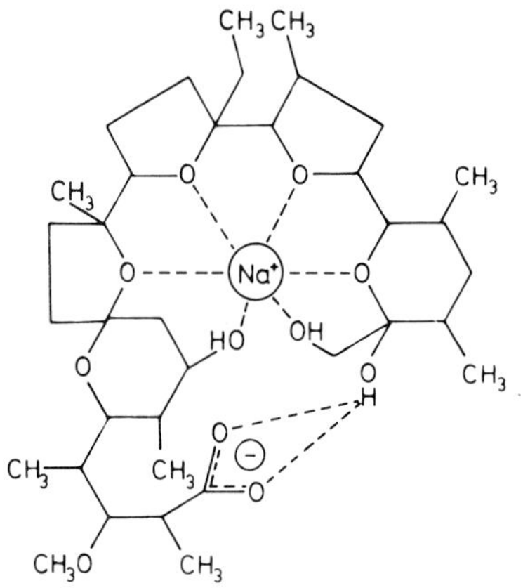

Monensin sodium

Fig. 9. Monensin, a drug that stimulates the formation of propionate in the rumen.

drug monensin (Fig. 9), a product of the fungus *Streptomyces cinnamonen-sis*. This ionophore compound already known for years as a coccidiostat, drastically increases the percentage of propionate in the rumen, even with concentrate diets. An inhibitory effect of monensin on methane production is only seen with high levels of the compound (≥ 30 ppm), is lost after feeding the drug for a few days, and cannot explain the increase in propionate seen with much lower levels (5 ppm) (Dinius *et al.*, 1976). Hydrogen gas does not accumulate. The shift in VFA is not reversed during long-term feeding of the drug. The 10% improvement noted in feed efficiency with monensin is probably at least partly due to the change in VFA, partly also to a lowered breakdown of proteins, since ammonia levels in the rumen are lowered by the drug (see Richardson *et al.*, 1976; Potter *et al.*, 1976). When the action of this antibiotic depends upon eliciting cyclic ion fluxes across biological membranes, as is the case with related antibiotics (e.g., valinomycin, nigericin), microbial growth would be impaired in the rumen.

Ethoxylated alcohols (Erwin and Marco, 1969), thiostrepton, and siomycin (Raun, 1974a), the antibiotics A477, A4696, vancomycin and oristocetin (Raun, 1974b), the compound bis-4-(3-dimethylaminopro-poxy)-2-methyl-5-*t*-butylphenyl sulfide · 2 HCl (Maplesden and Myers, 1972) reportedly increase propionate formation, but whether inhibition of methanogenesis occurs is not known.

In the body of mammals propylene glycol can be converted to glucose in various tissues including the liver. First, propylene glycol is primarily absorbed from the rumen as such and only partially fermented to propionate (Emery *et al.*, 1967; Hamada *et al.*, 1968). This conversion could be increased by adaptation of the rumen microflora to propanediol for 2 weeks. Clapperton and Czerkawski (1972) also concluded that a large portion of propylene glycol infused into the rumen of sheep (100 gm/day) was directly absorbed, but some was fermented in the rumen to lactic acid, while propanol was another product (Czerkawski and Breckenridge, 1973). Propionate was increased and the drop in acetic acid which was measured could not be explained. Furthermore, the increase in weight gain of lambs receiving 0.5 or 1.0 gm of propylene glycol per kg of body weight in their daily rations for 104 days, could not be explained by the effect of propylene glycol as a substrate alone. A change in the fermentation pattern was postulated (Shiga *et al.*, 1975). The extra effect of propylene glycol could have been the result of its antimethanogenic activity (Prins, 1970).

VI. RESEARCH NEEDS

It is to be expected that many additional investigations will be carried out in the near future on microbial metabolism of foreign compounds in the gastrointestinal tract and more will be learned about the toxicological and pharmacological consequences of these processes. It would be of interest to consider the nutritional implications as well, especially in those monogastric animals that cover a large part of their requirements for energy, protein, and vitamins by fermentation is the cecum and by coprophagy.

It is absolutely essential that we learn more about the way in which foreign chemicals are handled in the rumen. Both the pathways of drug degradation and the influences of drugs and their metabolites on the fermentative processes themselves have been studied in only a very few cases. The possible role of the rumen ciliate protozoa in the metabolism of pesticides and drugs is intriguing.

Research on the chemical manipulation of the fermentation in the rumen of growing ruminants could provide useful results in two ways. First, a drug that stimulates the formation of propionate directly or inhibits the enzyme hydrogenase in rumen microbes would seem preferable to the methane inhibitors discussed above, since their application often entails a loss of gaseous hydrogen. This not only represents a loss of energy to the animal, but results in a less efficient microbial growth (Demeyer and Van Nevel, 1975). Second, slowing down the rate of amino acid degradation in the rumen could improve the retention of nitrogen and increase growth rate by allowing more unfermented protein to escape from the forestomachs.

However, adaptation of the rumen microorganisms to such feed additives upon prolonged administration of the drugs is one of the most serious difficulties that could interfere with a successful practical application of such compounds. Inhibitors of methanogenesis which lose their effectiveness as a result of microbial adaptation still could be of value as orally administered therapeutics against ketosis, where a shift in the fermentation pattern is only desired for a short time. The tremendous capacity to adapt to all sorts of chemicals and feed compositions is a feature of the rumen fermentation that has been known for a long time and for which the ruminant has often been praised. Adaptation of the microorganisms to inhibitors naturally occurring in plants enables wild ruminants and other polygastric animals to consume toxic foods and to colonize nutritionally difficult environments (Moir, 1968; Freeland and Janzen, 1974).

Aside from the problem of microbial adaptation, it would seem that many of the desired nutritional changes in rumen metabolism can be attained by direct manipulation of the diet. Various treatments of food components are already used to meet the increased requirements in modern animal husbandry.

ACKNOWLEDGMENTS

I want to thank my colleagues D. I. Demeyer and C. J. Van Nevel for rewarding discussions and Mr. W. D. Brands for his assistance in preparing the figures. Mrs. J. A. H. Verweij-van Dijl is gratefully acknowledged for typing the manuscript.

REFERENCES

Abaza, M. A., Abou Akkada, A. R., and El-Shazly, K. (1975). Effect of rumen protozoa on dietary lipid in sheep. *J. Agric. Sci.* **85**, 135–143.
Abou Akkada, A. R., Bartley, E. E., Berube, R., Fina, L. R., Meyer, R. M., Henricks, D., and Julius, F. (1968). Simple method to remove completely ciliate protozoa of adult ruminants. *Appl. Microbiol.* **16**, 1475–1477.
Abou Akkada, A. R., Hassan, M. A., and Naga, M. A. (1973). Effect of some pesticides and herbicides on the rumen micro-organisms of sheep. *J. Agric. Sci.* **81**, 231–236.
Alexander, M. (1973). Nonbiodegradable and other recalcitrant molecules. *Biotechnol. Bioeng.* **15**, 611–647.
Anonymous. (1972). Excretion of methylmalonic acid by vitamin B_{12} deficient rats kept under germfree or conventional conditions. *Nutr. Rev.* **30**, 186–188.

Argenzio, R. A., Southworth, M., and Stevens, C. E. (1974). Sites of organic acid production and absorption in the equine gastrointestinal tract. *Am. J. Physiol.* **226,** 1042–1050.

Armstrong, B. K., and Curnow, D. H. (1967). The effect of streptomycin and erythromycin on vitamin B_{12} nutrition in rats in which coprophagy was prevented. *Br. J. Nutr.* **21,** 527–535.

Arnold, G. W., and Hill, J. L. (1972). Chemical factors affecting selection of food plants by ruminants. *In* "Phytochemical Ecology" (J. B. Harborne, ed.), pp. 71–101. Academic Press, New York.

Arvy, L. (1972). L'appendice vermiforme ou caecal. *Mammalia* **36,** Suppl., 1–68.

Barber, T. A., and Nagy, J. G. (1971). Effects of pesticides on mule deer rumen bacteria. *Trans. North Am. Wildl. Natur. Resour. Conf.* **36,** 153–162.

Barber, T. A., Schwartz, C. C., Nagy, J. G., and Streeter, C. L. (1970). Influence of pesticides on mule deer rumen bacteria. *J. Anim. Sci.* **31,** 235 (Abstr. No. 312).

Barrow, A., and Griffiths, L. A. (1974). Metabolism of the hydroxyethylrutosides. III. The fate of orally administered hydroxyethyl rutosides in laboratory animals; metabolism by rat intestinal microflora *in vitro. Xenobiotica* **4,** 743–754.

Bartley, E. E., Meyer, R. M., and Fina, L. R. (1975). Feedlot or grain bloat. *In* "Digestion and Metabolism in the Ruminant" (I. W. McDonald and A. C. I. Warner, eds.), pp. 551–562. Univ. of New England Publishing Unit, Armidale, Australia.

Bauchop, T. (1967). Inhibition of rumen methanogenesis by methane analogues. *J. Bacteriol.* **94,** 171–175.

Bauchop, T. (1971). Mechanism of hydrogen formation in *Trichomonas foetus. J. Gen. Microbiol.* **68,** 27–33.

Becker, E. R. (1929). Methods of rendering the rumen and reticulum of ruminants free from their normal infusorian fauna. *Proc. Natl. Acad. Sci. U.S.A.* **15,** 435–438.

Behmann, H. (1973). Vergleichend- und funktionell-anatomische Untersuchungen am Caecum and Colon myomorpher Nagetiere. *Z. Wiss. Zool.* **186,** 173–294.

Bell, E. A. (1972). Toxic amino acids in the leguminosae. *In* "Phytochemical Ecology" (J. B. Harborne, ed.), pp. 163–177. Academic Press, New York.

Bickel, M. H., Burkard, B., Meier-Strasser, E., and Van den Broek-Boot, M. (1974). Entero-bacterial formation of cyclohexylamine in rats ingesting cyclamate. *Xenobiotica* **4,** 425–439.

Blaxter, K. L., and Czerkawski, J. (1966). Modification of the methane production of the sheep by supplementation of its diet. *J. Sci. Food Agric.* **17,** 417–421.

Boyd, E. M. (1973). "Toxicity of Pure Foods." CRC Press, Cleveland, Ohio.

Braunberg, R. C., and Beck, V. (1968). Interaction of DDT and the gastrointestinal microflora of the rat. *J. Agric. Food Chem.* **16,** 451–453.

Broderick, G. A., and Smith, K. K. (1974). Inhibitors and measuring *in vitro* rumen proteolysis. *J. Anim. Sci.* **39,** 233 (Abstr. No. 365).

Buck, W. B. (1969). Untoward reactions encountered with medicated feeds. *In* "The Use of Drugs in Animal Feeds," pp. 196–217. Nat. Acad. Sci., Washington, D.C.

Bush, L. P., Boling, J. A., Allen, G., and Buckner, R. C. (1972). Inhibitory effects of perloline to rumen fermentation *in vitro. Crop Sci.* **12,** 277–279.

Cappenberg, T. E. (1974). Interrelations between sulfate-reducing and methane-producing bacteria in bottom deposits of a fresh-water lake. II. Inhibition experiments. *Antonie van Leeuwenhoek* **40,** 297–306.

Carleton, M. D. (1973). A survey of gross stomach morphology in New World Cricetinae (Rodentia, Muroidea), with comments on functional interpretations. *Misc. Publ., Mus. Zool., Univ. Mich.* **146,** 1–43.

Carlson, J. R., Dickinson, E. O., Yokoyama, M. T., and Bradley, B. (1975). Pulmonary edema and emphysema in cattle after intraruminal and intravenous administration of 3-methylindole. *Am. J. Vet. Res.* **36**, 1341–1347.

Casarett, L. J., and Doull, J. (1975). "Toxicology. The Basic Science of Poisons." Macmillan, New York.

Chalupa, W. (1975). Rumen bypass and protection of proteins and amino acid. *J. Dairy Sci.* **58**, 1198–1218.

Chalupa, W. and Scott, J. C. (1976). Protein nutrition of growing cattle. *In:* Tracer Studies on Non-protein Nitrogen III, pp. 13–25. IAEA, Vienna. Proceedings of a Research Coordination Meeting, Alexandria 15–18 March 1976.

Chalupa, W., Chow, A. W., and Parish, R. C. (1976). Chemical inhibition of amino acid degradation by rumen microbes. *Fed. Proc., Fed. Am. Soc. Exp. Biol.* **35**, 258 (Abstr. No. 295).

Chang, H. C., and Branen, A. L. (1975). Antimicrobial effects of butylated hydroxyanisole. *J. Food Sci.* **40**, 349–351.

Cheng, K.-J., Jones, G. A., Simpson, F. J., and Bryant, M. P. (1969). Isolation and identification of rumen bacteria capable of anaerobic rutin degradation. *Can. J. Microbiol.* **15**, 1365–1371.

Cheng, K.-J., Krishnamurty, H. G., Jones, G. A., and Simpson, F. J. (1971). Identification of products produced by the anaerobic degradation of naringin by *Butyrivibrio* sp. C$_3$. *Can. J. Microbiol.* **17**, 129–131.

Christiansen, W. C., Woods, W., and Burroughs, W. (1964). Ration characteristics influencing rumen protozoal populations. *J. Anim. Sci.* **23**, 984–988.

Chung, K.-T. (1976). Inhibitory effects of H$_2$ on growth of *Clostridium cellobioparum*. *Appl. Environ. Microbiol.* **31**, 342–348.

Clapperton, J. L. (1974). The effect of trichloroacetamide, chloroform and linseed oil into the rumen of sheep on some of the end-products of rumen digestion. *Br. J. Nutr.* **32**, 155–161.

Clapperton, J. L., and Czerkawski, J. W. (1971). The effect of tertiary branched-chain carboxylic acids on the energy metabolism of sheep. *Br. J. Nutr.* **26**, 459–468.

Clapperton, J. L., and Czerkawski, J. W. (1972). Metabolism of propane-1:2 diol infused into the rumen of sheep. *Br. J. Nutr.* **27**, 553–560.

Clark, D. E., Young, J. E., Younger, R. L., Hunt, L. M., and McLaran, J. K. (1964). The fate of 2,4-dichlorophenoxyacetic acid in sheep. *J. Agric. Food Chem.* **12**, 43–45.

Clarke, R. T. J., and Reid, C. S. W. (1969). Bloat in cattle. XXXI. The effect of dimetridazole on the rumen ciliate protozoa of dry and lactating cows. *N.Z. J. Agric. Res.* **12**, 437–445.

Clarke, R. T. J., Reid, C. S. W., and Young, P. W. (1969). Bloat in cattle. XXXII. Attempts to prevent legume bloat in dry and lactating cows by partial or complete elimination of the rumen holotrich protozoa with dimetridazole. *N.Z. J. Agric. Res.* **12**, 446–466.

Clemens, E., Woods, W., and Arthand, V. (1974). The effect of feeding unsaturated fats as influenced by gelatinized corn and by the presence or absence of rumen protozoa. II. Carcass lipid composition. *J. Anim. Sci.* **38**, 640–645.

Clemens, E. T., Stevens, C. E., and Southworth, M. (1975a). Sites of organic acid production and pattern of digesta movement in the gastrointestinal tract of swine. *J. Nutr.* **105**, 759–768.

Clemens, E. T., Stevens, C. E., and Southworth, M. (1975b). Sites of organic acid production and pattern of digesta movement in the gastrointestinal tract of geese. *J. Nutr.* **105**, 1341–1350.

Cottyn, B. G., Boucqué, C. V., Van Nevel, C. J., and Demeyer, D. I. (1973). Incorporation of linseed oil hydrolysate and sodium sulfite in rations for beef production. 1. Effect on digestibility and bull performance. Z. Tierphysiol., Tierernaehr. Futtermittelkd. **31**, 57–65.

Czerkawski, J. W. (1973). Effect of linseed oil fatty acids and linseed oil on rumen fermentation in sheep. J. Agric. Sci. **81**, 517–531.

Czerkawski, J. W., and Breckenridge, G. (1973). Dissimilation of 1,2-propane-diol by rumen microorganisms. Br. J. Nutr. **29**, 317–330.

Czerkawski, J. W., and Breckenridge, G. (1975a). New inhibitors of methane production by rumen micro-organisms. Development and testing of inhibitors in vitro. Br. J. Nutr. **34**, 429–446.

Czerkawski, J. W., and Breckenridge, J. G. (1975b). New inhibitors of methane production by rumen micro-organisms. Experiments with animals and other practical possibilities. Br. J. Nutr. **34**, 447–457.

Czerkawski, J. W., Blaxter, K. L., and Wainman, F. W. (1966). The metabolism of oleic, linoleic and linolenic acids by sheep with reference to their efforts on methane production. Br. J. Nutr. **20**, 349–362.

Czerkawski, J. W., Christie, W. W., Breckenridge, G., and Hunter, M. L. (1975). Changes in the rumen metabolism of sheep given increasing amounts of linseed oil in their diet. Br. J. Nutr. **34**, 24–44.

Dawson, R. M. C., and Hemington, N. (1974). Digestion of grass lipids and pigments in the sheep rumen. Br. J. Nutr. **32**, 327–340.

Dawson, R. M. C., and Kemp, P. (1969). The effect of defaunation on the phospholipids and on the hydrogenation of unsaturated fatty acids in the rumen. Biochem. J. **115**, 351–352.

Dearth, R. N., Dehority, B. A., and Potter, E. L. (1974). Rumen microbial numbers in lambs as affected by level of feed intake and dietary diethylstilbestrol. J. Anim. Sci. **38**, 991–996.

Demeyer, D. I. and Henderickx, H. (1966). The effect of unsaturated fatty acids upon in vitro methane production by mixed rumen bacteria. First World Congress on Animal Feeding. Vol. II, PP. 69–74. Madrid, 2–8 October 1966.

Demeyer, D. I., and Henderickx, H. K. (1967). The effect of C_{18} unsaturated fatty acids on methane production in vitro by mixed rumen bacteria. Biochim. Biophys. Acta **137**, 484–497.

Demeyer, D. I., and Van Nevel, C. J. (1975). Methanogenesis, an integrated part of carbohydrate fermentation, and its control. In "Digestion and Metabolism in the Ruminant" (I. W. McDonald and A. C. I. Warner, eds.), pp. 366–382. Univ. of New England Publishing Unit, Armidale, Australia.

Demeyer, D. I., Van Nevel, C. J., Henderickx, H. K., and Martin, J. (1969). The effect of unsaturated fatty acids upon methane and propionic acid in the rumen. In "Energy Metabolism of Farm Animals" (K. L. Blaxter, ed.), pp. 139–146. Oriel Press, Newcastle-upon-Tyne.

Dickinson, J. O., and Huber, W. G. (1972). Catabolism of orally administered histamine in sheep. Am. J. Vet. Res. **33**, 1789–1795.

Dinius, D. A., Simpson, M. E., and Marsh, P. B. (1976). Effect of monensin fed with forage on digestion and the ruminal ecosystem of steers. J. Anim. Sci. **42**, 229–234.

Dough, P. G. C., and Blair, S. S. B. (1975). The metabolism of foreign compounds in the cestode Moniezia expansa and the nematode Ascaris lumbricoides var. suum. Xenobiotica **5**, 279–292.

Drasar, B. S., and Hill, M. J. (1972). Intestinal bacteria and cancer. *Am. J. Clin. Nutr.* **25,** 1399–1404.

Drasar, B. S., and Hill, M. J. (1974). "Human Intestinal Flora." Academic Press, New York.

Drasar, B. S., Hill, M. J., and Williams, R. E. O. (1970). The significance of the gut flora in safety testing of food additives. *In* "Metabolic Aspects of Food Safety" (F. J. C. Roe, ed.), pp. 245–255. Blackwell, Oxford.

Dunlop, R. H. (1972). Pathogenesis of ruminant lactic acidosis. *Adv. Vet. Sci. Comp. Med.* **16,** 259–302.

Dunlop, R. H., and Hammond, P. B. (1965). D-Lactic acidosis in ruminants. *Ann. N.Y. Acad. Sci.* **119,** 1109–1130.

Eberhard, I. H., McNamara, J., Pearse, R. J., and Southwell, I. A. (1975). Ingestion and excretion of *Eucalyptus punctata* D.C. and its essential oil by the koala, *Phascolarctus cinereus* (Goldfuss). *Aust. J. Zool.* **23,** 169–179.

Edwards, D. I., and Mathison, G. E. (1970). The mode of action of metronidazole against *Trichomonas vaginalis. J. Gen. Microbiol.* **63,** 297–302.

Edwin, E. E., and Jackman, R. (1970). Thiaminase I in the development of cerebrocortical necrosis in sheep and cattle. *Nature (London)* **228,** 772–774.

Edwin, E. E., and Jackman, R. (1973). Ruminal thiaminase and tissue thiamine in cerebrocortical necrosis. *Vet. Rec.* **92,** 640–641.

Emery, R. S., Brown, R. E., and Black, A. L. (1967). Metabolism of DL-1,2-propanediol-2-^{14}C in a lactating cow. *J. Nutr.* **92,** 348–356.

Erwin, E. S., and Marco, G. J. (1969). Ruminant feeds. *Chem. Abstr.* **70,** 204 (Abstr. No. 86440y).

Eyssen, H. (1973). Role of gut microflora in metabolism of lipids and sterols. *Proc. Nutr. Soc.* **32,** 59–63.

Faruque, A. J. M. O., Jarvis, B. D. W., and Hawke, J. C. (1974). Studies on rumen metabolism. IX. Contribution of plant lipases to the release of free fatty acids in the rumen. *J. Sci. Food Agric.* **25,** 1313–1328.

Ferguson, K. A. (1975). The protection of dietary proteins and amino acids against microbial fermentation in the rumen. *In* "Digestion and Metabolism in the Ruminant" (I. W. McDonald and A. C. I. Warner, eds.), pp. 448–464. Univ. of New England Publishing Unit, Armidale, Australia.

Ferry, J. G., and Wolfe, R. S. (1976). Anaerobic degradation of benzoate to methane by a microbial consortium. *Arch. Microbiol.* **107,** 33–40.

Finegold, S. M. (1970). Interaction of antimicrobial therapy and intestinal flora. *Am. J. Clin. Nutr.* **23,** 1466–1471.

Fishbein, W. N., Carbone, P. P., and Hochstein, H. D. (1965). Acetohydroxamate: Bacterial urease inhibitor with therapeutic potential in hyperammonaemic states. *Nature (London)* **208,** 46–48.

Ford, E. J. H., and Gopinath, C. (1974). The excretion of phylloerythrin and bilirubin by the horse. *Res. Vet. Sci.* **16,** 186–198.

Francis, A. J., Spanggord, R. J., and Ouchi, G. I. (1975). Degradation of lindane by *Escherichia coli. Appl. Microbiol.* **29,** 567–568.

Freeland, W. J., and Janzen, D. H. (1974). Strategies in herbivory by mammals: The role of plant secondary compounds. *Am. Nat.* **108,** 269–289.

Freese, E., Sheu, C. W., and Galliers, E. (1973). Function of lipophylic acids as antimicrobial food additives. *Nature (London)* **241,** 321–325.

Fries, G. R., Marrow, G. S., and Gordon, C. H. (1969). Metabolism of *o, p'*- and *p,p'*- DDT by rumen microorganisms. *J. Agric. Fod Chem.* **17,** 860–862.

Froslie, A. (1974). Effects following intra-ruminal administration of DNOC and DNPB to sheep. *Acta Vet. Scand., Suppl.* **49**, 1–61.

Gedek, B. (1973). Futtermittelverderb durch Bakterien und Pilze und sein nachteiligen Folgen. *Uebers. Tierernaehr.* **1**, 45–56.

Golab, T., Herberg, R. J., Day, E. W., Rauw, A. P., Holzer, F. J., and Probst, G. W. (1969). Fate of carbon-14 trifluralin in artificial rumen fluid and in ruminant animals. *J. Agric. Food Chem.* **17**, 576–580.

Goldman, P., Peppercorn, M. A., and Goldin, B. R. (1974). Drugs metabolized by intestinal flora. *In* "Drug Interactions" (P. L. Morselli, S. Garattini, and S. N. Cohen, eds.), pp. 91–102. Raven, New York.

Gupta, J., and Nichols, R. E. (1962). A possible enzymatic cause of viscid ruminal contents—its relationship to legume bloat. *Am. J. Vet. Res.* **23**, 128–133.

Gutenmann, W. H., and Lisk, D. J. (1975). A feeding study with diphenylamine in a dairy cow. *Bull. Environ. Contam. Toxicol.* **13**, 177–180.

Gutenmann, W. H., Hardee, D. D., Holland, R. F., and Lisk, D. J. (1963a). Disappearance of 4-(2,4-dichlorophenoxybutyric)acid herbicide in the dairy cow. *J. Dairy Sci.* **46**, 991–992.

Gutenmann, W. H., Hardee, D. D., Holland, R. F., and Lisk, D. J. (1963b). Residue studies with 2,4-dichlorophenoxyacetic acid herbicide in the dairy cow and in a natural and artificial rumen. *J. Dairy Sci.* **46**, 1287–1288.

Haenel, H., and Bendig, J. (1975). Intestinal flora in health and disease. *Prog. Food Nutr. Soc.* **1**, 21–64.

Hamada, T., Tanji, K., Kim, K. S., Kameoka, K., and Morimoto, H. (1968). Utilization of DL-1,2-propanediol by young and adult goats. *Jpn. J. Zootech. Sci.* **39**, 536–542.

Hamilton-Miller, J. M. T. (1975). Antimicrobial agents acting against anaerobes. *J. Antimicrob. Chemother.* **1**, 273–289.

Hapke, H. J. (1975). "Toxikologie für Veterinärmediziner." Enke, Stuttgart.

Harmeyer, J. (1965). Zur Methodik experimenteller Untersuchungen an Pansenprotozoen. *Zentralbl. Veterinaer med., Reihe A* **12**, 841–880.

Harmeyer, J. (1973). Protozoologie des Pansens. *In* "Biologie und Biochemie der mikrobiellen Verdauung" (D. Giesecke and H. K. Henderickx, eds.), pp. 58–107. BLV Verlagsges., Munich.

Henderson, C. (1973). The effects of fatty acids on pure cultures of rumen bacteria. *J. Agric. Sci.* **81**, 107–112.

Hewitt, W. L. (1975). Clinical implications of the presence of drug residues in food. *Fed. Proc. Fed. Am. Soc. Exp. Biol.* **34**, 202–204.

Hill, K. J. (1971). The structure of the alimentary tract. *In* "Physiology and Biochemistry of the Domestic Fowl" (D. J. Bell and B. M. Freeman, eds.), Vol. 1 pp. 1–23. Academic Press, New York.

Hill, M. J. (1975). The etiology of colon cancer. *Crit. Rev. Toxicol.* **4**, 31–82.

Hino, T., Kametaka, M., and Kandatsu, M. (1973). The cultivation of rumen oligotrich protozoa. III. White clover factors which stimulate the growth of entodinia. *J. Gen. Appl. Microbiol.* **19**, 397–413.

Hoshino, S., and Sugiyama, S. I. (1974). Protein synthesis in a cell-free preparation from rumen protozoa. *Comp. Biochem. Physiol. B* **48**, 39–45.

Hungate, R. E. (1966). "The Rumen and its Microbes." Academic Press, New York.

Hungate, R. E. (1972). Relationships between protozoa and bacteria of the alimentary tract. *Am. J. Clin. Nutr.* **25**, 1480–1484.

Ibrahim, E. A., Ingalls, J. R., and Stanger, N. E. (1970). Effect of dietary diethylstilbestrol on population and concentrations of ciliate protozoa in dairy cattle. *Can. J. Anim. Sci.* **50,** 101–106.

Ings, R. M. J., McFadzean, J. A., and Ormerod, W. E. (1974). The mode of action of metronidazole in *Trichomonas vaginalis* and other microorganisms. *Biochem. Pharmacol.* **23,** 1421–1429.

Ivie, G. W. (1976). Epoxide to olefin: A novel biotransformation in the rumen. *Science* **191,** 959–961.

Ivie, G. W., Clark, D. E., and Rushing, D. D. (1974). Metabolic transformations of disugran by rumen fluid of sheep maintained on dissimilar diets. *J. Agric. Food Chem.* **22,** 632–634.

James, L. F., Allison, M. J., and Littledike, E. T. (1975). Production and modification of toxic substances in the rumen. *In* "Digestion and Metabolism in the Ruminant" (I. W. McDonald and A. C. I. Warner, eds.), pp. 576–590. Univ. of New England Publishing Unit, Armidale, Australia.

Jenkins, W. L. (1969). Effects of intraruminal administration of sulfadimidine to adult sheep. *J. S. Afr. Vet. Med. Assoc.* **40,** 159–176.

Jenkins, W. L., Davis, L. E., and Boulos, B. M. (1975). Transfer of drugs across the ruminal wall in goats. *Am. J. Vet. Res.* **36,** 1771–1776.

Jones, D. A. (1972). Cyanogenic glycosides and their function. *In* "Phytochemical Ecology" (J. B. Harborne, ed.), pp. 103–124. Academic Press, New York.

Jones, G. A. (1968). Influence of acetohydroxamic acid on some activities *in vitro* of the rumen microbiota. *Can. J. Microbiol.* **14,** 409–416.

Johnson, D. E. (1972). Effects of a hemiacetal of chloral and starch on methane production and energy balance of sheep fed a pelleted diet. *J. Anim. Sci.* **35,** 1064–1068.

Johnson, D. E., Wood, A. S., Stone, J. B., and Moran, E. T., Jr. (1972). Some effects of methane inhibition in ruminants (steers). *Can. J. Anim. Sci.* **52,** 703–712.

Kabara, J. J. (1975). Lipids as safe and effective antimicrobial agents for cosmetics and pharmaceuticals. *Cosmet. Perfum.* **90,** 21–25.

Krishnamurty, H. G., Cheng, K.-J., Jones, G. A., Simpson, F. J., and Watkin, J. E. (1970). Identification of products produced by the anaerobic degradation of rutin and related flavonoids by *Butyrivibrio* sp. C₃. *Can. J. Microbiol.* **16,** 759–767.

Kutches, A. J., and Church, D. C. (1971). DDT-¹⁴C Metabolism by rumen bacteria and protozoa *in vitro. J. Dairy Sci.* **54,** 540–543.

Kutches, A. J., Church, D. C., and Duryee, F. L. (1970). Toxicological effects of pesticides on rumen function *in vitro. Agric. Food. Chem.* **18,** 430–433.

Lanigan, G. W. (1970). Metabolism of pyrrolizidine alkaloids in the ovine rumen. II. Some factors affecting rate of alkaloid breakdown by rumen fluid *in vitro. Aust. J. Agric. Res.* **21,** 633–639.

Lanigan, G. W. (1971). Metabolism of pyrrolizidine alkaloids in the ovine rumen. III. The competitive relationship between heliotrine metabolism and methanogenesis in rumen fluid *in vitro. Aust. J. Agric. Res.* **22,** 123–130.

Lanigan, G. W. (1972). Metabolism of pyrrolizidine alkaloids in the ovine rumen. IV. Effects of chloral hydrate and halogenated methanes on rumen methanogenesis and alkaloid metabolism in fistulated sheep. *Aust. J. Agric. Res.* **23,** 1085–1091.

Lanigan, G. W., and Smith, L. W. (1970). Metabolism of pyrrolizidine alkaloids in the ovine rumen. I. Formation of 7α-hydroxy-1α-methyl-8α-pyrrolizidine from heliotrine and lasiocarpine. *Aust. J. Agric. Res.* **21,** 493–500.

Layrisse, M., and Vargas, A. (1975). Nutrition and intestinal parasitic infection. *Prog. Food Nutr. Sci.* **1,** 645–667.

Lindsay, D. R., and Kelly, R. W. (1970). The metabolism of phyto-oestrogens in sheep. *Aust. Vet. J.* **46**, 219–222.

Longhurst, W. M., Oh, H. K., Jones, M. B., and Kepner, R. E. (1968). A basis for the palatability of deer forage plants. *Trans. North Am. Wildl. Nat. Resour. Conf.* **33**, 181–189.

Maarse, H., and Kepner, R. E. (1970). Changes in composition of volatile terpenes in Douglas Fir needles during maturation. *J. Agric. Food. Chem.* **18**, 1095–1101.

McBee, R. H. (1971). Significance of intestinal microflora in herbivory. *Annu. Rev. Ecol. Syst.* **2**, 165–175.

McBride, B. C., and Wolfe, R. S. (1971). Inhibition of methanogenesis by DDT. *Nature (London)* **234**, 551–552.

McCalla, D. R., Olive, P., Tu, Y., and Fan, M. L. (1975). Nitrofurazone-reducing enzymes in *E. coli* and their role in drug activation *in vivo*. *Can. J. Microbiol.* **21**, 1484–1491.

McCoy, E. (1957). Changes in the host flora induced by chemotherapeutic agents. *Annu. Rev. Microbiol.* **8**, 257–272.

McDonald, I. W., and Warner, A. C. I., eds. (1975). "Digestion and Metabolism in the Ruminant." Univ. of New England Publishing Unit, Armidale, Australia.

McLeod, M. N. (1974). Plant tannins—their role in forage quality. *Nutr. Abstr. Rev.* **44**, 803–815.

Madella Amadei, D. (1966). Influenza dello Ziram (dimetil-di-thiocarbammato di zinco) sulla attività cellulolitica *in vitro* di liquido ruminale bovino. *Atti Soc. Ital. Sci. Vet.* **20**, 500–504.

Mahadevan, S., Sauer, F., and Erfle, J. D. (1976). Studies on bovine rumen bacterial urease. *J. Anim. Sci.* **42**, 745–753.

Maplesden, D. C., and Myers, G. S. (1972). Ruminant feed, additive, or veterinary compositions comprising a compound. *Chem. Abstr.* **77**, 267 (Abstr. No. 52328x).

Martin, A. K. (1975). Metabolism of aromatic compounds in the rumen. *Proc. Nutr. Soc.* **34**, 69A–70A.

Mathur, C. F., Smith, R. C., and Hawkins, G. E. (1976). Growth and morphology of *Streptococcus bovis* and of mixed rumen bacteria in the presence of aflatoxin B₁, *in vitro*. *J. Dairy Sci.* **59**, 455–458.

Mendel, J. L., and Walton, M. S. (1966). Conversion of *p,p'*-DDT to *p,p'*-DDD by intestinal flora of the rat. *Science* **151**, 1527–1528.

Mengel, C. E., and Klavins, J. V. (1967). Development of hemolytic anemia in rats fed methionine. *J. Nutr.* **92**, 104–110.

Menke, K. H., and Krampitz, G. (1973). Antibiotikawirkungen in nutritiver Dosierung. *Uebers. Tierernaehr.* **1**, 255–272.

Meyer, R. M., and Bartley, E. E. (1972). Bloat in cattle. XVI. Development and application of techniques for selecting drugs to prevent feedlot bloat. *J. Anim. Sci.* **34**, 234–240.

Midvedt, R. (1974). Microbial bile acid transformation. *Am. J. Clin. Nutr.* **27**, 1341–1347.

Milligan, L. D., Asplund, J. M., and Robblee, A. R. (1965). Effects of thiamine inhibitors on cellulose digestion and volatile fatty acid production in artificial rumen fermentations. *Can. J. Anim. Sci.* **45**, 99–104.

Mirvish, S. S. (1975). Formation of *N*-nitroso compounds: Chemistry, kinetics, and *in vivo* occurrence. *Toxicol. Appl. Pharmacol.* **31**, 325–351.

Miskus, R. P., Blair, D. P., and Casida, J. E. (1965). Conversion of DDT to DDD by bovine rumen fluid, lake water, and reduced porphyrins. *J. Agric. Food Chem.* **13**, 481–483.

Moir, R. J. (1968). Ruminant digestion and evolution. *Handb. Physiol., Sect. 6: Alim. Canal* Vol. 5 pp. 2673–2694.

246   R. A. Prins

Naga, M. A., Harmeyer, J. H., Holler, H., and Schaller, K. (1975). Suspected "B"-vitamindeficiency of sheep fed a protein-free urea containing purified diet. *J. Anim. Sci.* **40**, 1192–1198.

Nagy, J. G., and Tengerdy, R. P. (1967a). Antibacterial action of essential oils of *Artemisia* as on ecological factor. I. Antibacterial action of volatile oils of *Artemisia tridentata* and *Artemisia novo* on aerobic bacteria. *Appl. Microbiol.* **15**, 819–821.

Nagy, J. G., and Tengerdy, R. P. (1967b). Antibacterial action of essential oils of *Artemisia* as an ecological factor. II. Antibacterial action of the volatile oils or *Artemisia tridentata* (Big Sagebrush) on bacteria from the rumen of mule deer. *Appl. Microbiol.* **16**, 441–444.

Nagy, J. G., Steinhoff, H. W., and Ward, G. M. (1964). Effects of essential oils of sagebrush on deer rumen microbial function. *J. Wildl. Manage.* **28**, 785–790.

Neale, G., Gompertz, D., Schönsby, H., Tabaqchali, S., and Booth, C. C. (1972). The metabolic and nutritional consequences of bacterial overgrowth in the small intestine. *Am. J. Clin. Nutr.* **25**, 1409–1417.

Nichols, R. E. (1963). The control of experimental legume bloat with an enzyme inhibitor, alkyl aryl sulfonate sodium. *J. Am. Vet. Med. Assoc.* **143**, 998–999.

Nottle, M. C., and Beck, A. B. (1974). Urinary sediments in sheep feeding on oestrogenic clover. III. The identification of 4'-O-methyl equol as a major component of some sediments. *Aust. J. Agric. Res.* **25**, 509–514.

O'Brien, R. W., and Morris, J. G. (1972). Cited by Ings *et al.* (1974). O'Connor, J. J., Myers, G. S., Jr., Maplesden, D. C., and Van der Noot, G. W. (1970). Chemical additives in rumen fermentations *in vitro* effects of various drugs on rumen volatile fatty acids and protozoa. *J. Anim. Sci.* **30**, 812–818.

O'Connor, J. J., Myers, G. S., Jr., Maplesden, D. C., and Van der Noot, G. W. (1970). Chemical additives in rumen fermentations: *in vivo* effects of various drugs on rumen volatile fatty acids and protozoa. *J. Anim. Sci.* **30**, 812–818.

Oh, H. K., Sakai, T., Jones, M. B., and Longhurst, W. M. (1967). Effect of various essential oils isolated from Douglas fir needles upon sheep and deer rumen microbial activity. *Appl. Microbiol.* **15**, 777–784.

Oh, H. K., Jones, M. B., and Longhurst, W. M. (1968). Comparison of rumen microbial inhibition resulting from various essential oils isolated from relatively unpalatable plant species. *Appl. Microbiol.* **16**, 39–44.

Oh, H. K., Jones, M. B., Longhurst, W. M., and Connolly, G. E. (1970). Deer browsing and rumen microbial fermentation of Douglas fir as affected by fertilization and growth stage. *For. Sci.* **16**, 21–27.

Ørskov, E. R. (1975). Manipulation of rumen fermentation for maximum food utilization. *World Rev. Nutr. Diet.* **22**, 152–182.

Oyaert, W., and Bouckaert, J. H. (1959). Action of penicillin, chloral hydrate and chlorate on some metabolic aspects of ruminal flora. *Zentralbl. Veterinaermed.* **6**, 693–700.

Parish, R. C., and Trei, J. E. (1971). Compositions for improving the feed efficiency of ruminants comprising polyhalohemiacetal derivatives of saccharides. *Chem. Abstr.* **76**, 282 (Abstr. No. 44905x).

Parish, R. C., and Trei, J. E. (1972a). Improving feed utilization in ruminants with haloalkanoic acids, amides, or nitriles. *Chem. Abstr.* **76**, 68 (Abstr. No. 149223b).

Parish, R. C., and Trei, J. E. (1972b). Compositions utilizing bis (polyhalomethyl) derivatives to improve the feed efficiency of commercial ruminant animals. *Chem. Abstr.* **77**, 387 (Abstr. No. 60565n).

Parish, R. C., and Trei, J. E. (1973a). Improving the feed efficiency of ruminants using polyhaloaldehyde condensates. *Chem. Abstr.* **79**, 263 (Abstr. No. 114356g).

Parish, R. C., and Trei, J. E. (1973b). Improving the feed efficiency of ruminants using polyhaloalkamines. *Chem. Abstr.* **79,** 275 (Abstr. No. 52177p).

Patchett, A. A., Hoff, D. R., and Rooney, C. S. (1972a). Feed compositions for controlling the formation of methane in rumen fermentation. *Chem. Abstr.* **76,** 270 (Abstr. No. 23951u).

Patchett, A. A., Hoff, D. R., and Rooney, C. S. (1972b). Compositions for suppressing methane formation in a rumen fluid. *Chem. Abstr.* **77,** 344 (Abstr. No. 39251x).

Phillipson, A. T., ed. (1969). "Physiology of Digestion and Metabolism in the Ruminant." Oriel Press, Newcastle-upon-Tyne.

Phillipson, A. T. (1972). The protection of dietary components from rumen fermentations. *Proc. Nutr. Soc.* **31,** 159–164.

Polan, C. E., Huber, J. T., Young, R. W., and Osborne, J. C. (1969). Chronic feeding of s - [(2 - methoxy - 5 - oxo - Δ^2 - 1,3,4 - thiadiazonin - 4 - yl)methyl]O,O - dimethyl - phosphorodithioate (Supracide) to ruminating bull calves. *J. Agric. Food Chem.* **17,** 857–859.

Potter, E. L., Cooley, C. O., Richardson, L. F., Raun, A. P., and Rathmacher, R. P. (1976). Effect of monensin on performance of cattle fed forage. *J. Anim. Sci.* **43,** 665–669.

Prins, R. A. (1965). Action of chloral hydrate on rumen microorganisms *in vitro. J. Dairy Sci.* **48,** 991–993.

Prins, R. A. (1967). Some microbiological and biochemical aspects of rumen metabolism. Ph.D. Thesis, Utrecht, The Netherlands.

Prins, R. A. (1969). Effect of some antibiotics and sulphonamides on cellulose breakdown by mixed rumen microorganisms *in vitro. Br. Vet. J.* **125,** XVIII–XX.

Prins, R. A. (1970). Methanogenesis and propionate production in the rumen as influenced by therapeutics against ketosis. *Z. Tierphysiol., Tierernaehr. Futtermittelkd.* **26,** 147–151.

Prins, R. A. (1977). Biochemical activities of gut micro-organisms. *In* The Normal Flora of the Gut" (R. T. J. Clarke and T. Bauchop, eds.) Ch. 3, pp. 78–183. Academic Press, New York (in press).

Prins, R. A., and Prast, E. R. (1973). Oxidation of NADH is a coupled oxidase-peroxidase reaction and its significance for the fermentation in rumen protozoa of the genus *Isotricha. J. Protozool.* **20,** 471–477.

Prins, R. A., and Seekles, L. (1968). Effect of chloral hydrate on rumen metabolism. *J. Dairy Sci.* **51,** 882–887.

Prins, R. A., and van den Vorstenbosch, C. J. A. H. V. (1975). Interrelationships between rumen microorganisms. *Misc. Pap., Landbouwhoge-sch. Wageningen* **11,** 1–11.

Prins, R. A., and van der Meer, P. (1976). On the contribution of the acrylate pathway to propionate formation from lactate in the rumen of cattle. *Antonie van Leeuwenhoek* **42,** 25–31.

Prins, R. A., Van Nevel, C. J., and Demeyer, D. I. (1972a). Tetramisole: An anthelmintic drug without effect on the rumen fermentation. *Arch. Int. Physiol. Biochim.* **80,** 305–309.

Prins, R. A., Van Nevel, C. J., and Demeyer, D. I. (1972b). Pure culture studies of inhibitors for methanogenic bacteria. *Antonie van Leeuwenhoek* **38,** 281–287.

Prins, R. A., Lankhorst, A., van der Meer, P., and Van Nevel, C. J. (1975). Some characteristics of *Anaerovibrio lipolytica,* a rumen lipolytic organism. *Antonie van Leeuwenhoek* **41,** 1–11.

Quaghebeur, D., and Oyaert, W. (1971a). Effect of chloral hydrate and related compounds on the fermentation of glucose by rumen bacteria. *Zentralbl. Veterinaer med., Reihe A* **18,** 55–63.

Quaghebeur, D., and Oyaert, W. (1971b). Effect of chloral hydrate and related compounds

248   R. A. Prins

on the metabolism of lactic and pyruvic acid by rumen bacteria. *Zentralbl. Veterinaer med., Reihe A* **18,** 64–74.

Quaghebeur, D., and Oyaert, W. (1971c). Effect of chloral hydrate and related compounds on the activity of several enzymes in extracts of rumen microorganisms. *Zentralbl. Veterinaer med. Reihe A* **18,** 417–427.

Radeleff, R. D. (1970). "Veterinary Toxicology." Lea & Febiger, Philadelphia, Pennsylvania.

Radwan, M. A. (1972). Differences between Douglas fir genotypes in relation to browsing preference by black-tailed deer. *Can. J. For. Res.* **2,** 250–255.

Radwan, M. A. (1974). Natural resistance of plants to animals. In "Wildlife and Forest Management in the Pacific Northwest" (H. C. Black, ed.), pp. 85–94. School of Forestry, Oregon State University, Eugene.

Raun, A. P. (1974a). Ruminant feed utilization improvement. *Chem. Abstr.* **80,** 304 (Abstr. No. 107094n).

Raun, A. P. (1974b). Ruminant feed utilization improvement. *Chem. Abstr.* **81,** 340 (Abstr. No. 135092j).

Richardson, L. F., Raun, A. P., Potter, E. L., Cooley, C. O., and Rathmacher, R. P. (1976). Effect of monensin on rumen fermentation *in vitro* and *in vivo. J. Anim. Sci.* **43,** 657–664.

Roberts, G. W., and Boyd, J. W. (1974). Cerebrocortical necrosis in ruminants: Occurrence of thiaminase in the gut of normal and affected animals and its effect on thiaminase status. *J. Comp. Pathol.* **84,** 365–374.

Rosenberg, I. H., Beisel, W. R., Gordon, J. E., Katz, M., Keusch, G. T., Luckey, D., and Mata, L. J. (1974). Infant and child enteritis–malabsorption–malnutrition: The potential of limited studies with low-dose antibiotic feeding. *Am. J. Clin. Nutr.* **27,** 304–309.

Rossoff, I. S. (1974). "Handbook of veterinary drugs." Springer-Verlag, Berlin and New York.

Rowland, I. R., and Grasso, P. (1975). Degradation of N-nitrosamines by intestinal bacteria. *Appl. Microbiol.* **29,** 7–12.

Roxon, J. J., and Tesoriero, A. A. (1974). Effect of cysteine on cyclamate metabolism by rat intestinal microorganisms. *Aust. J. Pharm. Sci.* [N. S.] **3,** 26–28.

Rufener, W. H., Jr., and Wolin, M. J. (1968). Effect of CCl₄ on CH₄ and volatile fatty acid production in continuous cultures of rumen organisms and in a sheep rumen. *Appl. Microbiol.* **16,** 1955–1956.

Rumsey, T. S., Slyter, L. L., Shepherd, S. M., and Kern, D. L. (1970). Effect of p,p′-DDT on rumen ecology, EKG patterns and respiratory rate of beef steers. *J. Agric. Food chem.* **18,** 485–489.

Russell, G. R., and Smith, R. M. (1968). Reduction of heliotrine by a rumen microorganism. *Aust. J. Biol. Sci.* **21,** 1277–1290.

St. John, L. E., Jr., and Lisk, D. J. (1974). Feeding studies with Supracide in the dairy cow. *Bull. Environ. Contam. Toxicol.* **12,** 594–598.

Sakai, T., Maarse, H., Kepner, R. E., Jennings, W. G., and Longhurst, W. M. (1967). Volatile components of Douglas fir needles. *Agric. Food. Chem.* **15,** 1070–1072.

Salter, D. N. (1973). The influence of gut micro-organisms on utilization of dietary protein. *Proc. Nutr. Soc.* **32,** 65–71.

Satapathy, N., and Purser, D. B. (1967). Protozoan, bacterial, and volatile fatty acid changes associated with feeding tylosin. *Appl. Microbial.* **15,** 1417–1421.

Savage, D. C., and McAllister, J. S. (1971). Cecal enlargement and microbial flora in suckling mice given antibacterial drugs. *Infect. Immun.* **3,** 342–349.

Sawyer, M. S., Hoover, W. H., and Sniffen, C. J. (1974). Effects of a ruminal methane inhibitor on growth and energy metabolism in the ovine. *J. Anim. Sci.* **38**, 908-914.

Schaedler, R. W. (1973). The relationship between the host and its microflora. *Proc. Nutr. Soc.* **32**, 41-47.

Scheline, R. R. (1973). Metabolism of foreign compound by gastrointestinal microorganisms. *Pharmacol. Rev.* **25**, 451-523.

Schwartz, C. C. and Nagy, J. G. (1974). Pesticide effects on *in vitro* dry matter digestion in deer. *J. Wildl. Manage.* **38**, 531-534.

Schwartz, C. C., Nagy, J. G., and Streeter, C. L. (1973). Pesticide effect on rumen microbial function. *J. Anim. Sci.* **37**, 821-826.

Seinen, W., Winckels, H. W., and Prins, R. A. (1977). Toxicity of dioctyl tin dichloride in guinea pigs. (In preparation.)

Sharkey, M. J. (1971). Some aspects of coprophagy in rabbits and guinea pigs fed fresh lucerne. *Mammalia* **35**, 162-168.

Sheu, C. W., and Freese, E. (1973). Lipopolysaccharide layer protection of Gram-negative bacteria against inhibition by long-chain fatty acids. *J. Bacteriol.* **115**, 869-875.

Shiga, A., Shinozaki, K., and Kobayashi, Y. (1975). Effects of propylene glycol on growth and rumen volatile fatty acids of lambs. *Jpn. J. Zootech. Sci.* **46**, 334-341.

Shimbayashi, K., Obara, Y., Yonemura, T., Deguchi, N., and Nakanishi, M. (1973a). Effect of caprylohydroxamic acid on ruminal urease. *Jpn. J. Vet. Sci.* **35**, 327-334.

Shimbayashi, K., Yonemura, T., Deguchi, N., and Nakanishi, M. (1973b). Effect of caprylohydroxamic acid on rumen content of sheep and intestinal content of rat. *Jpn. J. Vet. Sci.* **35**, 425-432.

Shirley, E. K., and Schmidt-Nielsen, K. (1967). Oxalate metabolism in the pack rat, sand rat, hamster, and white rat. *J. Nutr.* **91**, 496-502.

Simpson, F. J., Jones, G. A., and Wolin, E. A. (1969). Anaerobic degradation of some bioflavonoids by microflora of the rumen. *Can. J. Microbiol.* **15**, 972-974.

Singh, Y. K., and Trei, J. E. (1971). Ruminal ammonia concentrations as influenced by methane inhibitors. *Fed. Proc., Fed. Am. Soc. Exp. Biol.* **30**, 404 (Abstr. No. 1180).

Singleton, A. G. (1972). The control of fermentation of carbohydrate. *Proc. Nutr. Soc.* **31**, 147-149.

Slyter, L. L. (1976). Influence of acidosis on rumen function. *J. Anim. Sci.* **43**, 910-929.

Slyter, L. L., and Wolin, M. J. (1967). Copper sulfate-induced fermentation changes in continuous cultures of the rumen microbial ecosystem. *Appl. Microbiol.* **15**, 1160-1164.

Slyter, L. L., Oltjen, R. R., Kern, D. L., and Blank, F. C. (1970). Influence of type and level of grain and diethylstilbestrol on the rumen microbial population of steers fed all-concentrate diets. *J. Anim. Sci.* **31**, 996-1002.

Small, J. D. (1968). Fatal enterocolitis in hamsters given lincomycin hydrochloride. *Lab. Anim. Care.* **18**, 411-420.

Smith, G. E., and Griffiths, L. A. (1974). Metabolism of *N*-acylated and *O*-alkylated drugs by the intestinal microflora during anaerobic incubation *in vitro. Xenobiotica* **4**, 477-487.

Smith, R. H. (1974). Kale poisoning. *Rep. Rowett Inst.* **30**, 112-131.

Southgate, D. A. T., and Durnin, J. V. G. A. (1970). Caloric conversion factors. An experimental reassessment of the factors used in the calculation of the energy value of human diets. *Br. J. Nutr.* **24**, 517-535.

Southwell, I. A. (1973). Variation in the leaf oil of *Eucalyptus punctata. Phytochemistry* **12**, 1341-1343.

Strand, L. P., and Scheline, R. R. (1975). The metabolism of vanillin and isovanillin in the rat. *Xenobiotica* **5**, 49–63.

Streeter, C. L., Oltjen, R. R., Slyter, L. L., and Fishbein, W. N. (1969). Urea utilization in wethers receiving the urease inhibitor acetohydroxamic acid. *J. Anim. Sci.* **29**, 88–93.

Sutton, J. D., Smith, R. H., McAllan, A. B., Storry, J. E., and Corse, D. A. (1975). Effect of variations in dietary protein and of supplements of cod-liver oil on energy digestion and microbial synthesis in the rumen of sheep fed hay and concentrates. *J. Agric. Sci.* **84**, 317–326.

Sykes, R. M., and Kirsch, E. J. (1972). Accumulation of methanogenic substrates in CCl_4 inhibited anaerobic sewage sludge digester cultures. *Water Res.* **6**, 41–55.

Tesoriero, A. A., and Roxon, J. J. (1975). [^{35}S]cyclamate metabolism: Incorporation of ^{35}S into proteins of intestinal bacteric *in vitro* and production of volatile ^{35}S-containing compounds. *Xenobiotica* **5**, 25–31.

Thiel, P. G. (1969). The effect of methane analogues on methanogenesis in anaerobic digestion. *Water Res.* **3**, 215–223.

Thomson, D. J. (1972). Physical form of the diet in relation to rumen fermentation. *Proc. Nutr. Soc.* **31**, 127–134.

Trei, J. E., Parish, R. C., Singh, Y. K., and Scott, G. C. (1971). Effect of methane inhibitors on rumen metabolism and feedlot performance of sheep. *J. Dairy Sci.* **54**, 536–539.

Trei, J. E., Scott, G. C., and Parish, R. C. (1972). Influence of methane inhibition on energetic efficiency in lambs. *J. Anim. Sci.* **34**, 510–515.

Trei, J. E., and Olson, W. A. (1969). Effect of chlorine containing analogues of methane on rumen fermentation. *J. Anim. Sci.* **29**, 173 (abstr.).

Tsai, C. G., and Jones, G. A. (1975). Isolation and identification of rumen bacteria capable of anaerobic phloroglucinol degradation. *Can. J. Microbiol.* **21**, 794–801.

Van Nevel, C. J. (1972). *In vitro* en *in vivo* studie over de remming der methaanproductie in de pensmaag van de herkauwer. Ph.D. Thesis, University of Ghent, Belgium.

Van Nevel, C. J., Henderickx, H. K., Demeyer, D. I., and Martin, J. (1969). Effect of chloral hydrate on methane and propionic acid in the rumen. *Appl. Microbiol.* **17**, 695–700.

Van Nevel, C., Demeyer, D. I., and Henderickx, H. K. (1970). Effect of chlorinated methane analogues on methane and propionic acid production in the rumen *in vitro.* *Meded. Fak. Landbouwwet., Rijksuniv. Gent.* **35**, 145–152.

Van Nevel, C. J., Demeyer, D. I., and Henderickx, H. K. (1971). Effect of fatty acid derivatives on rumen methane and propionate *in vitro.* *Appl. Microbiol.* **21**, 365–366.

Van Nevel, C. J., Demeyer, D. I., Coltyn, B. G., and Boucqué, C. V. (1973). Incorporation of linseed oil hydrolysate and sodium sulfite in rations for beef production. *Z. Tierphysiol., Tierernaehr. Futtermittelkd.* **31**, 66–71.

Van Nevel, C. J., Prins, R. A., and Demeyer, D. I. (1974). On the inverse relationship between methane and propionate in the rumen. *Z. Tierphysiol., Tierernaehr. Futtermittelkd.* **33**, 121–125.

Vervaeke, I. J., Decuypere, J. A., and Henderickx, H. K. (1975). Continuous culture study of the small intestinal bacterial activity of pigs: Influence of a nutritional dose virginiamycin. *Proc. Int. Symp. Gnotobiol., 5th, 1975* (Abstract).

Visek, W. J. (1972). Effects of urea hydrolysis on cell life-span and metabolism. *Fed. Proc., Fed. Am. Soc. Exp. Biol.* **31**, 1178–1193.

Walker, R. (1973). The influence of gut micro-organisms on the metabolism of drugs and food additives. *Proc. Nutr. Soc.* **32**, 73–78.

Walton, J. R. (1975). Indirect consequences of low-level use of antimicrobial agents in animal feeds. *Fed. Proc., Fed. Am. Soc. Exp. Biol.* **34**, 205–208.

Walton, J. R., and Bird, R. G. (1975). A possible mechanism to explain the growth promotion effect of feed antibiotics in farm animals: Zinc bacitracin induced cell wall damage in *Escherichia coli in vitro. Zentralbl. Veterinaer med., Reihe B* **22**, 318–325.
Watson, M., Pharaoh, B., Wyllie, J., and Benson, W. W. (1975). Metabolism of low oral doses of DDT and DDE by tame mule deer fawns. *Bull. Environ. Contam. Toxicol.* **13**, 316–323.
Weigand, E. (1974). Zur biologischen Wirkung von Sulfit im Futter beim Wiederkäuer. *Uebers. Tierernaehr.* **2**, 29–58.
Willard, F. L., and Kodras, R. (1967). Survey of chemical compounds tested *in vitro* against rumen protozoa for possible control of bloat. *Appl. Microbiol.* **15**, 1014–1019.
Williams, P. P., and Dinusson, W. E. (1973). Ruminal volatile fatty acid concentrations and weight gains of calves reared with and without ruminal ciliated protozoa. *J. Anim. Sci.* **36**, 588–591.
Williams, P. P., and Feil, V. J. (1971). Identification of trifluralin metabolites from rumen microbial cultures. Effect of trifluralin on bacteria and protozoa. *J. Agric. Food Chem.* **19**, 1199–1204.
Williams, P. P., and Stolzenberg, R. L. (1972). Ruminal bacterial degradation of benzo-(b)-thien-4-yl-methylcarbamate (Mobam) and effect of Mobam on ruminal bacteria. *Appl. Microbiol.* **23**, 745–749.
Williams, P. P., Robbins, J. D., Gutierrez, J., and Davis, R. E. (1963). Rumen bacterial and protozoal responses to insecticide substrates. *Appl. Microbiol.* **11**, 517–522.
Williams, P. P., Davison, K. L., and Thacker, E. J. (1968). *In vitro* and *in vivo* rumen microbiological studies with 2-chloro-4,6-bis (isopropylamino)-*S*-triazine (Propazine). *J. Anim. Sci.* **27**, 1472–1476.
Williams-Smith, H. (1967). Observations on the flora of the alimentary tract of animals and factors affecting its composition. *J. Pathol. Bacteriol.* **89**, 95–122.
Wolfe, R. S. (1971). Microbial formation of methane. *Adv. Microb. Physiol.* **6**, 107–146.
Wolin, M. J. (1974). Metabolic interactions among intestinal microorganisms. *Am. J. Clin. Nutr.* **27**, 1320–1328.
Wolin, M. J. (1975). Interactions between the bacterial species in the rumen. *In* "Digestion and Metabolism in the Ruminant" (I. W. McDonald and A. C. I. Warner, eds.), pp. 134–148. Univ. of New England Publishing Unit, Armidale, Australia.
Yokoyama, M. T., Carlson, J. R., and Dickinson, E. O. (1975). Ruminal and plasma concentrations of 3-methyl-indole associated with tryptophan-induced pulmonary edema and emphysema in cattle. *Am. J. Vet. Res.* **36**, 1349–1352.
Zintzen, H. (1973). Vitamin B₁(Thiamin) in der Ernährung des Wiederkäuers. *Uebers. Tierernaehr* **1**, 273–323.

8

Interactions of Drugs and Intestinal Mucosal Endoplasmic Reticulum

RAJENDRA S. CHHABRA and J. MICHAEL TREDGER

I. INTRODUCTION

Until recently it was thought that the role of intestinal mucosa in xenobiotic disposition was limited primarily to the absorption of drugs and foreign chemicals (xenobiotics). However, in recent years, development of sensitive analytical methodology has revealed that drugs may interact with intestinal mucosal endoplasmic reticulum during the absorptive process. This interaction may lead to "activation" or "inactivation" (toxication–detoxication) of drugs, thus affecting their toxicity or therapeutic effectiveness.

Intestinal absorptive cells contain a moderate amount of endoplasmic reticulum consisting of two components—rough-surfaced endoplasmic reticulum composed of membranes whose outer surface is studded with ribosomes, and smooth-surfaced endoplasmic reticulum which is devoid of ribosomes. When the cell is disrupted mechanically or chemically, the endoplasmic reticulum is transformed to different-sized vesicles. These vesicles, both rough and smooth, are known as the microsomal fraction of the cell (tissue). In this chapter, endoplasmic reticulum is referred to as the microsomal fraction.

It is well established that hepatic endoplasmic reticulum contains a group of nonspecific enzymes termed as "microsomal drug-metabolizing enzymes" which biotransform a wide variety of chemicals, including drugs, pesticides, carcinogens, herbicides, food additives, and industrial organic solvents, as well as endogenous substrates such as fatty acids and steroids. These enzyme systems have in common several properties, including their location in the endoplasmic reticulum and the requirement of NADPH, molecular oxygen, and an electron transport system consisting of NADPH-cytochrome c reductase, lipid, and a carbon monoxide binding pigment generally known as cytochrome P-450. Compounds metabolized by these systems are usually quite lipid-soluble prior to metabolism. The reaction products are less lipid-soluble and are excreted as such or after conjugation. The rates of toxication–detoxication of drugs are affected by a number of factors, including age, sex, species, strain, disease, nutritional status, and foreign chemicals. Consideration of these various factors is an important criterion for assessment of the overall capacity of an organism to biotransform drugs. The details of hepatic drug metabolism are well documented (Fouts, 1962; Conney, 1967; Gillette, 1971; Remmer, 1972; Mannering, 1971; Gillette et al., 1972). The metabolism of drugs by the gastrointestinal tract has been reviewed by Hartiala (1973) and a number of articles have been published by Wattenberg on intestinal metabolism of benzpyrene (Wattenberg, 1970, 1971a,b, 1972).

The purpose of this paper is to report current research in our and other laboratories showing a number of similarities and some dissimilarities between in vitro hepatic and intestinal biotransformation of drugs and the factors modifying these systems.

II. DISTRIBUTION OF DRUG-METABOLIZING ENZYMES IN THE INTESTINE

Distribution of microsomal drug-metabolizing enzymes along the entire length of the intestine is such that the enzyme activity is highest in the proximal part of the small intestine and then progressively decreases towards the distal end. Wattenberg *et al.* (1962) showed that, in rat, aryl hydrocarbon hydroxylase (AHH) or benzpyrene hydroxylase activity was highest in the proximal portion of the small intestine. Hietanen and Vainio (1973) found a similar pattern of distribution of AHH in mice, guinea pigs, and rabbits. In rats treated with 3-methylcholanthrene (3-MC), the AHH activity increased throughout the small intestine but the magnitude of induction was higher in the proximal than in the distal part of the small intestine (Wattenberg *et al.*, 1962). In mice, the dealkylation of 7-ethoxycoumarin was found to be highest in the jejunum between 4 and 12 cm distal to the pylorus. We studied (Chhabra and Fouts, 1976) the distribution of ethylmorphine N-demethylase, aniline hydroxylase and AHH activities, and cytochrome P-450 content in 30 cm segments of the proximal 150 cm segment of rabbit small intestine. The activities of all drug-metabolizing enzymes were highest in the proximal 60 cm of the small intestine and progressively declined thereafter. However, cytochrome P-450 contents were approximately the same in all segments from the first 120 cm of small intestine, although there was a decrease in cytochrome P-450 content in the last 30 cm segment. Recently, Hoensch *et al.* (1975) have reported that AHH, 4-nitroanisole O-demethylase, and cytochrome P-450 activities are highest in the upper small intestine of rat and decline progressively towards the ileum. Distribution studies among mucosal cell populations showed mature tip cells contained 6–10 times more cytochrome P-450 and drug-metabolizing enzyme activity per mg of microsomal protein than epithelial crypt cells.

The treatment of laboratory animals with phenobarbital causes a proliferation of endoplasmic reticulum in the liver and an increase in the synthesis of drug-metabolizing enzymes. Similarly, proliferation of intestinal endoplasmic reticulum in the apical part of the absorptive cell in phenobarbital-pretreated rats has been reported by Thomas *et al.* (1972) and Menard *et al.* (1974). However, there seems to be a species difference in the proliferation of endoplasmic reticulum since human intestinal absorptive cells did not show a proliferation of endoplasmic reticulum after the administration of phenobarbital (Tytgat *et al.*, 1973).

III. BIOCHEMICAL PROPERTIES OF SOME INTESTINAL MICROSOMAL DRUG-METABOLIZING ENZYMES

Comparison of rabbit intestinal and hepatic microsomal metabolism of various drug substrates shows that rates of metabolism are generally lower in intestine (Table I). In our studies (Chhabra and Fouts, 1976) we

TABLE I
Metabolism of Various Drug Substrates and Cytochrome Contents in Rabbit Hepatic and Intestinal Microsomes[a]

Assay	Liver (Mean ± S.E.)	Intestine (Mean ± S.E.)	Liver/intestine (Mean ± S.E.)
Aminopyrine[b]	82.0 ± 5.2	12.4 ± 1.3	6.6
Benzphetamine[b]	116.2 ± 11.8	16.7 ± 1.7	7.0
Ethylmorphine[b]	26.3 ± 3.4	8.5 ± 1.0	3.1
p-Chloro-N-methylaniline[b]	48.1 ± 6.5	25.9 ± 2.6	1.9
[14]C-Benzene[c]	38.0 ± 3.7	Not detectable	—
[14]C p-Xylene[c]	211.5 ± 21.8	70.0 ± 6.5	3.0
7-Ethoxycoumarin[c]	23.0 ± 0.9	1.2 ± 0.08	19.2
Biphenyl[c]	35 ± 1.1	2.3 ± 0.2	15.2
Styrene oxide[c]	84 ± 13.5	43.5 ± 10.5	1.9
Benzpyrene[c]	8.5 ± 0.5	1.0 ± 0.05	8.4
p-Nitrophenol[d]	219.0 ± 24	313.5 ± 16.5	0.7
Cytochrome c[e]	2.73 ± 0.12	1.5 ± 0.06	1.8
Cytochrome P-450[f]	1.38 ± 0.07	0.60 ± 0.03	2.3
Cytochrome b_5[f]	1.02 ± 0.08	0.46 ± 0.03	2.0

[a] Data compiled from Chhabra and Fouts (1976), Tredger et al. (1976), and James et al. (1976). Reproduced with permission © 1976, American Society for Pharmacology and Experimental Therapeutics. The Williams and Wilkins Co.
[b] nMoles of formaldehyde formed/mg of microsomal protein/15 minutes.
[c] nMoles of product formed/mg of microsomal protein/15 minutes.
[d] nMoles of p-nitrophenol glucuronide.
[e] μMoles of cytochrome c reduced/mg of microsomal protein/15 minutes.
[f] nMoles of cytochrome/mg of microsomal protein.

found that the rates of all the enzymatic reactions studied, with the one exception of glucuronidation of 4-nitrophenol, were lower in intestine and varied from 15 to 50% of those observed in hepatic microsomal fractions. UDP-Glucuronyltransferase activity was slightly higher in intestine than in liver. The only qualitative difference noted was the absence of benzene hydroxylase in small intestine.

When the total organ activity of aminopyrine N-demethylase in small intestine and liver was compared, the activity in the small intestine was only 1.5–2% of that in the liver. With styrene oxide as substrate, epoxide hydrase activity in the whole small intestine was about 3–3.5% of total hepatic activity (James et al., 1976). However, this low rate of metabolism in the small intestine does not rule out the importance of this tissue in the activation–inactivation of drugs since the surface area of the small intestine and the duration of a foreign chemical's residence in the small intestine may be the determining factors in the contribution of the small intestine to the overall metabolism of foreign chemicals in animals. Our studies have also shown that, like the liver, intestinal microsomal aminopyrine N-demethylase, aniline hydroxylase, and AHH activities in rabbit require NADPH and O_2 for maximum activity. Previously Lehrmann et al. (1973) have shown this requirement for the O-dealkylation of 7-ethoxycoumarin by mouse small intestinal microsomes. This requirement of the small intestinal enzymes for NADPH and O_2 classifies them in the mixed-function oxidase category (Mason, 1957). The intestinal enzyme activities are inhibited by the in vitro addition of cytochrome c, SKF 525A, and by incubation under CO— suggesting that the flavoprotein NADPH-cytochrome c reductase and hemoprotein cytochrome P-450 are the components of the intestinal electron transport system. The similarities in the properties of the mixed-function oxidases of rabbit liver and intestine were also emphasized because both tissues had comparable patterns of protein activity, time activity, substrate activity, and pH activity relationships. Similar properties of the enzyme catalyzing the O-dealkylation of 7-ethoxycoumarin were reported by Lehrmann et al. (1973).

The hepatic microsomal CO-binding pigments from control and 3-MC-treated rats differ in their properties. When reduced, the CO-binding pigment from untreated animals has an absorption peak at 450 nm, whereas in 3-MC-treated animals this peak shifts to 448 nm and is designated as P-448 or P_1-450. The cytochrome P-450-containing microsomal fraction is relatively nonspecific and catalyzes the metabolism of a variety of drug substrates while the cytochrome P-448-containing fraction is more specific and biotransforms a limited number of drug substrates—especially polycyclic hydrocarbons. Zampaglione and Mannering (1973) have proposed that intestinal and pulmonary microsomes from control or 3-MC-treated rats contain primarily the P_1-450 or P-448 AHH system and they believe that this cytochrome predominates in the portals of drug entry (intestine, lung, and skin). However, our studies (Chhabra et al., 1974a; Chhabra and Fouts, 1976; Bend et al., 1972) in rabbit show that, like liver, intestinal and pulmonary microsomes contain predominately cytochrome P-450 whose reduced CO-binding absorption spectra closely resemble that of hepatic cytochrome P-450. Moreover, so far we have been unable to induce cytochrome P-448 in rabbit intestinal microsomes with 3-MC pretreatment. This suggests that Zampaglione and Mannering's hypothesis may not hold in species other than rat.

The in vitro addition of drug substrates to liver microsomes produces typical binding spectra (Schenkman et al., 1967). In our studies (Chhabra and Fouts, 1976) we have shown that the in vitro addition of benzphetamine and aniline to hepatic and intestinal microsomes pro-

TABLE II

Comparison of Absorption Maxima, Minima, and ΔA_{max} of Aniline and Benzphetamine Added *in Vitro* in Rabbit Hepatic and Intestinal Microsomes[a]

		Absorption		
Ligand	Tissue	Maximum	Minimum	$\Delta A_{max} \times 10^3$ [Mean $\pm$ SE (N=3)]
Benzphetamine	Liver	388	422	24.3 $\pm$ 1.3
	Small intestine	385–388	422–423	6.3 $\pm$ 0.3
Aniline	Liver	431	393–395	45 $\pm$ 7.0
	Small intestine	431	396–400	11.6 $\pm$ 1.9

[a] The microsomes were suspended in 0.1 M HEPES buffer, pH 7.6, to give a final concentration of 2 mg of protein per ml. Benzphetamine (4.14 mg/ml) or aniline (39 mg/ml) were added to sample cuvettes in 2–10 μl volumes, the reference cuvette received equal amounts of distilled water. The spectra were recorded on Aminco DW2 Spectrophotometer. The ΔA_{max} were calculated from the difference in absorbance between peak and trough and is expressed in terms of Δ O.D. ($\times 10^{-3}$) per 2 mg of microsomal protein per ml. Table taken from Chhabra and Fouts (1976). Reproduced with permission © 1976, American Society for Pharmacology and Experimental Therapeutics. The Williams and Wilkins Co.

duced typical type I and type II binding spectra, respectively. The wavelengths of maximum and minimum absorption are shown in Table II. ΔA_{max} values for both type I and II ligands were about four times higher in liver microsomes than in intestinal microsomes. Schenkman *et al.* (1973) have suggested that the *in vitro* addition of organic solvents to liver microsomes produces a reverse type I spectral change, possibly due to the displacement of *in vivo* bound endogenous substrates. In our studies the *in vitro* addition of ethanol induced a distinct reverse type I spectrum in liver microsomes but produced negligible spectral changes in intestinal microsomes. This shows that perhaps intestinal cytochrome P-450 does not bind endogenous substrate *in vivo* or that ethanol cannot displace substrate bound *in vivo* to intestinal cytochrome P-450.

IV. FACTORS AFFECTING INTESTINAL DRUG METABOLISM

A. Species Differences in Intestinal Microsomal Drug-Metabolizing Enzymes

There is very little information available on species differences in intestinal drug-metabolizing enzymes. Wattenberg *et al.* (1962) have reported AHH activities in intestinal mucosa of mouse, guinea pig, rabbit, hamster, dog, monkey, baboon, and man. AHH activity was found to be lowest in man and highest in monkey (about 40 times that in man), whereas other species had 3–12 times AHH activity of man. Recently, we have published a comparative study of a number of intestinal and hepatic drug-metabolizing enzyme activities in various laboratory species (Chhabra *et al.*, 1974a). Rats, mice, hamsters, guinea pigs, and rabbits were used in this study. The enzyme reactions investigated included the hydroxylation of aniline, biphenyl and benzpyrene, and the N-demethylation of ethylmorphine. NADPH-cytochrome c reductase activity and cytochrome P-450 contents were measured as components of the microsomal electron transport system. These enzyme activities were present in the livers of all the species (Table III) and varied in magnitude over a two to sixfold range among species for any given enzyme activity. In the intestines from mice, rats, guinea pigs, and hamsters, some of the enzymatic activities were either absent or had very low activities which would require very sensitive methods of detection. The rabbit emerged as the best animal in which to study intestinal drug metabolism, since all drug-metabolizing enzyme activities studied were present in easily measurable amounts.

The interspecies differences in intestinal drug metabolism are mostly due to genetic factors but may also result from the induction of drug-metabolizing enzyme activities in the small intestine by chemicals ingested with the food. The animal diets vary in their composition. Hietanen and Vainio (1973) observed that feeding rats with rabbit or guinea pig pellets increased rat duodenal AHH activity almost fivefold, suggesting that diet may be contributing in part towards interspecies variation in intestinal toxication–detoxication of zenobiotics.

B. Age

Studies on the variations which age imposes on intestinal microsomal enzyme activities are few and appear to be limited to those investigations of mixed-function oxidases in the immediate postnatal period. In a previous report, we demonstrated that several drug-metabolizing enzyme activities in the intestine of rabbits do not attain adult activities for at least 10 weeks after birth (Tredger *et al.*, 1976). Three phases are apparent during the developmental process. First is a 3-week period after birth when activities are initially detectable but remain low; second is a period (20–30 days postpartum) when activities increase rapidly and reach adult values and, finally, there is a prolonged third stage during which activities exhibit a transient fall (around 50 days of age) before adult activities are ultimately achieved. Typical developmental patterns

TABLE III
Species Variations in Hepatic and Intestinal Microsomal Drug-Metabolizing Enzymes and Cytochrome P-450 Content[a]

Enzyme	Tissue	Species				
		Rabbit	Guinea pig	Rat	Mouse	Hamster
Ethylmorphine-N-demethylase (nmoles of HCHO formed/mg of microsomal protein in 15 minutes ± S.E.)	Liver	60.3 ± 22.8	37.7 ± 3.4	188.6 ± 8.9	101.3 ± 9.6	110.8 ± 15.1
	Intestine	11.2 ± 1.6	8.8 ± 0.3	ND	ND	ND
Biphenyl hydroxylase (nmoles of 4-hydroxybiphenyl formed/mg of microsomal protein in 15 minutes ± S.E.)	Liver	58.1 ± 1.6	77.9 ± 1.8	34.4 ± 1.4	95.3 ± 10.0	47.4 ± 3.0
	Intestine	8.2 ± 0.6	12.8 ± 2.9	3.2 ± 0.3	8.6 ± 0.7	3.2 ± 0.5
Aryl hydrocarbon hydroxylase (relative fluorescence units/mg of microsomal protein in 15 minutes ± S.E.)	Liver	2775 ± 191	995 ± 37	3009 ± 211	1705 ± 172	579 ± 41
	Intestine	835 ± 39	372 ± 86	138 ± 8	101 ± 21	33 ± 6
Aniline hydroxylase (nmoles of p-aminophenol formed/mg of microsomal protein in 15 minutes ± S.E.)	Liver	9.8 ± 2.3	10.6 ± 1.0	15.0 ± 0.9	24.1 ± 1.9	19.1 ± 1.3
	Intestine	2.0 ± 0.2	2.1 ± 0.7	ND	ND	ND
NADPH-Cytochrome c reductase (nmoles of cytochrome c reduced/mg microsomal protein/minute ± S.E.)	Liver	185.0 ± 15.5	55.4 ± 2.8	118.3 ± 18.3	113.0 ± 6.8	44.3 ± 4.1
	Intestine	140.0 ± 23.0	43.6 ± 4.6	49.7 ± 7.3	90.0 ± 1.6	36.9 ± 2.6
Cytochrome P-450 content (nmoles/mg microsomal protein ± S.E.)	Liver	1.1 ± 0.32	1.45 ± 0.16	0.84 ± 0.07	1.1 ± 0.07	1.26 ± 0.07
	Intestine	0.38 ± 0.07	0.18 ± 0.02	See ref.[b]	0.04 ± 0.01	0.16 ± 0.01

[a] Data compiled from Chhabra et al. (1974a). Reproduced with permission © 1974, American Society for Pharmacology and Experimental Therapeutics. The Williams and Wilkins Co.
[b] Read details in Chhabra et al. (1974a).

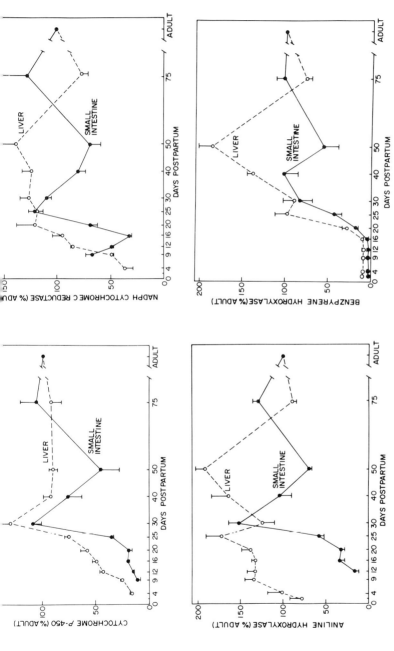

Fig. 1. Postnatal development of mixed function oxidase activities in rabbit liver and intestine. Each value is the mean ± S.E. for at least four separate determinations. All enzyme activities are expressed as a percentage of the adult activity at the corresponding time point in liver (○– – –○) and small intestine (●——————●). The normal range of activities in adult male rabbits is presented in Table I with their units. From Tredger & Chhabra (1976). Reproduced with permission © 1976, American Society for Pharmacology and Experimental Therapeutics. The Williams and Wilkins Co.

261

for intestinal cytochrome P-450 content, NADPH-cytochrome c reductase, aniline hydroxylase, and AHH activities are shown in Fig. 1 and are compared with the corresponding patterns in neonatal rabbit liver. Some differences between the developmental profiles in intestinal and hepatic tissues are apparent and mainly reflect the better correlation between drug-metabolizing enzyme activities and cytochrome P-450 content in intestinal than in hepatic microsomes. This correlation was also apparent in the findings of Short and his colleagues (Short et al., 1972) who examined the postnatal development of mixed-function oxidases in the intestine and other tissues from swine.

C. Circadian Variation

In the liver, many microsomal enzymes involved in intermediary metabolism and in drug metabolism exhibit a readily detectable circadian periodicity in their activities (Hardeland et al., 1973). However, few comparable studies reporting the presence of rhythmic changes in intestinal microsomal enzyme activities have been published, although circadian variations in the intestinal absorption of amino acids and carbohydrates (Furuya and Yugari, 1974) and in the activities of various digestive enzymes in the small intestine (Saito et al., 1975; Stevenson et al., 1975) have been reported. Perhaps the most relevant published work is that of Edwards et al. (1972) who described a rhythmic variation in sterol synthesis in rat intestine, but who did not monitor the activity of a particular enzyme in this tissue.

Recently, work performed in our own laboratory has indicated that intestinal microsomal drug-metabolizing enzyme activities may exhibit rhythmic variations (Tredger and Chhabra, 1977). Figure 2 illustrates data obtained using rats and rabbits and measuring AHH activity over a 24 hour period. In the intestine of both species, two peaks in activity were apparent, one in the early morning and the second during the late afternoon. This rhythmic pattern (containing two peaks in activity) was also observed for AHH activity in rabbit liver (Fig. 2). However, in rat liver, a single peak in the activity of AHH during the early morning was detected (Fig. 2), as has been noted by previous authors (Radzialowski and Bousquet, 1968; Lake et al., 1976). Consequently, species differences in the daily rhythmic pattern of hepatic AHH activity may exist in the rat and rabbit. Moreover, the rhythmic pattern in hepatic enzyme activities in either species may not be identical with that found in extrahepatic tissues.

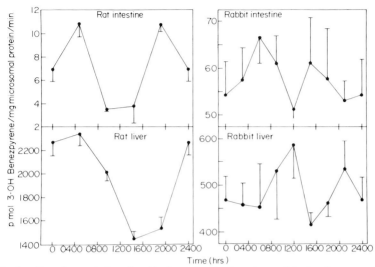

Fig. 2.   Circadian variation of aryl hydrocarbon hydroxylase activity in microsomes from the liver and intestine of rats and rabbits. Each point is the mean ± S.E. for the determinations. AHH activity ws stored and assayed as described elsewhere (Tredger and Chhabra, 1976). Values at 2400 (●) hr are shown twice for the sake of clarity and continuity. Animals were maintained on a 12-hour alternating light/dark cycle (0800–2000 hour Eastern Standard Time with light).

D.   Hormones

The effects of various steroid and peptide hormones on intestinal microsomal enzyme activities have been recently reviewed by Hartiala (1973). Consequently, only the major and more recent aspects of hormonal interactions with drug metabolism are considered here (Table IV).

Sex hormones appear to play an important regulatory role in the control of mixed-function oxidase activities in rat liver. In male rats, hepatic drug-metabolizing enzyme activities are usually higher than in females (Chhabra and Fouts, 1974; Quinn *et al.*, 1958). This does not appear to be the case in the intestine (Hartiala *et al.*, 1964; Feuer *et al.*, 1971; Chhabra and Fouts, 1974) although, in contrast to these results, one report has described higher AHH activities in the intestines of male rats than in females (Hietanen, 1974). Castration did not substantially affect intestinal drug-metabolizing enzyme activities (Hietanen, 1974) in contrast to its effect in liver.

Glucocorticoids may be important in the control of mixed-function oxidase activities in rat tissues. For example, the adrenalectomy of male rats resulted in lower drug-metabolizing enzyme activities in the intes-

TABLE IV
Interactions between Steroid Hormones and Microsomal Enzyme Activities in the Small Intestine

Pretreatment	Enzymatic activity	Effect[a]	Reference
Cortisone	Ethylmorphine N-demethylase	0	Thomas et al., 1972
Adrenalectomy	Benzpyrene hydroxylase	−	Nebert and Gelboin, 1969
Differences due	Benzpyrene hydroxylase	>	Hietanen, 1974
to endogenous	Benzpyrene hydroxylase	=	Chhabra and Fouts, 1974
sex hormones	UDP-glucuronyltransferase	=	Hartiala et al., 1964;
			Chhabra and Fouts, 1974
	Aniline 4-hydroxylase,	=	Feuer et al., 1971
	hexobarbital oxidase, amino-		
	pyrine N-demethylase		
Castration	Benzpyrene hydroxylase,	−	Hietanen, 1974
	UDP-glucuronyltransferase		

[a] Key to symbols: −, a decrease in activity followed pretreatment; 0, no effect; >, activity in males is greater than in females; =, male and female activities are similar.

tine as well as in the liver (Nebert and Gelboin, 1969). The same effect was observed after hypophysectomy (Nebert and Gelboin, 1969). Nonetheless, Thomas *et al.* (1972) reported that the administration of cortisone had no effect on intestinal ethylmorphine demethylase activity. In contrast, we have noted increases in intestinal benzphetamine demethylase, benzpyrene hydroxylase, NADPH-cytochrome *c* reductase activities, and in cytochrome *P*-450 content after the administration of dexamethasone by intraperitoneal injection to 20-day-old rabbits (Chhabra, R. S. and Tredger, J. M. unpublished).

E. Diet

Much of the pioneering work identifying the importance of dietary components as potential effectors of intestinal mixed-function oxidase activities was performed by Wattenberg and his colleagues. This work and the major contributions made by other investigators are summarized in Table V.

Following the observation that starvation decreased AHH activity in the small intestine of rats (Wattenberg *et al.*, 1962), Wattenberg and co-authors showed that various dietary manipulations could affect this intestinal enzyme activity. These manipulations included the feeding of different commercial chow diets (Wattenberg, 1971b) and the feeding of semi-purified diets (Wattenberg *et al.*, 1962; Wattenberg, 1971a,b; Billings and Wattenberg, 1972). The results from these experiments led to the proposal that much of the AHH activity in the small intestine of rats is due to exogenous inducers in the diets (Wattenberg, 1972). This proposal was supported by the finding that the addition of various vegetables to a semi-purified diet caused increases in intestinal AHH activity in rats (Wattenberg, 1971a,b). It was further endorsed by the observation that compounds (especially indoles) isolated from chemical extracts of vegetables of the Brassicacae family could induce AHH activity in the liver and intestine when administered to rats (Loub *et al.*, 1975). Work from other laboratories using starvation, different commercial chow diets (Hietanen and Vainio, 1973), and semi-purified diets (Hoensch *et al.*, 1975; Pantuck *et al.*, 1975) has provided additional evidence of the importance of dietary components in determining AHH activities in the small intestine.

It is noteworthy that all the above-mentioned studies have been performed using rats as the experimental animal. To our knowledge, the only comparable study in another animal species is that of James *et al.* (1976) using rabbits. In this work and in our own preliminary studies, also using rabbits (Chhabra, R. S. and Tredger, J. M. unpublished), no

TABLE V

The Effects of Various Dietary Modifications on Microsomal Enzyme Activities in the Small Intestine

Dietary manipulation	Enzymatic activity	Effect[a]	Reference
Starvation (> 48 hours)	3-Methyl-4-methylaminoazobenzene-N-demethylase	−	Billings and Wattenberg, 1972
	Benzpyrene hydroxylase	−	Hietanen and Vainio, 1973; Wattenberg, 1970; Wattenberg et al., 1962
	UDP-Glucuronyltransferase	−	Hietanen and Vainio, 1973
	UDP-Glucuronyltransferase	0	Marselos and Laitinen, 1975
	β-Glucuronidase	+	Marselos and Laitinen, 1975
Cholesterol-rich (2%) diet	Benzpyrene hydroxylase, UDP-glucuronyltransferase, NADPH-cytochrome c reductase	+	Hietanen et al., 1975a
Lipid-supplemented diet	UDP-glucuronyltransferase; benzpyrene hydroxylase	0	Hietanen et al., 1975b
Fat-free diet	Benzpyrene hydroxylase	−	Wattenberg et al., 1962
Comparisons of different commercial chow diets	Benzpyrene hydroxylase; UDP-glucuronyltransferase	Variable	Hietanen and Vainio, 1973; Wattenberg 1971a,b
		Variable	Hietanen and Vainio, 1973
Semi-purified diets (compared with laboratory chow)	Epoxide hydrase, benzphetamine demethylase	0	James et al., 1976
	Phenacetin O-deethylase	−	Pantuck et al., 1975
	Cytochrome P-450, benzpyrene hydroxylase, 4-nitroanisole O-demethylase	−	Hoensch et al., 1975
	Cytochrome b_5	+	Hoensch et al., 1975

Low iron content diet	Cytochrome P-450, benzpyrene hydroxylase	−	Hoensch et al., 1975
	4-nitroanisole O-demethylase, cytochrome b_5	0	Hoensch et al., 1975
	Benzpyrene hydroxylase	+	Wattenberg, 1971a,b
Additions of various vegetables to semi-purified diet in descending order of potency:			
Brussel sprouts			
Cabbage			
Turnips			
Broccoli			
Alfalfa			
Cauliflower			
Spinach			
Dill			

[a] Key to symbols: −, decrease in activity observed; +, increase in activity observed; 0, no effect.

changes in the intestinal microsomal enzyme activities were noted after feeding semi-purified diet. The reasons for this apparent species difference are not immediately obvious but may be of considerable importance should a regulatory role be envisioned for diet in the control of enzyme activities in the intestine of all mammals, including man.

Factors other than dietary contaminants are undoubtedly important in regulating enzyme activities in the small intestine. For example, the amount of dietary iron (Hoensch *et al.*, 1975) and the quantity and quality of dietary lipid (Wattenberg *et al.*, 1962; Hietanen and Vainio, 1973; Hietanen *et al.*, 1975a,b,) have been shown to influence intestinal microsomal enzyme activities in rats. The effects of various drugs on these activities are considered in the following section.

F. Xenobiotics

The administration of drugs by the oral route, the passage of many inhaled particulate compounds into the intestine, and the intake of environmental contaminants and food additives in the diet are the three major means by which the intestinal mucosa may be exposed to drugs, environmental pollutants, and other xenobiotics. Many investigators have examined the effects of administration of various chemicals on microsomal enzyme activities in the intestinal mucosa, although most of this work has been confined to studies on the mixed-function oxidase system. Table VI summarizes these findings.

Polycyclic and polychlorinated hydrocarbons have been frequently used in studying interactions between xenobiotics and the intestinal endoplasmic reticulum and, possibly because of its high sensitivity, benzpyrene hydroxylase (AHH) activity is the microsomal component most usually assayed. After pretreatment of rats (Gelboin and Blackburn, 1964; Pantuck *et al.*, 1973, 1974; Lake *et al.*, 1973; Nebert and Gelboin, 1969; Aitio, 1974; Wattenberg, 1970; Zampaglione and Mannering, 1973), mice (Gentil and Sims, 1971; Nebert and Gelboin, 1969; Wiebel *et al.*, 1973; Watanabe *et al.*, 1975a,b; Niwa *et al.*, 1975; Gielen *et al.*, 1972), and hamsters (Nebert and Gelboin, 1969) with various polycyclic hydrocarbons administered by the oral or intraperitoneal route, increases in AHH activity were frequently observed. Only in some strains of mice (e.g., DBA/2, AKR/N, NZW/BLN, NZB/BLN) genetically "resistant" to the induction of AHH by polycyclic hydrocarbons were no increases in intestinal AHH activity noted after the administration of polycyclic hydrocarbons (Nebert and Gelboin, 1969; Niwa *et al.*, 1975). While hepatic AHH activity was also unchanged after the administration of polycyclic hydrocarbons to the same strains of mice (Nebert and Gelboin, 1969; Niwa *et al.*, 1975), the activity could be induced in both liver and intestine using 2,3,7,8-tetrachlorodibenzo-*p*-dioxin (TCDD), an extremely potent polychlorinated hydrocarbon (Chhabra *et al.*, 1974b, 1976b; Poland *et al.*, 1974).

Increases in AHH activity in rat and mouse liver after polycyclic hydrocarbon treatment are usually associated with a blue shift to 448 nm in the peak of the CO-dithionite reduced versus dithionite reduced difference spectrum of microsomal supensions, indicating the formation of a new cytochrome species (*P*-448). In mouse intestine, Poland *et al.* (1974) have shown that the same generation of cytochrome *P*-448 occurs after the administration of TCDD to both "resistant" and "susceptible" strains of mice and after the administration of 3-MC to only susceptible strains. However, in rats, Zampaglione and Mannering (1973) showed quantitative increases, but no qualitative change, in intestinal cytochrome *P*-450 after 3-MC administration. These authors proposed that the constitutive terminal oxidase in control rat intestinal drug-metabolizing enzyme systems was cytochrome *P*-448 and not cytochrome *P*-450 (Zampaglione and Mannering, 1973). At the present time, no corroboration of this observation is available despite publications from several authors who have measured the cytochrome *P*-450 content of rat intestinal microsomes (Hoensch *et al.*, 1975; Chhabra *et al.*, 1974a; Correia and Schmid, 1975).

Although polycyclic hydrocarbons appear to act as potent inducers of AHH and cytochrome *P*-448 activities in the intestines of rats and mice, in keeping with the findings of studies using the liver (Mannering, 1971), their effects are less pronounced when most other mixed-function oxidase activities are considered. Thus, Lake *et al.* (1973) could detect no changes in the intestinal activities of biphenyl 4-hydroxylase, biphenyl 2-hydroxylase, or 4-chloro-*N*-methylaniline-*N*-demethylase in rats pretreated with 3-MC. The lack of induction of biphenyl 2-hydroxylase is somewhat surprising considering its response to polycyclic hydrocarbons in rat liver (Creaven *et al.*, 1965).

Polycyclic hydrocarbons occur naturally in both cigarette smoke and charcoal-broiled beef. The feeding of charcoal-broiled beef to rats resulted in a substantial increase in the rate of phenacetin dealkylation in the intestine (Pantuck *et al.*, 1975). Phenacetin and benzpyrene were also metabolized more rapidly in the intestine after the exposure of rats to cigarette smoke (Welch *et al.*, 1972). However, these effects of cigarette smoke were not reproducible in later work (Van Cantfort and Gielen, 1975; Abramson and Hutton, 1975).

Other chemicals seem far less potent than the polycyclic hydrocarbons in affecting intestinal mixed-function oxidase activities. For example,

TABLE VI

The Effects of Xenobiotics on Microsomal Enzyme Activities in the Small Intestine

Active agent	Enzymatic activity	Effect[a]	References
Polycyclic and polychlorinated hydrocarbons			
3-Methylcholanthrene	Benzpyrene hydroxylase	+	Aitio, 1974; Gelboin and Blackburn, 1964, Gentil and Sims, 1971; Gielen *et al.*, 1972; Lake *et al.*, 1973; Nebert and Gelboin, 1969; Poland *et al.*, 1974; Watanabe *et al.*, 1975a,b; Wattenberg *et al.*, 1962; Zampaglione and Mannering, 1973
	3-Methyl-4-methylaminoazobenzene N-demethylase	+	Billings and Wattenberg, 1972
	Cytochrome *P*-450	+	Poland *et al.*, 1974; Zampaglione and Mannering, 1973
	Biphenyl 4-hydroxylase	0	Lake *et al.*, 1973
	Biphenyl 2-hydroxylase	0	Lake *et al.*, 1973
	4-Chloromethylaniline-N-demethylase	0	Lake *et al.*, 1973
	Phenacetin O-deethylase	+	Welch *et al.*, 1972
Charcoal-broiled Beef	Phenacetin O-deethylase	+	Pantuck *et al.*, 1975
	Benzpyrene hydroxylase	+	Wattenberg and Leong, 1965
3-4-Benzpyrene	Benzpyrene hydroxylase	+	Wattenberg *et al.*, 1962
	Phenacetin O-deethylase	+	Pantuck *et al.*, 1973, 1974
1,2-Benzanthracene	Benzpyrene hydroxylase	+	Wattenberg *et al.*, 1962; Wiebel *et al.*, 1973
1,2,5,6-Dibenzanthracene	Benzpyrene hydroxylase	+	Wattenberg *et al.*, 1962
5,6-Naphthoflavone	Benzpyrene hydroxylase	+	Niwa *et al.*, 1975; Watanabe *et al.*, 1975a,b
7,8-Naphthoflavone	Benzpyrene hydroxylase	+	Watanabe *et al.*, 1975b
Cigarette smoke	Benzpyrene hydroxylase	+	Welch *et al.*, 1972
	Phenacetin O-deethylase	+	Welch *et al.*, 1972
	Benzpyrene hydroxylase	0	Abramson and Hutton, 1975; Van Cantfort and Gielen, 1975
Polychlorinated biphenyl	Benzpyrene hydroxylase	+	Hietanen *et al.*, 1975a
2,3,7,8-Tetrachlorodibenzo-*p*-dioxin	Benzpyrene hydroxylase	+	Poland *et al.*, 1974
	Cytochrome *P*-450	+	Poland *et al.*, 1974

Drugs

Phenobarbital	Benzpyrene hydroxylase	0	Lake *et al.*, 1973; Nebert and Gelboin, 1969; Poland *et al.*, 1974
	Benzpyrene hydroxylase	+	Watanabe *et al.*, 1975a
	Aniline 4-hydroxylase	0	Feuer *et al.*, 1971
	Hexobarbital oxidase	0	Feuer *et al.*, 1971; Franklin and Kyegombe, 1973
	Aminopyrine *N*-demethylase	0	Feuer *et al.*, 1971
	7-Ethoxycoumarin *O*-deethylase	+	Lehrmann *et al.*, 1973; Scharf and Ullrich, 1973, 1974; Ullrich and Weber, 1974
	NADPH-Cytochrome *c* reductase	+	Lehrmann *et al.*, 1973; Scharf and Ullrich, 1973, 1974
	Cytochrome *P*-450	+	Lehrmann *et al.*, 1973; Scharf and Ullrich, 1973, 1974
	Ethylmorphine *N*-demethylase	+	Thomas *et al.*, 1972
	UDP-Glucuronyltransferase	0	Franklin and Kyegombe, 1973
	Glucose-6-phosphatase	−	Menard *et al.*, 1974
	Proliferation of endoplasmic reticulum (e.r.)	0	Tytgat *et al.*, 1973
Marijuana			
Others	Proliferation of endoplasmic reticulum	0	Tytgat *et al.*, 1973
Piperonyl butoxide	Benzpyrene hydroxylase	+	Lake *et al.*, 1973
	Biphenyl 4-hydroxylase	0	Lake *et al.*, 1973
	Biphenyl 2-hydroxylase	0	Lake *et al.*, 1973
	4-Chloromethylaniline-*N*-demethylase	0	Lake *et al.*, 1973
Isosafrole	Benzpyrene hydroxylase	+	Lake *et al.*, 1973
	Biphenyl 4-hydroxylase	0	Lake *et al.*, 1973
	Biphenyl 2-hydroxylase	0	Lake *et al.*, 1973
	4-Chloromethylaniline-*N*-demethylase	0	Lake *et al.*, 1973
Indole derivatives	Benzpyrene hydroxylase	+	Loub *et al.*, 1975
Cobalt; hemoglobin	Cytochrome *P*-450	+	Correia and Schmid, 1975
	Benzpyrene hydroxylase	+	Correia and Schmid, 1975

[a] Key to symbols: +, an increase in activity followed pretreatment; −, a decrease in activity followed pretreatment; 0, no effect.

phenobarbital is a potent inducer of hepatic mixed-function oxidases (Conney, 1967) but has been reported to have no effect on intestinal AHH (Lake *et al.*, 1973; Nebert and Gelboin, 1969; Gielen *et al.*, 1972), aniline hydroxylase (Feuer *et al.*, 1971), hexobarbital oxidase (Feuer *et al.*, 1971; Franklin and Kyegombe, 1973), aminopyrine demethylase (Feuer *et al.*, 1971), and UDP-glucuronyltransferase activities (Franklin and Kyegombe, 1973), nor on smooth endoplasmic reticulum proliferation (Tytgat *et al.*, 1973). Nonetheless, some reports have indicated that phenobarbital can induce intestinal microsomal enzyme activities in mice or rats (Lehrmann *et al.*, 1973; Thomas *et al.*, 1972; Ullrich and Weber, 1974; Scharf and Ullrich, 1973, 1974). In addition, various phenothiazine derivatives (Wattenberg and Leong, 1965), piperonyl butoxide and isosafrole (Lake *et al.*, 1973), various indoles (Loub *et al.*, 1975), and cobalt and heme (Correia and Schmid; 1975) have been shown to increase some mixed-function oxidase activities in rat intestine. Whether such effects are species-specific is not presently known. However, we have noted that 3-MC or phenobarbital pretreatment did not affect various drug-metabolizing enzyme activities in the intestines of 20-day-old rabbits and that the same compounds, TCDD and DDT, also had no inducing effects in adult rabbits (Chhabra, R. S. and Tredger, J. M. unpublished).

V. CONCLUSIONS AND RESEARCH NEEDS

Comparison of drug-metabolizing enzymes in rabbit small intestine and liver shows mainly quantitative differences; most of the activities are two to seven times higher in the liver than in the intestine. These enzymes, in both tissues, require NADPH and O_2 for maximum activity and are inhibited by cytochrome c, SKF-525A, and CO. The *in vitro* addition of drug substrates to microsomal fractions of both tissues produced typical type I and type II binding spectra. In general, the hepatic and intestinal drug-metabolizing enzymes have a similar pattern of development. Comparison of the relationships between activities and pH, duration of incubation, substrate, and protein concentration further suggests that rabbit intestinal and hepatic drug-metabolizing enzymes have similar characteristics.

We suggest the need for further research on the following aspects of intestinal endoplasmic reticulum and drug interactions which are listed below.

1. So far, studies have been generally confined to the *in vitro* metabolism of drug substrates by microsomal fractions of intestine. A comparison of *in vitro* and *in vivo* drug–membrane interactions is neces-

sary to fully appreciate the role of the intestinal mucosa in the biotransformation of foreign chemicals.

2. The controversy that the rat intestinal enzyme system is predominantly dependent on cytochrome P-448 in untreated and 3-MC-pretreated animals should be resolved. Rat intestinal microsomal cytochrome P-448 or P-450 should be purified from untreated and 3-MC- or phenobarbital-pretreated rats and the biochemical properties of the system(s) should be studied.

3. There should be more studies on species variations in metabolism of foreign chemicals by the intestine. The study of human intestinal enzymes is necessary to establish its resemblance, if any, to animal species. Although instability of microsomal enzymes is one of the deterrents for human studies, we have recently shown that if tissue samples from laboratory animals are stored under liquid nitrogen, there is no loss in the activities of drug-metabolizing enzymes (Chhabra et al., 1976a; Tredger and Chhabra, 1976). This technique may be useful for storage of human biopsy or even, on some occasions, postmortem tissue samples for later processing.

4. The role of the nutritional status of an animal in biotransformation of drugs by the intestinal enzymes should be investigated further. Previous studies have been largely limited to one enzyme system (AHH) and only in one species (rat). Furthermore, there are hardly any studies on the effect of deficient or supplemented diets on the intestinal drug-metabolizing enzymes. Since the nutritional status of an animal is one of the most important factors which could influence the therapeutic value or toxicity of a drug, research on this aspect is needed.

5. There seem to be species differences in the induction of intestinal drug-metabolizing enzymes. Rabbit intestinal enzymes do not respond to pretreatment by a number of foreign chemicals but are increased when rabbits are pretreated with the synthetic glucocorticoid, dexamethasone. The varying response of different species to the induction of intestinal drug-metabolizing enzymes by environmental chemicals may help in extrapolating the results to man.

6. The interaction of drugs with other functions of the endoplasmic reticulum, such as the transport of lipids, is another important area to be investigated. Studies in this direction should aid in explaining the role of drugs in the malabsorption of nutrients.

ACKNOWLEDGMENTS

The authors are indebted to Dr. James R. Fouts for his encouragement, advice, and support of the research undertaken in our laboratory.

REFERENCES

Abramson, R. K., and Hutton, J. J. (1975). Effects of cigarette smoking on aryl hydrocarbon hydroxylase activity in lungs and tissues of inbred mice. *Cancer Res.* **35**, 23–29.

Aitio, A. (1974). Different elimination and effect on mixed-function oxidase of 20-methyl-cholanthrene after intragastric and intraperitoneal administration. *Res. Commun. Chem. Pathol. Pharmacol.* **9**, 701–710.

Bend, J. R., Hook, G. E. R., Easterling, R. E., Gram, T. E., and Fouts, J. R. (1972). A comparative study of the hepatic and pulmonary microsomal mixed-function oxidase systems in the rabbit. *J. Pharmacol. Exp. Ther.* **183**, 206–217.

Billings, R. E., and Wattenberg, L. W. (1972). The effects of dietary alterations on 3-methyl-4-methylaminoazobenzene *N*-demethylase activity. (36254). *Proc. Soc. Exp. Biol. Med.* **139**, 865–867.

Chhabra, R. S., and Fouts, J. R. (1974). Sex differences in the metabolism of xenobiotics by extrahepatic tissue in rats. *Drug Metab. Dispos.* **2**, 375–379.

Chhabra, R. S., and Fouts, J. R. (1976). Biochemical properties of some microsomal xenobiotic-metabolizing enzymes in rabbit small intestines. *Drug. Metab. Dispos.* **4**, 208–214.

Chhabra, R. S., Pohl, R. J., and Fouts, J. R. (1974a). A comparative study of xenobiotic metabolizing enzymes in liver and intestine of various animal species. *Drug. Metab. Dispos.* **2**, 443–447.

Chhabra, R. S., Tredger, J. M., Philpot, R. M., and Fouts, J. R. (1974b). Selection of inducers: An important factor in characterizing genetic differences to induction of aryl hydrocarbon hydroxylase in strains of mice. *Life Sci.* **15**, 123–130.

Chhabra, R. S., Tredger, J. M., and Fouts, J. R. (1976a). The effect of freezing and storage in liquid nitrogen on drug-metabolizing enzyme activities in rodent tissue preparations. *Fed. Proc., Fed. Am. Soc. Exp. Biol.* **35**, 244.

Chhabra, R. S., Tredger, J. M., Philpot, R. M., and Fouts, J. R. (1976b). Relationship between aryl hydrocarbon hydroxylase induction and *de novo* synthesis of cytochrome *P*-448 (*P*₁-450). *Chem.-Biol. Interact.* **15**, 21–31

Conney, A. H. (1967). Pharmacological implications of microsomal enzyme induction. *Pharmacol. Rev.* **19**, 317–366.

Correia, M. A., and Schmid, R. (1975). Effect of cobalt on microsomal cytochrome *P*-450: Differences between liver and intestinal mucosa. *Biochem. Biophys. Res. Commun.* **65**, 1378–1384.

Creaven, P. J., Parke, D. V., and Williams, R. T. (1965). A fluorimetric study of the hydroxylation of biphenyl *in vitro* by liver preparations of various species. *Biochem. J.* **96**, 879–885.

Edwards, P. A., Muroya, H., and Gould, R. G. (1972). *In vivo* demonstration of the circadian rhythm of cholesterol biosynthesis in the liver and intestine of the rat. *J. Lipid Res* **13**, 396–401.

Feuer, G., Sosa-Lucero, J. C., Lumb, G., and Moddel, G. (1971). Failure of various drugs to induce drug-metabolizing enzymes in extrahepatic tissues of the rat. *Toxicol. Appl. Pharmacol.* **19**, 579–589.

Fouts, J. R. (1962). Interaction of drugs and hepatic microsomes. *Fed. Proc., Fed. Am. Soc. Exp. Biol.* **21**, 1107–1111.

Franklin, C. S., and Kyegombe, D. B. (1973). The distribution and induction of some drug-metabolizing enzymes in man. *Br. J. Pharmacol.* **47**, 616P.

Furuya, S., and Yugari, Y. (1974). Daily rhythmic changes of L-histidine and glucose absorption in rat small intestine *in vivo*. *Biochim. Biophys. Acta* **343**, 558–564.

Gelboin, H. V., and Blackburn, N. R. (1964). The stimulatory effect of 3-methylcholanthrene on benzpyrene hydroxylase activity in several rat tissues: Inhibition by actionomycin D and puromycin. *Cancer Res.* **24,** 356–360.

Gentil, A., and Sims, P. (1971). The metabolism of 7,12-dimethylbenz[α]anthracene by homogenates of the stomach and small intestine of mice. *Z. Krebsforsch.* **76,** 223–230.

Gielen, J. E., Goujon, F. M., and Nebert, D. W. (1972). Genetic regulation of aryl hydrocarbon hydroxylase induction. II. Simple Mendelian expressions in mouse tissues *in vivo. J. Biol. Chem.* **247,** 1125–1137.

Gillette, J. R. (1971). Effect of various inducers on electron transport system associated with drug metabolism by liver microsomes. *Metab., Clin. Exp.* **20,** 215–227.

Gillette, J. R., Davis, D. W., and Sasame, H. AL (1972). Cytochrome *P*-450 and its role in drug metabolism. *Annu. Rev. Pharmacol.* **12,** 57–84.

Hardeland, R., Hohmann, D., and Rensing, L. (1973). The rhythmic organization of rodent liver. A review. *J. Interdiscip. Cycle Res.* **4,** 89–118.

Hartiala, K. (1973). Metabolism of hormones, drugs, and other substances by the gut. *Physiol. Rev.* **53,** 496–534.

Hartiala, K. J. W., Pulkkinen, M. O., and Savola, P. (1964). Beta-D-glucosiduronic acid conjugation by the mucosa of various organs. *Nature (London)* **201,** 1036.

Hietanen, E. (1974). Effect of sex and castration on hepatic and intestinal activity of drug-metabolizing enzymes. *Pharmacology* **12,** 84–89.

Hietanen, E., and Vainio, H. (1973). Interspecies variations in small intestinal and hepatic drug hydroxylation and glucuronidation. *Acta Pharmacol. Toxicol.* **33,** 57–64.

Hietanen, E., Laitinen, M., Lang, M., and Vainio, H. (1975a). Inducibility of mucosal drug-metabolizing enzymes of rats fed on a cholesterol-rich diet by polychlorinated biphenyl, 3-methylcholanthrene, and phenobarbitone. *Pharmacology* **13,** 287–296.

Hietanen, E., Laitinen, M., Vainio, H., and Hanninen, O. (1975b). Dietary fats and properties of endoplasmic reticulum. II. Dietary lipid-induced changes in activities of drug-metabolizing enzymes in liver and duodenum of rat. *Lipids* **10,** 467–472.

Hoensch, H., Woo, C. H., and Schmid, R. (1975). Cytochrome *P*-450 and drug metabolism in intestinal villous and crypt cells of rats: Effect of dietary iron. *Biochem. Biophys. Res. Commun.* **65,** 399–406.

James, M. O., Fouts, J. R., and Bend, J. R. (1976). Hepatic and extrahepatic metabolism *in vitro* of an epoxide (8-^{14}C-styrene oxide) in the rabbit. *Biochem. Pharmacol.* **25,** 187–193.

Lake, B. G., Hopkins, R., Chakraborty, J., Bridges, J. W., and Parke, D. V. (1973). The influence of some hepatic enzyme inducers and inhibitors on extrahepatic drug metabolism. *Drug Metab. Dispos.* **1,** 342–349.

Lake, B. G., Tredger, J. M., Burke, M. D., Chakraborty, J., and Bridges, J. W. (1976). The circadian variation of hepatic microsomal drug and steroid metabolism in the golden hamster. *Chem.-Biol. Interact.* **12,** 81–90.

Lehrmann, C., Ullrich, V., and Rummel, W. (1973). Phenobarbital inducible drug monooxygenase activity in the small intestine of mice. *Naunyn-Schmiedeberg's Arch Pharmacol.* **276,** 89–98.

Loub, W. D., Wattenberg, L. W., and Davis, D. W. (1975). Aryl hydrocarbon hydroxylase induction in rat tissues by naturally occurring indoles of cruciferous plants. *J. Natl. Cancer Inst.* **54,** 985–988.

Mannering, G. J. (1971). Properties of cytochrome *P*-450 as affected by environmental factors: Qualitative changes due to administration of polycyclic hydrocarbons. *Metab., Clin. Exp.* **20,** 228–245.

Marselos, M., and Laitinen, M. (1975). Starvation and phenobarbital treatment effects on drug hydroxylation and glucuronidation in the rat liver and small intestinal mucosa. *Biochem. Pharmacol.* **24,** 1529–1535.

Mason, H. S. (1957). Mechanisms of oxygen metabolism. *Science* **125,** 1185–1188.

Menard, D., Bertleloot, A., and Hugon, J. S. (1974). Action of phenobarbital on the ultrastructure and the enzymatic activity of the mouse intestine and mouse liver. *Histochemistry* **38,** 241–252.

Nebert, D. W., and Gelboin, H. V. (1969). The *in vivo* and *in vitro* induction of aryl hydrocarbon hydroxylase in mammalian cells of different species, tissues, strains, and developmental and hormonal states. *Arch. Biochem. Biophys.* **134,** 76–89.

Niwa, A., Kumaki, K., Nebert, D. W., and Poland, A. P. (1975). Genetic expression of aryl hydrocarbon hydroxylase activity in the mouse. Distinction between the "responsive" homozygote and heterozygote at the Ah locus. *Arch. Biochem. Biophys.* **166,** 559–564.

Pantuck, E. J., Hsiao, K.-C., Maggio, A., Kakamura, K., Kuntzman, R., and Conney, A. H. (1973). Effect of cigarette smoking on phenacetin metabolism. *Clin. Pharmacol. Ther.* **15,** 9–17.

Pantuck, E. J., Hsiao, K.-C., Kaplan, S. A., Kuntzman, R., and Conney, A. H. (1974). Effects of enzyme induction on intestinal phenacetin metabolism in the rat. *J. Pharmacol. Exp. Ther.* **191,** 45–52.

Pantuck, E. J., Hsiao, K.-C., Kuntzman, R., and Conney, A. H. (1975). Intestinal metabolism of phenactin in the rat: Effect of charcoal-broiled beef in rat chow. *Science* **187,** 744–745.

Poland, A. P., Glover, E., Robinson, J. R., and Nebert, D. W. (1974). Genetic expression of aryl hydrocarbon hydroxylase activity: Induction of mono-oxygenase activities and cytochrome *P*-450 formation by 2,3,7,8-tetrachlorodibenzo-*p*-dioxin in mice genetically "non-responsive" to other aromatic hydrocarbons. *J. Biol. Chem.* **249,** 5599–5606.

Quinn, G. P., Axelrod, J., and Brodie, B. B. (1958). Species, strain, and sex differences in metabolism of hexobarbitone, amidopyrine, anit-pyrene, and aniline. *Biochem. Pharmacol.* **1,** 152–158.

Radzialowski, F. M., and Bousquet, W. F. (1968). Daily rhythmic variation in hepatic drug metabolism in the rat and mouse. *J. Pharmacol. Exp. Ther.* **163,** 229–238.

Remmer, H. (1972). Induction of drug-metabolizing enzyme system in the liver. *Eur. J. Clin. Pharmacol.* **31,** 116–136.

Saito, M., Murakami, E., Nishida, T., Fujisawa, Y., and Suda, M. (1975). Circadian rhythms in digestive enzymes in the small intestine of rat. 1. Patterns of the rhythms in various regions of the small intestines. *J. Biochem. (Tokyo)* **78,** 475–480.

Scharf, R., and Ullrich, V. (1973). *In vitro* induction of drug monooxygenase activity by phenobarbital in the isolated mouse jejunum. *Naunyn-Schmiedeberg's Arch. Pharmacol.* **278,** 329–332.

Scharf, R., and Ullrich, V. (1974). *In vitro* induction by phenobarbital of drug monooxygenase activity in mouse isolated small intestine. *Biochem. Pharmacol.* **23,** 2127–2137.

Schenkman, J. B., Remmer, H., and Estabrook, R. W. (1967). Spectral studies of drug interaction with hepatic microsomal cytochrome. *Mol. Pharmacol.* **3,** 113–123.

Schenkman, J. B., Cinti, D. L., Moldeus, P. W., and Orrenius, S. (1973). Newer aspects of substrate binding to cytochrome *P*-450. *Drug Metab. Dispos.* **1,** 111–120.

Short, C. R., Maines, M. D., and Westfall, B. A. (1972). Postnatal development of drug-metabolizing enzyme activity in liver and extrahepatic tissue of swine. *Biol. Neonate* **21,** 54–68.

Stevenson, N. R., Ferrigni, F., Parnicky, K., Day, S., and Fierstein, J. S. (1975). Effect of changes in feeding schedule on the diurnal rhythms and daily activity of intestinal brush border enzymes and transport systems. *Biochim. Biophys. Acta* **406**, 131–145.

Thomas, F. B., Baba, N., Greenburger, N. J., and Salsburey, D. (1972). Effect of phenobarbital on small intestinal structure and function in the rat. *J. Lab. Clin. Med.* **80**, 548–558.

Tredger, J. M., and Chhabra, R. S. (1976). Preservation of various microsomal drug-metabolizing components in tissue preparation from the livers, lungs, and small intestines of rodents. *Drug Metab. Dispos.* **4**, 451–459.

Tredger, J. M. and Chhabra, R. S. (1977). Circadian variations in microsomal drug-metabolizing activities in liver and extrahepatic tissues from rat and rabbit. *Xenobiotica.* **7**, 481–489.

Tredger, J. M., Chhabra, R. S., and Fouts, J. R. (1976). Postnatal development of mixed-function oxidation as measured in microsomes from the small intestine and liver of rabbits. *Drug. Metab. Dispos.* **4**, 17–23.

Tytgat, G. N., Saunders, D. R., and Rubin, C. E. (1973). Failure of phenobarbital and marijuana to stimulate the smooth endoplasmic reticulum in the human intestinal absorptive cell. *Eur. J. Clin. Invest.* **3**, 363–370.

Ullrich, V., and Weber, P. (1974). A direct test for monooxygenase activity of intact small intestine using surface reflectance fluorimetry. *Biochem. Pharmacol.* **23**, 3309–3315.

Van Cantfort, J., and Gielen, J. (1975). Organ specificity of aryl hydrocarbon hydroxylase induction by cigarette smoke in rats and mice. *Biochem. Pharmacol.* **24**, 1253–1256.

Watanabe, M., Konno, K., and Sato, H. (1975a). Effect of feeding and lighting on the regulation of aryl hydrocarbon (benzo[α]pyrene) hydroxylase activity in the liver, small intestine, and lung of mice. *Gann* **66**, 123–132.

Watanabe, M., Watanabe, K., Konno, K., and Sato, H. (1975b). Genetic differences in the induction of aryl hydrocarbon hydroxylase and benzo[α]pyrene carcinogenesis in C_3H/He and DBA/2 strains of mice. *Gann* **66**, 217–226.

Wattenberg, L. W. (1970). The role of the portal of entry in inhibition of tumorigenesis. *Prog. Exp. Tumor Res.* **14**, 89–104.

Wattenberg, L. W. (1971a). Studies of polycyclic hydrocarbon hydroxylases of the intestine possibly related to cancer. *Cancer* **28**, 99–102.

Wattenberg, L. W. (1971b). Enzymatic reactions and carcinogenesis. *Collect. Pop. Annu. Symp. Fundam. Cancer Res.* **24**, 241–254.

Wattenberg, L. W. (1972). Dietary modification of intestinal and pulmonary aryl hydrocarbon hydroxylase activity. *Toxicol. Appl. Pharmacol.* **23**, 741–748.

Wattenberg, L. W., and Leong, J. L. (1965). Effects of phenothiazines on protective systems againat polycyclic hydrocarbons. *Cancer Res.* **25**, 365–370.

Wattenberg, L. W., Leong, J. L., and Strand, P. J. (1962). Benzpyrene hydroxylase activity in the gastrointestinal tract. *Cancer Res.* **22**, 1120–1125.

Welch, R. M., Cavallito, J., and Loh, A. (1972). Effect of exposure to cigarette smoke on the metabolism of benzo[α]pyrene and acetophenetidin by lung and intestine of rats. *Toxicol. Appl. Pharmacol.* **23**, 749–758.

Wiebel, F. J., Leutz, J. C., and Gelboin, H. V. (1973). Aryl hydrocarbon (benzo[α]pyrene) hydroxylase: Inducible in extrahepatic tissues of mouse strains not inducible in liver. *Arch. Biochem. Biophys.* **154**, 292–294.

Zampaglione, N. G., and Mannering, G. J. (1973). Properties of benzpyrene hydroxylase in the liver, intestinal mucosa, and adrenal of untreated and 3-methylcholanthrene-treated rats. *J. Pharmacol. Exp. Ther.* **183**, 676–685.

9

Drug Effects on Gastric Mucosa

KEVIN J. IVEY

This review will concentrate on current knowledge of the damaging effects of drugs on the gastric mucosa, particularly in man. The pathophysiology of these drugs will be detailed. Drugs used in the treatment of mucosal damage will be discussed with emphasis on their actions on pathogenetic mechanisms. While numerous excellent direct histological studies have been carried out on the ulcerogenic effects of drugs in animals, very few similar studies have been carried out in man. Assessment of damage in man has depended on less direct assessment such as radiology and stool blood loss and hence our knowledge is much less exact. Research needs in this area and in therapy of mucosal damage will be outlined.

I. PATHOGENESIS

A. Acid

Acid plays a major role in the pathogenesis of peptic ulceration occurring spontaneously in man. This is more obvious in the case of duodenal ulcer where the average acid output is greater than normal. It is not as apparent with gastric ulcer where the average acid output is less than normal. Nevertheless, acid is necessary for the development of the great majority, if not all, of peptic ulcers in man (Ivey, 1974a).

Most of the ulcerogenic drugs which cause damage to the gastric mucosa in animals and in some cases man, have little or no stimulating effect on acid secretion. Such drugs include aspirin, indomethacin, phenylbutazone, smoking and nicotine. Those drugs which stimulate acid secretion, e.g., caffeine, reserpine, corticosteroids, and possibly ethanol, are moderate to mild stimulators only. Once mucosal damage has been initiated by a drug, all evidence indicates that this damage is increased in the presence of acid. It appears, however, that most ulcerogenic drugs initiate mucosal damage by a mechanism other than acting through acid alone.

B. Mucus

It has been proposed that mucus is not only a lubricant to the stomach but a protective barrier to damaging agents including acid. It seems, however, that mucus is only weakly alkaline and offers very little barrier to the movement of hydrogen ions which diffuse right through it (Heatley, 1959). Aspirin, corticosteroids, phenylbutazone and indomethacin (Menguy, 1969) decrease the amount of mucus secreted as well as alter its composition. It is difficult to determine if this effect is primary, or secondary to drug damage to surface mucus secreting cells. The latter view is more widely held.

In 1914 George Milton Smith noted that if acid and bile were placed in the stomach of cats he produced severe mucosal damage. He was unable to produce similar damage in the dog stomach which he attributed to the large amount of mucus present and which appeared to be stimulated by the presence of bile and acid. Thus, there may be a mechanism by which mucus protects the mucosa by physically separating the damaging agent from it.

C. Cell Renewal

Corticosteroids decrease the rate of renewal of mucosal cells and reduce the rate of loss (Max and Menguy, 1970). It has been postulated that this is their mechanism of action in producing mucosal damage. While it is hard to explain immediate drug-induced cell damage on this basis, it could possibly account for longer term damage as in chronic gastritis or peptic ulcer. On the other hand, carbenoxolone, which increases healing rate of gastric ulcer in man (Doll, 1964) also causes a delay in cell renewal and a reduction in cell exfoliation (Lipkin, 1971). It seems hard to attribute both damage and healing to the same mechanism.

Aspirin, on the other hand, has no effect on mitotic frequency but both aspirin and phenylbutazone increase the rate of exfoliation of surface epithelial cells (Max and Menguy, 1970). This latter effect is probably nonspecific damage to those cells.

D. Gastric Mucosal Barrier

For many years, the pathogenesis of peptic ulcer and other mucosal lesions has been considered to be a balance between acid output and gastric mucosal resistance.

Peptic ulcer = Acid secretion × Mucosal resistance

Attempts at measuring mucosal resistance in terms of mucus or cell renewal rates have not met with much success and studies of these modalities in man have met with limiting technical difficulties. In recent years it has been realized that:

Gastric acid output = Acid secretion − Acid absorption

The concept of back-diffusion of hydrogen ions was introduced by Teorell in 1933 (Teorell, 1933, 1939). After ligating a cat's stomach at the proximal and distal ends he introduced a known volume of hydrochloric acid. With time, the volume remained constant as did chloride (Cl^-) concentration, but H^+ concentration decreased while Na^+ increased (Fig. 1). Teorell interpreted this as back-diffusion of hydrogen ions from the lumen across the gastric mucosa in exchange for sodium ions from the mucosa (Fig. 2). In the normal stomach while the gradient between hydrogen ions in the gastric lumen at pH 1.0 and those in blood at pH 7.4 is over 2 million to 1, there is normally little movement of hydrogen ions back into the mucosa. This unique ability of the stomach

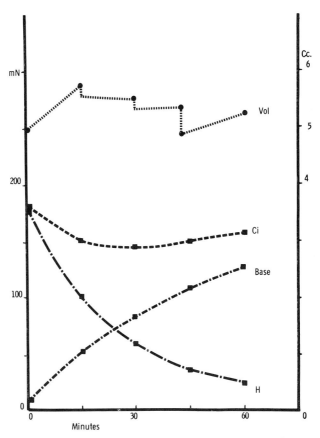

Fig. 1. Introduction of isotonic hydrochloric acid into a cat's stomach. Note the "exponential" decrease of the acidity (H) and the simultaneous increase of alkali cations (base) without appreciable volume change, indicating an exchange diffusion process (see Fig. 2). (From Teorell, 1939, with permission.)

to limit movement of these ions has been termed the gastric mucosal barrier to hydrogen and sodium ion movement (Ivey, 1971a, 1973, 1974b). Other intestinal surfaces such as the small intestine lack this ability so that acid diffuses into these mucosae to a much greater extent producing cell damage.

The gastric mucosal barrier concept was popularized by Horace Davenport working in Charles Code's Laboratory, Mayo Clinic. Davenport, in a series of experiments beginning in 1964, demonstrated the ability of certain drugs such as aspirin to increase back-diffusion of hydrogen ions into gastric mucosa (Davenport, 1964, 1965a,b,c, 1967a,b,

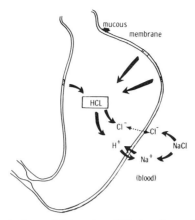

Fig. 2. Sketch schematically explaining the "diffusion theory." The gastric juice is secreted mainly as pure HCl (about isotonic with blood). There is a continuous outward diffusion of HCl and a simultaneous inward diffusion of NaCl—strictly speaking, an ionic exchange between H^+ and Na^+. The reduction of acidity and variation of amount of chloride take place in this manner. (From Teorell, 1939, with permission.)

1968, 1970a,b, 1971; Davenport *et al.*, 1964). At the same time more sodium ions move into the lumen. The degree of damage to the mucosa as manifested by bleeding and protein loss was proportional to the amount of hydrogen ions diffusing back into the mucosa (Davenport, 1964, 1965a, 1970b).

In the intact stomach, aspirin-induced damage produces an acute gastritis predominantly in the acid-secretory area (the body) of the stomach. Microscopically superficial erosions are produced, usually not extending deeper than the muscularis mucosae (Lynch *et al.*, 1964; Ivey *et al.*, 1975a; Baskin *et al.*, 1976).

Thus far, the gastric mucosal barrier has not been localized anatomically but this function appears to be performed by or via the apical plasma membrane of the surface epithelial cells. Electron microscopic studies carried out in the mouse (Hingson and Ito, 1971) and man (Ivey *et al.*, 1975a; Baskin *et al.*, 1976) after damage to the mucosa by aspirin indicate that the apical membrane of the surface cells may be completely destroyed while the tight junctions between cells remain intact. Aspirin-induced changes in ionic permeability and mucosal cell damage are not permanent and recovery begins within an hour (Ivey *et al.*, 1975a; Baskin *et al.*, 1976).

In Tables I and II are listed drugs known to alter or not to alter the gastric mucosal barrier. Of the common ulcerogenic drugs, only aspirin,

TABLE I
Drugs Which Damage the Gastric Mucosal Barrier

Aspirin and salicylic acid
Alcohol and other aliphatic acids, e.g., butanol
Bile salts
Indomethacin[a]
16-16-dimethyl PGE_2
Short-chain fatty acids, e.g., acetic, propionic
Hypertonic solutions of glucose, sucrose, urea
Eugenol
Diethylaminoethyl
Acetazolamide
Sodium fluoride
Decyl sulfate
Lysolecithin
Phospholipase
Digitonin
Oxethazaine
Promethazine hydrochloride
Mersalyl
Dithiothreital
N-ethylmaleimide iodoacetamide
Thiocyanate
2,3-Dimercaptopropranol
p-Chloromercuribenzoate
Pancreatic juice

[a] Heidenhain (fundic) pouches in dogs.

TABLE II
Drugs Which Do Not Damage the Gastric
Mucosal Barrier

Corticosteroids
Phenylbutazone
Indomethacin[a]
Nicotine
Caffeine
Cimetidine
15-Methyl PGE_2
Atropine
Carbenoxolone
Gastrin
Antidiuretic hormone
N-Acetylcysteine

[a] Antral pouches in dogs.

alcohol (in a concentration greater than 8%), and possibly indomethacin, damage the gastric mucosal barrier. Phenylbutazone does not affect the gastric mucosal barrier. Corticosteroids do not alter the gastric mucosal barrier when given alone in man (Ivey *et al.*, 1975b) or animals (Chung *et al.*, 1970; Chvasta and Cooke, 1972). When given to animals for prolonged periods with drugs which do affect the barrier, such as aspirin or acetic acid, corticosteroids augment the back-diffusion of hydrogen ions caused by these drugs alone (Aubrey and Burns, 1972; Chung *et al.*, 1970). While cigarette smoking has been associated with peptic ulceration and gastritis in man, neither it nor nicotine given orally or intravenously affects mucosal permeability (Ivey *et al.*, 1973). Bile acids, however, destroy the normal barrier in man (Ivey *et al.*, 1970a,b) and recent studies suggest that cigarette smoking increases bile reflux into the stomach (Read and Grech, 1973). Thus, it may indirectly cause increased back-diffusion of hydrogen ions across gastric mucosa. Cigarette smoking and nicotine may exert their main action in producing duodenal ulcer by inhibiting pancreatic bicarbonate secretion, thus reducing neutralization of duodenal acid (Konturek *et al.*, 1971).

So far only chemical methods of measuring electrolyte fluxes have been mentioned in determining the integrity of the gastric mucosal barrier. Measurement of the potential difference (PD) across the gastric mucosa provides a simple and alternative method (Andersson and Grossman, 1965; Ivey, 1971a). Hogben (1955) has shown that gastric PD in the frog's stomach *in vitro* is dependent on active transport of chloride ions into the lumen, i.e., against their concentration gradient which is from lumen to mucosa. The permeability of the upper gastrointestinal tract to chloride ions is in the following order: duodenum > antrum > fundus. Therefore, one would expect the PD in the fundus (where the chloride ion "leak" is least) to be greater than in the antrum, and that of the antrum to be greater than in the duodenum. This has been found to be the case (Andersson and Grossman, 1965; Durbin, 1967; Geall *et al.*, 1970). If mucosal permeability to chloride ions is increased, gastric PD will be reduced. Geall *et al.* (1970) employing peripheral venous blood for the reference electrode, found a marked reduction in gastric PD after intragastric instillation of bile, aspirin (70–140 mM) and alcohol. In each case the drop in PD began within 3 minutes, reaching a peak within 30 minutes, and was followed by gradual recovery.

Good correlation has been found between changes in net ionic fluxes and PD after ulcerogenic drugs in the dog (Chvasta and Cooke, 1972). In man mucosal cell damage induced by aspirin and recovery has been found to correlate well with changes and recovery of PD (Ivey *et al.*, 1975a; Baskin *et al.*, 1976).

NORMAL

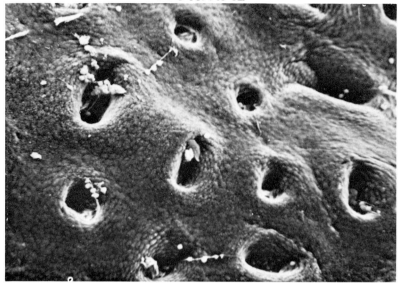

ASPIRIN

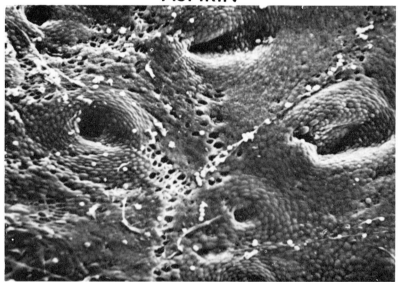

Fig. 3. Scanning electron microscopic (SEM) appearance of normal human gastric mucosa before and 10 minutes after two 300 mg aspirin tablets. The ten large holes in the top picture are the gastric pits. The numerous small holes affecting approximately 25% of the surface epithelial cells situated between the gastric pits are the result of aspirin damage.

286

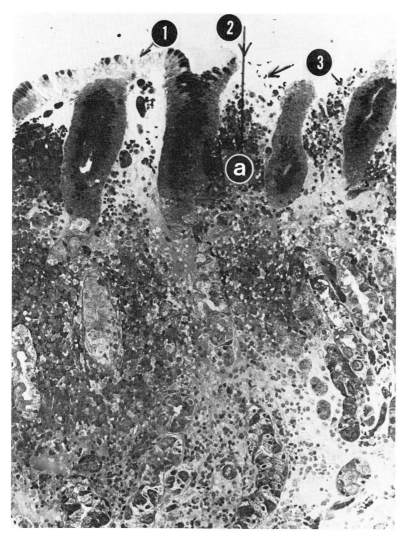

Fig. 4. Light microscopic appearance of an adjacent area in the same subject showing more extensive mucosal damage. The arrowed sections illustrate: (1) loss of mucus granules in surface epithelial cells. This appearance would correspond with the SEM appearance of aspirin damage in Fig. 3. (2) Accumulation of red blood cells below the surface where they could easily move through the damaged surface into the lumen to cause macroscopic bleeding. (3) Loss of epithelial lining cells or microscopic erosion.

In man, aspirin is known to be associated with peptic ulcer disease epidemiologically, to be clinically associated with major hemorrhage from acute hemorrhagic gastritis, and in normal doses to produce gastric erosions endoscopically (Thorsen *et al.*, 1968; Baskin *et al.*, 1976) in 50% of subjects when given with HCl, to increase stool blood loss in 70% subjects (Grossman *et al.*, 1961), and to produce microscopic cell damage in 100% of normal subjects (Baskin *et al.*, 1976) (Figs. 3 and 4). Thus studies of the gastric mucosal barrier and its relationship to aspirin assume marked clinical significance.

Davenport's animal studies with aspirin showed that aspirin did not produce damage unless there was acid present and the amount of damage increased with the amount of acid present. Practical application of this in therapy or prevention of aspirin-induced damage is to raise the pH of gastric contents, preferably to neutral pH 7 but certainly to above pH 3.5. Aspirin is a weak acid with a pK_a of 3.5. Below pH 3.5 the majority of the drug exists in the lipid-soluble undissociated state whence it easily penetrates gastric mucosal cells to initiate damage; above pH 3.5 it is in the nonlipid soluble dissociated state which does not penetrate cell membranes.

Studies in man supporting this theory are the absence of increased stool blood loss with well-buffered aspirin compared to unbuffered (Leonards and Levy, 1969); the absence of gastric erosions on gastroscopy when aspirin is given buffered with bicarbonate compared to acid (Thorsen *et al.*, 1968); and the reduction of microscopic cell damage after two aspirin tablets from 20% to 8% when acid secretion is inhibited by the histamine H_2(type II)-receptor antagonists (MacKercher *et al.*, 1976).

In a related study on stress ulcers (acute hemorrhagic gastritis) in burn patients, McAlhany and associates (1976) divided patients into two groups—a control and a group given intense therapy with antacids to maintain gastric pH around 7.0. Only one of twenty-four patients receiving antacid developed significant upper gastrointestinal bleeding, while seven of twenty-four receiving no antacid experienced hemorrhage with or without gastric ulcer perforation ($p < 0.02$).

II. DRUG TREATMENT OF GASTRIC MUCOSAL DAMAGE

Drug therapy for peptic ulcer and gastric mucosal disease consists mainly of therapy with one or more of the following agents: antacids, anticholinergics, carbenoxolone, prostaglandins, and the histamine type II-receptor antagonists.

A. Antacids

The mechanism of action of the antacids is purely by neutralization of gastric contents. Because of rapid gastric emptying, and an alkaline pH increases gastric emptying, enormous doses have to be frequently given, e.g., half-hourly or less to achieve this. This is only practical for a limited period of time in extenuating circumstances, e.g., patients bleeding with acute hemorrhagic gastritis (Ivey, 1971b).

Nevertheless, the medical profession has "felt" that antacid therapy, if it did not heal peptic ulcer, certainly relieved symptoms, though no controlled studies were ever performed to show this. Unfortunately, two double-blind crossover studies presented recently failed to show a significant difference between antacid and placebo in relief of duodenal ulcer pain. The results were the same whether a potent (*in vitro* buffering capacity 135 mEq HCl) or less potent (buffering of 30 mEq HCl) antacid was used (Sturdevant *et al.*, 1976).

Large doses of liquid antacids (equivalent to 30 ml Mylanta I or Maalox) given one and three hours after a meal and at bed time, do reduce gastric pH for considerable periods (Fordtran *et al.*, 1973). Using this antacid regimen, a recent double blind endoscopic study showed significantly greater healing by antacid than placebo (Peterson, 1977) in patients with duodenal ulcer.

B. Anticholinergics

The mechanism of action of the anticholinergics is by reduction of gastric acid secretion. These agents have no effect on ionic permeability (the gastric mucosal barrier) in animal (Overholt *et al.*, 1969) or man (Ivey and Clifton, 1971).

Like antacids, they have been used for many years in treatment of peptic ulcer disease because everybody "felt" they worked, there was no other effective medical therapy, and they were, if nothing else, "logical placebos". The effect of oral administration of these drugs on gastric acid secretion, relief of ulcer pain, and healing of peptic ulcer has recently been extensively reviewed (Ivey, 1975). In the doses routinely recommended by the manufacturers there is very little evidence that these agents had any effect on secretion, pain relief, or ulcer healing. In maximally recommended doses the evidence is very equivocal at best for any effect. In order to achieve any effectiveness, these drugs have to be given in doses usually well above those recommended by the manufacturers. Such doses are usually not tolerated well for long because of the common side effects of dry mouth and blurring of vision.

C. Carbenoxolone

This drug has been shown in a majority of trials published from England to increase the healing rate of gastric ulcers in ambulatory but not hospitalized patients (Doll *et al.*, 1962). A collaborative study of United States investigators has failed to confirm this finding. The drug suffers from an aldosteronelike action of causing hypertension and hypokalemia in a considerable percentage of patients, so that all patients on the drug need frequent monitoring of blood pressure and serum electrolytes. Its mechanism of action is unknown. Carbenoxolone does not appear to affect gastric acid secretion (Berstad *et al.*, 1970; Cocking and MacCraig, 1969) or protect the gastric mucosal barrier in man (Ivey and Gray, 1973a,b) or animal (Simons and Moody, 1975; Gordon *et al.*, 1975). It does reduce surface epithelial cell renewal and turnover rate in restrained mice (Lipkin, 1970). The significance of this is uncertain as corticosteroids do this also in animals. Max and Menguy (1970) have postulated that this is the mechanism of the ulcerogenic action of corticosteroids.

D. Prostaglandins (PG)

Since this ubiquitous group of hormones was shown to reduce gastric secretion, high hopes have been held for their use in the therapy of gastric ulcer disease. PGE and PGA analogues have the most antisecretory effect though, in man, $PGF_{2\alpha}$ in large doses also has an inhibitory effect (Newman *et al.*, 1975).

The development of orally effective agents 15-methyl PGE_2 and 16,16-dimethyl PGE_2, with respect to inhibition of acid secretion in man, has been a promising development. In animal studies (Robert *et al.*, 1976) prostaglandins were able to prevent steroid and secretagogue-induced ulcers. When given orally vomiting was a prominent side effect. As this did not occur when the drug was given intrajejunally or parenterally it suggests a local irritant effect.

Prostaglandins do suffer from having multiple effects on different organs. Depending on the analogue used, nausea, vomiting, and/or diarrhea have been frequent side effects. Whether any of the prostaglandin analogues could ever be safely used in women of childbearing age is a serious question.

While no studies of the effect of these agents have been carried out in man, Bolton and Cohen (1976) recently reported that 16,16-dimethyl PGE_2 but not 15-methyl PGE_2 altered the gastric mucosal barrier in dog by increasing permeability to hydrogen and sodium ions and reducing gastric mucosal potential difference.

It appears that more research studies on the effects of prostaglandins in man are required before their use in therapy of peptic ulcer disease in man can be assessed.

E. Histamine Type II-Receptor Antagonists

The development of these agents, which has been reviewed elsewhere, appears to be a pharmacological dream come true (Ivey, 1974c). With supporting animal studies, these agents have already been clearly shown to inhibit acid secretion whether basal (Ivey *et al.*, 1975c) or stimulated by either a meal (Henn *et al.*, 1975), caffeine (Cano *et al.*, 1976), pentagastrin, histamine or the vagal nerve (Konturek *et al.*, 1974). The duration of action of a single dose of the latest derivative cimetidine appears to be about 6 hours. To date, cimetidine has been given to over 1000 patients without any serious side effects being recorded. This is a major advantage over the anticholinergics and prostaglandins. The only side effects to date with cimetidine have been small increases in serum SGOT and creatinine, and five cases of (reversible) gynecomastia have been reported in the first 1000 patients continued on the drug.

Metiamide, the first available orally effective H_2-blocker, or its successor, cimetidine, has already been shown in controlled studies to relieve significantly, pain of peptic ulcer disease (Pounder *et al.*, 1975), and to increase the healing rate of peptic ulcers using endoscopic evaluation (Anonymous, 1975).

A number of case reports have already attested to the successful use of these agents in treating patients with the most severe ulcer diathesis—the Zollinger–Ellison syndrome (Richardson and Walsh, 1976). At a symposium organized by Smith, Kline and French in Chicago in 1975, some forty-five cases of severe peptic ulcer diathesis due to Zollinger–Ellison syndrome, systemic mastocytosis or short bowel syndrome were presented. In nearly all cases the patients' acid output had been reduced to normal or below, ulcer symptoms relieved, and in many cases intractable ulcers healed on therapy with the oral H_2-blocker, metiamide. Such cases had not been followed long enough to determine whether the effect of the drug might become less with time. It has been shown in Zollinger-Ellison patients that the combination of a histamine type II-blocker plus an anticholinergic drug in maximally recommended doses reduces acid secretion after a single dose for approximately 2 hours longer than does the H_2-blocker alone (Richardson and Walsh, 1976).

In an uncontrolled study MacDonald and associates (1976) from Canada recently reported cessation of major upper gastrointestinal bleeding in all of eleven patients with acute stress ulcers (hemorrhagic gastritis). These were generally ill patients with underlying conditions such as postrenal transplantation or immunosuppressive therapy. Remarkably, the bleeding stopped in almost all cases after the first oral dose of the drug.

MacKercher and associates (1976) found that a 300 mg tablet of cimetidine given 1 hour before 600 mg of aspirin orally, significantly reduced aspirin-induced gastric mucosal damage. Without cimetidine, mean percentage of surface epithelial cells damaged 10 minutes after aspirin administration was 20%. With prior cimetidine therapy the percentage of cells damaged at 10 minutes was only 4%. A possible reason for the remarkable therapeutic efficacy of the H_2-blockers may be that they have a protective effect on gastric mucosa independent of their acid inhibitory action. Ivey and associates (1975c) noted that cimetidine caused a significant elevation in gastric transmucosal potential difference in man. The rise in PD seemed greater than could be accounted for by a simple liquid-junction potential due to the rise in pH to 7.0. Moreover, addition of acid to the gastric lumen caused no fall in PD. Some animal studies suggest that the H_2 blockers have an effect on ionic permeability (Fromm et al., 1976) or mucosal protection (Bugajski et al., 1976) independent of their acid inhibitory effect.

III. RESEARCH NEEDS

A. Pathogenesis

1. Pathogenicity of Ulcerogenic Drugs

a. **Peptic Ulcer.** Controlled prospective studies need to be carried out to determine which drugs are ulcerogenic in man. Of drugs known to be ulcerogenic in animals, such as aspirin, corticosteroids, phenylbutazone, indomethacin, alcohol, and nicotine, only aspirin appears to be clearly associated with peptic ulceration in man. Even this association is based on epidemiological studies rather than direct assessment (Gillies and Skyring, 1969). Likewise an indirect role has been attributed to cigarette smoking and nicotine on the basis of an increased healing rate with cessation of smoking (Doll, 1964). While there are no good prospective studies to show that corticosteroids, phenylbutazone, or indomethacin are ulcerogenic in man, there are also no good trials to show they are not.

b. **Acute Mucosal Damage.** Studies need to be carried out as to whether the ulcerogenic drugs produce acute mucosal damage in man.

Again only for aspirin is the evidence clear cut (Ivey *et al.*, 1975a; Baskin *et al.*, 1976). In the case of aspirin, histological assessment shortly after aspirin intake proved the most accurate method of assessment. This showed cellular damage in all normal subjects given two aspirin tablets. All subjects also showed a drop in potential difference, showing an excellent correlation with morphological change with this drug. Direct morphological assessment appears more accurate than indirect assessment by blood loss studies (70% positive for aspirin; Matsumoto and Grossman, 1956; Grossman *et al.*, 1961; Croft and Wood, 1955) or endoscopic assessment by macroscopic changes (50% positive or less for aspirin; Thorsen *et al.*, 1968). Such morphological studies have not been carried out for corticosteroids, indomethacin, or phenylbutazone.

c. Acute Hemorrhagic Gastritis. Aspirin again is the only drug clearly associated with this life-threatening clinical entity in man (Valman *et al.*, 1968) though there is a strong clinical impression that alcohol is a factor in many cases. Why does aspirin, however, produce this entity in some few patients and not in the great majority of others? Why do these same patients who have bled severely from acute hemorrhagic gastritis after ulcers react in a normal manner to the drug after recovery (Parry and Wood, 1967)?

2. Pathogenetic Mechanisms

a. Gastric Mucosal Barrier. It is clearly not desirable to biopsy all subjects in order to assess drug-induced damage if an alternate method can be found. Changes in the gastric mucosal barrier appear to correlate well with aspirin-induced histological damage in man (Ivey *et al.*, 1975a; Baskin *et al.*, 1976). Changes in ionic permeability have only been carried out for aspirin (Ivey *et al.*, 1972a,b), prednisolone (Ivey *et al.*, 1975b), cigarette smoking and nicotine (Ivey *et al.*, 1973) in man. Of these only aspirin altered ionic permeability. Similarly, aspirin caused a fall in PD while prednisolone (Ivey *et al.*, 1975b), nicotine and cigarette smoking (Ivey *et al.*, 1973), phenylbutazone, and indomethacin did not (Murray *et al.*, 1974). Alcohol caused a fall in PD when given in high concentrations in man (Geall *et al.*, 1970). Its effect in lower concentrations on PD has not been studied, while no studies have been carried out on its effect on ionic permeability in man.

Because PD is easier to measure in man than ionic permeability, its use may have wider application. PD is however affected by factors other than mucosal damage. For example, highly acid (Ivey *et al.*, 1976) and neutral pH solutions will both raise PD in man (Ivey, K. J. unpublished studies).

294   Kevin J. Ivey

Further studies need to be done to assess all factors affecting PD in man in order to allow interpretation of changes in PD in relation to histological damage.

b. Mucus. George Milton Smith's 1914 observation that mucus protected gastric mucosa from bile and acid in the dog should be tested further in man.

c. Cell Renewal. It has been observed in both animals (Hingson and Ito, 1971) and man (Ivey *et al.*, 1975a; Baskin *et al.*, 1976) that histological recovery from aspirin-induced damage has largely taken place within an hour. Previously, it had been thought that this required days based on cell regeneration and migration times. This would not make sense, however, in an organ constantly exposed to possible irritants such as spices in foods, alcohol, extremes of temperature from hot coffee and tea to ices, as well as ulcerogenic drugs. Studies need to be made of the mechanism for immediate cell movement to replace those lost or damaged. Do the large cell-rich gastric pits act as storehouses for cellular replacement of surface damaged cells?

B. Treatment

1. *Antacids and Anticholinergics*

Further controlled studies need to be done to determine if these relatively expensive drugs do make any difference to either symptoms or healing of peptic ulcer disease. For example, few if any studies with anticholinergics have utilized endoscopy. Senator E. Kefauver's Drug Amendment Act of 1962 put the onus directly on the manufacturers to prove the efficacy of their drugs as well as safety.

2. *Prostaglandins*

The safety and efficacy of these drugs need to be shown in man. It needs to be shown whether they damage gastric mucosa in man, by physiological studies of ionic permeability and potential difference, and histological studies.

3. *Histamine H_2-Receptor Antagonists*

All studies to date indicate that these drugs are efficacious and safe. These agents do not damage gastric mucosa histologically (Ivey, K. J.) and cause a rise in PD (Ivey *et al.*, 1975c). Preliminary studies from Ebgland show these drugs significantly relieve symptoms of peptic ulcer and increase healing (Anonymous, 1975; Pounder *et al.*, 1975, 1976).

Further large scale double-blind cooperative studies are currently being held throughout the United States.

Long-term studies with cimetidine will need to be carried out to assess the effect of this drug on the recurrence rate of peptic ulcer. Will continued use of the drug be necessary during remissions? How will long-term therapy with H_2 blockers compare with surgery for gastric and/or duodenal ulcer, or even the Zollinger–Ellison syndrome? Will long-term studies show the drug to be completely free of side effects, particularly, bone marrow depression attributed to the thiourea side chain in the earlier derivative, metiamide? Will gastric secretion of intrinsic factor be inhibited along with acid secretion? What will be the long-term effect of achlorhydria on iron absorption and a variety of other physiological parameters, e.g., intestinal and pancreatic function? Will this drug prove equally efficacious in other forms of acid-peptic disease such as peptic esophagitis and postoperative gastritis?

These are exciting questions, but with rapid advances in our understanding of the pathophysiology of drug damage to gastric mucosa and the application of these principles to therapy, the answers lie just around the corner.

ACKNOWLEDGMENTS

This work was supported in part by the Medical Research Service of the Veterans Administration, and grants from Smith, Kline and French laboratories and the Clinical Research Center of the University of Missouri.

REFERENCES

Andersson, S., and Grossman, M. I. (1965). Profile of pH, pressure, and potential difference at gastroduodenal junction in man. *Gastroenterology* **49,** 364–371.

Anonymous. (1975). A multicentre trial. *Lancet* **2,** 779–781.

Aubrey, D. A., and Burns, G. P. (1972). Effect of acetic acid on antral phase of gastric secretion after prolonged systemic administration of prednisolone. *Am. J. Surg.* **124,** 325–330.

Baskin, W. N., Ivey, K. J., Krause, W. J., Jeffrey, G. E., and Gemmell, R. T. (1976). Aspirin-induced ultrastructural changes in human gastric mucosa. Correlation with potential difference. *Ann. Intern. Med.* 85:299–303.

Berstad, A., Peterson, H., and Myren, J. (1970). The effect of intraduodenal carbenoxolone sodium on gastric and duodenal secretion in man. In "Carbenoxolone Sodium" (J. H. Baron and F. M. Sullivan, eds.), pp. 69–73. Butterworth, London.

Bolton, J. P., and Cohen, M. M. (1976). Permeability effects of E_2 prostaglandins on canine gastric mucosa. Gastroenterology **70,** 865.

Bugajski, J., Hano, J., and Danek, L. (1976). Effect of metiamide, a histamine H_2-receptor antagonist, on the development of gastric stress ulcers and acid secretion. *Eur. J. Pharm.* **36,** 237–240.

Cano, R., Isenberg, J. I., and Grossman, M. I. (1976). Cimetidine inhibits caffeine-stimulated gastric acid secretion in man. *Gastroenterology* **70,** 1055–1057.

Chung, R., Field, M., and Silen, W. (1970). Gastric permeability to H$^+$; effects of prednisolone and acetylsalicylic acid on the coefficient of H$^+$ diffusion. Gastroenterology 58:1038.

Chvasta, T. E., and Cooke, A. R. (1972). The effect of several ulcerogenic drugs on the canine gastric mucosal barrier. *J. Lab. Clin. Med.* **79,** 302–315.

Cocking, J. B., and MacCraig, J. N. (1969). Effect of low dosage of carbenoxolone sodium on gastric ulcer healing and acid secretion. *Gut* **10,** 219–223.

Croft, D. N., and Wood, P. H. N. (1955). Gastric mucosa and susceptibility to occult gastrointestinal bleeding caused by aspirin. *Br. Med. J.* **1,** 137–141.

Davenport, H. W. (1964). Gastric mucosal injury by fatty and acetylsalicylic acids. *Gastroenterology* **46,** 245–253.

Davenport, H. W. (1965a). Damage to the gastric mucosa: Effects of salicylates and stimulation. *Gastroenterology* **49,** 189–196.

Davenport, H. W. (1965b). Potassium fluxes across the resting and stimulated gastric mucosa: Injury by salicylic and acetic acids. *Gastroenterology* **49,** 238–245.

Davenport, H. W. (1965c). Is the apparent hyposecretion of acid by patients with gastric ulcer a consequence of a broken barrier to diffusion of hydrogen ions into the gastric mucosa. *Gut* **6,** 513.

Davenport, H. W. (1967a). Ethanol damage to canine oxyntic glandular mucosa. *Proc. Soc. Exp. Biol. Med.* **126,** 657–662.

Davenport, H. W. (1967b). Salicylate damage to the gastric mucosal barrier. *N. Engl. J. Med.* **276,** 1307–1312.

Davenport, H. W. (1968). Destruction of the gastric mucosal barrier by detergents and urea. *Gastroenterology* **54,** 175–181.

Davenport, H. W. (1970a). Back diffusion of acid through the gastric mucosa and its physiological consequences. *Prog. Gastroenterol.* **2,** 42–56.

Davenport, H. W. (1970b). Effect of lysolecithin, digitonin, and phospholipase A upon the dog's gastric mucosal barrier. *Gastroenterology* **59,** 505–509.

Davenport, H. W. (1971). Protein-losing gastropathy produced by sulfhydryl reagents. *Gastroenterology* **60,** 870–879.

Davenport, H. W., Warner, H. A., and Code, C. F. (1964). Functional significance of gastric mucosal barrier to sodium. *Gastroenterology* **47,** 142–152.

Doll, R. (1964). Medical treatment of gastric ulcer. *Scott. Med. J.* **9,** 183–197.

Doll, R., Hill, I. D., Hutton, C., and Underwood, D. J. (1962). Clinical trial of a triterpenoid liquorice compound in gastric and duodenal ulcer. *Lancet* **2,** 793–795.

Durbin, R. P. (1967). Electrical potential difference of the gastric mucosa. *Handb. Physiol., Sect. 6: Aliment. Canal* Vol. 2, Chapter 49, pp. 879–888.

Fordtran, J. S., Morawski, S. G., and Richardson, C. T. (1973). In vivo and in vitro evaluation of liquid antacids. *N. Engl. J. Med.* **288,** 923–928.

Fromm, D., Silen, M., and Robertson, R. (1976). Histamine effects on H$^+$ permeability by isolated gastric mucosa. *Gastroenterology* **70,** 1076–1081.

Geall, M. G., Phillips, S. E., and Summerskill, W. H. (1970). The profile of gastric potential difference in man: Effects of aspirin, alcohol, bile and endogenous acid. *Gastroenterology* **58,** 437–443.

Gillies, M. A., and Skyring, A. P. (1969). Gastric and duodenal ulcer: The association between aspirin ingestion, smoking and family history of ulcer. *Med. J. Aust.* **1,** 280–284.

Gordon, M. J., O'Brien, P., Skillman, J. J., Silen, W. (1975). The effect of carbenoxolone on changes in canine and human gastric mucosa caused by taurocholate and ethanol. *Surgery* **77,** 707-714.

Grossman, M. I., Matsumoto, K. K., and Lichter, R. J. (1961). Fecal blood loss produced by oral and intravenous administration of various salicylates. *Gastroenterology* **40,** 383-388.

Heatley, N. G. (1959). Muco-substance as a barrier to diffusion. *Gastroenterology* **37,** 313-317.

Henn, R. M., Isenberg, J. I., Maxwell, V., and Sturdevant, R. A. L. (1975). Inhibition of gastric acid secretion by cimetidine in patient's with duodenal ulcer. *N. Engl. J. Med.* **293,** 371-375.

Hingson, D. J., and Ito, S. (1971). Effect of aspirin and related compounds on the fine structure of mouse gastric mucosa. *Gastroenterology* **61,** 156-177.

Hogben, C. A. M. (1955). Active transport of chloride by isolated frog gastric epithelium: Origin of the gastric mucosal potential. *Am. J. Physiol.* **180,** 641-649.

Ivey, K. J. (1971a). Gastric mucosal barrier. *Gastroenterology* **61,** 247-257.

Ivey, K. J. (1971b). Acute hemorrhagic gastritis–modern concepts based on pathogenesis. *Gut* **12,** 750-754.

Ivey, K. J. (1973). Gastric mucosal barrier—recent advances. *Acta Hepato-Gastroenterol.* **20,** 524-531.

Ivey, K. J. (1974a). Pathogenesis of peptic ulcer. *Aust. N.Z. J. Med.* **4,** 71-74.

Ivey, K. J. (1974b). Gastritis. *In* "Recent Advances in Gastrointestinal Physiology and Clinical Application," pp. 1289-1304. Med. Clin. North Am., Philadelphia, Pennsylvania.

Ivey, K. J. (1974c). Control of gastric acid secretion by histamine H_2-receptor antagonists; a pharmacological dream come true? *Aust. N.Z. J. Med.* **4,** 521-524.

Ivey, K. J. (1975). Anticholinergics. Do they work in peptic ulcer? *Gastroenterology* **68,** 154-166.

Ivey, K. J., and Clifton, J. A. (1971). Ionic movement across the gastric mucosa of man: Reproducibility and effect of intravenous atropine. *J. Lab. Clin. Med.* **78,** 753-764.

Ivey, K. J., and Gray, C. (1973a). Effect of carbenoxolone on ionic fluxes across normal gastric mucosa and that associated with gastric ulcer. *Aust. N.Z. J. Med.* **3,** 451-456.

Ivey, K. J., and Gray, C. (1973b). Effect of carbenoxolone on the gastric mucosal barrier in man after administration of taurocholic acid. *Gastroenterology* **64,** 1101-1105.

Ivey, K. J., Clifton, J. A., and DenBesten, L. (1970a). Effect of bile salts and atropine on ionic movement across human gastric mucosa. *Gut* **59,** 203-205.

Ivey, K. J., DenBesten, L., and Clifton, J. A. (1970b). Effect of bile salts on ionic movement across the human gastric mucosa. *Gastroenterology* **59,** 683-690.

Ivey, K. J., Morrison, S., and Gray, C. (1972a). Effects of salicylates on the gastric mucosal barrier in man. *J. Appl. Physiol.* **33,** 81-85.

Ivey, K. J., Morrison, S., and Gray, C. (1972b). Effect of intravenous salicylates on the gastric mucosal barrier in man. *Am. J. Dig. Dis.* **17,** 1055-1064.

Ivey, K. J., Parsons, C., and Trigg, T. (1973). Effect of cigarette smoking and nicotine on gastric ionic permeability in man. *Proc. Aust. Soc. Med. Res.* **3,** 144.

Ivey, K. J., Jeffrey, G. E., Krause, W., and Baskin, W. N. (1975a). Aspirin-induced ultrastructural changes in human gastric mucosa. Correlation with potential difference. *Clin. Res.* **23,** 519A.

Ivey, K. J., Parsons, C., and Weatherby, R. (1975b). Effect of prednisolone and salicylic acid on ionic fluxes across the human stomach. *Aust. N.Z. J. Med.* **5,** 408-412.

Ivey, K. J., Baskin, W. N., and Jeffrey, G. E. (1975c). Effect of cimetidine on gastric potential difference in man. *Lancet* **2,** 1072-1073.

Ivey, K. J., Krause, W., MacKercher, P., Baskin, W., and Jeffrey, G. E. (1976). Effect of acid on aspirin-induced ultrastructure and potential difference changes in human gastric mucosa. *Clin. Res.* **24**, 287A.

Konturek, S. J., Solomon, T. E., McCreight, W. G., Johnson, L. R., and Jacobsen, E. D. (1971). Effects of nicotine on gastrointestinal secretions. *Gastroenterology* **60**, 1098–1102.

Konturek, S. J., Biernat, J., and Oleksy, J. (1974). Effect of metiamide, a histamine H_2-receptor antagonist, on gastric response to histamine, pentagastrin, insulin, and peptone meal in man. *Am. J. Dig. Dis.* **19**, 609–616.

Leonards, J. R., and Levy, G. (1969). Reduction or prevention of aspirin-induced occult gastrointestinal blood loss in man. *Clin. Pharmacol. Ther.* **10**, 571–575.

Lipkin, M. (1970). Carbenoxolone sodium and the rate of extrusion of gastric epithelial cells. *In* "Carbenoxolone Sodium" (J. H. Baron and F. M. Sullivan, eds.), pp. 11–17. Butterworth, London.

Lipkin, M. (1971). In "defence" of the gastric mucosa. *Gut* **12**, 599–603.

Lynch, A., Shaw, H., and Milton, G. W. (1964). Effect of aspirin on gastric secretion. *Gut* **5**, 230–236.

McAlhany, J. C., Czaja, A. J., and Pruitt, B. A. (1976). Antacid control of acute gastroduodenal disease. *8th Annu. Meet. Am. Burn Assoc.* p. 15.

MacDonald, A. S., Steele, B. J., and Bottomley, M. G. (1976). Treatment of stress-induced upper gastrointestinal haemorrhage with metiamide. *Lancet* **1**, 68–70.

MacKercher, P. A., Ivey, K. J., Baskin, W. N., Krause, W., and Jeffrey, G. E. (1976). Effect of cimetidine on aspirin-induced human gastric mucosal damage. *Gastroenterology* **70**, 912.

Matsumoto, K. K., and Grossman, M. I. (1956). Quantitative measurement of gastrointestinal blood loss during ingestion of aspirin. *Proc. Soc. Exp. Biol. Med.* **102**, 119–128.

Max, M., and Menguy, R. (1970). Influence of adrenocorticotrophin, cortisone, aspirin and phenylbutazone on the rate of exfoliation and the rate of renewal of gastric mucosal cells. *Gastroenterology* **58**, 329–333.

Menguy, R. (1969). Gastric mucus and the gastric mucosal barrier. *Am. J. Surg.* **117**, 806–812.

Murray, H. S., Strottman, M. P., and Cooke, A. R. (1974). Effect of several drugs on gastric potential difference in man. *Br. Med. J.* **1**, 19–21.

Newman, A., de Moraes-Filho, J. P. P., Philippakos, D., and Misiewicz, J. J. (1975). The effect of intravenous infusions of prostaglandins E_2 and $F_{2\alpha}$ on human gastric function. *Gut* **16**, 272–276.

Overholt, B. F., Brodie, D. A., and Chase, B. J. (1969). Effect of the vagus nerve and salicylate administration on the permeability characteristics of the rat gastric mucosal barrier. *Gastroenterology* **56**, 651–658.

Parry, D. J., and Wood, P. H. N. (1967). Relationship between aspirin taking and gastroduodenal haemorrhage. *Gut* **8**, 301–305.

Peterson, W. L. (1977). Effect of an antacid regimen on the healing and pain of duodenal ulcer (DU). A cooperative study. *Gastroenterology* **72**, 1112.

Pounder, R. E., Williams, J. G., Milton-Thompson, G. J., and Misiewicz, J. J. (1975). Relief of duodenal ulcer symptoms by oral metiamide. *Br. Med. J.* **2**, 307–309.

Pounder, R. E., Hunt, R. H., Stekelman, M., Milton-Thompson, G. J., and Misiewicz, J. J. (1976). Healing of gastric ulcer during treatment with cimetidine. *Lancet* **1**, 337–339.

Read, N. W., and Grech, P. (1973). Effect of cigarette smoking on competence of the pylorus: Preliminary study. *Br. Med. J.* **3**, 313–316.

Richardson, C. T., and Walsh, J. H. (1976). The value of a histamine H_2-receptor antagonist in the management of patients with the Zollinger–Ellison syndrome. *N. Engl. J. Med.* **294**, 133–135.

Robert, A., Schultz, J. R., Nezamis, J. E., and Lancaster, C. (1976). Gastric antisecretory and anti-ulcer properties of PGE_2, 15-methyl PGE_2, and 16-16-dimethyl PGE_2. Intravenous, oral and intrajejunal administration. *Gastroenterology* **70**, 359–370.

Simons, M., and Moody, F. G. (1975). Carbenoxolone effects on gastric mucosal permeability and blood flow. *Gastroenterology* **68**, 957.

Smith, G. M. (1914). An experimental study of the relation of bile to ulceration of the mucous membrane of the stomach. *J. Med. Res.* **30**, 147–183.

Sturdevant, R. A. L., Isenberg, J. I., Secrist, D., and Ansfield, J. J. (1976). Controlled trials of antacid (AA) versus placebo (P) on duodenal ulcer (DU) pain. *Gastroenterology* **70**, A-83.

Teorell, T. (1933). Untersuchungen über die Magensaftsekretion. *Skand. Arch. Physiol.* **66**, 225–230.

Teorell, T. (1939). On the permeability of the stomach for acids and some other substances. *J. Gen. Physiol.* **23**, 263–274.

Thorsen, W. B., Western, D., Tanaka, Y., Morrissey, J. F. (1968). Aspirin injury to the gastric mucosa. *Arch. Intern. Med.* **121**, 499–506.

Valman, H. B., Parry, D. J., and Coghill, N. F. (1968). Lesions associated with gastroduodenal haemorrhage, in relation to aspirin intake. *Br. Med. J.* **4**, 661–663.

Section II

NUTRITIONAL EFFECTS ON DRUG METABOLISM AND ACTION

10

Nutrients in Drug Detoxication Reactions

R. T. WILLIAMS

I. INTRODUCTION

In this paper it is proposed to describe the metabolic reactions of drugs in the animal body and to indicate what nutrients are required so that these reactions can be carried out successfully. The details of the effects of specific nutrients are dealt with in succeeding papers in this symposium.

The Nutritive Requirement of the Body

Any text book of nutrition will give one the information that the nutrients required by the body are carbohydrates, fats, proteins, mineral salts, vitamins, and water. It is taken for granted that oxygen is also required. These substances are used to provide energy for the body and materials for growth in young animals, for regeneration of tissues in adults, and for the production of essential hormones and catalysts which are necessary for the proper functioning of the multitude of anabolic and catabolic reactions which make up the living organism. Since drug detoxication reactions are mainly enzymatic and the formation of metabolites require the participation of compounds provided by the body, it is reasonable to assume that all the accepted nutrients of the body are likely to be used in these reactions.

II. THE METABOLIC REACTIONS OF DRUGS

Drugs and other foreign compounds are usually metabolized in two phases whereby lipid-soluble compounds are converted into polar, water-soluble, excretory products. In the first phase the drug undergoes reactions which can be classified as oxidations, reductions and hydrolyses and during these reactions the drug acquires OH, COOH, NH_2, or SH groups which enable it to undergo the second phase consisting of synthetic reactions or conjugations. This concept can be summarized in reaction (1).

$$
\text{Drug} \quad \xrightarrow{\text{phase I}} \quad
\begin{array}{l}
\text{oxidation} \\
\text{reduction} \\
\text{hydrolysis} \\
\text{products}
\end{array}
\quad \xrightarrow{\text{phase II}} \quad
\begin{array}{l}
\text{synthetic} \\
\text{or} \\
\text{conjugation} \\
\text{products}
\end{array}
\qquad (1)
$$

Both phase I and II reactions are usually catalyzed by enzymes which are proteins. Therefore, proteins are required for the synthesis of these enzymes and therefore any nutritional state which reduces the availability of amino acids could be expected to reduce the amounts of drug metabolizing enzymes. This can occur when the calorie intake is low, that is, of carbohydrate, fat, and protein, since under these conditions protein will be catabolized and used as a source of energy reducing the availability of amino acids for enzyme synthesis.

III. NUTRIENTS REQUIRED IN PHASE I REACTIONS

A. Oxidative Reactions

There are many types of oxidative reactions and they include epoxidation, aromatic hydroxylation, aliphatic hydroxylation, oxidative dealkylation, N-oxidation, S-oxidation, P-oxidation, and replacement of S by O (see Williams and Millburn, 1975). They can be summarized in reactions (2)—(9b).

$$-HC{=}CH \longrightarrow -HC\overset{O}{\underset{\diagdown}{\diagup}}CH- \qquad (2)$$

$$ArH \longrightarrow ArOH \qquad (3)$$

$$RH \longrightarrow ROH \qquad (4)$$

$$ROR \longrightarrow ROH \qquad (5a)$$

$$RNHR \longrightarrow RNH_2 \qquad (5b)$$

$$RSR \longrightarrow RSH \qquad (5c)$$

$$RNH_2 \longrightarrow RNHOH \qquad (6a)$$

$$R_2NH \longrightarrow R_2NOH \qquad (6b)$$

$$R_3N \longrightarrow R_3NO \qquad (6c)$$

$$\diagup\hspace{-0.3em}S \longrightarrow \diagup\hspace{-0.3em}SO \longrightarrow \diagup\hspace{-0.3em}SO_2 \qquad (7)$$

$$\diagup\hspace{-0.3em}P \longrightarrow \diagup\hspace{-0.3em}PO \qquad (8)$$

$$\diagup\hspace{-0.3em}C{=}S \longrightarrow \diagup\hspace{-0.3em}C{=}O \qquad (9a)$$

$$\diagup\hspace{-0.3em}P{=}S \longrightarrow \diagup\hspace{-0.3em}P{=}O \qquad (9b)$$

Where Ar = aromatic ring, R = aliphatic group, and R is Ar or R.

Most of these reactions occur in the endoplasmic reticulum of the cells of various organs, especially the liver. The oxidizing system is a mixed-function oxidase system consisting of a membrane-bound multicomponent system, the constituents of which are NADPH-cytochrome c (or P-450) reductase, cytochrome P-450, and a lipid. These constituents function during oxidation of a substrate (RH) shown in Scheme 1 as proposed by Coon *et al.* (1975) where R OH is the oxidized substrate and C is an unidentified electron acceptor.

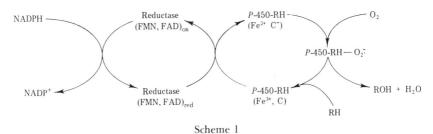

Scheme 1

The nutrients (see Table I) used in this system are nicotinamide for NADPH, riboflavine for FMN and FAD in NADPH-cytochrome P-450 reductase and glycine, pantothenic acid, iron and copper for the synthesis of the heme of cytochrome P-450. Ascorbic acid is also known to be necessary for cytochrome P-450 in certain species such as the guinea pig. Pantothenic acid is a component of acetyl-CoA which is used in the synthesis of δ-aminolevulinic acid (ALA) from glycine, and copper is necessary for the activity of ferrochelatase in converting protoporphyrin IX to heme (Wagner and Tephly, 1975). Proteins and amino acids are also needed for the apoenzymes of cytochrome P-450 and of NADPH-

TABLE I
Nutrients in Phase I Oxidation Reactions

Nutrients	Component of oxidizing system requiring nutrient
Nicotinic acid	NADPH
Riboflavin (vitamin B_2)	FMN and FAD in NADPH–cytochrome c reductase
Glycine	Heme (in Cyt-P-450)
Pantothenic acid	CoA (ALA synthesis)
Fe	Heme
Cu	Ferrochelatase in heme synthesis
Protein	Apo-enzymes
Ascorbic acid (vitamin C) in some species	?
Ca	Maintenance of
Zn	membranes
Mg	

cytochrome P-450 reductase. There is also evidence that the maintenance of the membranes on which the oxidizing system is bound needs
the presence of calcium, zinc, and magnesium.

Lipid also plays an important role in microsomal oxidation; phosphatidylcholine has been identified as an essential lipid (Strobel *et al.*,
1970).

B. Reductive Reactions

There are several reductive reactions of drugs in the body and they
include azo reduction, nitro reduction, the reduction of ketones, aldehydes, carbon— carbon double bonds, of pentavalent to trivalent arsenic, of disulfide bonds to sulfydryl groups and of sulfoxides and
N-oxides to the corresponding divalent sulfur compounds and tertiary
amines, respectively. These are summarized in (10)–(18)

$$-N{=}N- \longrightarrow -NH-NH- \longrightarrow -NH_2 \ + \ -NH_2 \qquad (10)$$

$$-NO_2 \longrightarrow -NO \longrightarrow -NHOH \longrightarrow -NH_2 \qquad (11)$$

$$R_2CO \longrightarrow R_2CHOH \qquad (12)$$

$$RCHO \longrightarrow RCH_2OH \qquad (13)$$

$$-HC{=}CH- \longrightarrow -H_2C-CH_2^- \qquad (14)$$

$$AsO{\cdot}OH \longrightarrow AsO \qquad (15)$$

$$RS-SR \longrightarrow 2\ RSH \qquad (16)$$

$$R_2SO \longrightarrow R_2S \qquad (17)$$

$$R_3NO \longrightarrow R_3N \qquad (18)$$

In azo reduction the enzyme appears to be NADPH-cytochrome c
reductase for which the nutrients nicotinic acid and riboflavin, apart
from protein, are needed. Azo reductase occurs in the cytosol and in the
microsomal fraction of liver cells. Nitro reductase activity also occurs in
the cytosol and microsomes. The enzymes involved require NADPH,
FMN, and FAD; one form of nitro reductase also requires cytochrome
P-450 (see reviews by Walker, 1970; Mitchard, 1971). The nutrient requirements for azo and nitro reduction are therefore much the same as
those required for microsomal oxidation.

The enzymes reducing ketones require NADH and NADPH and
therefore are dependent upon the nutrient, nicotinic acid. Little is

known of the enzymatic details of other reductions, but they no doubt depend upon nutrients similar to those of azo and nitro reduction.

C. Hydrolytic Reactions

The hydrolytic reactions which occur in the body include the hydrolysis of carboxylic esters, carbamates, amides, and phosphoric esters including thio esters, and the addition of water to epoxides. These reactions are catalyzed by a variety of enzymes which occur not only in the liver but also in other tissues. These enzymes vary widely from tissue to tissue and with species and strain. The reactions include those shown below where R and R' may be aryl or alkyl groups.

Carboxylic esters

$$RCOOHR' \rightarrow RCOOH + R'OH$$

Carbamates

$$RNHCOOR' \rightarrow RNHCOOH + R'OH$$

Amides

$$RCONHR' \rightarrow RCOOH + NH_2R'$$

Phosphoric esters

$$e.g., (RO)_2POOR \rightarrow (RO)_2POOH + ROH$$

Epoxides

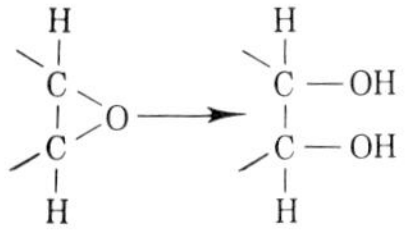

Apart from proteins for enzyme synthesis, and mineral salts which may be needed for enzyme activity, it is not clear what nutrients are used in these reactions.

It should be mentioned that organophosphoric triesters can be de-esterified by three mechanisms, hydrolysis as shown in the reaction for phosphoric esters above, which is probably the most common. The other two reactions are not hydrolyses, one being an oxidative de-arylation and is microsomal and may therefore require the NADPH–P-450 system, and the other, glutathione transferase-catalyzed. These reactions may occur during the metabolism of parathion (Hutson, 1975), shown in (19) and (20) below.

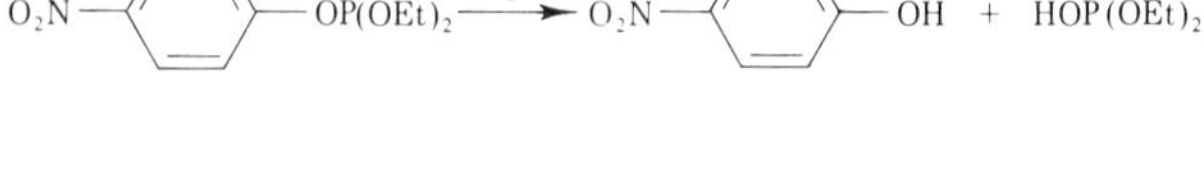

(19)

$$O_2N-\langle\ \rangle-\overset{\overset{S}{\|}}{OP(OEt)_2} \ + \ GSH \longrightarrow O_2N-\langle\ \rangle-SG \ + \ HO\overset{\overset{S}{\|}}{P}(OEt)_2$$

(20)

IV. NUTRIENTS IN PHASE II REACTIONS OR CONJUGATIONS

Foreign compounds containing suitable chemical groups such as OH, NH_2, COOH and SH, phase I metabolites of drugs, and many natural metabolites of the body can undergo synthetic reactions called conjugations and, usually, as a result of these syntheses, such compounds are detoxicated and their biological activity diminished or abolished. Conjugation means the union or coupling of two substances in the body and in this context the two substances are the drug or its phase I metabolite and a compound provided by the body, the conjugating agent. This agent is derived ultimately from the nutrients supplied to the body.

In man, there are eight major conjugation reactions (see Table II) involving the provision by the body, as conjugating agents, glucuronic acid from its carbohydrate resources, glycine, cysteine, glutamine, glutathione, and methionine from its amino acid resources, sulfate and sulfur also from amino acid resources, and acetyl radicals from any source, fat, carbohydrate or protein, that will supply them via acetyl-CoA.

In addition to the above conjugations, there are others which may occur in man to a minor extent and some which occur specifically in certain species. Thus in certain birds and reptiles ornithine is a conjugating agent whereas in insects glucose is used instead of glucuronic acid. These minor and sometimes rare conjugations (Williams and Millburn, 1975) may utilize taurine, serine, arginine, certain peptides, glucose, glucosamine, ribose, formate and succinate, all of which are supplied

TABLE II
Major Conjugations in Man

Glucuronic acid conjugation
Glycine conjugation or hippuric acid synthesis
Glutamine conjugation
Mercapturic acid synthesis (glutathione conjugation)
Methylation
Acetylation
Sulfate conjugation
Thiocyanate synthesis

from the organism's sources of carbohydrates, fats, proteins, or minerals.

V.   GENERAL MECHANISM OF CONJUGATION AND NUTRIENTS REQUIRED

Conjugations are synthetic reactions and need a source of energy for their accomplishment. This energy is supplied through ATP which is formed from the energy yielding nutrients of the body.

Conjugations are characterized by the formation of an active intermediate which in most cases is a nucleotide. A transferring enzyme is also necessary to catalyze the reaction between the activated intermediate and the conjugating agent or drug. There are two kinds of conjugation reactions depending upon whether the conjugating agent (Type A) or the drug (Type B) is activated as shown below:

Type A

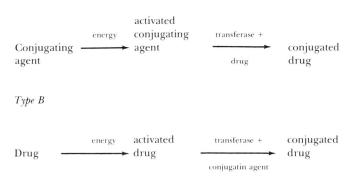

Of the eight reactions given in Table II, the glucuronic acid and sulfate conjugations, methylation, acetylation, and thiocyanate synthesis are Type A, whereas glycine and glutamine conjugations and mercapturic acid synthesis are Type B. The active intermediates are nucleotides in the cases of the glucuronic acid, sulfate, glycine, and glutamine conjugations and methylation and acetylation, whereas they are reactive simple inorganic or organic compounds in the cases of the thiocyanate and mercapturic acid syntheses, as shown in Table III.

The role of nutrients in Phase II reactions is summarized in Table IV and the place of each nutrient in these reactions can be located by exam-

TABLE III
Mechanism of Conjugation

Conjugating agent	Activated conjugating agent	Transferase
Type A		
Glucuronic acid	Uridine diphosphate glucuronic acid (UDPGA)	Glucuronyltransferase
Sulfate	Phosphoadenosine phosphosulfate (PAPS)	Sulfotransferase
Methyl group	S-Adenosylmethionine	Transmethylase
Acetyl group	Acetyl-CoA	Transacetylase
Sulfur	Thiosulfate [$H_2S(S)O_3$]	Thiosulfate sulfurtransferase

Drug	Activated drug	Conjugating agent
Type B		
Aromatic acid (Ar COOH)	Aroyl-CoA	Glycine
Arylacetic acid (ArCH$_2$COOH)	Arylacetyl-CoA	Glutamine
Aromatic ring	Epoxide	Glutathione

ining the mechanism of each reaction (Williams, 1967) in the order given in Table II.

A. Glucuronic Acid Conjugation

The steps in glucuronide formation are shown in Scheme 2.

Precursors in food → glycogen → glucose 1-phosphate

$\xrightarrow{\text{uridine triphosphate}}$ uridine diphosphate glucose $\xrightarrow[\text{dehydrogenase}]{\text{DPN}^+}$ UDP-glucuronic acid $\xrightarrow[\text{transferase}]{\text{drug + glucuronyl}}$ β-glucuronide + uridine diphosphate.

Scheme 2

As suggested in Table IV, nicotinic acid and carbohydrate are needed for the production of UDPGA.

B. Glycine Conjugation

Glycine conjugation occurs according to the following steps shown in Scheme 3.

TABLE IV
Nutrients Utilized in Phase II Reactions

Nutrient	Use	Phase II reaction
Carbohydrates		
Glucose	Synthesis of UDPGA, N-acetylglucosamine, ribose, glucose	Glucuronide synthesis Rare conjugations
Proteins and derivatives		
Glycine	Conjugating agent	Hippuric acid synthesis
Glutamine	Conjugating agent	Glutamine conjugation (man and monkeys)
Glutathione	Conjugating agent	Mercapturic acid synthesis
Cysteine and cystine	Source of S for thiosulfate and sulfate; source of taurine	Cyanide detoxication; sulfate conjugation; taurine conjugation
Methionine	Synthesis of adenosylmethionine	Methylation
Ornithine	Conjugating agent	Ornithuric acid synthesis (birds and reptiles)

Taurine Serine Aspartic acid Arginine Alanine Glutamic acid Certain peptides	Rare conjugating agents	Conjugations found occasionally in certain species with specific compounds
Tryptophan	Source of formylkynurenine	Formylation (a rare reaction)
Fats		
Acetyl (can also be derived from carbohydrate and protein)	Synthesis of acetyl-CoA	Acetylation
Vitamins		
Pantothenic acid	Synthesis of CoA	Hippuric acid synthesis, glutamine conjugation; acetylation.
Lipoic acid	Synthesis of aroyl-CoA and arylacetyl CoA	Hippuric acid synthesis; glutamine conjugation
Folic acid	Synthesis of 5-methyl-tetrahydrofolic acid Methyl-B_{12}?	Certain methylations, e.g. of dopamine Certain methylations, e.g. of Hg?
Vitamin B_{12}	Hydroxocobalamin	Cyanide detoxication
Nicotinic acid	For DPN needed for many enzymes, e.g., synthesis of UDPGA	Glucuronide synthesis

Aromatic acid + ATP → aroyladenylate + pyrophosphate

Aroyladenylate + CoA-SH → aroyl-CoA + adenylic acid

Aroyl-CoA + glycine $\xrightarrow[N\text{-acylase}]{\text{glycine}}$ aroylglycine + CoA-SH

Scheme 3

These reactions require at least three nutrients: the vitamins, lipoic acid for the activation of the aromatic acid catalyzed by octanoic thiokinase, and pantothenic acid for the synthesis of CoA, and then the amino acid glycine as the conjugating agent which is derived from protein. The rate at which glycine is produced in the body from protein is limited and varies from species to species.

C. Glutamine Conjugation

The mechanism of this conjugation is believed to be similar to that of glycine conjugation and one simply has to replace "aromatic acid" by "arylacetic acid" and "aroyl" by "arylacetyl" in the above reactions of glycine conjugation. The two mechanisms probably differ in the enzyme involved in the last step shown in reaction (21).

$$\text{Arylacetyl-CoA + glutamine} \rightarrow \text{arylacetylglutamine + CoA-SH} \quad (21)$$

This enzyme is species-specific, occurring only in man and probably monkeys. The nutrient requirement of this conjugation is similar to glycine conjugation except that glutamine is needed instead of glycine.

D. Mercapturic Acid Synthesis

The synthesis of mercapturic acids occurs with a large variety of foreign compounds and the initial step consists of the combination of the compound (XH) or an active metabolite of it such as an epoxide, with glutathione catalyzed by one of the numerous glutathione S-transferases. This is illustrated in Scheme 4.

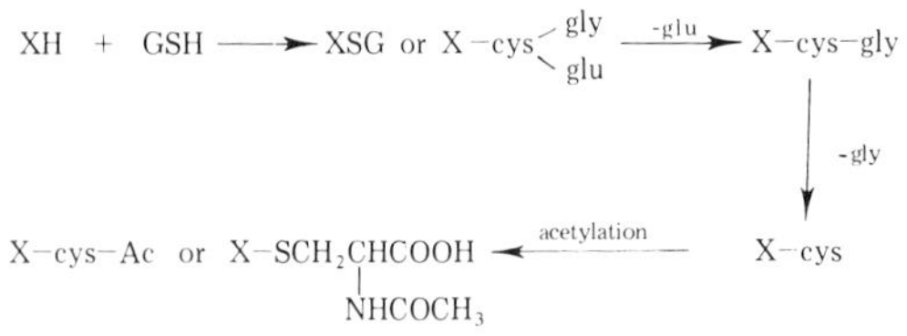

$$\text{XH + GSH} \longrightarrow \text{XSG or X}-\text{cys} \begin{matrix} \text{gly} \\ \text{glu} \end{matrix} \xrightarrow{\text{-glu}} \text{X}-\text{cys}-\text{gly}$$

$$\downarrow \text{-gly}$$

$$\text{X}-\text{cys}-\text{Ac or X}-\text{SCH}_2\text{CHCOOH} \xleftarrow{\text{acetylation}} \text{X}-\text{cys}$$
$$\qquad\qquad\qquad\qquad\quad |$$
$$\qquad\qquad\qquad\quad \text{NHCOCH}_3$$

Scheme 4

The nutrients required in this conjugation are glutathione (γ-L-glutamyl-L-cysteinylglycine) and pantothenic acid as a component of acetyl-CoA which is involved in the final step of acetylation.

E. Methylation

There are numerous forms of methylation which include (1) the methylation of nitrogen in primary, secondary, and tertiary amines and of secondary and tertiary nitrogen in N-heterocycles, (2) the methylation of oxygen in OH groups particularly in catechols and (3) the methylation of sulfur in certain compounds containing SH groups.

The mechanism is relatively simple and follows in Scheme 5, where X = N, O or S.

$$\text{ATP + methionine} \rightarrow S\text{-adenosylmethionine} + P_i + Pp_i$$

$$S\text{-Adenosylmethionine + RXH} \xrightarrow{\text{methyltransferase}} \text{RXMe} + S\text{-adenosylhomocysteine}$$

Scheme 5

There are several methyltransferases and specificity in methylation depends on the nature of the enzyme. The main nutrient involved in methylation is the essential amino acid methionine from which the methyl group is derived.

F. Acetylation

Acetylation is mainly a reaction of drugs which contain amino groups and include aliphatic and aromatic amines, hydrazines and hydrazides, amino acids and the sulphonamide group ($-SO_2NH_2$). The mechanism of acetylation is relatively straightforward as is shown in reactions (22) and (23).

$$\text{CH}_3\text{CO-Don + CoA-SH} \rightarrow \text{H-Don + CoA-S—COCH}_3 \qquad (22)$$

$$\text{CoA-S-COCH}_3 + \text{H-Acc} \xrightarrow{\text{transacetylase}} \text{CoA-SH + CH}_3\text{CO-Acc} \qquad (23)$$

where $\text{CH}_3\text{CO-Don}$ is the acetyl donor and H-Acc the acetyl acceptor. From the point of view of nutrients, the acetyl donor source may be fat, carbohydrate or protein. The other nutrient needed is pantothenic acid for the provision of CoA. Protein is also needed for the enzymes, the transacetylases, of which there are several.

G. Sulfate Conjugation

The conjugating agent used in this process is inorganic sulfate and the conjugation is mainly with phenolic OH groups. Aliphatic OH groups and aromatic NH_2 groups can also conjugate with sulfate but usually these are minor processes. However, inorganic sulfate is not utilized directly but in the form of the nucleotide, 3'-phosphoadenosine 5'-phosphosulfate (PAPS), which is synthesized from inorganic sulfate and ATP shown in reactions (24)–(26).

$$\text{ATP} + \text{SO}^{2-}_4 \rightarrow \text{Adenosine 5'-phosphosulfate (APS)} + \text{PP}_i \qquad (24)$$

$$\text{APS} + \text{ATP} \rightarrow \text{PAPS} + \text{ADP} + \text{H}^+ \qquad (25)$$

$$\text{PAPS} + \text{ROH} \rightarrow \text{ROSO}^-_3 + \text{3'-phosphoadenosine 5'-phosphate(PAP)} \quad (26)$$

Apart from the nucleotides, the body has to provide sulfate which is apparently limited in supply. In the body much of this sulfate is derived from sulfur-containing amino acids although exogenous inorganic sulfate can also be utilized. The nutrients utilized in sulfate conjugation are therefore cysteine, cystine, and probably methionine.

H. Thiocyanate Synthesis

This reaction is specific for the cyanide ion. The reaction is a simple one catalyzed by the widely distributed enzyme, thiosulfate sulfurtransferase, which transfers the labile sulfur in thiosulfate to the cyanide ion [see reaction (27)].

$$\text{CN}^- + \text{S}{=}\text{SO}^{2-}_3 \xrightarrow{\text{transferase}} \text{SCN}^- + \text{SO}^{2-}_3 \qquad (27)$$

For this reaction the body has to provide, apart from protein for the enzyme, the thiosulfate. This is apparently derived from cystine or cysteine, two molecules of cysteine being required to make one of thiosulfate.

VI. CONCLUSION

It is thus clear that all the reactions of drug metabolism are dependent upon the nutrient supply of the body. Some of these nutrients such as amino acids and vitamins are in short supply and detoxication reactions depending upon amino acids are of limited capacity. Nutrients such as carbohydrates are normally in good supply and this may be the reason why, under normal circumstances, the glucuronic acid conjugation mechanism is so versatile and widespread.

The mention of the glucuronic acid mechanism, however, recalls the case of the cat which has a defect in this mechanism. This defect is not a lack of the conjugating agent, glucuronic acid, or of the nucleotide, uridine diphosphate glucuronic acid (UDPGA), but of the right form of the enzyme transferring glucuronic acid from UDPGA to certain foreign compounds. Benzoic acid and phenol are more toxic to the cat than to many other species. The poisoning of cats by benzoate present in meat given as food has been reported by Bedford and Clarke (1971, 1972). Benzoic acid is detoxicated in several species by conjugation with glycine which is limited in supply and when the glycine is exhausted conjugation with glucuronic acid takes place. In the cat, however, conjugation of benzoic acid with glucuronic acid does not occur (Bridges *et al.*, 1970) and poisoning ensues when the dose of benzoic acid exceeds that which can be detoxicated by the available glycine. In the case of phenol, detoxication occurs by conjugation with sulfate for small doses and with glucuronic acid for large doses (Capel *et al.*, 1972). In the cat, glucuronic acid conjugation of phenol does not occur and therefore only the sulfate conjugation, which is of limited capacity, is available for detoxication. Glucuronic acid conjugation of certain compounds, however, does occur in the cat, since diphenylacetic acid and hydratropic acid are highly conjugated with glucuronic acid in this animal (J. C. Caldwell, P. A. F. Dixon, and R. L. Smith, unpublished data).

REFERENCES

Bedford, P. G. C., and Clarke, E. G. C. (1971). Suspected benzoic acid poisoning in the cat. *Vet. Rec.* **88,** 599–601.
Bedford, P. G. C., and Clarke, E. G. C. (1972). Experimental benzoic acid poisoning in the cat. *Vet. Rec.* **90,** 53–58.
Bridges, J. W., French, M. R., Smith, R. L., and Williams, R. T. (1970). The fate of benzoic acid in various species. *Biochem. J.* **118,** 47–51.
Capel, I. D., French, M. R., Millburn, P., Smith, R. L., and Williams, R. T. (1972). The fate of (^{14}C)phenol in various species. *Xenobiotica* **2,** 25–34.
Coon. M. J., van der Hoeven, T. A., Haugen, D. A., Guengerich, F. P., Vermilion, J. L., and Ballou, D. P. (1975). Biochemical characterization of highly purified cytochrome P-450 and other components of the mixed function oxidase system of liver microsomal membranes. *In* "Cytochromes P-450 and b$_5$" (D. Y. Cooper *et al.*, eds.), pp. 25–46. Plenum, New York.
Hutson, D. H. (1975). *In* "Foreign Compound Metabolism in Mammals," Vol. 3, p. 526. Chem. Soc. London.
Mitchard, M. (1971). Bioreduction of organic nitrogen. *Xenobiotica* **1,** 469–481.
Strobel, H. W., Lu, A. Y. H., Heidema, J., and Coon, M. J. (1970). Phosphatidylcholine requirement in the enzymatic reduction of hemoprotein P-450 and in fatty acid, hydrocarbon, and drug hydroxylation. *J. Biol. Chem.* **245,** 4851.

Wagner, G. S., and Tephly, T. R. (1975). A possible role of copper in the regulation of heme biosynthesis through ferrochelatase. In "Cytochromes P-450 and b$_5$" (D. Y. Cooper et al, eds), pp. 343–354. Plenum, New York.

Walker, R. (1970). The metabolism of azo compounds: A review of the literature. Food Cosmet. Toxicol. **8,** 659–676.

Williams, R. T. (1967). Biogenesis of conjugation and detoxication products. In "Biogenesis of Natural Compounds" (P. Bernfeld, ed.), 2nd ed., pp. 589–639. Pergamon, Oxford.

Williams, R. T., and Millburn, P. (1975). Detoxication mechanisms. In "Physiological and Pharmacological Biochemistry" (H. F. K. Blaschko, ed.), pp. 211–266. Butterworth, London.

11

Diet–Drug Interactions and Incompatibilities

DAPHNE A. ROE

I. INTRODUCTION

In any consideration of the incompatibilities of drugs and food, we should remember that this is a subject which has been known to the medical profession since the time when drugs were first used, and before the era of rational therapy. Ancient writers were much preoccupied with the need to give instructions about when a medicine should be administered in relation to food. Pharmacology in ancient Babylonia and Assyria was based on the theory that disease is due to the entry of a demon into the patient's body, and this being the belief, nauseous drugs were given before food, in order to make the demon come out (Kocher, 1952–1953; Levey, 1961; Mettler, 1947).

319

Traditional directions for drug usage have included the term ante cibus (a.c.) and post cibus (p.c.), and these terms may denote some innate understanding that a state of fasting or feasting could promote or diminish the pharmacological function of particular drugs or drug mixtures. It has been generally accepted that if a drug is to be rapidly absorbed it should be given on an empty stomach. This would infer that food under these circumstances is incompatible with the optimal functioning of that particular medicinal agent (Adams, 1844).

Utilization of food substances or beverages as antidotes to drug poisoning has been a common practice for many years. Emesis has been induced by mustard and water or by concentrated salt solutions, raw eggs, boiled starch or flour, and milk. These so-called demulcents were considered to diminish toxic drug absorption as was hot strong tea which was frequently given to precipitate apomorphine, cinchona alkaloids, strychnine, veratrine, digitalis, antipyrine, colchicine, as well as heavy metals (Boyd, 1958).

Adverse effects of drugs on the body's ability to absorb nutrients have only been described in the past 50 years. The first studies of drug-induced malabsorption, arising from the presence of the drug in the gastrointestinal tract, are of effects of mineral oil on the uptake of fat soluble vitamins and carotene.

II. INFLUENCE OF FOOD AND OTHER DIETARY CONSTITUENTS ON DRUG ABSORPTION (TABLE I)

Koch-Weser (1974) has suggested that effects of food on drug absorption may involve the water and lipid solubility of the drug, the nature and temperature of the food, formation of drug–food precipitates, as well as the effect of food on the gastrointestinal pH, motility, and blood flow.

Gastric absorption of any drug, but particularly acidic drugs, is reduced after food. Intake of food decreases blood levels of concomitantly administered aspirin derivatives (Wood, 1967). It has long been known that alcohol is better tolerated when taken with food, and it is generally agreed that this is due to the delaying effect of food in the stomach on gastric emptying and the absorption of alcohol. Protein, carbohydrate, and fat have each separately been shown to have a retarding effect on acute alcohol intoxication, though a mixed meal is considered to be most efficient (Tuovenin, 1930; Goldberg, 1943; Elbel and Schleyer, 1956; Kalant, 1971). Mellanby (1919) first demonstrated the influence of milk in reducing the effects of alcohol, and this has since been confirmed by

TABLE I
Influence of Food on Drug Absorption

Drug	Intake status promoting absorption	
	Fasting	Fed
Ethanol	↑	
Aspirin	↑	
Barbiturates		
Penicillins (other than ampicillin)	↑	
Tetracycline	↑	Milk and milk products only ↓
Demethylchlortetracycline	↑	Milk and milk products only ↓
Nitrofurantoin (macrocrystalline)		↑
Griseofulvin		↑ Fat
Theophylline	↑	
Propantheline bromide	↑	

Miller *et al.* (1966). The effectiveness of food in reducing alcohol absorption varies inversely with the time between the meal and the intake of the alcoholic beverages (Herbich and Prokop, 1963). Mildly acidic drugs, including aspirin and the barbiturates, become more ionized and less well absorbed as the pH of the medium increases. Hence they are absorbed better from the stomach than from the small intestine (Albert, 1967). In the postprandial state, acute barbiturate poisoning may be delayed because of a buffering effect of food components, including protein, on stomach acidity.

The intestinal absorption of many drugs is slowed by concurrent food intake, either because of delayed gastric emptying or because of dilution of the drug in the intestinal contents.

Very many studies have been carried out on the effect of food on the absorption of antibiotics. If food is taken one-half to one hour before crystalline penicillin K, benzyl penicillin G, oxacillin or 2-biphenylylpenicillin, a decline is noted in the blood levels of these antibiotics (Heatley, 1956; Klein *et al.*, 1963; Sabath *et al.*, 1963). Absorption of ampicillin, as indicated by serum levels after oral doses, is only slightly affected by food intake (Klein and Finland, 1963). Food has been shown to significantly decrease and delay the absorption of lincomycin. It should be noted that only low levels of this antibiotic are attained in the serum after oral doses, due either to excretion into the bile or from the intestinal mucosa, with the effect of significant fecal loss. Parenteral drug administration has been advocated in order to avoid inefficient uptake of this drug, both because of the food factor and the intestinal loss (McCall *et al.,* 1967).

Calcium, magnesium, aluminum, and iron salts can interfere with the absorption of tetracycline (Kunin and Finland, 1961; Prescott, 1969). Neuvonen *et al.* (1970) showed that when organic iron was given with tetracyclines, lower blood levels of these antibiotics resulted. In their studies subjects received a therapeutic dose of a tetracycline drug alone, or that same tetracycline with 40 mg iron. When this dosage of iron was given with the antibiotics, it resulted in lower blood levels of tetracycline, oxytetracycline, methacycline, and doxycycline. Reduction in the blood levels of these antibiotics varied from 50% in the case of tetracycline, to 90% in the case of doxycycline. Greenberger (1973), in reviewing this investigation, suggests that it might be a good idea to withdraw supplemental iron preparations when people are receiving oral tetracyclines. Data, however, hardly justify the withholding of iron when it is needed, but rather that it be given at times of the day when tetracycline is not being administered. The iron–tetracycline incompatibility has considerable practical importance because of the prevalent practice of giving iron to young women to prevent or treat iron deficiency, and also to give them tetracyclines to control acne. A number of studies have indicated that ingestion of milk or milk products at the same time as therapeutic doses of tetracycline reduces the absorption of the drug as well as its clinical efficiency. In a study by Scheiner and Oltemeier (1962), ingestion of whole milk, as well as buttermilk or cottage cheese, induced a significant decrease in the blood levels of orally administered demethylchlortetracycline (Declomycin). These authors found that if there were no milk or milk products included in the meal, then there was no lowering effect of food on serum antibiotic concentrations. The suggestion was made that the effect of the milk products might be because of a chelation of the demethylchlortetracycline by calcium caseinate (Krondl, 1970). Antacids containing divalent or trivalent cations such as calcium, magnesium, and aluminum impair the absorption of tetracyclines when these are orally administered. Whereas this has been attributed to chelation of the cation by the tetracycline, it is possible that, as with sodium bicarbonate, there is also an inhibiting effect on the dissolution of the tetracycline in gastric fluid by these antacids (Barr *et al.,* 1971; Hansten, 1973; Shils, 1962).

Absorption of certain other antibacterial agents may be delayed or impaired by concomitant intake of food or specific nutrients. Simultaneous ingestion of food with certain sulfa drugs including sulfadimethoxine, sulfamethoxypyridazine, and sulfisoxazole reduces the absorption of these drugs (MacDonald *et al.*, 1967). Sulfasalazine, formerly known as salicylazosulfapyridine, is cleaved by colonic bacteria yielding 5-aminosalicylate and sulfapyridine. The sulfapyridine is absorbed and the 5-aminosalicylate remains in the colon and is excreted in the feces. The amounts of the active metabolites of the drug depend on the characteristics of the intestinal flora, and these in turn may be altered by variation in the diet. It has been suggested that alterations in intestinal transit time might alter the distribution of this drug and its metabolites. In view of the current interest in increasing the intake of dietary fiber, one wonders whether this might have an effect on the metabolism of sulfasalazine. If iron salts, such as ferrous sulfate, are given at the same time as sulfasalazine, decreased drug levels result. It is unclear whether variation in iron intake alters the blood levels of this drug. However, since this is the drug of choice in ulcerative colitis and granulomatous colitis, in which iron deficiency anemia is common, it is important to understand this particular drug nutrient incompatibility (Das and Eastwood, 1973; Goldman and Peppercorn, 1975; Peppercorn and Goldman, 1972).

Under certain conditions and with specific drugs, food or food components can enhance drug absorption. The broad-spectrum antibacterial agent, nitrofurantoin, is used in the treatment of urinary infections. Several studies have shown that the dissolution rate, absorption, and bioavailability of this drug are dependent upon its particulate size (Conklin and Hailey, 1969; Paul *et al.*, 1967; Stoll *et al.*, 1973). Two commercial forms of this drug are available, a macrocrystalline form in a capsule and a tablet form containing the drug in a microcrystalline formulation. It has been suggested by the manufacturers that both forms be taken with food in order to minimize side effects which include nausea and vomiting. Bates *et al.* (1974) studied the effect of food on the absorption and excretion of both of these products of nitrofurantoin. When the drug was taken immediately following a breakfast of cornflakes, buttered toast, and milk, the maximum excretion rate of the drug, after administration of the macrocrystalline form, was increased, as against the urinary excretion of the same product when taken with the subject in the fasting state. However, this effect was not obtained when the microcrystalline form of the drug was administered; that is, with this product there was no difference in maximal excretion rate between fasting and fed subjects. There was no difference in the excretion of the two forms of the drug when either was given to subjects who had had the standard breakfast. It has been reported that, in the fasting state, less nitrofurantoin is absorbed. Whereas food appears to increase the bioavailability of the drug as reported in these studies of Bates *et al.*, only four subjects were studied by the investigators, and it would appear that further investigations are necessary. More particularly, it would be important to know whether the effects of food on the excretion of this drug into the urine are similar in normal subjects and in patients with urinary infections. It has been suggested, but not confirmed, that the increases in the bioavailability of nitrofurantoin induced by food may be due to an increased gastric emptying time so that the drug may be more efficiently dissolved in gastric fluids before its passage into the duodenum, where absorption of the drug is most efficient (Conklin, 1972). More information is needed on the particular kinds of food which affect nitrofurantoin absorption and utilization as an antibacterial agent in the urine.

Crouse (1961) found that ingestion of a high fat meal enhanced the absorption of the systemic antifungal agent, griseofulvin. It was previously thought that higher serum levels of griseofulvin following administration of a meal high in fats could be due either to increased absorption of the drug or perhaps to a decreased rate of clearance of the drug from a lipemic serum. However, when an intravenous fat emulsion (Lipomul) was used, it had no effect on griseofulvin levels in the blood.

In studies by Kabasakalian *et al.* (1970) the urinary excretion of 6-demethylgriseofulvin was used as an index of griseofulvin absorption in a single human subject. Effects of the time of drug administration, fat intake, dietary modification, dose level, and particle size of the drug on metabolite excretion were followed. Absorption was lowest in the morning following an overnight fast. Absorption was at a maximum when the drug was administered at noon. A high fat breakfast enhanced drug absorption, but this effect was not elicited when a high fat supper was given. Addition of fried foods and nuts to the diet also increased drug absorption.

The percentage of the drug absorbed was independent of dose level, but microsize griseofulvin products were better absorbed than large particle size products. The effect of time of administration on griseofulvin absorption appears to be real in that the same pattern was followed when the drug was given a month after the initial experiment. It is suggested by the authors that perhaps there is a circadian rhythm either of intestinal motility or biliary excretion which affects griseofulvin absorption. In a wider context, it is clear from these studies that the influence of food and dietary pattern on drug absorption is complex and that there may be interaction from other gastrointestinal variables.

In my own rather extensive experience of therapeutic use of the microcrystalline form of griseofulvin, I have found that a single 250-mg tablet or capsule of this drug, given to anyone with cholecystitis or cholelithiasis will evoke acute gall bladder pain, this effect being magnified by concomitant intake of a fatty meal. Indeed, this abdominal pain, evoked by griseofulvin, can be used as a diagnostic test for gall bladder disease (D. A. Roe, unpublished). It would be interesting to know whether griseofulvin stimulates cholecystokinin release, thus causing contraction of the gall bladder.

The lowering effect of food on the bioavailability of certain other drugs may seriously reduce therapeutic efficacy when the drug is given by the oral route. It is well known that the absorption of the drug, theophylline, commonly used in the management of asthma, is markedly reduced by food (Piafsky and Ogilvie, 1975). In studies conducted by Welling *et al.* (1975), it was found that the absorption of theophylline was faster when it was given after a high protein meal rather than a high fat or high carbohydrate meal. Peak levels of theophylline in these studies were highest when the solid form of the drug was given, dissolved in 500 ml of water and taken fasting.

Propantheline bromide (Pro-banthine) is mainly used as an anticholinergic, antispasmodic in the treatment of peptic ulceration. It is also used to diminish sweat secretion and pharmacologically has inhibitory effects upon exocrine function. Studies by Gibaldi and Grundhoffer (1975) showed that, using salivary flow rate as an index of anticholinergic response, diminution in salivary flow rate was greater when propantheline was given to subjects in the fasting condition than when the same dose was given after a standard breakfast. Whereas this finding might be interpreted to mean that a side effect of propantheline therapy, namely dryness of the mouth, might be diminished by eating, nevertheless it also implies that the desired therapeutic effect of the drug, that is, diminished gastric secretion, may also be lessened by food intake, and that therefore it is preferable that the drug be taken between meal times.

III. VITAMIN INTAKES AND DRUG RESPONSES (TABLE II)

Information is available showing that intake of specific vitamins, above that normally occurring in the diet, can lower blood levels of drugs with which these nutrients interact. Under these circumstances, desired therapeutic effects may not be obtained.

It has been shown that folic acid decreases blood levels of diphenylhydantoin and phenobarbital, and that fit frequency and severity in drug-treated epileptics may be increased by therapeutic doses of this vitamin

TABLE II
Effects of High Vitamin Intake on Blood Levels of Drugs and Drug Responses

		Effects	
Drug	Interacting vitamin	Blood level of drug	Clinical change or response
Diphenylhydantoin (DPH)	Folic acid	↓	Fit frequency
Phenobarbital (PB)			and severity ↑
DPH	Pyridoxine	↓	
PB	(Vitamin B$_6$)		
Isonicotinic acid	Pyridoxine		Anti-Tb
hydrazide			activity ↓
L-Dopa	Pyridoxine		Parkinsonian
			rigidity ↑
Coumarin			
anticoagulants	Vitamin K		Hyprothrombinemia ↓

(Bayless *et al.*, 1971; Jensen and Oleson, 1970; Mattson *et al.*, 1973). It has been suggested that the hydroxylase enzyme metabolizing diphenylhydantoin is folate-dependent (Maxwell *et al.*, 1972).

Recently Hansson and Sillanpaa (1976) reported that serum concentrations of diphenylhydantoin and phenobarbital are reduced by pyridoxine at doses of 400 mg/day. These authors have considered that this drug–nutrient interaction may be explained by increased activity of pyridoxal phosphate-dependent enzymes which might be involved in metabolism of these drugs. No suggestion has been made that high intake of pyridoxine could inhibit absorption of anticonvulsants.

Megadoses of pyridoxine have been shown to inhibit the activity of isonicotinic acid and hydrazide (INH) against tuberculosis in mice (McCune *et al.*, 1957). This may be understood in that pyridoxal, a vitamer of pyridoxine, forms a Schiff base with INH which is then excreted in the urine. Pyridoxine administration can also obviate or reduce the therapeutic efficacy of L-dopa in Parkinson's disease (Cotzias, 1969; Jameson, 1970; Duvoison *at al.*, 1969). A Schiff base between L-dopa and pyridoxine has been described, and formulation of this product may prevent delivery of L-dopa to the brain (Evered, 1971).

Vitamin K antagonizes the inhibitory effect of coumarin anticoagulants on the synthesis of vitamin K-dependent hepatic clotting proteins. High doses of vitamin K decrease the hypoprothrombinemic effect of coumarin drugs and lessen their clinical effectiveness (Koch-Weser and Sellers, 1971). In general this field has not been well explored and there is a real need to investigate blood levels of drugs with and without concurrent vitamin intake as also to ascertain the role of vitamins in accounting for inadequate drug responses.

IV. DRUG-INDUCED MALNUTRITION (TABLE III)

Drugs can impair nutrient absorption when they are taken with food or shortly after food. Reported effects include adsorption of a nutrient onto a drug polymer, solution of a nutrient, alterations in gut motility, as well as maldigestion induced by pharmacologic agents. The anion-exchange resin, cholestyramine, which has been utilized for its property of sequestering bile acids, also has the capacity to interfere with nutrient absorption either because bile salts are no longer available for optimal absorption of fat soluble vitamins of A, D, E and K, or because the resin actually binds or adsorbs nutrients. In 1963, Hashim and van Italie demonstrated that cholestyramine at a dosage of 30 gm/day could produce steatorrhea in normal human subjects. In some of these subjects who received vitamin A with an olive oil formula meal, cholestyramine administration caused a significant suppression of peak levels of this vitamin. Impaired absorption of vitamin K due to cholestyramine has been shown in dogs, chicks, and also in patients receiving the drug

TABLE III
Effects of Drugs on Nutrient Absorption

Drug	Nutrient malabsorption
Cholestyramine	Fat
	Vitamins A, D, and K, folacin
	Vitamin B_{12}
Cellulose phosphate	Calcium, magnesium
Antacids (aluminum hydroxide)	Phosphorus, calcium
Laxatives	
Mineral oil	Vitamins A, D, K
Phenolphthalein	Fat, vitamin D
Neomycin	Fat, nitrogen, cholesterol,
	sugars, carotene, vitamin B_{12}
	iron
Colchicine	Fat, nitrogen, sugars
p-Aminosalicylic acid	Vitamin B_{12}
Biguanides	Vitamin B_{12}
(metformin, phenformin)	
Potassium chloride	Vitamin B_{12}
Ethanol	Thiamine, folacin

(Robinson *et al.*, 1964; Whiteside *et al.*, 1965; Visintine *et al.*, 1961). Impaired absorption of vitamin D has been shown in rats fed cholestyramine and this drug has also been shown to increase fecal calcium losses. Osteomalacia developed in one patient, a woman who had had an ileal resection, and who subsequently was given cholestyramine (Harkins and Hagerman, 1965; Heaton *et al.*, 1972; Thompson and Thompson, 1969). In a recent study by West and Lloyd (1975) of 18 children with familial hypercholesterolemia who received cholestyramine as long-term therapy, there was a significant decrease in the mean serum concentrations of vitamins A and E, and of inorganic phosphorus over the first 2 years of treatment, although values remained well within the normal range. Folate depletion also occurred in these children with reductions in both serum and red cell folate levels. The authors suggest that dietary phosphate may be bound to the cholestyramine resins and that also polyglutamates of folacin may be bound to resins, since these are anionic.

Cellulose phosphate decreases the absorption of calcium (as 47-calcium) and magnesium (Berstad *et al.*, 1975). Cellulose phosphate is generally considered to be an ion-exchange resin with special affinity for divalent cations (Pack, 1973). It may be useful in the prevention of renal calculi because of a reduction in urinary calcium excretion, although large amounts of the drug would have to be taken as well as a magnesium supplement to prevent magnesium depletion.

Syndromes of phosphorus depletion induced by intake of antacids have recently aroused concern. Earlier reports of single cases of osteomalacia in patients taking antacids were believed to be the result of abuse of these medications. Bloom and Flinchum (1960) described a case of osteomalacia resulting from antacid-induced phosphorus depletion, the antacid being aluminum hydroxide. A similar case of osteomalacia was reported by Lotz *et al.* in 1964, in which a patient taking excessive quantities of a nonabsorbable antacid developed debility, osteomalacia, and marked alterations in calcium and phosphorus metabolism. In 1974, Baker *et al.* described a patient receiving regular dialysis who developed hypophosphatemia due to aluminum hydroxide therapy which then resulted in osteomalacia and severe proximal myopathy. Both the osteomalacia and the myopathy responded to treatment of the hypophosphatemia by stopping the aluminum hydroxide therapy and the administration of a neutral phosphate mixture. Vitamin D therapy was not given.

Lotz *et al.* (1968) investigated the effects of antacids on three normal volunteers, two patients with hypoparathyroidism and one patient with pseudohypoparathyroidism. Metabolic studies of one of the normal patients showed that during antacid therapy when the subject was receiving aluminum hydroxide at a level of 90 ml/day, fecal phosphorus excretion increased, serum phosphorus levels decreased, and evidence was obtained of increased calcium absorption. By the seventy-fifth day of treatment, she complained of severe weakness and anorexia, to an extent that she remained in bed. In the patients with hypoparthyroidism, antacid treatment extending over 130 days led to increased fecal excretion of phosphorus, negative phosphorus balance, increased urinary calcium levels, and negative calcium balance, mainly attributable to hypercalciuria. In the case of pseudohypoparathyroidism, antacid therapy over a 16-day period resulted in decreases in urinary phosphorus excretion, increases in fecal phosphorus loss, and evidence of an increase in calcium absorption. All of the subjects who were treated with antacids for prolonged periods entered a state of debility, associated with weakness, anorexia, and malaise. These symptoms were correlated with decreases in serum phosphorus levels. It is pointed out that this syndrome of phosphorus depletion may develop in patients taking antacids as prophylaxis or treatment for peptic ulcer, or in patients receiving corticosteroids who also take antacids to minimize the risk of developing peptic ulcer.

Bone disease associated with intake of both corticosteroids and antacids would predictably consist in an association of osteoporosis and osteomalacia. We may well be concerned that states of phosphorus depletion are more common than is generally realized, because antacids are freely available as over the counter drugs and they may be taken shortly after food, thus diminishing the absorption of dietary phosphorus. It is to be remembered that whereas cereals are often considered to be a major source of phosphorus in the diet, much of the phosphorus present in such foods is present as phytate (inositol hexophosphate), which is only available after hydrolysis by intestinal phytase. Intestinal phytase activity, at least in laboratory animals, is correlated directly with the vitamin D content of the diet, and therefore decreased availability of dietary phosphorus would be associated with low vitamin D intakes (Editorial, 1968; Steenbock et al., 1953).

Factitious diarrhea associated with abuse of laxatives or cathartics can increase nutrient losses via the gut to an extent to produce malabsorption syndromes. Signs and symptoms are reminiscent of chronic pancreatitis, and patients may be erroneously diagnosed as having pancreatic disease whereas, in fact, they are taking cathartics in a self-abusive, neurotic manner, either to gain attention or to escape dreaded constipation (Cummings et al., 1974). Osteomalacia has been described in patients taking phenolphthalein as a laxative (Frame et al., 1971). Since this drug has not been shown to produce a specific toxic effect on the absorptive mucosa of the small intestine, it is presently assumed that malabsorption may be due at least in part to an increase in the rate of passage of nutrients through the intestinal lumen. Magnesium sulfate ingestion decreased intestinal transit time but only has a modest effect on nutrient absorption producing small increases in the fecal excretion of sodium, potassium, nitrogen, and fat (Race et al., 1970). We would infer, though as yet there is no experimental proof in human subjects, that malabsorption induced by laxatives and similar drugs would be intensified by their administration with or shortly after food.

A number of drugs are known to produce a state of maldigestion. Among these are neomycin, which interferes with the action of bile salts and decreases pancreatic lipase activity (Faloon, 1966; Mehta et al., 1964). Neomycin also produces a reversible malabsorption syndrome through its direct toxic effect upon the intestinal mucosa. Neomycin decreases fat absorption, as well as the absorption of cholesterol, carotene, vitamin B_{12}, iron, and sugars. The latter effect is due to an inhibition of intestinal disaccharidase activity. Fecal fat, nitrogen, calcium, sodium, and potassium are increased by neomycin (Faloon, 1970; Gordon et al., 1968; Jacobson et al., 1960).

Colchicine produces both maldigestion and malabsorption, mainly through a rapid and direct toxic effect on the villi and microvilli, though additionally digestion may be decreased by rapid transit of the intestinal contents. This drug, like neomycin, inhibits or impairs intestinal disaccharidase activity, presumably because of the destruction of the brush border where these enzymes are located (Race et al., 1970). Many other drugs may produce intestinal malabsorption, which can affect one or more nutrients. Alcohol inhibits both folate and thiamine absorption (Halsted et al., 1967; Tomasulo et al., 1968). Other drugs which have been documented as producing malabsorption in some patients include tetracycline and other broad spectrum antibiotics, p-aminosalicylic acid (PAS), biguanides used as oral hypoglycemic agents, potassium chloride and the folate antagonist, methotrexate. Selective malabsorption of vitamin B_{12}, due to interference with the ilial receptor has been induced by intake of PAS, of the biguanides, metformin and phenformin, and by potassium chloride (Dobbins, 1968; Heinivaara and Palva, 1964; Tomkin et al., 1971; Palva et al., 1972).

It should be noted that although a number of drugs have been documented as causing malabsorption of nutrients detectable by laboratory tests, clinical evidence of malabsorption is usually associated either with intensive and prolonged therapy, or added abuse of alcohol, which also can cause malabsorption.

V. SYSTEMIC REACTIONS INDUCED BY DRUG-FOOD INCOMPATIBILITIES (TABLE IV)

Since 1961 there have been many reports of acute hypertensive attacks developing in patients receiving drugs which are monamine oxidase inhibitors. Monamine oxidase inhibitor drugs including phenelzine, isocarboxazide, pargyline, and tranylcypromine were introduced into therapeutic use as mood elevating agents for the treatment of severe depression. These drugs elevate norepinephrine and serotonin levels in the central nervous system, and potentiate the cardiovascular facts of simple phenylethylamines such as tyramine. Asatoor *et al.* (1963) observed that toxic reactions to cheese might occur in patients on these drugs, resembling those associated with the paroxysmal release of catecholamines from a pheochromocytoma. Attacks are characterized by transient hypertension, headaches, palpitations, nausea, and vomiting, and cases of cerebral hemorrhage have been documented. The severity of the attacks has been related not only to the drug dosage but also to the level of tyramine in particular foods or food samples.

A number of foods were shown to evoke hypertensive crises in patients receiving monoamine oxidase inhibitors, but there was great vari-

TABLE IV
Systemic Reactions due to Drug–Food Incompatibilities

Drug or drug group	Foods inducing reaction	"Toxic" food/beverage component	Acute effect
Monamine oxidase inhibitors, e.g., tranylcypromine procarbazine	Cheese, yeast, broad beans, pickled herring, chicken liver, wine	Tyramine Dopamine	Hypertensive crises
Tetraethylthiuram disulfide [disulfiram (Antabuse)]		Ethanol	"Acetaldehyde reactions"
Metronidazole	Liqueur desserts, wine sauces and wine-containing casseroles	Ethanol	
Oral hypoglycemic agents		Ethanol	Hypoglycemic attacks

ability in the severity of the reactions related to the tyramine content of various foods consumed prior to the attack. The tyramine content of cheeses was shown to vary with their tyrosine content and their content of tyrosine decarboxylase. Cheeses with a high tyramine content were those which were allowed to mature and undergo bacterial putrefaction. Thus, intake of unmatured cheeses by persons receiving these drugs was more innocuous than comparable intake of cheeses long matured and of high flavor. Blackwell and Mabbit (1965) estimated the tyramine content of a number of cheeses and found the highest values among cheddar cheeses to be in those samples with acid or rancid flavors. Whereas cheese was the most common food to produce the pressor effects in patients on these drugs, a number of other foods and beverages were incriminated as well as amines other than tyramine. Several patients had attacks of hypertension and severe headaches after eating the British yeast extract, Marmite. Blackwell *et al.* (1965) showed that Marmite contains tyramine which was apparently responsible for the hypertensive effects and also histamine which could have caused flushing, another side effect of ingestion of this product by persons on monamine oxidase inhibitors.

Other foods which have been recognized to produce hypertensive effects in those patients on these drugs are broad beans, pickled herring, chickens' liver and certain wines, as for example, the Italian wine, Chiante. In broad beans the amino acid dopa, or its amine derivative dopamine, have been incriminated (Blomley, 1964). These amines which escape oxidative deamination are believed to enter the general circulation and to release norepinephrine from local stores in nerve endings and also to prolong the action of this catecholamine on adrenergic receptors (Sapeika, 1969). It seems that the drugs inhibit the monamine oxidase either in the intestine or in the liver or both (Thomas, 1963). Reactions usually occur within one-half to one hour within ingestion of the offending food or drink.

In a patient on tranylcypromine described by Nuessle and Norman (1965), a hypertensive attack as well as severe precordial chest pain developed in 45 minutes after the man had eaten a piece of Schmaltz herring.

The interaction between tranylcypromine and cheddar cheese was actually utilized to treat two patients with severe postural hypotension. When given this drug at a dose of 70 mg/day and 90 mg cheddar cheese daily, equivalent to 26 mg of tyramine per day, the blood pressure rose and the patients were able to sit up and stand for a period of about 6 hours/day (Diamond *et al.*, 1969).

The severity of drug-nutrient reactions evoked by the MAO inhibitor antidepressants has greatly limited their usage in recent years. Procarbazine, a drug of choice in the chemotherapy of Hodgkins disease, is also a weak MAO inhibitor. Hypertension has been described in patients eating tyramine containing foods while on procarbazine therapy (Spivak, 1974).

Tetraethylthiuram disulfide, known either as Disulfiram or Antabuse, is commonly used as an alcohol deterrent drug in alcoholics. If alcohol is consumed after this drug is taken, unpleasant symptoms occur including severe headache, flushing, nausea and vomiting, hypotension, weakness, vertigo, blurred vision, and convulsions. The reaction begins within 5–10 minutes of drinking the alcohol and may be evoked by intake of as little as 6–7 ml of alcohol in sensitive people. Similarly, this reaction to Disulfiram will occur when patients take such foods as wine-containing sauces or casseroles, desserts containing liquor, or wine vinegar. Collectively the symptoms have been termed the "acetaldehyde syndrome" and are due to the fact that the drug inhibits the enzyme aldehyde dehydrogenase which oxidases acetaldehyde derived from alcohol. This same syndrome has been produced by injection of acetaldehyde (Hald et al., 1948; Hald and Jacobsen, 1948; Murdoch Ritchie, 1965).

Alcohol and alcohol-containing foods may produce Disulfiram-like reactions of varying severity in diabetics receiving oral hypoglycemic agents of the sulfonylurea group as well as in patients receiving metronidazole. Reactions are most severe in patients receiving chlorpropamide. Cases of alcohol-precipitated acute lactic acidosis have been described, developing in people on the biguanide phenformin. Alcohol may also produce a hypoglycemic reaction in patients on chlorpropamide (Harris, 1971; Carulli, 1971; Pryor, 1960; Food and Drug Administration, 1970).

VI. ADVERSE EFFECTS OF FOOD CONSTITUENTS ON NUTRIENT AVAILABILITY (TABLE V)

Let us confuse the issue by going back to a simple definition. If we are to consider that a drug is an agent with a pharmacologic action, then certain nutrients as well as non-nutrient constituents of food fall in this category. Among the non-nutrient constituents of food which impair nutrient absorption, we must include tannates, as in tea, coffee, phytates and certain elements of dietary fiber. We must be concerned that nutrients may be prescribed therapeutically, and that their adequate absorp-

TABLE V
Adverse Effects of Food Constituents
on Mineral Absorption

Interacting food or beverage and active constituent	Specific effect on mineral uptake
Tea (tannates)	Ferric chloride ↓
Bran (phosphate)	Ferrous sulfate ↓
(phytate)	
Milk, cheese (phosphate)	Zinc sulfate ↓
Brown bread (phytate)	
Coffee	
Bran (phytate)	Calcium salts ↓

tion and utilization is dependent upon noninterference by food components. It is known, however, that tea can impair the absorption of
nonheme iron and could therefore contribute to impaired utilization of
iron given to correct an iron deficiency. Disler *et al.* (1975) studied the
effect of tea drinking on the absorption of iron among Indian house-
wives living near Durban. The drinking of tea without milk was found to
inhibit the absorption of iron from a solution of ferric chloride and also
from a solution of ferrous sulfate containing ascorbic acid. Tea mixed
with milk produced about the same effect on the absorption of iron from
a solution of ferrous sulfate with ascorbic acid as did tea without milk.
Tea also significantly inhibited the absorption of heme iron from a solution of uncooked rabbit hemoglobin in tomato juice. Further, and this is
significant, tea had no significant effect on the absorption of heme iron
from cooked ground lamb mixed with a rabbit hemoglobin gravy. It was
therefore concluded that tea did not inhibit the absorption of hemoglobin iron if it had been cooked. The authors considered it likely that the
inhibition induced by tea on iron absorption was due to the formation of
tannates, which were nonabsorbable. It is known that the formation of
such iron complexes within the intestinal lumen may diminish iron absorption. Preliminary observations by the same authors, as yet unpublished, indicate that coffee has a similar effect though the mechanism is
unknown.

In recent years, zinc salts have been used to promote wound healing,
but it is known that certain foodstuffs such as dairy products including
milk and cheese, as well as brown bread, decrease zinc absorption as
shown by significant lowering of peak serum zinc levels. Schelling *et al.*

(1973) showed that the absorption of zinc sulfate after a breakfast was less than when the same dose was given to subjects in the fasting state. Pécoud *et al.* (1975) administered zinc sulfate to volunteer subjects with water, coffee, various breakfasts, with sodium phytate or with a high dose of sodium phosphate. Peak serum zinc levels were reduced by coffee drinking and serum zinc levels did not rise when zinc was given with meals containing milk and cheese, rich in calcium, phosphorus, and protein. When the zinc salt was given with meals containing brown bread, with an equivalent of 102 mg phytic acid, a slight rise in serum zinc concentrations was found, but a much greater rise in the zinc levels was obtained when similar meals were given containing white bread equivalent to 4 mg phytic acid. When zinc was given without a sodium phytate or phosphate, either at a low or high dosage, the rise in serum zinc was lower than when the zinc was given with water alone. While zinc has been given with meals in order to diminish gastric irritation, it is clear from these studies that this may impair absorption unless the characteristics of the meal are carefully monitored.

According to Payler *et al.* (1975), intestinal transit time became faster in subjects receiving about 20 gm of bran/day who had an initial transit time of 3 days or more, but this same bran intake caused a slowing of their transit time when the initial transit was in the order of 1 day. While wheat bran significantly altered transit time in these subjects, oatmeal had no significant effect. Bjorn-Rasmussen (1974) has found that bran reduces iron absorption. In a careful study of iron absorption from breads he found that even a small amount of bran in bread has significantly reduced iron absorption. He has commented that the inhibitory effect of bran on iron absorption may be due to the high phytate content. While this may be true, bran also has a high phosphate content which could also inhibit the absorption of iron. Evidence has been obtained that phytates, while reducing the absorption of nonheme iron, have no significant effect on heme iron absorption (Hallberg and Solvell, 1967). It should be remembered that these studies stemmed from the consideration of McCance *et al.* (1943), who first considered that high phytate and phosphate contents of bran bread might make iron unavailable for absorption. Callender and Warner (1970), on the other hand, have produced some evidence in human subjects that iron may be more available from brown bread than from white bread similarly enriched with iron. There is no question that, in the past, confusion about the relative iron absorption from brown bread and white bread, or from products containing bran and high levels of phytate to those containing lower levels of these ingredients, have resulted from differing experimental methodologies.

Jenkins *et al.* (1975) studied the male student volunteers with respect to the effects of ingestion of wheat fiber on hematologic status, fecal steroid output, and serum levels of cholesterol and triglycerides. Fecal weights were significantly increased by the daily intake of 36 gm of wheat fiber. There was a decrease in fecal neutral steroid concentration which was significant statistically. Fasting cholesterol, triglyceride, and blood sugar were unchanged after the feeding of the wheat fiber. However, during the wheat fiber regime, serum iron levels were reduced and when the wheat fiber intake was increased, there was a significant fall in mean corpuscular volume and mean corpuscular hemoglobin.

There are also several publications suggesting or showing that serum calcium levels may be reduced by the feeding of bran (Heaton and Pomare, 1974; Reinhold *et al.*, 1973). In these studies, phytate present in the bran or in breads in which the bran is present, caused precipitation of the calcium phytate in the intestinal lumen so that it could not be absorbed. The effect of high dietary phytic acid intake on plasma calcium has also been studied by Wills and Fairney (1972) in rats. The rats were unable to maintain plasma calcium concentrations when ingesting a high dietary content of phytic acid, even though they were given an adequate vitamin D intake. Indeed, increasing intake of vitamin D_3 did not overcome the effects of the phytic acid in the diet.

While high intakes of dietary fiber are being advocated as a prophylactic measure to minimize the risk of constipation, diverticulosis, and diverticulitis, as well as chronic cancer, we should be cognizant with the implications of these studies in that they indicate that bran can affect adsorption of certain minerals adversely. Whether these effects are transient and adaptation to the changing diet occurs is presently unclear. The situation is further complicated by the fact that we are as yet unclear about many of the mechanisms which might diminish nutrient absorption when the intake of dietary fiber is increased. The use of such terms as bran and dietary fiber without qualification is confusing and it seems that many people are misled into equating possible adsorptive properties of fiber elements with the affects of other components in the bran such as phytates. A recent plea for better nomenclature with respect to dietary plant fibers is timely (Schaller, 1975). Very little information had been obtained on the effects of specific dietary fiber components on nutrient absorption other than in relation to the minerals which have been discussed.

Ershoff (1974), reviewing a number of studies in laboratory animals on the effects of plant fiber on the toxicity of foreign compounds, has concluded that "various drugs, chemicals, and food additives are highly toxic when fed to rats and mice in conjunction with a purified low fiber diet at dosages that are without deleterious effect when fed with diets that are high in dietary fiber." This author has further noted that different plant fibers may vary significantly from one another in their ability to counteract the toxic effects of foreign compounds.

VII. NUTRIENT–NUTRIENT INCOMPATIBILITIES (TABLE VI)

It has recently been shown that the practice of taking megadoses of vitamins as a home remedy may induce adverse nutritional effects. It is known that excess intake of vitamin E by animals can cause a prolongation of the prothrombin time with an associated hemorrhagic state, indicative of vitamin K deficiency (Doisy, 1961; March *et al.*, 1973; Mellette and Leone, 1960). In vitamin K-deficient animals treated with vitamin E, vitamin K-dependent coagulation factors are further depressed. Corrigan and Marcus (1974) reported that a man receiving Warfarin sodium after pulmonary infarction developed ecchymoses on the legs and arms during the period of concomitant intake of vitamin E. During a test period when he took vitamin E in addition to Warfarin sodium, there was a decline in the level of his vitamin K-dependent clotting factors II, VII, IX, X, whereas these levels returned towards the pre-vitamin E levels when the vitamin E therapy treatment was discontinued. The case is of considerable interest, but the implications of the combination of Warfarin sodium and vitamin E are somewhat unclear since this patient was also on clofibrate therapy.

Murphy and Zelman (1965) observed that four out of nine paraplegics taking 1 gm ascorbic acid daily to keep their urine acid had low serum vitamin B_{12} levels. The destructive effect of ascorbic acid on vitamin B_{12} was first reported by Hutchins *et al.* (1956). Herbert and Jacob (1974) investigated the effect of 0.1, 0.25, and 0.5 gm of ascorbic acid on the

TABLE VI
Effects of Megadose Vitamin Intake on the Availability
of Other Vitamins

Megadose vitamin	Interacting vitamins	Effect on vitamin status
C	B_{12}	Serum B_{12} ↓ ?
E	K	Vitamin K↓ (Coumarin anticoagulant effect ↑)

vitamin B_{12} content of hospital meals. The food was from meals used for delivery to individual patients on the wards. Food was homogenized and incubated with ascorbic acid at 37°C for 30 minutes. The vitamin B_{12} content of homogenized meals was determined in those that had no ascorbic acid added, as well as in meals which had ascorbic acid added at the stated levels. Ascorbic acid was shown by the technique of these investigators to cause destruction of the vitamin B_{12} in the food, the degree of this destruction being dependent on the amount of ascorbic acid added, as well as the character of the meals. The authors suggest that this may mean that various ingredients in different foods may either augment or reduce the destructive effect of the ascorbate, perhaps because of their oxidative or reducing capacity.

Deleterious effects of ascorbic acid on vitamin B_{12} in food have been questioned by Newmark et al. (1976). They determined the vitamin B_{12} content of foods by microbiological and radiometric assay and could find no significant destruction of vitamin B_{12} induced by adding ascorbic acid to their samples. They consider that Herbert and Jacob did not extract all the vitamin B_{12} from samples during preparations for assay (Newmark et al., 1976). The clinical association of megadosage ascorbic acid therapy and vitamin B_{12} depletion requires further study.

VIII. SUMMARY AND CONCLUSIONS

In considering the wide range of interactions between food and drugs, and between nutrients in foods and nutrients given for rational or empirical therapeutic purposes, it is necessary to consider practical implications. Prescriptions indicating that a drug should be taken three or four times a day often do not indicate whether the drug is to be taken intermediately between meals, just before meals, at meals, or immediately after meals. Indeed, with the changing life styles so that many small snack meals may be consumed it is difficult to find the appropriate time at which drugs should be given in order not to interact with foods or food components. Yet desirable serum levels of particular drugs may not be reached if their absorption is diminished by the presence of food in the gastrointestinal tract. We have further to consider the hazard of drug-induced nutrient malabsorption which may have clinical implications in the production of nutritional deficiency because the very people who take drugs at high dosage and/or for a prolonged period of time may also be those who by virtue of their disease may be in a state of marginal deficiency prior to drug intake. Acute toxic reactions resulting from food–drug incompatibilities should be predictable and avoidable.

Little is known as yet about the effect of dietary fiber on nutrient or drug absorption and virtually no research has been directed toward the important subject of whether non-nutrient food additives may decrease or increase the bioavailability of drugs. While we know that the public have been led to believe that meganutrient self-treatment is desirable and that vitamins are perhaps the best drugs, it is our responsibility to assess the various hazards of such self-treatment because pharmacological doses of single nutrients can either reduce the availability of food factors or interfere with the drug regimens. While guidelines are available to define the foreign compounds which can safely be added to food, we are not yet in a position to offer similar guidelines on the appropriateness or otherwise of taking drugs and food together. Research in this area will require the combined efforts of pharmacologists and nutritionists; development of suitable animal models; and data retrieval from comprehensive drug surveillance programs. As yet, however, the information gathered by such programs is too limited to indicate the complexity of food–drug interference. The absorbed fraction of a drug dose or of a nutrient determine disposition to the tissues. We must remind ourselves that pharmacokinetics and nutritional physiology are bedfellows, and that rational therapeutics depends on a knowledge of both disciplines.

IX. RESEARCH NEEDS

The research needs which have been identified are listed below.

1. Systemic investigation of effects of food components on the bioavailability of drugs.

2. Development of animal models for the study of drug-induced malabsorption.

3. Investigations of the nutritional requirements of persons and populations on long-term drugs.

4. Design of diet studies to be incorporated into protocols for new drug testing in animals and clinical trials.

5. Expansion of comprehensive drug surveillance information to include diet and nutritional parameters as well as documentation of systemic reactions induced by drug–food incompatibilities.

6. Studies of the effect of dietary fiber on nutrient and drug absorption.

7. Investigation of the impact of therapeutic or megadose nutrient supplements on availability of nutrients in the diet and on drug absorption or response.

8. Development of drug labeling system and manuals to indicate drug-nutrient interactions and incompatibilities.

REFERENCES

Adams, F. (1844). "The Seven Books of Paulus Aegineta," Vol. 1, pp. 1–5, 376–385, 507–511, and 520–523. Printed for the Sydenham Society, London.

Albert, A. (1967) Patterns of metabolic disposition of drugs in man and other species. *Drug Responses Man, Ciba Found. Vol., 1966* p. 57.

Asatoor, A. M., Levi, A. J., and Milne, M. D. (1963). Tranylcypromine and cheese. *Lancet* **2**, 733–734.

Baker, L. R. I., Ackrill, P., Cattell, W. R., Stamp, T. C. B., and Watson, L. (1974). Iatrogenic osteomalacia and myopathy due to phosphate depletion. *Br. Med. J.* **3**, 150–152.

Barr, W. H., Adir, J., and Barrettson, L. (1971). Decrease of tetracycline absorption in man by sodium bicarbonate. *Clin. Pharmacol. Ther.* **12**, 779–784.

Bates, T. R., Sequeira, J. A., and Tembo, A. V. (1974) Effect of food on nitrofurantoin absorption. *Clin Pharmacol. Ther.* **16**, 63–68.

Bayless, E. M., Crowley, J. M., Preece, J. M., Sylvester, P. E., and Marks, V. (1971). Influence of folic acid on blood phenytoin levels. *Lancet* **1**, 62–64.

Berstad, A., Jørgensen, J., Frey, H., and Vogt, J. H. (1975). The acute effect of sodium cellulose phosphate on intestinal absorption and urinary excretion of calcium in man. *Acta Med. Scand.* **197**, 361–365.

Bjorn-Rasmussen, D. (1974). Iron absorption from wheat bread. Influence of various amounts of bran. *Nutr. Metab.* **16**, 101–110.

Blackwell, B., and Mabbit, L. A. (1965). Tyramine in cheese related to hypertensive crises after monoamine oxidase inhibition. *Lancet* **1**, 938–940.

Blackwell, B., Marley E., and Mabbit, L. A. (1965). Effects of yeast extract after monamine oxidase inhibition. *Lancet* **1**, 940–943.

Blomley, B. J. (1964). Monamine oxidase inhibitors. *Lancet* **2**, 1181–1182.

Bloom, W. L., and Flinchum, D. (1960). Osteomalacia with pseudofractures caused by ingestion of aluminum hydroxide. *J. Am. Med. Assoc.* **174**, 1327–1330.

Boyd, E. N. (1958). Drugs acting on mucous membranes and skin. *In* "Pharmacology in Medicine" (V. A. Drill, ed.), 2nd ed., pp. 691–695. McGraw-Hill, New York.

Callender, S. T., and Warner, G. T. (1970). Iron absorption from brown bread. *Lancet* **1**, 546–547.

Carulli, N. (1971). Alcohol–drugs interaction in man: alcohol and tolbutamide. *Eur. J. Clin. Invest.* **1**, 421–424.

Conklin, J. D. (1972). Biopharmaceutics of nitrofurantoin. *In* "Bioavailability of Drugs" (B. B. Brodie and W. M. Heller, eds.), pp. 178–181. Karger, Basel.

Conklin, J. D., and Hailey, S. J. (1969). Urinary drug excretion in man during oral dosage of different nitrofurantoin formulations. *Clin. Pharmacol.Ther.* **10**, 534–539.

Corrigan, J. J., and Marcus, F. I. (1974). Coagulopathy associated with vitamin E ingestion. *J. Am. Med. Assoc.* **230**, 1300–1301.

Cotzias, G. C. (1969). Metabolic modification of some neurologic disorders. *J. Am. Med. Assoc.* **210**, 1255–1262.

Crounse, R. G. (1961). Human pharmacology of griseofulvin: The effect of fat intake on gastrointestinal absorption. *J. Invest. Dermatol.* **37**, 529–533.

Cummings, J. H., Sladen, G. E., James, O. F. W., Sarner, M., and Misiewicz, J. J. (1974). Laxative-induced diarrhea: A continuing clinical problem. *Br. Med. J.* **1,** 537–541.

Das, K. M., and Eastwood, M. A. (1973). Effect of iron and calcium on salicylazosulfapyridine metabolism. *Scott. Med. J.* **18,** 45–50.

Diamond, M. A., Murray, R. H., and Schmid, P. (1969). Treatment of idiopathic postural hypertension with oral tyramine (TY) and monamine oxidase inhibitor (MI). *J. Clin. Res.* **17,** 237.

Disler, P. B., Lynch, S. R., Charlton, R. W., Torrance, J. D., Bothwell, T. H., Walker, R. B., and Mayet, F. (1975). The effect of tea on iron absorption. *Gut* **16,** 193–200.

Dobbins, W. O. (1968). Drug-induced steatorrhea. *Gastroenterology* **54,** 1193–1195.

Doisy, E. A., Jr. (1961). Nutritional hypoprothrombinemia and metabolism of vitamin K. *Fed. Proc., Fed. Am. Soc. Exp. Biol.* **20,** 989–994.

Duvoisin, R. C., Yahr, M. D., and Cole, L. D. (1969). Reversal of the "dopa effect" in parkinsonism by pyridoxine. *Trans. Am. Neurol. Assoc.* **94,** 81–84.

Editorial. (1968). Food, feces and phosphorus. *N. Engl. J. Med.* **278,** 451–452.

Elbel, H., and Schleyer, F. (1956). "Blutalkohol. Die Wissenschaftlichen Grundlagen der Beurtteilung von Blutalkoholbefinden bei Strassenverkehrsdelikten," 2nd ed. Thieme, Stuttgart.

Ershoff, B. H. (1974). Antitoxic effects of plant fiber. *Am. J. Clin. Nutr.* **27,** 1395–1398.

Evered, D. F. (1971). L-dopa as a vitamin-B_6 antagonist. *Lancet* **1,** 914.

Faloon, W. W. (1966). Effect of neomycin and kanamycin upon intestinal absorption. *Ann. N.Y. Acad. Sci.* **132,** 879–887.

Faloon, W. W. (1970). Drug production of intestinal malabsorption. *N.Y. State J. Med.* **70,** 2189–2192.

Food and Drug Administration. (1970). "Reports of Suspected Adverse Reactions to Drugs," No. 700301-064-01001. FDA, Washington, D.C.

Frame, B., Guiang, H. L., Frost, H. M., and Reynolds, W. A. (1971). Osteomalacia induced by laxative (phenolphthalein) ingestion. *Arch. Intern. Med.* **128,** 794–796.

Gibaldi, M., and Grundhofer, B. (1975). Biopharmaceutic influences on the anticholinergic effects of propantheline. *Clin. Pharmacol. Ther.* **18,** 457–461.

Goldberg, L. (1943). Quantitative studies on alcohol tolerance in man. The influence of ethyl alcohol on sensory, motor and psychological functions referred to blood alcohol in normal and habituated individuals. *Acta Physiol. Scand.* **5,** Suppl. 16, 1.

Goldman, P., and Peppercorn, M. A. (1975). Sulfasalazine. *N. Engl. J. Med.* **293,** 20–23.

Gordon, C. P. T., Haro, E. N., Paes, I. C., and Faloon, W. W. (1968). Studies of malabsorption and calcium excretion induced by neomycin sulfate. *J. Am. Med. Assoc.* **204,** 127–134.

Greenberger, N. J. (1973). Effects of antibiotics and other agents on the intestinal transport of iron. *Am. J. Clin. Nutr.* **26,** 104–112.

Hald, J., and Jacobsen, E. (1948). A drug sensitizing the organism to ethyl alcohol. *Lancet* **2,** 1001–1004.

Hald, J., Jacobsen, E., and Larsen, V. (1948). The sensitizing effect of tetraethylthiuramdisulfide (Antabuse) to ethylalcohol. *Acta Pharmacol. Toxicol.* **4,** 285–296.

Hallberg, L., and Solvell, L. (1967). Absorption of hemoglobin iron in man. *Acta Med. Scand.* **181,** 335–354.

Halsted, C. H., Griggs, R. C., and Harris, J. W. (1967). The effect of alcoholism on the absorption of folic acid (H^3-PGA). Evaluated by plasma levels and urine excretion. *J. Lab. Clin. Med.* **69,** 116–131.

Hansson, O., and Sillanpaa, M. (1976). Pyridoxine and serum concentration of phenytoin and phenobarbitone. *Lancet* **1,** 256.

Hansten, T. D. (1973). "Drug Interactions," 2nd ed., p. 147. Lea & Febiger, Philadelphia, Pennsylvania.

Harkins, R. W., and Hagerman, L. M. (1965). Retention of dietary fats in experimental steatorrhea induced by cholestyramine. Fed. Proc., Fed. Am. Soc. Exp. Biol. 24, 357 (abstr.).

Harris, E. L. (1971). Adverse reactions to oral antidiabetic agents. Br. Med. J. 3, 29–30.

Hashim, S. A., and van Italie, T. B. (1963). Experimental steatorrhea in human subjects in malabsorption syndromes. World Congr. Gastroenterol. [Proc.], 2nd, 1962 pp. 26–30.

Heatley, N. G. (1956). Comparative serum concentration and excretion experiments with benzylpenicillin (G) and phenoxymethyl penicillin (V) on single subject. Antibiot. Med. 2, 33–41.

Heaton, K. W., and Pomare, E. W. (1974). Effect of bran on blood lipids and calcium. Lancet 1, 49.

Heaton, K. W., Lever, J. V., and Barnard, D. (1972). Osteomalacia associated with cholestyramine therapy for post ileectomy diarrhea. Gastroenterology 62, 642–646.

Heinivaara, O., and Palva, I. P. (1964). Malabsorption of vitamin B_{12} during treatment of paraaminosalicylic acid. A preliminary report. Acta Med. Scand. 175, 469–471.

Herbert, V., and Jacob, E. (1974). Destruction of vitamine B_{12} by ascorbic acid. J. Am. Med. Assoc. 230, 241–242.

Herbich, J., and Prokop, L. (1963). Studies on the influence of food and fluid ingestion on the blood alcohol level (Ger) Wien. Klin. Wochenschr. 75, 421–427.

Hutchins, H. H., Cravioto, P. J., and Macek, T. J. (1956). A comparison of the stability of cyanocobalamin and its analogs in ascorbate solution. J. Am. Pharm. Assoc. 45, 806–808.

Jacobson, E. D., Prior, J. T., and Faloon, W. W. (1960). Malabsorptive syndrome induced by neomycin: Morphologic alterations in the jejunal mucosa. J. Lab. Clin. Med. 56, 245–250.

Jameson, H. D. (1970). Pyridoxine for levodopa-induced dystonia. J. Am. Med. Assoc. 211, 1700.

Jenkins, D. J. A., Hill, M. S., and Cummings, J. H. (1975). Effect of wheat fiber on blood lipids, fecal steroid excretion and serum iron. Am. J. Clin. Nutr. 28, 1408–1411.

Jensen, O. N., and Oleson, O. V. (1970). Subnormal serum folate due to anticonvulsive therapy. A double blind study of the effect of folic acid treatment in patients with drug-induced subnormal serum folates. Arch. Neurol. (Chicago) 22, 181–182.

Kabasakalian, P., Katz, M., Rosenkrantz, B., and Townley, E. (1970). Parameters affecting absorption of griseofulvin in a human subject using urinary metabolite excretion data. J. Pharm. Sci. 59, 595–600.

Kalant, H. (1971). Absorption, diffusion, distribution and elimination of ethanol: Effects on biological membranes. In "The Biology of Alcoholism 1: Biochemistry" (B. Kissin and H. Begleiter, eds.), p. 10. Plenum, New York.

Klein, J. O., and Finland, M. (1963). Ampicillin. Activity in vitro and absorption and excretion in normal young men. Am. J. Med. Sci. 245, 544–555.

Klein, J. O., Sabath, L. D., and Finland, M. (1963). Laboratory studies of oxacillin. Am. J. Med. Sci. 245, 399–412.

Kocher, F. (1952–1953). Ein Akkadischer medizinischer Schülertext aus Bogaskoy. Arch. Orientforsch. 16, 47–56.

Koch-Weser, J. (1974). Bioavailability of drugs. (First of 2 parts.) N. Engl. J. Med. 291, 233–237.

Koch-Weser, J., and Sellers, E. M. (1971). Drug interactions with coumarin anticoagulants (first of two parts). N. Engl. J. Med. 285, 487–498.

Krondl, A. (1970). Present understanding of the interaction of drugs and food during absorption. *Can. Med. Assoc. J.* **103**, 360–364.

Kunin, C. M., and Finland, M. (1961). Clinical pharmacology of the tetracycline antibiotics. *Clin. Pharmacol. Ther.* **2**, 51–69.

Levey, M. (1961). Some objective factors of Babylonian medicine in the light of new evidence. *Bull. Hist. Med.* **35**, 61–70.

Lotz, M., Ney, R., and Bartter, F. C. (1964). Osteomalacia and debility resulting from phosphorus depletion. *Trans. Assoc. Am. Physicians* **77**, 281–295.

Lotz, M., Zisman, E., and Bartter, F. C. (1968). Evidence for a phosphorus depletion syndrome in man. *N. Engl. J. Med.* **278**, 409–415.

McCall, C. E., Steigbigel, N. H., and Finland, M. (1967). Lincomycin: Activity in vitro and absorption and excretion in normal young men. *Am. J. Sci.* **254** 144–155.

McCance, R. A., Edgecomb, C. N., and Widdowson, E. M. (1943). Phytic acid and iron absorption. *Lancet* **2**, 126–128.

McCune, R., Deuschle, K., and McDermott, W. (1957). The delayed appearance of isoniazid antagonism by pyridoxine in vivo. *Am. Rev. Tuberc.* **76**, 1106–1109.

MacDonald, H., Place, V. A., Falk, H., *et al.* (1967). Effect of food on absorption of sulfonamides in man. *Chemotherapia* **12**, 282–285.

March, B. E., Wong, E., Seier, L., Sim, J., and Biely, J. (1973). Hypervitaminosis E in the chick. *J. Nutr.* **103**, 371–377.

Mattson, R. H., Gallagher, B. B., Reynolds, E. H., and Glass, D. (1973). Folate therapy in epilepsy. A controlled study. *Arch. Neurol. (Chicago)* **29**, 78–81.

Maxwell, J. D., Hunter, J., Stewart, D. A., Ardeman, S., and Williams, R. (1972). Folate deficiency after anticonvulsant drugs. An effect of hepatic enzyme induction. *Br. Med. J.* **1**, 297–299.

Mehta, S. K., Wesser, E., and Sleisenger, M. A. (1964). The in vitro effect of bacterial metabolites in antibiotics on pancreatic lipase activity. *J. Clin. Invest.* **43**, 1252 (abstr.).

Mellanby, E. (1919). Alcohol: Its absorption into and disappearance from the blood under different conditions. *Med. Res. Counc. (G.B.), Spec. Rep. Ser.* **SRS-31.**

Mellette, S. J., and Leone, L. A. (1960). Influence of age, sex, strain of rat and fat soluble vitamins on hemorrhagic syndromes in rats given irradiated beef. *Fed. Proc., Fed. Am. Soc. Exp. Biol.* **19**, 1045–1049.

Mettler, C. C. (1947). "History of Medicine," p. 174. McGraw-Hill (Blackiston), New York.

Miller, D. S., Sterling, J. L., and Udkin, J. (1966). Effect of ingestion of milk on concentrations of blood alcohol. *Nature (London)* **212**, 1051.

Murdoch Ritchie, J. (1965). The aliphatic alcohols. In "The Pharmacological Basis of Therapeutics" (L. S. Goodman and A. Gilman, eds.), 3rd ed., pp. 155–156. Macmillan, New York.

Murphy, F. J., and Zelman, S. (1965). Ascorbic acid as a urinary acidifying agent. I. Comparison with the ketogenic effect of fasting. *J. Urol.* **94**, 297–299.

Newmark, H. L., Schemer, J., Marcus, M., and Prabhudesai, M. (1976). Stability of vitamin B$_{12}$ in the presence of ascorbic acid. *Am. J. Clin. Nutr.* **29**, 645–649.

Neuvonen, P. J., Gothoni, G., Hackman, R., and Björksten, K. (1970). Interference of iron with the absorption of tetracyclines in man. *Br. Med. J.* **4**, 532–534.

Nuessle, W. F., and Norman, F. C. (1965). Pickled herring and tranylcypromine reaction. *J. Am. Med. Assoc.* **192**, 726–727.

Pack, C. Y. C. (1973). Sodium cellulose phosphate. Mechanism of action and effect on mineral metabolism. *J. Clin. Pharmacol.* **13**, 15.

Palva, I. P., Salokannel, S. J., Timonen, T., and Palva, H. L. A. (1972). Drug-induced malabsorption of vitamin B_{12}, IV. Malabsorption and deficiency of B_{12} during treatment with slow release potassium chloride. *Acta Med. Scand.* **191**, 355–357.

Paul, H. E., Kenyan, J. H., Paul, M. F., and Borgmann, A. R. (1967). Laboratory studies with nitrofurantoin-relationship between crystal size, urinary excretion in the rat and man and emesis in dogs. *J. Pharm. Sci.* **56**, 882–885.

Payler, D. K., Pomare, E. W., Heaton, K. W., and Harvey, R. F. (1975). The effect of wheat bran on intestinal transit. *Gut* **16**, 209–213.

Pécoud, A., Donzel, P., and Schelling, J. L. (1975). Effect of foodstuffs on the absorption of zinc sulfate. *Clin. Pharmacol. Ther.* **17**, 469–474.

Peppercorn, M. A., and Goldman, P. (1972). The role of intestinal bacteria in the metabolism of salicylazosulfapyridine. *J. Pharmacol. Exp. Ther.* **181**, 555–562.

Piafsky, K. M., and Ogilvie, R. I. (1975). Dosage of theophylline in bronchial asthma. *N. Engl. J. Med.* **292**, 1218–1222.

Prescott, L. F. (1969). Pharmacokinetic drug interactions. *Lancet* **2**, 1239–1243.

Pryor, D. S. (1960). Hypoglycaemic effect of chlorpropamide. *Med. J. Aust.* **2**, 539–540.

Race, T. F., Paes, I. C., and Faloon, W. W. (1970). Intestinal malabsorption induced by oral colchicine. Comparison with neomycin and cathartic agents. *Am. J. Med. Sci.* **259**, 32–41.

Reinhold, J. G., Nasr, K., Lahimgarzadeh, A., and Hedayati, H. (1973). Effect of purified phytate and phytate-rich bread upon metabolism of zinc calcium, phosphorus and nitrogen in man. *Lancet* **1**, 283.

Robinson, H. J., Keley, K. L., and Lehman, E. G. (1964). Effect of cholestyramine, a bile acid binding polymer, on vitamin K absorption on dogs. *Proc. Soc. Exp. Biol. Med.* **115**, 112–115.

Sabath, L. D., Klein, J. O., and Finland, M. (1963). Ancillin (2-biphenylylpenicillin) antibacterial activity and clinical pharmacology. *Am. J. Med. Sci.* **246**, 129–146.

Sapeika, N. (1969). "Food Pharmacology," pp. 93–94. Thomas, Springfield, Illinois.

Schaller, D. (1975). Plant fibers in nutrition: Need for better nomenclature. *Am. J. Clin. Nutr.* **28**, 1347.

Scheiner, J., and Oltemeier, W. A. (1962). Experimental study of factors inhibiting absorption and effective therapeutic levels of declomycin. *Surg. Gynecol. Obstet.* **114**, 9–14.

Schelling, J. L., Muller-Hess, S., and Thonney, F. (1973). Effect of food on zinc absorption. *Lancet* **2**, 283–284.

Shils, M. E. (1962). Some metabolic aspects of tetracycline. *Clin. Pharmacol. Ther.* **3**, 321–339.

Spivack, S. D. (1974). Procarbazine. *Ann. Intern. Med.* **81**, 795–800.

Steenbock, H., Krieger, C. H., Wiest, W. G., and Pileggi, V. J. (1953). Vitamin D and intestinal.phytase. *J. Biol. Chem.* **205**, 993–999.

Stoll, R. G., Bates, T. R., and Swarbrick, J. (1973). *In vitro* dissolution and *in vivo* absorption of nitrofurantoin from deoxycholic acid coprecipitates. *J. Pharm. Sci.* **62**, 55–68.

Thomas, J. C. S. (1963). Monamine oxidase inhibitors in cheese. *Br. Med. J.* **2**, 1406.

Thompson, W. B., and Thompson, G. R. (1969). Effect of cholestyramine on the absorption of vitamin D and calcium. *Gut* **10**, 717–722.

Tomasulo, R. M. G., Kater, M. V., and Iber, F. L. (1968). Impairment of thiamine absorption in alcoholism. *Am. J. Clin. Nutr.* **21**, 1341–1344.

Tomkin, G. H. (1973). Malabsorption of vitamin B_{12} in diabetic patients treated with phenformin: A comparison with metformin. *Br. Med. J.* **3**, 673–675.

Tomkin, G. H., Hadden, D. R., Weaver, J. A., and Montgomery, D. A. D. (1971). Vitamin B_{12} status of patients on long-term metformin therapy. *Br. Med. J.* **2**, 685–687.

Tuovenin, P. I. (1930). Uber den Alkoholgehalt des Blutes unter verschiedenen Bedingungen. *Skand. Arch. Physiol.* **60,** 1.

Visintine, R. E., Michaels, G. D., Fukayama, G., Conklin, J. D., and Kinsell, L. W. (1961). Xanthomatous biliary cirrhosis treated with cholestyramine. *Lancet* **2,** 341-343.

Welling, P. G., Lyons, L. L., Craig, W. A., and Trochta, G. A. (1975). Influence of diet and fluid on bioavailability of theophylline. *Clin. Pharmacol. Ther.* **17,** 475-480.

West, R. J., and Lloyd, J. K. (1975). The effect of cholestyramine on intestinal absorption. *Gut* **16,** 93-98.

Whiteside, C. H., Harkins, R. W., Fluckiger, H. B., and Sarett, H. P. (1965). Utilization of fat soluble vitamins by rats and chicks fed cholestyramine, a bile acid sequestrant. *Am. J. Clin. Nutr.* **16,** 309-314.

Wills, M. R., and Fairney, A. (1972). Effect of increased dietary phytic acid on cholecalciferol requirements in rats. *Lancet* **3,** 406-408.

Wood, J. H. (1967). Effect of food on aspirin absorption. *Lancet* **2,** 212.

12

Ascorbic Acid and Drug Metabolism

V. G. ZANNONI, P. H. SATO, and L. E. RIKANS

I. INTRODUCTION

Drug metabolism can be markedly influenced by many factors such as age, sex, strain and species, stress, hormones, drugs, environmental chemicals, as well as the nutritional status of the animal. With regard to ascorbic acid, most of the previous *in vivo* studies showed decreased metabolism of a variety of pharmacological agents in vitamin C-deficient animals but there is little information to date about the underlying biochemical basis for the action of the vitamin. The mechanism involved in hepatic drug metabolism is complex, involving an electron transport system. Our current knowledge of the microsomal pathway responsible for the detoxification of many pharmacological agents is shown in Fig. 1. The type of reactions which utilize this system include *O*-demethylation, *N*-demethylation, hydroxylation, nitro reduction as well as the hydroxy-

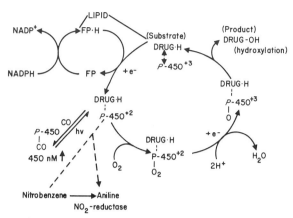

Fig. 1. Liver microsomal electron transport system responsible for the metabolism of drugs, steroids, and foreign chemicals.

lation of steroids, including cholesterol. The electron transport system contains a heme protein, cytochrome P-450, which is reduced by NADPH via a flavoprotein, cytochrome P-450 reductase. For oxidative metabolic reactions, cytochrome P-450, in its reduced state (Fe^{+2}), incorporates one atom of oxygen into the drug substrate and another into water. Many metabolic reductive reactions also utilize this system. In addition, there is a lipid component, phosphatidylcholine, which is associated with the electron transport and is an obligatory requirement for drug metabolism. It is obvious that in such a complex series of events the vitamin could participate at a variety of levels.

In 1941, Richards *et al.* found that pentobarbital-sleeping time was prolonged in scorbutic guinea pigs which could be reversed when ascorbic acid was administered. In 1954, Axelrod *et al.* observed a threefold increase in the plasma half-life of such compounds as acetanilide, aniline, and antipyrine in ascorbic acid-deficient guinea pigs and upon repleting the animals with ascorbic acid the half-life of the drugs returned to normal levels. In 1961, Conney *et al.* demonstrated that vitamin C-deficient guinea pigs with no obvious signs of scurvy were sensitive to the muscle relaxant, zoxazolamine, and that the increased duration of action of the drug *in vivo* correlated with a decrease in its liver microsomal oxidation *in vitro*. In 1965, Degkwitz and Staudinger observed that the *p*-hydroxylation of acetanilide as well as the hydroxylation of coumarin decreased in scorbutic animals, and the diminished hydroxylation of coumarin was reversed when the deficient animals were given ascorbic acid (Degkwitz *et al.*, 1968). The effect of ascorbic acid deficiency on the activities of ethoxycoumarin demethylase, benzo(a)-pyrene hydroxylase, and epoxide hydrase were examined in guinea pig lung, intestine, and liver by Kuenzig *et al.* (1976). Ethoxycoumarin demethylase activity in liver and lung decreased to 50% of control activity by day 10; in contrast, intestinal ethoxycoumarin demethylase remained unchanged. Furthermore, ascorbic acid deficiency had no effect on benzo(a)pyrene hydroxylase or epoxide hydrase activity in liver, lung, or intestine. These workers conclude that the effect of ascorbic acid deficiency on microsomal enzyme activity is substrate- and tissue-dependent in the guinea pig.

An effect of ascorbic acid on *in vitro* drug oxidation has also been demonstrated. Leber *et al.* (1969) reported that liver microsomes from scorbutic animals had significant decreases in the demethylation of aminopyrene, hydroxylation of acetanilide, and cytochrome P-450 content, but not cytochrome b_5 content. They also showed that phenobarbital and 3-methylcholanthrene (inducers of the microsomal electron transport system) caused an increase in the mixed-function oxygenases in the scorbutic animal, which could be blocked by the prior administration of ethionine. Kato *et al.* (1969) studied the metabolism of a variety of compounds such as aniline, hexobarbital, zoxazolamine, aminopyrine, diphenhydramine, meperidine, p-nitroanisole, p-nitrobenzoic acid, and p-dimethylaminobenzene in microsomes prepared from ascorbic acid-deficient adult guinea pigs maintained on a deficient diet for 12 days. In contrast to some of the previous studies, these investigators showed that although the metabolism of aniline, hexobarbital, and zoxazolamine decreased, the metabolism of the other drugs examined was unaltered. Furthermore, there was no significant decrease in microsomal electron transport components, such as cytochrome P-450 or cytochrome b_5, or in the activity of NADPH cytochrome c reductase or NADPH oxidase. They concluded that the effect of vitamin C deficiency is rather specific on hydroxylation reactions only and involves the "terminal oxidase" component of the electron system. In contrast to the above findings, *in vitro* studies in our laboratory (Zannoni *et al.*, 1972) using young guinea pigs weighing 200–250 gm indicated a substantial decrease in drug oxidation reactions such as aniline hydroxylation, aminopyrine N-demethylation and p-nitroanisole O-demethylation. In addition, there was a significant decrease in the quantity of cytochrome P-450 and NADPH cytochrome P-450 reductase. However, the decreased activities occurred only when the microsomal ascorbic acid had reached 30% of normal values. Recent studies by Sikic *et al.* (1976) indicate that both cytochrome P-450 and aminopyrine N-demethylation decreased to 60% of control values in liver microsomes at 21 and 25 days of deficiency, whereas there were no significant changes in other organs such as lung and kidney. Glutathione S-aryltransferase activity was decreased in scorbutic liver and unchanged in lung. On the other hand, N-acetylation of p-aminobenzoic acid, a nonmicrosomal drug detoxification reaction, was increased in kidneys of deficient animals with no changes in the other two organs. Repletion with ascorbic acid resulted in complete recovery of liver microsomal metabolism by day 7. The latter finding is in keeping with our studies in that we found that it required at least 6 days for various drug metabolism activities to return to normal levels upon replenishing the diet of deficient animals with ascorbic acid.

II. *IN VIVO* EFFECTS OF ASCORBIC ACID

The effect of vitamin C deficiency on drug enzymes and electron transport components in young male guinea pigs (200–250 gm) maintained on a deficient diet for 10 or 21 days is shown in Table I. Aniline hydroxylation, aminopyrine N-demethylation, and p-nitroanisole O-demethylation were not altered after 10 days but were significantly decreased in animals on the deficient diet for 21 days. Similar results were found with the electron transport components in that the quantity of cytochrome P-450 and P-450 reductase were significantly depressed in 21-day-deficient animals. At this time the concentration of liver ascorbic acid was approximately 30% of normal; the animals had lost at most 5% of their body weight and were not frankly scorbutic. In addition, fasted animals which were supplemented with the vitamin and had lost between 25% to 30% of their body weight had either normal or higher drug oxidation activity, indicating that the decrease observed in the ascorbic acid-deficient animals was not due to reduced caloric intake.

A more dramatic effect of the *in vivo* requirement of ascorbic acid was obtained when animals undergoing rapid growth such as weanling guinea pigs, (90–100 gm, 1–2 weeks of age) were placed on a vitamin C-deficient diet for a relatively short period of time, 8 or 15 days. In addition, and importantly, an increased dietary intake of ascorbic acid in these animals resulted in a concomitant increase in a variety of drug oxidative reactions and electron transport components (Table II). Microsomal NADPH cytochrome P-450 reductase, N-demethylase and O-demethylase increased as much as 200, 60 and 300%, respectively, compared to the activities in microsomes isolated from 15-day-deficient animals. Under these conditions the increase in the quantity of cytochrome P-450 was less than 45%. However, when animals were placed on a normal chow diet and supplemented with 1 mg/ml of ascorbic acid in

Effect of Vitamin C Deficiency (10 and 21 Days) on Drug Enzymes and Electron Transport Components in Guinea Pig Liver Microsomes[a]

	Activity[b]			
	Normal[c]	Vitamin C-deficient (10 days)	Vitamin C-deficient (21 days)	Decrease (%)
Aniline hydroxylase	1.6 ± 0.2	1.3 ± 0.1	0.8 ± 0.2 $p < 0.001$	50
Aminopyrine N-demethylase	3.9 ± 0.1	3.3 ± 0.4	1.7 ± 0.3 $p < 0.001$	56
p-Nitroanisole O-demethylase	3.2 ± 0.4	3.0 ± 0.2	1.1 ± 0.2 $p < 0.001$	66
Cytochrome P-450	0.05 ± 0.01	0.05 ± 0.001	0.03 ± 0.003 $p < 0.01$	40
NADPH cytochrome P-450 reductase	0.80 ± 0.2	0.87 ± 0.33	< 0.10	85
NADPH cytochrome c reductase	124 ± 21	167 ± 20	83 ± 11 $p < 0.05$	33
Cytochrome b_5	0.03 ± 0.004	0.03± 0.003	0.02 ± 0.006 $p > 0.05$	33
Liver ascorbic acid Supernatant fraction 15,000 g(mg/100 gm wet weight)	19.4 ± 2.9	6.2 ± 1.5	2.5 ± 1.5	
Microsomal fraction (mg/100 gm wet weight)	1.1 ± 0.38	0.6 ± 0.09	0.35 ± 0.20	

[a] Mean = SE of 10 animals per group. Data obtained from Zannoni et al. (1972).

[b] Activity of aniline hydroxylase, aminopyrine N-demethylase, and p-nitroanisole O-demethylase equals μmoles of product formed/hour/100 mg of microsomal protein at 27°C. Cytochrome P-450 equals μmoles/100 mg microsomal protein; NADPH cytochrome P-450 reductase equals μmoles reduced/hour/100 mg microsomal protein at 27°C.

[c] Normal animals (200–250 gm) were maintained on a vitamin C-deficient diet supplemented with 50 mg of ascorbic acid in their drinking water/day.

TABLE II
Stimulation of Drug Metabolism by Ascorbic Acid in Weanling Guinea Pigs[a,b]

Treatment	Liver ascorbic acid (mg/100 gm)	P-450	P-450 reductase	O-Demethylase	N-Demethylase
Deficient diet (15-day) (6)	<1.0	0.047 ± 0.002	3.4 ± 0.4	2.6 ± 0.2	10.0 ± 0.8
Deficient diet (8-day) (8)	2.5	0.061 ± 0.003	5.3 ± 0.9	6.2 ± 0.6	11.8 ± 0.8
Ascorbate (7 mg) (5)[c]	6	0.060 ± 0.004	7.0 ± 0.8	7.5 ± 0.5	14.1 ± 0.9
Ascorbate (25 mg) (6)[d]	8	0.060 ± 0.004	7.5 ± 0.8	8.0 ± 0.5	15.9 ± 2.3
Ascorbate (75 mg) (5)[e]	14	0.066 ± 0.006	8.9 ± 1.4	9.0 ± 0.5	15.6 ± 0.8
Chow[f]	27	0.068 ± 0.002	10.2 ± 0.7	10.5 ± 1.0	15.7 ± 0.4

[a] Data modified from Sato and Zannoni (1974).

[b] Units of activity: cytochrome P-450, μmoles/100 mg of microsomal protein; P-450 reductase, μmoles P-450 reduced/hour/100 mg of microsomal protein at 27°C; O-demethylase, μmoles p-nitrophenol formed/hour/100 mg of microsomal protein at 27°, N-demethylase, μmoles formaldehyde formed/hour/100 mg of microsomal protein at 27°. Mean ± S.E. per group is given. Number in parentheses is number of animals in each group.

[c] Ascorbate, 7 mg: vitamin C-deficient diet, and 7 mg ascorbic acid/day, orally, for 8 days.

[d] Ascorbate, 25 mg: vitamin C-deficient diet, and 25 mg ascorbic acid/day, orally, for 8 days.

[e] Ascorbate, 75 mg: vitamin C-deficient diet and 75 mg ascorbic acid/day, orally, for 8 days.

[f] Chow: chow diet supplemented three times/week with greens for 8 days.

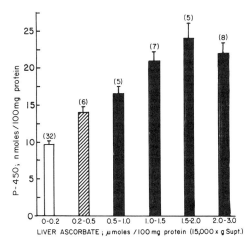

LIVER ASCORBATE ; μ moles / 100 mg protein (15,000 x g Supt.)

Fig. 2. Relationship between cytochrome P-450 and ascorbic acid concentration. Cytochrome P-450 and ascorbic acid were determined in the liver 15,000 × g supernatant fraction from guinea pigs maintained on an ascorbic acid-deficient diet (open bar), normal chow diet (cross-hatched bar) or chow plus 1 mg ascorbic acid/ml in the drinking water daily (solid bars). Animals were divided up into groups according to the concentration of ascorbic acid in their livers. One μ mole of ascorbic acid/100 mg protein equals 19 mg % (L. E. Rikans and V. G. Zannoni, unpublished data).

their drinking water, there was a marked increase in cytochrome P-450 (Fig. 2). The quantity of cytochrome P-450 increased 250% compared to deficient animals and 180% compared to animals on a normal chow diet without ascorbic acid supplements.

Studies with fetal guinea pig livers also showed a correlation between drug metabolism activities, the quantity of electron transport components, and liver ascorbic acid concentration. Fetal livers with ascorbic acid concentrations of 4.5 mg/100 gm liver had no detectable cytochrome P-450 or O-demethylase activity. On the other hand, fetal livers with an ascorbic acid concentration of 17.5 mg/100 gm liver, a level approaching that of the dams, had comparable cytochrome P-450 and O-demethylase activities, while livers with intermediate levels of ascorbic acid had intermediate levels of P-450 and O-demethylase activity (Zannoni and Sato, 1975).

III. SPECIFICITY STUDIES

The results of *in vivo* specificity studies with other reducing agents such as reduced 2,6-dichlorophenolindophenol dye, glutathione,

TABLE III
Effect of Various Reducing Agents in Drug Metabolism, *In Vivo* [a]

	Liver ascorbic acid (mg%)	Cytochrome P-450	NADPH cytochrome P-450 reductase	p-Nitroanisole O-demethylase	Aminopyrine N-demethylase
Chow diet	27.0	0.070	10.3	10.6	15.7
Ascorbic acid-deficient diet	2.0	0.060	5.6	6.0	10.8
+ ascorbate	13.5	0.067	8.7	9.1	15.6
+ reduced 2,6-DCPP	3.8	0.056	6.0	5.4	13.5
+ reduced GSH	1.2	0.064	8.9	6.0	13.6
+ D-isoascorbate	5.7	0.058	4.6		11.3
+ ascorbyl palmitate	10.8	0.069	6.7	8.3	13.0

[a] Treatment: Groups of weanling guinea pigs were fed as follows: Chow diet: Chow guinea pig diet supplemented with greens. 8-day ascorbic acid-deficient: Ascorbic acid-deficient guinea pig diet. Reduced 2,6-dichlorophenolindophenol dye: 2 mg/day given to guinea pigs on ascorbic acid-deficient diet, treated for 8 days. Reduced glutathione: 10 mg/day given to guinea pigs on ascorbic acid-deficient diet, treated for 8 days. D-Isoascorbate: 200 mg/day given to guinea pigs on ascorbic acid-deficient diet, treated for 8 days. Ascorbyl palmitate: 50 mg/day supplemented to guinea pigs on ascorbic acid-deficient diet, treated for 8 days.

Activities of cytochrome P-450 reductase, O-demethylase and N-demethylase equals μmoles of product formed/hour/100 mg of microsomal protein at 27°C. Cytochrome P-450 = μmoles/100 mg protein. Data obtained from Zannoni et al. (1974).

d-isoascorbic acid, and a more lipophilic analogue of ascorbic acid, ascorbyl palmitate, are shown in Table III. These compounds were not as effective as ascorbic acid in protecting drug metabolism activities. However, 2,6-dichlorophenolindophenol dye showed some protection of aminopyrine N-demethylase activity as did reduced glutathione. Also, the animals receiving glutathione had in the order of 60% more NADPH cytochrome P-450 reductase activity compared to 8-day-deficient animals. Ascorbyl palmitate could replace L-ascorbic acid when compared on an equal molar basis and d-isoascorbic acid was not as effective as the vitamin unless given more than one time per day. Under these conditions cytochrome P-450 and N-demethylase activity were increased to normal levels. The effect of d-isoascorbic acid can be explained, in part, by the difficulty in obtaining adequate tissue concentrations since it is rapidly excreted by the kidney. Similar results were observed by Degkwitz and Kim (1973) who, in addition, found that 5-oxo-D-gluconate could replace ascorbic acid in that the quantity of cytochrome P-450 and b_5 were about the same as in animals supplied with equal amounts of ascorbic acid (Table IV). These investigators suggest that since 5-oxo-D-gluconate cannot participate in an oxidation–reduction capacity that a possible function for ascorbic acid in drug metabolism is one other than an oxidation–reduction role. In addition, they not only found de-

TABLE IV

Effect of L-Ascorbate, 5-Oxo-D-Gluconate, and D-Arabino-Ascorbate on the Amounts of Cytochromes P-450 and b_5 in 14-Day Ascorbic Acid-Deficient Guinea Pigs[a]

Administration to deficient guinea pigs	Specific cytochrome concentration [nmole/mg protein] cytochrome P-450	Cytochrome b_5	Number of animals
None	0.65 ± 0.06	0.58 ± 0.04	10
Sodium L-ascorbate			
5 × /24 hours ip	1.00 ± 0.05	0.74 ± 0.07	6
5 × /24 hours per os	0.82 ± 0.09	0.57 ± 0.09	6
15 × /72 hours per os	1.52 ± 0.18	1.07 ± 0.13	5
Potassium 5-oxo-D-gluconate			
5 × /24 hours per os	0.89 ± 0.09	0.77 ± 0.14	5
Sodium D-arabino-ascorbate			
5 × /24 hours ip	0.93 ± 0.09	0.68 ± 0.09	5
5 × /24 hours per os	0.72 ± 0.17	0.62 ± 0.07	4
10 × /48 hours per os	0.72 ± 0.06	0.58 ± 0.06	4
15 × /72 hours per os	0.86 ± 0.18	0.55 ± 0.12	9

[a] Data modified from Degkwitz and Kim (1973).

creased levels of cytochrome P-450, P-454 and b_5 in liver microsomes prepared from vitamin C-deficient guinea pigs but also in adrenals, kidneys, and spleen (Degkwitz et al., 1974).

Additional in vitro dialysis studies with microsomes prepared from normal animals indicated that ascorbic acid was more effective than glutathione or d-isoascorbic acid in protecting cytochrome P-450 and drug enzyme activities from the detrimental effects of dialysis (Table V). Upon dialysis, microsomal ascorbic acid decreased from 0.08 to 0.03 μmoles per 100 mg of microsomal protein; cytochrome P-450 decreased from 0.05 to 0.02 while O-demethylase activity decreased about 90% (from 6.6 to 0.8 μmoles of p-nitrophenol formed per hour per 100 mg of microsomal protein). With prior addition of ascorbic acid to the dialysate (3.0 × 10^{-4} M), cytochrome P-450 was protected 33%, and O-demethylase activity was protected 93%. Glutathione at a concentration of 3.0 × 10^{-4} M was not an effective protective agent but, at five times the concentration of ascorbic acid, it protected cytochrome P-450 by 67% and O-demethylase activity by 91%. In addition, ascorbic acid sulfate of gulonolactone at a concentration of 3.0 × 10^{-4} M were not protective. Moreover, the in vitro addition of ascorbic acid to dialyzed microsomes did not activate O-demethylase, or increase the ability of cytochrome P-450 to bind carbon monoxide.

TABLE V
Loss of Cytochrome P-450 and O-Demethylase Activity on Dialysis in Normal Guinea Pig Microsomes and Protection by Ascorbic Acid[a]

	Ascorbic[b] acid	P-450[c]	O-demethylase[d]
Undialyzed microsomes	0.08	0.05	6.6
Dialyzed microsomes	0.03	0.02	0.8
Dialyzed versus ascorbic acid	0.25	0.042	6.2
Dialyzed versus d-isoascorbic acid	0.29	0.03	6.2
Dialyzed versus glutathione	0.04	0.02	1.4

[a] One ml of liver microsomes (20 mg protein/ml) from normal guinea pigs were dialyzed against 1 liter of 0.25 M sucrose (pH 7.5) for 3.5 days at 4°C, with stirring. Other dialyses were carried out in 0.25 M sucrose containing ascorbic acid, or d-isoascorbic acid, or glutathione at a concentration of 3.0 × $10^{-4} M$, pH 7.5, for 3.5 days at 4°C with stirring. Control undialyzed microsomes were stored at 4°C for 3.5 days. Data from Sato (1976).
[b] Ascorbic acid; μmoles/100 mg microsomal protein
[c] P-450; μmoles/100 mg microsomal protein
[d] O-demethylase; μmoles of p-nitrophenol formed/hour/100 mg microsomal protein at 27°C.

IV. *IN VIVO* REVERSAL OF DRUG METABOLISM AND CYTOCHROME *P*-450 TURNOVER IN DEFICIENT GUINEA PIGS

Drug enzyme activities and the microsomal electron transport components required from 6 to 10 days to return to normal levels in 21-day vitamin C-deficient animals replenished with ascorbic acid in spite of the fact that the quantity of liver ascorbic acid reached normal levels within 3 days (Zannoni *et al.*, 1972). These findings are in keeping with the *in vivo* studies of Axelrod *et al.* (1954) who found that the plasma half-life of such compounds as aniline, antipyrine, and acetanilide in vitamin C-deficient guinea pigs was increased by 60% and took from 5 to 8 days to return to normal when the animals were given ascorbic acid. Also, Sikic *et al.* (1976) showed that although partial recovery from decreases in drug metabolism occurred in 3 days, complete recovery required 7 days. Degkwitz and Kim (1973) found that cytochrome *P*-450 and cytochrome b_5 returned to normal levels in a shorter period of time, from 1 to 1.5 days, after the liver ascorbic acid concentration had reached normal levels. They gave the vitamin intraperitoneally 5 times per day and to animals on a deficient diet for shorter periods, 14 days. However, it required up to 3 days after the liver ascorbic acid concentration had reached normal levels for cytochrome *P*-450 and cytochrome b_5 to return to normal levels when the vitamin was given orally on the repeated dosage schedule.

The time required for the reestablishment of adequate drug metabolism activity in deficient animals could be due to the time needed for the resynthesis of specific proteins associated with drug enzymes. To test this, several laboratories using drug enzyme inducers such as phenobarbital or 3-methylcholanthrene have shown that the protein synthesizing machinery involved in the microsomal electron transport is not substantially jeopardized and is operable in vitamin C deficiency (Kato *et al.*, 1969; Zannoni *et al.*, 1972; Avenia, 1972). For example, in animals pretreated with phenobarbital, it was found that aniline hydroxylase, aminopyrine *N*-demethylase and *p*-nitroanisole *O*-demethylase, as well as cytochrome *P*-450, NADPH *P*-450 reductase, and NADPH cytochrome *c* reductase were induced to the same extent in ascorbic acid-deficient compared to normal animals; the fold increase in specific activity was the same order of magnitude in both groups (Table VI). It appears from these studies that ascorbic acid is not involved in general protein synthesis but the possibility that it could participate more specifically in heme synthesis was also investigated. Luft *et al.* (1972) reported

TABLE VI
Phenobarbital Induction of Drug Enzymes and Electron Transport Components in Normal and Vitamin C-Deficient Guinea Pigs[a]

	Activity[b]					
	Normal[c]			Vitamin C-deficient[c]		
	No Rx	PB Rx	Fold increase	No Rx	PB Rx	Fold increase
Aniline hydroxylase	1.6	2.3	1.4	0.8	1.7	2.1
Aminopyrine N-demethylase	3.9	9.6	2.5	1.7	7.6	4.5
p-Nitroanisole O-demethylase	3.2	11.1	3.5	1.1	6.5	5.9
Cytochrome P-450	0.05	0.11	2.2	0.03	0.06	2.0
NADPH P-450 reductase	0.8	2.6	3.3	<0.10	2.8	28.0
NADPH cytochrome c reductase	124.0	288.0	2.3	83.0	250.0	3.0
Cytochrome b_5	0.03	0.03	1.0	0.02	0.02	1.0

[a] Phenobarbital treatment: guinea pigs received 1 mg sodium phenobarbital/ml for 4 days in drinking water; 30–40 ml consumed per day. Data modified from Zannoni *et al.* (1972).

[b] Activity equals µmoles of product formed/hour/100 mg of microsomal protein at 27°C.

[c] Liver ascorbic acid: normal induced, 195 µg/gm wet weight (15,000 × g supernatant fraction), 19 µg/gm wet weight (microsomal fractin); vitamin C-deficient induced, 71 µg/gm wet weight (15,000 × g supernatant fraction), 5 µg/gm wet weight (microsomal fraction).

TABLE VII

Effect of δ-Aminolevulinic Acid on the Content of Cytochrome *P*-450 in the Liver of Ascorbic Acid-Deficient Guinea Pigs[a]

	Number of animals	Ascorbic acid (μg/gm liver)	Cytochrome *P*-450 (nmole/mg protein)	Cytochrome b_5 (nmole/mg protein)
21 Days ascorbic acid-deficient guinea pigs	12	<10	0.46 ± 0.11	0.47 ± 0.12
+ Ascorbic acid	6	271 ± 76	0.81 ± 0.07	0.45 ± 0.11
+ δ-Aminolevulinic acid	6	<10	0.90 ± 0.16	0.65 ± 0.12
+ Ascorbic acid and δ-aminolevulinic acid	7	209 ± 47	0.99 ± 0.14	0.54 ± 0.08
+ δ-Aminolevulinic acid and actinomycin D	7	<10	0.60 ± 0.07	0.46 ± 0.03

[a] Data modified from Luft *et al.* (1972).

that the administration of a precursor of heme, d-aminolevulinic acid (ALA), to vitamin C-deficient guinea pigs caused an increase in the quantity of cytochrome P-450 (Table VII) and suggested that ascorbic acid may be involved in the formation of this essential metabolite of heme synthesis. The synthesis of heme is given below in Scheme 1.

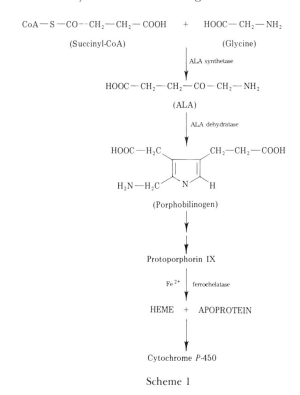

Scheme 1

In view of these findings, it was important to determine if vitamin C deficiency affected the activity of ALA synthetase, the rate-limiting enzyme in heme synthesis (Kappas *et al.*, 1968). Studies in our laboratory indicate that although the cytochrome P-450 content in livers from guinea pigs on a vitamin C-deficient diet was markedly decreased compared to control livers (10.3 compared with 17.9 nmole/100 mg supernatant protein), there were no significant differences in ALA synthetase activity, neither in whole cell homogenate (18.1 versus 16.5 nmole/hour/100 mg protein) nor in mitochondria (720 versus 680 nmole/hour/100 mg protein) (Table VIII). Thus, it appears that ascorbic acid deficiency does not affect the initial step in heme biosynthesis. However, the possibility that one of the other enzymes in heme synthesis may be

TABLE VIII

Cytochrome P-450 Content and the Activities of ALA Synthetase in Control and Ascorbic Acid-Deficient Guinea Pigs[a]

Treatment	Cytochrome[b] P-450 (nmole/100 mg)	ALA synthetase[c] homogenate (nmole/hour/100 mg)	ALA synthetase[c] mitochondria (nmole/hour/100 mg)
Normal[d]	19.2 ± 1.1 (12)	16.5 ± 2.3 (12)	680 ± 50 (5)
Ascorbate-deficient[d]	9.5 ± 0.7 (11)	18.1 ± 1.9 (11)	720 ± 90 (5)

[a] Values are mean ± S.E.; number in parentheses equals animals. Data from L. E. Rikans, C. R. Smith, and V. G. Zannoni (1977).

[b] Cytochrome P-450 was determined in the liver 15,000 g supernatant fraction; $p < 0.01$.

[c] Activity equals nmol ALA formed/hour/100 mg of whole cell homogenate or sonicated mitochondrial protein at 37°.

[d] Ascorbic acid was determined in the liver 15,000 g supernatant fraction and was 1740 nmoles/100 mg protein in normal and 99 nmoles/100 mg protein in deficient animals.

affected in vitamin C depletion should be considered. For example, there could be differences in ferrochelatase activity, since iron must be maintained in its ferrous state for incorporation into protoporphorin IX (Burnham, 1968), and ascorbic acid might be involved at this level. Furthermore, it would be of interest to examine the degradation of cytochrome P-450, since a reduction of P-450 content in ascorbic acid-deficient livers could also be the result of an increased breakdown of the cytochrome.

V. DRUG–CYTOCHROME P-450 BINDING AND K_m STUDIES

A qualitative difference in drug cytochrome P-450 binding spectra occurs in vitamin C-deficient guinea pig microsomes with type II substrates such as aniline (Zannoni *et al.*, 1972). The spectrum is atypical in that the trough is at 405 nm instead of 390 nm and the peak at 440 nm instead of 430 nm. There is also a decrease in the absorption intensity, which correlated with the decrease in the quantity of cytochrome P-450 in the deficient animals. The addition of ascorbic acid or other reducing agents such as glutathione or reduced 2,6-dichlorophenolindophenol did not reverse the altered aniline–cytochrome P-450 binding. However, ascorbyl palmitate, a more lipophilic analogue of ascorbic acid, did restore atypical aniline–cytochrome P-450 binding spectra but the absorption intensity at 450 nm was still depressed. Gundermann *et al.* (1973)

also found differences in drug cytochrome P-450 binding in that the type I hexobarbital binding spectra required higher concentrations of the barbiturate to achieve half maximal spectral changes.

Kinetic studies from a variety of laboratories indicate no significant changes in the apparent K_m of overall drug metabolism reactions such as aminopyrine N-demethylation, p-nitroanisole O-demethylation, or hexobarbital hydroxylation (Zannoni et al., 1972; Zannoni and Sato, 1975; Avenia, 1972; Gundermann et al., 1973). The data in Table IX gives the K_m values of aminopyrine N-demethylase and p-nitroanisole O-demethylase with microsomes isolated from 8 and 15-day ascorbic acid-deficient animals, animals receiving 50 mg/day of ascorbic acid for 8 days, and animals receiving a normal diet of chow pellets. As can be observed, the apparent Michaelis-Menten affinity constants were not significantly altered in any of the groups. Gundermann et al. (1973) also found no apparent change in the K_m of hexobarbital in normal and ascorbic acid deficient microsomes, $6.2 \times 10^{-3} M$ versus $5.0 \times 10^{-3} M$.

VI. LIPID PEROXIDATION AND PHOSPHATIDYLCHOLINE IN NORMAL AND DEFICIENT ANIMALS

It is known that lipid peroxidation is detrimental to drug metabolism and antioxidants which inhibit peroxidation, such as N,N'-diphenyl-

TABLE IX
Apparent K_m of Liver Microsomal Aminopyrine N-Demethylase and p-Nitroanisole O-Demethylase of Weanling Guinea Pigs on Various Ascorbic Acid Regimens[a]

	N-Demethylase[b] (K_m)	O-Demethylase[b] (K_m)	Liver ascorbate (mg/100 gm)
Chow diet	$1.67 \times 10^{-3} M$	$5.40 \times 10^{-4} M$	27.0
Deficient diet plus ascorbate (50 mg/day/8 days)	$1.57 \times 10^{-3} M$	$4.35 \times 10^{-4} M$	9.9
Deficient diet for 8 days	$1.67 \times 10^{-3} M$	$4.43 \times 10^{-4} M$	2.0
Deficient diet for 15 days	$1.82 \times 10^{-3} M$	$2.10 \times 10^{-4} M$	<1.0

[a] Data modified from Sato and Zannoni (1974, 1976).
[b] Microsomal N-demethylase and O-demethylase were determined by incubating 6 concentrations of aminopyrine ($8.0 \times 10^{-3} M$–$6.7 \times 10^{-4} M$) and 7 concentrationsn of p-nitroanisole ($1.0 \times 10^{-3} M$–$1.5 \times 10^{-4} M$) with microsomes prepared from the various groups of animals. The apparent K_m values were calculated form reciprocal plots of 1| velocity versus 1| substrate concentration.

TABLE X
Lipid Peroxidation in Normal and Vitamin C-Deficient Microsomes[a]

		Activity[b]	
	Oxygen uptake	Malonaldehyde formed	NADPH disappearance
Normal[c]	160	0.33	10.3
Vitamin C-deficient[d]	118 (74%)	0.23 (70%)	7.9 (77%)

[a] Data obtained from Sato and Zannoni (1976).
[b] Activity; μmoles/hour/100 mg microsomal protein at 27°C.
[c] Normal (chow diet plus greens); liver ascorbic acid = 27.7 mg/100 gm liver.
[d] Vitamin C deficient (15 days); liver ascorbic acid = 4.3 mg/100 gm liver.

enediamine, protect drug enzyme activities (Carpenter, 1972). The possibility existed that ascorbic acid through its property as an antioxidant could be functioning by inhibiting lipid peroxidation. Table X gives results on the rate of lipid peroxidation in normal and deficient guinea pig microsomes using three methods of assay, oxygen consumption, NADPH disappearance, and malonaldehyde formation (Sato and Zannoni, 1976). The rate of lipid perioxidation was, in fact, somewhat lower in microsomes deficient of the vitamin compared to control microsomes and it is unlikely that the decrease in drug metabolism activities and quantity of electron transport components observed in vitamin C deficiency can be accounted for via this mechanism. Furthermore, analysis of the quantity of the essential lipid component involved in drug metabolism, phosphatidylcholine, in normal, vitamin C-deficient, and starved animals indicate that the ascorbic acid-deficient microsomes showed only an 18% decrease in the quantity of phosphatidylcholine compared to nondeficient microsomes (Table XI). However, in fasted animals given ascorbic acid, the quantity of phosphatidylcholine was even lower than in vitamin C-deficient animals, despite the fact that the concentration of ascorbic acid in livers of the starved animals was adequate (42.6 mg/100 gm wet weight liver) and they had normal drug metabolism activities (Sato and Zannoni, 1974). In addition, there was no significant difference in the chromatographic migration of either phosphatidylcholine or its precursor, phosphatidylethanolamine in normal or vitamin C-deficient animals (Sato and Zannoni, 1976); authentic phosphatidylcholine, R_f = 0.64, normal R_f = 0.68, vitamin C-deficient R_f = 0.66; authentic phosphatidylethanolamine, R_f = 0.80, normal R_f = 0.84, vitamin C-deficient R_f = 0.82.

TABLE XI
Phosphatidylcholine in Normal, Vitamin C-Deficient and Starved Guinea Pigs[a]

	Phosphatidylcholine (μmoles/100 mg microsomal protein)	Microsomal protein (mg/ml)	Body weight (gm)	Liver weight (gm)	$\frac{\text{Liver}}{\text{body}}$ (%)
Normal[b]	27.2	34.8	249	10.6	4.3
Vitamin C-deficient[c]	22.4	32.2	236	13.0	5.5
Starved[d]	19.2	23.0	155	5.5	3.5

[a] Data obtained from Sato and Zannoni (1976).
[b] Normal; chow diet plus greens; ascorbic acid = 51.1 mg/100 gm liver
[c] Vitamin C-deficient; 15 days; ascorbic acid = 3.6 mg/100 gm liver
[d] Starved; 3 days plus 17 mg ascorbic acid/ml in drinking water; ascorbic acid = 42.6 mg/100 gm liver

VII. COMPARATIVE PHYSICOCHEMICAL PROPERTIES OF CYTOCHROME P-450 IN NORMAL AND ASCORBIC ACID-DEFICIENT MICROSOMES

The properties of hepatic microsomal cytochrome P-450 prepared from normal and ascorbic acid-deficient animals did not differ with respect to storage at $5°$, treatment with sodium cholate, treatment with glycerol, and microsomal protein concentration. In addition, the quantity of microsomal cytochrome b_5, and cytochrome P-420, the inactive form of cytochrome P-450 was not significantly different (Sato and Zannoni, 1976). However, some physicochemical differences were found and include behavior upon sonication or dialysis. The time required to inactivate 50% of cytochrome P-450 prepared from normal animals was 180 seconds compared to 78 seconds for deficient guinea pigs. The addition of ascorbic acid (2.0 mM) did not protect the microsomes from either group from the effects of sonication. Furthermore, dialysis of microsomes from normal guinea pigs for 60 hours resulted in less of a decrease in the quantity of cytochrome P-450 and O-demethylase activity compared to the decrease obtained with ascorbic acid-deficient microsomes. Cytochrome P-450 prepared from deficient animals decreased 87% compared to 18% in the normal microsomes and O-demethylase activity decreased 74% compared to 28%. The presence of ascorbic acid $(1.7 \times 10^{-3} M)$ protected both cytochrome P-450 and O-demythlase activity (up to 90%). D-Isoascorbic acid $(3.0 \times 10^{-4} M)$ could replace L-ascorbic acid in that cytochrome P-450 was protected 33%, and O-demethylase activity was protected 93%. Glutathione, ascorbic acid sulfate, or gulonolactone at a concentration of $3.0 \times 10^{-4} M$ were ineffective (<5% protection).

Determination of the concentration of liver microsomal ascorbic acid and cytochrome P-450 indicated that there is a relatively consistent quantitative relationship of ascorbic acid to cytochrome P-450. The ratio of liver ascorbic acid to cytochrome P-450 was in the order of 2.0 in both ascorbic acid-deficient and normal microsomes. Similar results were also obtained in adrenal tissue. In addition, various fractions obtained with partial purification by ammonium sulfate and calcium phosphate gel of cytochrome P-450 from normal and ascorbic acid-deficient guinea pig livers had ratios of ascorbic acid to total CO-binding heme protein from 1.3 to 3.7 (in the normal) and from 1.2 to 3.0 (in the ascorbic and acid-deficient). These experiments suggested that ascorbic acid may be more directly associated with the heme protein, perhaps with the iron. In keeping with this concept, $\alpha\alpha'$-dipyridyl, a ferrous iron chelator, was found to inhibit the CO-binding spectra of cytochrome P-450 resulting in a decrease in the cytochrome P-450–CO absorption spectrum at 450 nm. The cytochrome P-450–CO binding decreased in the order of 50% in the presence of 12.8 mM α,α'-dipyridyl. Importantly, the decrease of the cytochrome P450–CO spectrum by the chelator could be prevented by 22.7 mM ascorbic acid. In addition, o-phenanthroline, another inhibitor with a high affinity for ferrous iron, inhibited the cytochrome P-450–CO binding spectrum to the same extent as was found with α,α'-dipyridyl and its action was also prevented by the vitamin. The decreased formation of the CO–cytochrome P-450 spectrum by α,α'-dipyridyl and o-phenanthroline can be accounted for since these metal chelators can bind to the reduced ferrous iron of cytochrome P-450 resulting in a spectrum which has an absorption maximum at the same wavelength as the cytochrome P-450–CO ligand, i.e., at 450 nm (Sato and Zannoni, 1976). Table XII summarizes the inhibition of cytochrome P-450–CO spectrum formation by α,α'-dipyridyl as well as other metal chelators in guinea pig microsomes. Of the chelators tested only ferrous iron chelators, such as α,α'-dipyridyl and o-phenanthroline significantly inhibited the cytochrome P-450–CO spectrum (55% inhibition). Ascorbic acid at a concentration of 22.7 mM protected against this inhibition. The apparent affinity constants of α,α'-dipyridyl for inhibition of cytochrome P-450–CO ligand formation in normal microsomes was 2.99×10^{-4} M, and 3.14×10^{-4} M in deficient microsomes. Ascorbic acid was protective in both cases and had an affinity constant of 4.98×10^{-4} M

TABLE XII
Inhibition of Cytochrome P-450–CO Ligand Formation by Metal Chelators in Normal Guinea Pig Microsomes[a]

	Cytochrome P-450 (μmoles/100 mg microsomal protein)	Inhibition (%)	Cytochrome b_5 (μmoles/100 mg microsomal protein)
No inhibitor	0.085	—	0.043
α,α'-Dipyridyl	0.038	55	0.039
o-Phenanthroline	0.038	55	0.038
8-Hydroxyquinoline sulfonate	0.091	−6	0.039
Bathocuproine[b]	0.096	−13	0.034
Diethyldithiocarbamate	0.082	3	0.041

[a] Washed microsomes (4.0 mg protein/ml) were incubated with the various metal chelators at concentration of 12.8 mM for 3 days at 4°C. Data obtained from Sato and Zannoni (1976).

[b] Bathocuproine and diethyldithiocarbamate converted cytochrome P-450 to cytochrome P-4 The value for P-450 with bathocuproine represents 44% cytochrome P-420 and the value for P-4 with diethyldithiocarbamate represents 17% cytochrome P-420.

TABLE XIII
Inhibition of Aniline Hydroxylase and Cytochrome P-450–CO Ligand by α,α'-Dipyridyl and Protection by Ascorbic Acid[a]

		Days of treatment		
		0	2	3
Untreated[b]	Aniline hydroxylase[c]	1.33	1.16	0.89
	Cytochrome P-450–CO[d]	0.068	0.069	0.061
+ α,α'-	Aniline hydroxylase	2.20	1.03	0.50
Dipyridyl	Cytochrome P-450–CO	0.067	0.042	0.031
+ α,α'-	Aniline hydroxylase	1.75	1.35	1.03
Dipyridyl and ascorbic acid	Cytochrome P-450–CO	0.068	0.072	0.073

[a] Washed microsomes (4.0 mg protein/ml) from normal guinea pig livers were treated with α,α'-dipyridyl (2.7 mM) for 2 and 3 days at 4°C; other microsomal preparations were treated with α,α'-dipyridyl (2.7 mM) plus ascorbic acid (22.7 mM). Aliquots (0.5 ml) of the microsomes were assayed for aniline hydroxylase in an incubation volume of 3.0 ml. Aliquots of the α,α'-dipyridyl-treated microsomes were diluted 1:10 with 0.05 M sodium phosphate, $1 \times 10^{-3} M$ EDTA, pH 7.4, for determination of cytochrome P-450–CO. Data obtained from Sato and Zannoni (1976).

[b] Untreated microsomes with added ascorbic acid (22.7 mM) did not differ significantly in aniline hydroxylase activity and amount of cytochrome P-450–CO found in untreated microsomes with no ascorbic acid added.

[c] Aniline hydroxylwse; μmoles p-aminophenol formed/hour/100 mg microsomal protein.

[d] Cytochrome P-450–CO; μmole/100 mg microsomal protein.

in normal and $4.83 \times 10^{-4} M$ in deficient microsomes (Sato and Zannoni, 1976). Glutathione was less effective than ascorbic acid in its protective ability and had an affinity constant of $20.8 \times 10^{-4} M$. In contrast to $\alpha\alpha'$-dipyridyl and o-phenanthroline, structurally related chelators with high affinity for copper, such as 8-hydroxyquinoline sulfonate, bathocuproine, or diethyldithiocarbamate did not significantly inhibit cytochrome P-450–CO spectrum formation (<5%). The metal chelators, in general, showed slight inhibition on the microsomal heme protein cytochrome b_5 and 22.7 mM ascorbic acid had no protective effect on this cytochrome. *In addition*, the effect of α,α'-dipyridyl on microsomal hydroxylation reactions is shown in Table XIII. The degree of reduction of aniline hydroxylase activity corresponded to the amount of cytochrome P-450-$\alpha\alpha'$-dipyridyl ligand formed, and the inhibition by $\alpha\alpha'$-dipyridyl was averted when ascorbic acid was added to the microsomal preparations. Thus, ascorbic acid was effective in protecting not only the cytochrome P-450–CO spectrum formation but also the hydroxylase activity from $\alpha\alpha'$-dipyridyl inhibition.

VIII. RESEARCH NEEDS

In vivo studies have been shown that the liver microsomal drug metabolism system as well as steroid and cholesterol metabolism have decreased activity in ascorbic acid deficiency and are enhanced when high supplements of the vitamin are given to guinea pigs. Drug metabolizing activities and microsomal electron transport components could be reversed by *in vivo* repletion of ascorbic acid to vitamin C-deficient animals. It required, in most cases, from 3 to 6 days. Studies with drug enzyme inducers indicate that *de novo* protein synthesis is operable in vitamin C deficiency and the activity of the initial enzymatic step in heme synthesis is not compromised. Kinetic studies with typical drug enzymes such as N-demethylase and O-demethylase indicate that there is no significant change in the affinity of these enzymes for their substrates in normal, ascorbic acid-deficient, or in animals given high supplements of the vitamin. In addition, the decrease in drug metabolism activity observed in ascorbic acid deficiency is not due to increased lipid peroxidation or a quantitative change in the essential phospholipid component involved in drug metabolism, i.e., phosphatidylcholine.

Differences which exist between normal and ascorbic acid-deficient microsomes include: less stability of ascorbic acid-deficient microsomes to sonication, dialysis, and treatment with ferrous iron metal chelators such as α,α'-dipyridyl and o-phenanthroline. The decrease in cytochrome P-450 and O-demethylase activity with dialysis could be prevented by ascorbic acid. Furthermore, a quantitative relationship of ascorbic acid to microsomal cytochrome P-450 was found in liver and adrenal tissue during dialysis of both normal and deficient microsomes and during partial purification of the cytochrome. In addition, ascorbic acid protected cytochrome P-450 from inhibition by ferrous iron chelators. These studies suggest that there is an interaction between ascorbic acid and cytochrome P-450 involving the heme iron.

The requirement for vitamin C in the metabolism of drugs, steroids, and cholesterol in humans may be important, especially during growth periods. Those individuals with insufficient intake of the vitamin may show sensitivity and possible toxicity to pharmacological agents. This would be the case, for example, if increased formation of drug metabolites is necessary to insure an adequate rate of drug detoxification. In this regard increasing the intake of ascorbic acid in humans above the recommended daily allowance to observe if there is an effect on the biological plasma half-life of a variety of drugs, steroids, and cholesterol would be of clinical interest.

ACKNOWLEDGMENTS

This study was supported, in part, by Grant No. 23007 from Hoffmann–La Roche, Inc.

REFERENCES

Avenia, R. W. (1972). Studies on the role of ascorbic acid in the metabolism of drugs by the guinea pig hepatic microsomal mixed-function oxidase system. Ph.D. Thesis, Cornell University Library, Ithaca, New York.

Axelrod, J., Udenfriend, S., and Brodie, B. B. (1954). Ascorbic acid in aromatic hydroxylation. III. Effects of ascorbic acid on hydroxylation of acetanilid, aniline, and antipyrine *in vivo. J. Pharmacol. Exp. Ther.* **111**, 176–181.

Burnham, B. (1968). The chemistry of the porphyrine. *Semin. Hematol.* **5**, 296–321.

Carpenter, M. P. (1972). Vitamin E and microsomal drug hydroxylations. *Ann. N.Y. Acad. Sci.* **203**, 81–92.

Conney, A. H., Bray, G. A., Evans, C., and Burns, J. J. (1961). Metabolic interactions between L-ascorbic acid and drugs. *Ann. N.Y. Acad. Sci.* **92**, 115–127.

Degkwitz, E., and Kim, K. S. (1973). Comparative studies on the influence of L-ascorbate, D-arabino-ascorbate and 5-oxo-D-gluconate on the amounts of cytochrome P-450 and b_5 in liver microsomes of guinea pigs. *Hoppe-Seyler's Z. Physiol. Chem.* **354**, 555–561.

Degkwitz, E., and Staudinger, H. (1965). Untersuchungen zur Hydroxylierung von Acetanilid mit Lebermikrosomen normaler und skorbutischer Meerschweinchen. *Hoppe-Seyler's Z. Physiol. Chem* **342**, 63–72.

Degkwitz, E., Luft, D., Pfeiffer, U., and Staudinger, H. (1968). Untersuchungen über microsomale Enzymaktivitäten (Cumarinhydroxylierung, NADPH-Oxidation, Glucose-6-Phosphatase und Cytochromgehalte (P-450 und b_5) bei normalen, skorbutischen und hungernden Meerschweinchen. *Hoppe-Seyler's Z. Physiol. Chem.* **349**, 465–471.

Degkwitz, E., Walsch, S., and Dubberstein, M. (1974). Influence of L-ascorbate on the concentrations of microsomal cytochrome P-450 and cytochrome b_5 in adrenals, kidney, and spleen on guinea pigs. *Hoppe-Seyler's Z. Physiol. Chem.* **355**, 1152–1158.

Gundermann, K., Degkwitz, E., and Staudinger, H. (1973). Mixed-function oxygenation of $(+)$ and $(-)$ hexobarbital and spectral changes of cytochrome P-450 in liver of guinea pigs fed without L-ascorbic acid. *Hoppe-Seyler's Z. Physiol. Chem.* **354**, 238–242.

Kappas, A., Levere, R. D., and Granick, S. (1968). The regulation of porphyrin and heme synthesis. *Semin. Hematol.* **5**, 323–334.

Kato, R., Takanaka, A., and Oshima, T. (1969). Effect of vitamin C deficiency on metabolism of drugs and TPNH-linked electron transport system in liver microsomes. *Jpn. J. Pharmacol.* **19**, 25–33.

Kuenzig, W., Tkaczevski, V., Kamm, J. J., Conney, A. H., and Burns, J. J. (1976). Ascorbic acid deficiency and extrahepatic metabolism of drugs and carcinogens. *Fed. Proc., Fed. Am.* **35**, 666.

Leber, H., Degkwitz, E., and Staudinger, H. (1969). Untersuchungen zum Einfluss der Ascorbinsäure auf die Aktivität und die Biosynthese mischfunktioneller Oxygenasen sowie den Gehalt an Hämoproteiden in der Mikrosomenfraktion der Meerschweinchenleber. *Hoppe-Seyler's Z. Physiol. Chem.* **350**, 439–445.

Luft, D., Degkwitz, E., Hochli-Kaufmann, L., and Staudinger, H. (1972). Einfluss von

d-Aminolävulinsäure auf den Gehalt an Cytochrom P-450 in der Leber ascorbin-
säurefrei ernährter Meerschweinchen. *Hoppe-Seyler's Z. Physiol. Chem.* **353,** 1420–
1422.

Richards, R. K., Keuter, K., and Klatt, T. I. (1941). Effects of vitamin C deficiency on
action of different types of barbiturates. *Proc. Soc. Exp. Biol. Med.* **48,** 403–409.

Rikans, L. E., Smith, C. R., and Zannoni, V. G. (1977). Ascorbic acid and heme synthesis in
deficient guinea pig liver. *Biochem. Pharmacol.* **26,** 797–799.

Sato, P. H. (1976). Ascorbic acid and hepatic microsomal drug metabolism. Ph.D. Thesis,
New York University, New York.

Sato, P. H., and Zannoni, V. G. (1974). Stimulation of drug metabolism by ascorbic acid in
weanling guinea pigs. *Biochem. Pharmacol.* **23,** 3121–3128.

Sato, P. H., and Zannoni, V. G. (1976). Ascorbic acid and hepatic drug metabolism. *J.
Pharmacol. Exp. Ther.* **198,** 295–307.

Sikic, B. I., Mimnaugh, E. G., Litterst, C. L., and Gram, T. E. (1976). The effects of
ascorbic acid deficiency and repletion on pulmonary, renal, and hepatic drug
metabolism in the guinea pig. *Fed. Proc., Fed. Am. Soc. Exp. Biol.* **35,** 408.

Zannoni, V. G., and Sato, P. H. (1975). Effects of ascorbic acid on microsomal drug
metabolism. *Ann. N. Y. Acad. Sci.* **258,** 119–131.

Zannoni, V. G., Flynn, E. J., and Lynch, M. M. (1972). Ascorbic acid and drug metabolism.
Biochem. Pharmacol. **21** 1377–1392.

Zannoni, V. G., Lynch, M. M., and Sato, P. H. (1974). Effect of ascorbic acid on drug-
metabolizing systems in the neonatal guinea pig. *In* "Perinatal Pharmacology: Problems and Priorities" (J. Dancis and J. C. Hwang, eds.), pp. 131–147. Raven, New
York.

13

Dietary Minerals and Drug Metabolism

GEORGE C. BECKING

I. INTRODUCTION

As shown by Becking (1976), the effect of dietary minerals on the metabolism of compounds foreign to the body (drugs, pesticides, food additives, etc.) has been intensely investigated during the last decade. Research in this area was markedly accelerated when it became evident that the same qenzyme system was responsible for the metabolism of foreign compounds as well as endogenous steroids.

Many enzymatic reactions are involved in the metabolism of foreign compounds (Table I). One of the most widely studied systems is the

371

TABLE I
Some Enzymatic Reactions Involved in Mammalian Drug Metabolism

Microsomal cytochrome P-450-dependent enzyme systems
(Liver, lung, skin, kidney, placenta, intestine, adrenal)
  N-Dealkylation
  O-Dealkylation
  S-Dealkylation
  Aliphatic oxidation
  Aromatic hydroxylation
  Oxidative deamination
  Reductases (azo and nitro)
Microsomal non-P-450-dependent systems
  Hydrolytic (esterases, phosphatases)
  Conjugation (glucuronyl transferase)
Nonmicrosomal enzymes
  Soluble esterases and amidases
  Alcohol and aldehyde oxidation
  Amine oxidases
  Dehalogenation

microsomal cytochrome P-450 mixed-function oxidases found in liver, kidney, lung, and several other tissues. This enzyme system may be broken down into three components: a characteristic cytochrome termed cytochrome P-450, a cytochrome reductase (P-450 reductase), and a lipid–phospholipid component). This mixed-function oxidase requires oxygen and NADPH for activity (Williams, 1975). The reader is referred to the latter article as well as the succinct overview of the types of reactions carried out by this enzyme system which is presented in Chapter 10 in this treatise by Professor Williams.

Dietary minerals could change the activity of this complex enzyme system by: altering the binding of the substrate, altering the rate of synthesis or degradation of the various components, or an alteration or change in the physiological activity of the phospholipid membrane of the endoplasmic reticulum. Such changes may be brought on by the deficiency or excess of one dietary mineral, the effect of two or more minerals or the effect of the dietary mineral acting in concert with some other dietary component known to alter hepatic drug metabolism, for example, vitamins (Becking, 1973; Catz *et al.*, 1970).

Man is continually exposed to environmental chemicals, and chemical therapeutic agents are widely used. The role of diet in the physiological disposition of these chemicals becomes a matter of great concern, since any alteration in the metabolism of such foreign compounds could lead to a grossly exaggerated toxic response and possibly to an increased rate of chemical carcinogenesis. The effect of diet on the metabolism of chemical carcinogens has recently been reviewed by Clayson (1975) and Wattenburg (1975). Marginal mineral deficiencies are known to occur in developed countries such as the United States and Canada (Karp *et al.*, 1974; Gortner, 1975) and cases of zinc deficiency (Halsted, 1973; Hambridge *et al.*, 1972; Sandstead *et al.*, 1967) and copper deficiency (Al-Rashid and Spangler, 1971; Dunlap *et al.*, 1974) have been documented in humans. We must also be concerned with the effect of the dietary levels of the so-called nonessential or toxic metals on drug metabolism. Such minerals might effect drug metabolizing systems directly or accentuate a marginal deficiency of some other essential nutrient.

Information on the alteration of drug metabolism by both essential and nonessential trace minerals is increasing rapidly (Table II), but additional research must be carried out on the interaction of one or more dietary minerals with the complex systems metabolizing drugs. More emphasis must be placed on the study of the effects of dietary components on the metabolism of drugs in other tissues such as skin, lung, kidney, etc. This review will concentrate on the effects of dietary minerals on the hepatic mixed-function oxidase system only.

TABLE II
Some Minerals Reported to Alter Mixed-Function Oxidase Reactions[a]

Mineral	Species	Route of administration	Reference
Beryllium	Rat	Intratracheal	Jacques and Witschi (1973)
Cadmium	Rat	Diet	Hadley *et al.* (1974)
	Mouse	Intraperitoneal	Unger and Clausen (1973)
Cerium	Rat	Intravenous	Arvela and Karki (1971)
Copper	Rat	Diet	Moffitt and Murphy (1973a)
Iron	Rat	Diet	Becking (1972)
	Mouse		Catz *et al.* (1970)
	Rat	Intravenous	Alvares *et al.* (1972)
Lead	Rat	Per os (gavage)	Norpath *et al.* (1974)
	Rat	Diet	Alvares *et al.* (1976)
Magnesium	Rat	Diet	Becking and Morrison (1970b)
Mercury	Rat	Diet	Wagstaff (1973a)
	Mouse	Subcutaneous	Lucier *et al.* (1973)
Selenium	Rat	Diet	Burk and Masters (1975)
Zinc	Rat	Diet	Becking and Morrison (1970a)

[a] Similar to that reported by Becking (1976a).

II. ESSENTIAL MINERALS

Readers are referred to standard nutrition texts such as Underwood (1971) for a discussion of basic nutrition principles involved in dietary mineral research. A Technical Report Series by the World Health Organization Expert Committee (1973) is an excellent source of information on the role of trace elements in human nutrition.

A. Magnesium

Magnesium has been shown to be an essential requirement for optimal *in vitro* enzyme activity of the mixed-function oxidase system. Magnesium deficiency has also been reported in humans and the effect of such deficiencies on drug metabolism should be studied.

The data summarized in Tables III and IV indicate that magnesium-deficient rats metabolize foreign chemicals at a slower rate, both *in vitro* and *in vivo*, than control animals. Previous studies by Becking and Morrison (1970b) have shown that the metabolism of aminopyrine is also lower in magnesium-deficient animals whereas the oxidation of pentobarbital, pentobarbital sleeping times, and the reduction of p-nitrobenzoic acid are not affected by the dietary regimen. Data in Table IV show unaltered microsomal protein synthesis during these studies. The synthesis of specific proteins could have been altered and not detected by the analytical techiques utilized. Earlier studies by Menaker

TABLE III
Metabolism *In Vitro* and *In Vivo* of Aniline during Magnesium Depletion[a]

		In vitro[b]	*In vivo*[c]
Diet	Days on test	p-Aminophenol (nmoles/mg protein/hour)	Total p-aminophenol excreted (mg/24 hour)
Mg-deficient	12	66.1 ± 2.4[d]	4.7 ± 0.3[d]
Control (Isocaloric)		122.4 ± 8.2	6.5 ± 0.3
Mg-deficient $\pm$ Mg	12 ± 14	84.3 ± 8.0	6.5 ± 0.3
Control (Isocaloric)		92.0 ± 7.3	6.7 ± 0.2

[a] Reprinted from *Federation Proceedings*, **35**: 2480–2485, 1976.

[b] Results are expressed as the mean value obtained with 6 rats $\pm$ S.E.M. Microsomal drug metabolism *in vitro* was reported as nmoles p-aminophenol formed/mg microsomal protein/hour.

[c] Drug metabolism *in vivo* was reported as milligrams of p-aminophenol excreted/24 hours after an intraperitoneal dose of 50 mg aniline hydrochloride/kg.

[d] Significantly different from control values ($p < 0.05$).

TABLE IV

Microsomal Protein and Cytochrome P-450 Content and NADPH Cytochrome c Reductase Activity during Magnesium Depletion[a,b]

Diet	Days on test	Protein (mg/gm wet liver)	Cytochrome	
			P-450 (nmoles/mg protein)	c reductase (nmoles cytochrome[c] reduced/mg protein/minute)
Mg-deficient	12	25.5 ± 1.1	0.65 ± 0.07[c]	49.5 ± 1.4[c]
Control (Isocaloric)		26.8 ± 0.9	0.88 ± 0.05	73.1 ± 4.0
Mg-deficient + Mg	12 + 14		0.85 ± 0.09	65.7 ± 3.4
Control (Isocaloric)			0.92 ± 0.05	69.1 ± 2.3

[a] Results are expressed as the mean value obtained with 6 rats ± S.E.M.
[b] Reprinted from *Federation Proceedings*, **35**: 2480–2495, 1976.
[c] Significantly different from control values ($p < 0.05$).

(1954) had shown that magnesium-deficient rats exhibit lower protein synthesis than control animals. The lower level of cytochrome P-450 in magnesium-deficient rats and the concomitant decreased cytochrome c reductace activity may explain, at least in part, the lower rate of drug metabolism, but the results of previous studies must be adequately explained. That is, why were two metabolic pathways (pento-barbital oxidase and nitro reductase) unaltered during magnesium depletion? Since all enzymatic activities returned to essentially control levels, when formerly deficient animals were fed the magnesium-containing diet, it is apparent that all metabolic alterations described by Becking and Morrison (1970b) and those reported at this time are indeed due to the lower level of magnesium in the diet.

Since magnesium-deficient rats were shown to have unaltered glucose-6-phosphate dehydrogenase and isocitrate dehydrogenase activities, one cannot explain the altered *in vivo* drug metabolism by a lower rate of NADPH production.

Magnesium deficiency may alter drug metabolism directly or via some alteration in the tissue content of other metals. The effect of magnesium depletion on tissue metal content was determined. Since the dietary regimen used did not alter serum calcium levels (G. C. Becking, unpublished), hypocalcemia, a nutritional stress known to alter drug metabolism (Dingell *et al.*, 1966) and to co-exist with hypomagnemsia (MacIntyre, 1967), does not play a significant role in the alteration of drug metabolism by low dietary levels of magnesium.

Fouts and Pohl (1971) postulated that changes in the level of cytochrome P-450 reductase activity caused by changes in tissue metal concentrations may explain, at least in part, the alterations in drug metabolism found during studies of mineral deficiencies. Under dietary conditions causing decreased tissue levels of the appropriate cation this hypothesis might be valid, but during our magnesium depletion studies total liver magnesium and microsomal magnesium, copper, and zinc levels were essentially unaltered. An alternate mechanism for the noted changes in drug metabolism must be found.

The following unpublished, preliminary experiments indicate that the effects of magnesium depletion on drug metabolism are more complex than previously described by Becking and Morrison (1970b). A possible interplay between dietary magnesium and the thyroid, and perhaps phospholipid metabolism, is slowly emerging. Plasma thyroxine levels in magnesium-depleted animals have been shown to be significantly lower than controls, as expected from earlier studies of Humphrey and Heaton (1972). Thyroxine values of 4.3 μ/100 ml were found in deficient animals compared to control values of 7.3 μ/100 ml. Kato and Takahashi (1968) reported decreased drug metabolism in thyroidectomized male rats. Unlike thyroidectomized animals, magnesium-deficient rats exhibit unaltered barbiturate oxidase and nitroreductase activities. Thyroid hormone levels in magnesium-depleted animals are probably only a part of the reason for the noted changes in drug metabolism.

Consideration must be given to the effect of magnesium depletion on phospholipid metabolism. Besides a decrease in serum thyroxine levels, the magnesium-deficient diet has been shown to cause a marked decrease in serum inorganic phosphate. Slightly decreased levels of microsomal phosphatidylcholine and a marked decrease in microsomal lysophosphatidylcholine levels were noted after 12 days on the magnesium-deficient diet. Coon et al. (1971) have shown that the rat liver mixed-function oxidase system is highly dependent on the phosphatidylcholine content of the microsomal fraction. Whether magnesium depletion alters drug metabolism via effects on the thyroid, thus altering phospholipid levels in liver microsomes, remains unanswered. A recent paper by Saenger et al. (1976) describing the alteration of in vivo drug metabolism in children with thyroid disorders, would seem to support the hypothesis that the effect of magnesium depletion on hepatic drug metabolism is mediated in some way by thyroid hormone levels.

B. Potassium

The possible effect of dietary potassium on rat liver drug metabolism was studied for the following reasons: potassium deficiency has been reported in man (Katsikas and Goldsmith, 1971); renal changes are found in both magnesium and potassium-depleted rats (Welt, 1964); such renal lesions may play a role in altering the physiological disposition of drugs and other foreign chemicals in addition to any effect dietary magnesium and potassium may have on hepatic drug metabolism; potassium and magnesium, major intracellular cations, play important roles in maintaining *in vivo* membrane integrity which is essential for optimal microsomal drug metabolism.

Studies reported by Becking (1974), and summarized in Table V, show that a large decrease in the dietary intake of potassium does not alter drug metabolism in a similar fashion to that found during magnesium depletion studies. Neither oxidative nor reductive pathways were altered during potassium depletion (Table V). Glucuronyl transferase, a non-*P*-450 dependent microsomal enzyme, was found to be more active in potassium-deficient rats, but no satisfactory explanation of the physiological significance of this *in vitro* observation is possible at this time.

The *in vitro* enzyme results shown in Table V are consistent with the amounts of cytochrome *P*-450 in the livers of potassium-deficient rats (Becking, 1974). No effect of potassium depletion on cytochrome *P*-450 content and cytochrome *c* reductase activity was noted, nor was there an alteration in microsomal protein content. It is evident that the decreased drug metabolism noted during magnesium depletion studies was not due to concomitant hypokalemia, since *in vitro* drug metabolism was not altered during potassium depletion and was altered during magnesium depletion.

TABLE V

Microsomal Drug Metabolism *In Vitro* during Potassium Depletion[a]

		Drug-metabolizing activity[b]		
Diet	Days on test	Aniline hyroxylation	Aminopyrine demethylation	*p*-Nitrobenzoic acid reduction
Deficient	18	59.2 ± 2.2	59.8 ± 2.0	13.7 ± 0.6
Control		58.2 ± 3.4	53.4 ± 2.7	14.4 ± 1.2
Deficient	35	46.1 ± 3.1	48.3 ± 1.8	11.1 ± 0.8
Control		50.7 ± 4.3	51.0 ± 1.5	12.2 ± 1.0
Deficient + potassium	38 + 18	54.3 ± 2.3	54.3 ± 2.6	13.6 ± 0.9
Control		55.4 ± 1.9	51.9 ± 3.0	12.9 ± 1.3

[a] Reprinted from *Federation Proceedings*, **35:** 2480–2485, 1976.
[b] Drug-metabolizing activity is expressed as nmoles of product formed by the 17,500 × g rat liver supernatant/mg microsomal protein/hour. Results are expressed as the mean value obtain with 8 rats S.E.M.

TABLE VI
Effect of Potassium Depletion on Pentobarbital[a] Sleeping Times and *In Vivo* Metabolism of Aminopyrine[b]

Diet	Days on test	Sleeping time (minutes)	Plasma Aminopyrine half-life (minutes)	4-Aminoantipyrine[c] (μg/ml)
Deficient		142 ± 11[d]	122 ± 6[d]	12.9 ± 1.1
Control	38	90 ± 8	80 ± 4	10.0 ± 0.9
Deficient + potassium		101 ± 12	90 ± 7	9.8 ± 1.5
Control	38 + 18	83 ± 7	84 ± 5	9.2 ± 1.1

[a] Administered as an ip dose of 40 mg/kg to groups of 20 rats.
[b] Administered as an ip dose of 80 mg/kg to 6 groups of 5 rats. Results are expressed as the mean volume ± S.E.M.
[c] Total 4-aminoantipyrine in plasma was determined 2 hours after drug administration to 6 rats on each diet. Results are expressed as the mean value ± S.E.M.
[d] Significantly different from control values ($p < 0.05$).

Although potassium depletion failed to alter the rate of *in vitro* drug metabolism, it is apparent from the data shown in Table VI that potassium-deficient diets markedly altered the *in vivo* disposition of pentobarbital and aminopyrine. It is evident that the plasma half-life of the weakly basic drug aminopyrine is much greater in potassium-depleted rats than controls. The physiological processes responsible for this change in plasma half-life are reversible, as indicated by the effect of dietary repletion with potassium chloride. Since no alteration in the *in vitro* metabolism of aminopyrine was noted (Table V), it is not surprising that the plasma level of the major metabolite 4-aminoantipyrine was not significantly different in potassium-deficient rats and controls 2 hours after drug injection. Possibly renal changes during potassium depletion alter the physiological disposition of drugs. A better protocol for the studies would have been to follow the plasma level of 4-aminoantipyrine simultaneously with aminopyrine, thus showing the effect of potassium depletion on the excretion of the more basic metabolite, 4-aminoantipyrine, as well as the parent compound. This would have given more definitive information on the possible effects of dietary potassium on renal excretion of drugs.

Another indicator of *in vivo* drug metabolism, pentobarbital sleeping times, were found to be prolonged in potassium-deficient rats (Table VI). Repletion with potassium chloride again shows that this effect is due solely to a lack of potassium in the diet and not to some other unknown factor.

Changes in plasma half-lives and barbiturate sleeping times depend on many factors, some of which are: metabolism; blood:tissue distribution; renal function. From the results presented at this time, and those published by Hirsch (1974), it appears likely that the prolonged plasma half-life for aminopyrine is due to an altered renal clearance. Possibly, this might also explain the increased pentobarbital sleeping times found in potassium-deficient rats, but drug:tissue distribution, as it relates to the absorption and excretion of drugs from the central nervous system, probably plays a major role in determining the pharmacological effect of barbiturates. Such processes could conceivably be markedly altered in potassium-depleted animals, thus leading to a prolongation of drug action. Some of these questions could have been answered if brain levels of pentobarbital had been determined during potassium depletion studies. The exact role of dietary potassium in drug metabolism remains unanswered. The effect of magnesium depletion on renal function (Smith et al., 1962) would indicate the possibility of a similar mechanism of action for dietary magnesium and potassium. From the results of experiments carried out to date, magnesium and potassium appear to alter drug disposition by distinctly different modes of action. Magnesium exerts its effect on the metabolic process probably via some effect on thyroid activity and/or phospholipid metabolism, whereas the major effect of dietary potassium appears to be on renal function. Magnesium may also alter renal function, thus adding to the in vivo effects noted, but its major effect appears to be on the microsomal enzyme system rather than on kidney function.

The studies reported by Becking (1974) would have been of more value if in vivo studies had been carried out at an earlier time within the experimental protocol. The severe hypokalemic state of the animals at 38 days on test bears little relevance to the human situation. In view of the early renal lesions noted by Toback et al. (1976), in vivo drug metabolism studies in mildly hypokalemic rats and, if possible, humans, should be carried out. Changes in the phospholipids of the kidney during early potassium depletion (Toback et al., 1976) suggest that drug metabolism in kidney may be altered and this possibility should be investigated.

C. Iron

Iron appears to be one of the dietary constituents commonly found to be marginal deficient in man's diet (Gortner, 1975). Besides studying the possible effect of dietary deficiency on drug metabolism, one must watch for an alteration in drug metabolic activity caused by an increased intake

TABLE VII
Effects of Varying Dietary Iron Levels on *In Vitro* Drug Metabolism

| Diet | Days on test | *In vitro* metabolic activity[a] | | |
		Aniline hydroxylase	Aminopyrine demethylase	Pentobarbital oxidase
High-Fe		27.3 ± 1.9	—	104.1 ± 7.0
Minus-Fe	25	43.3 ± 2.5[b]	52.3 ± 6.4	141.9 ± 16.7
Control		25.8 ± 2.3	43.8 ± 3.2	119.4 ± 7.4
High-Fe		21.3 ± 1.9	44.4 ± 3.1	96.0 ± 9.4
Minus-Fe	35	39.1 ± 1.8[b]	58.8 ± 4.6[b]	107.6 ± 10.2
Control		20.4 ± 1.3	40.1 ± 3.6	88.9 ± 7.3
Minus-Fe+Fe	40 + 7	30.2 ± 3.1	36.9 ± 4.7	—
Control	47	26.5 ± 1.6	38.2 ± 5.4	—

[a] Drug-metabolizing activity is expressed as nmoles of product formed by the $17,500 \times g$ supernatant/mg microsomal protein/hour. Results are expressed as the mean value obtained with 4 rats ± S.E.M.

[b] Significantly different from control values ($p < 0.05$).

of iron, largely due to self-medication with iron-containing protein and cytochrome P-450, and the number of people found marginally iron-deficient in the United States and Canada, make it important to consider the effect of dietary iron levels on hepatic drug metabolism.

The results of studies carried out in rats (Becking, 1972) are summarized in Tables VII and VIII. *In vitro* microsomal metabolism of aminopyrine and aniline was markedly increased during iron depletion, but was unaltered after 35 days on a diet containing 1.5 times the normal iron content. The metabolism of pentobarbital was unaltered by the iron-deficient or high iron diet. It should be noted that nitroreductase activity also was unaltered by dietary iron levels. All rats in these studies were monitored clinically for iron status by the determination of hemoglobin and hematocrit values. Significant increases in all oxidative drug metabolic reactions studied were noted when hemoglobin levels had decreased to 50% of control. Aniline (a type II substrate) was metabolized at an increased rate when hemoglobin values had dropped to only 65–70% of controls.

A reasonable correlation between *in vitro* and *in vivo* drug metabolism was noted when aniline and aminopyrine metabolism was studied (Tables VII and VIII). No such correlation was noted in the metabolism of pentobarbital. This again points out the danger of relying on the measurement of barbiturate sleeping times as the sole index of *in vivo* drug metabolism. Sleeping times not only are a measure of *in vivo* metabolic

TABLE VIII
Effect of Iron Depletion on *In Vivo* Drug Metabolism

Substrate[a] (days on test)	Diet	Sleeping time (minutes)	Plasma half-life (minutes)	*In vivo* metabolic activity[b] Plasma metabolite (μg/ml) p-Aminophenol[c]	4-Aminoantipyrine[d]
Aniline (25)	Minus-Fe		58 ± 4[e]	14.7 ± 2.0[e]	
	Control		89 ± 6	6.9 ± 2.2	
Aminopyrine (40)	Minus-Fe		107 ± 8[e]		15.9 ± 1.9[e]
	Control		138 ± 6		9.8 ± 0.9
Pentobarbital (35)	Minus-Fe	86 ± 8[e]	78 ± 3		
	Control	63 ± 7	70 ± 2		

[a] Chemicals were administered in *n*-saline as an ip dose of: aniline, 50 mg/kg; aminopyrine, 80 mg/kg and pentobarbital, 35 mg/kg.

[b] Results are expressed as the mean value obtained with 5 rats (10 for sleeping times) ± S.E.M.

[c] Total *p*-aminophenol in plasma was determined 1.5 hour after drug administration.

[d] Total 4-aminoantipyrine in plasma was determined 2 hours after drug administration.

[e] Significantly different from control values ($p < 0.05$).

activity, but are related closely to changes in the physiology of the central nervous system. Data presented in Table VIII substantiate the idea that serum metabolite levels and/or plasma half-lives are much more accurate indicators of *in vivo* drug metabolism than sleeping times. It is evident from the data in Table VIII that a good correlation was obtained between the *in vitro* drug metabolism of aniline and aminopyrine and the respective half-lives and serum metabolite concentration, whereas no change in the *in vitro* metabolism of pentobarbital was found although sleeping times were prolonged in iron-deficient rats.

Species variation to dietary iron was evident comparing the results in rats reported by Becking (1972) to those in mice obtained by Catz *et al.* (1970). Catz *et al.* (1970) noted an increased rate of metabolism of aminopyrine and hexabarbital (type I substrates), whereas under her experimental conditions no alteration in the rate of aniline metabolism was noted. Aniline hydroxylase activity was the most sensitive parameter to dietary iron levels in rats (Becking, 1972). The poor correlation between the rate of *in vitro* barbiturate metabolism and sleeping times was also noted by Catz *et al.* (1970), but these authors did not measure plasma half-life values or metabolite concentrations.

No attempt was made by Becking (1972) to measure tissue iron, as well as other metals, in iron-depleted and/or rats exposed to high dietary iron intake. The findings of Symes *et al.* (1969) that iron depletion in rats results in decreased hepatic iron and increased copper levels may be relevant to the present studies in rats. It has been shown by Fouts and Pohl (1971) that ferric ion inhibits cytochrome P-450 reductase activity *in vitro,* and ferrous ions stimulate this same enzyme, one of the rate-limiting steps in hepatic microsomal drug metabolism. The oxidation of the ferric iron in ferritin to ferrous iron could possibly lead to local concentrations of ferrous iron which could stimulate hepatic microsomal drug metabolism. Although a possible explanation for the altered metabolic reactions found in rat liver, the findings of Catz *et al.* (1970) indicate that no alteration in the iron content of liver subfractions is noted in iron-deficient mice. It is tempting to speculate from some recent *in vitro* studies (G. C. Becking, unpublished) that tissue ferritin levels may alter the rate of hepatic drug metabolism as well as play a role in controlling iron metabolism (Crichton, 1973). It has been found that ferritin, added at 400 μg/ml to *in vitro* digests inhibits aniline hydroxylase and aminopyrine demethylase activities approximately 50%.

Because of widespread marginal iron deficiency, the clinical significance in humans of these animal experiments must be ascertained. O'Malley and Stevenson (1973) made an attempt to study the effect of severe iron deficiency in humans on drug metabolism. No effect on the plasma half-life of antipyrine was noted in seven patients. No attempt was made to study males and females separately and only two subjects were anemic from low dietary iron intake. Although strongly suggestive that drug metabolism in humans is unaltered in iron anemia, it is difficult to compare results from patients anemic from hormonal imbalance and/or drug overdoses to results from animals, anemic solely from a low dietary intake of iron.

Hoensch *et al.* (1975) have shown that iron-deficient diets cause a marked decrease in intestinal drug metabolism within 2 days. If found applicable to humans, such findings may be of more importance to man than the increased hepatic drug metabolism noted in rats after 18–35 days on iron-deficient diets. Wattenberg (1975) has reviewed the role of intestinal arylhydroxylases in protecting against the carcinogenic potential of such compounds as benzpyrene. The level of iron in the diet at which the intestinal cells lose their drug-metabolizing activity, and thus their potential for protecting against carcinogenic aromatic hydrocarbons, should be determined. Attempts could then be made to relate this to the various iron levels found in man's diet.

D. Copper

Considering the physiological interrelationships of copper and iron (Seelig, 1972; Hedges and Kornegay, 1973), and reports of copper deficiency in humans (Al-Rashid and Spangler, 1971; Dunlap *et al.*, 1974), it is important to determine the effect of dietary copper on mammalian drug metabolism.

Although Underwood (1971) described the principal effects of copper deficiency and copper toxicity in animals, such subtle effects as alterations in microsomal drug metabolism are not well studied. Sharpless (1946) presented data indicating a possible role for dietary copper in the microsomal metabolism of foreign compounds. This study showed that a dietary supplement of copper decreased the hepatocarcinogenicity of *p*-dimethylaminoazobenzene.

Moffitt and Murphy (1973a,b) investigated the effects of dietary levels of copper on hepatic drug metabolism and some of their data are presented in Table IX. The overall pattern of effects of dietary copper on drug metabolism is extremely varied. Note in Table IX the different effect of copper depletion on aniline hydroxylase (decreased activity) and benzpyrene hydroxylase (increased activity). Also note that rats fed a copper-deficient diet metabolized hexobarbital at a much lower rate than control animals and exhibited a marked prolongation in hexobarbital sleeping times. All changes were due solely to the lack of copper in

TABLE IX

Effect of Daily Copper Intake on Microsomal Drug Metabolism in the Rat[a]

Copper status	N	Days on test	In vitro activity[b]				Hexobarbital[c] sleeping time (minutes)
			Aniline hydroxylase	Benzpyrene hydroxylase	Hexobarbital oxidase		
Dietary							
Minus-Cu	14	0	1.70 ± 0.10	3.60 ± 0.15	7.02 ± 0.66		13.0 ± 1.5
	6	42	0.66 ± 0.10[d]	4.74 ± 0.27[d]	2.04 ± 0.52[d]		32.3 ± 1.5[d]
Minus-Cu+Cu	6	42 + 14	1.86 ± 0.16	3.90 ± 0.33	7.54 ± 0.39		15.0 ± 2.7
Copper in Water							
50 ppm	5	30	1.01 ± 0.05	2.74 ± 24			
150 ppm	5	30	0.95 ± 0.10	2.79 ± 0.21			
Controls	10	30	1.18 ± 0.08	2.82 ± 0.39			

[a] Data represent a summary from Becking (1976a), previously calculated from Moffitt and Murphy (1973b).

[b] Values represent mean ± S.E.M. of N animals per group. Respective enzyme activities are reported as: μmoles p-aminophenol/gm/hour (aniline hydroxylase); pmoles 3-hydroxybenzpyrene/gm/hour (benzpyrene hydroxylase); and μmoles hexobarbital metabolized/gm/hour (hexobarbital oxidase).

[c] Hexobarbital, 100 mg/kg, administered intraperitoneally.

[d] Significantly different from control values ($p < 0.05$).

the diet as evidenced by the return to essentially control enzyme activities after copper repletion studies. The dietary regimen utilized by Moffitt and Murphy (1973a,b) in these studies did not alter the hepatic concentrations of zinc and manganese but did lower the total hepatic copper levels to $3.81 \, \mu g/gm$ from a control value of $5.58 \, \mu g/gm$.

I have not included in Table IX results of experiments where rats were given water containing 450 ppm copper for 30 days. As shown in Table IX no significant adverse effects on hepatic drug metabolism were noted in rats after 30 days consuming water containing 150 ppm copper. It should be noted that Moffitt and Murphy (1973a) did show a marked decrease in aniline hydroxylase activity on the 450 ppm copper regimen, whereas benzpyrene hydroxylase was essentially unaltered.

As postulated by Fouts and Pohl (1971), alterations in hepatic drug metabolism in response to varying dietary levels of copper may be due to inhibition or activation of cytochrome P-450 reductase by intracellular cation concentrations. *In vitro* studies by Peters and Fouts (1970) have shown a copper level of 0.2 mM inhibited cytochrome c reductase activity. If the increased copper content of microsomes, due to the high copper intake, altered *in vivo* drug metabolism by an inhibition of cytochrome c reductase, we must explain why all mixed-function oxidase reactions are not altered by the high copper regimen.

Moffitt and Murphy (1973a) postulated that copper-deficient diets caused an alteration in drug metabolism by interfering with the substrate binding in the microsomes. These same authors have shown that microsomal copper levels were unaltered during copper depletion. It would seem that other mechanisms will be needed to explain the effect of dietary copper levels on drug metabolism.

Although a definitive mechanism by which cdietary copper levels alter the rate of hepatic drug metabolism has not been formulated, some evidence of the possible heterogeneity of microsomal aromatic hydroxylases is evident from studies on the pharmacological action of parathion, 3,4-dichloraniline, and zoxazolamine (Moffitt and Murphy, 1973a,b).

Parathion, normally detoxified by microsomal enzymes to p-nitrophenol or activated to paraoxon by the same enzyme system, was found to be much more toxic in copper-deficient mice. These findings correlate with the finding that rats fed copper-deficient diets had a markedly lower rate of parathion metabolism to p-nitrophenol.

The production of methemoglobinemia by 3,4-dichloroaniline depends on the hydroxylation of this compound by microsomal enzymes. One would expect a much less severe toxic response to this compound, both in copper-loaded animals, since aniline hydroxylase activity was lower in both animal groups. Experimental results verified this hypothesis.

Zoxazolamine is converted to 6-hydroxyzoxazolamine, a compound having little or no muscle relaxant activity. Copper depletion of rats increased the paralysis time and decreased the rate of *in vitro* metabolism of zoxazolamine. Copper loading had no effect on either parameter.

The variable effects of dietary copper levels on *in vitro* metabolism and *in vivo* pharmacological activity of several compounds in rats support the hypothesis that at least two microsomal enzymes are available for the hydroxylation of aromatic compounds. The increased benzpyrene hydroxylase activity in copper-deficient animals and the unaltered benzpyrene metabolism in copper-loaded rats gives support for a third distinct hepatic system available for aryl hydroxylation reactions.

E. Zinc

Marginal deficiency of zinc, an essential nutrient for animals and man (Underwood, 1971), is probably more widespread than previously considered (Pal, 1974). The studies of Sanstead *et al.* (1967) on zinc-deficient humans in the Middle East are well known, while other reports suggestive of marginal human zinc deficiency have also been published (Hambridge *et al.,* 1972; Halsted, 1973; Kubota *et al.,* 1968).

Zinc depletion in rats has been shown to alter hepatic drug metabolism (Becking and Morrison, 1970a). From data given in Table X it is evident that rat liver microsomal enzymes exhibited variable sensitivity to zinc depletion. Becking and Morrison (1970a) reported no alteration in aromatic hydroxylase activity (both aniline and zoxazolamine as substrates) after 58 days on the zinc-deficient regimen, whereas it is evident (Table X) that the oxidation of pentobarbital is extremely sensitive to dietary zinc levels. The N-demethylation of aminopyrine was also lower in zinc-deficient animals but this reaction was not as sensitive to alterations in dietary zinc as was the oxidative metabolism of pentobarbital. No alteration in nitroreductase activity was noted during these studies.

It is difficult to account for the decrease in *in vitro* and *in vivo* drug metabolism during zinc depletion on the basis of decreased levels of cytochrome P-450. Microsomal protein levels remained unaltered during zinc depletion and the rate of NADPH production was found to be unaltered (Becking and Morrison, 1970a). No attempt was made to measure cytochrome c reductase or cytochrome P-450 reductase activities during zinc depletion experiments. Therefore, it is not known whether alterations in cytochrome P-450 activity could account, at least in part, for the changes found in hepatic drug metabolism.

TABLE X
Effect of Zinc Depletion on Microsomal Drug Metabolism

Diet	Days on test	*In vitro* metabolism [a]			Sleeping [b] time (minutes)	Cytochrome *P*-450 (nmoles/mg protein)
		Aminopyrine demethylase	Pentobarbital oxidase			
Ad lib control			113.9 ± 18.9		49 ± 4	0.93 ± 0.04
Isocaloric control	38		78.0 ± 9.2		47 ± 3	0.84 ± 0.02
Minus-Zn			51.6 ± 3.9		70 ± 5	0.69 ± 0.02^c
Isocaloric control			89.1 ± 11.3		41 ± 4	0.77 ± 0.01
Minus-Zn + Zn	$44 + 14$		103.0 ± 7.9		46 ± 5	0.81 ± 0.04
Isocaloric control	46	61.8 ± 7.3				0.80 ± 0.03
Minus-Zn		37.6 ± 4.9^c				0.70 ± 0.03^c
Minus-Zn + Zn	$46 + 14$	55.9 ± 3.5				0.84 ± 0.02

[a] Results are expressed as the mean value obtained with 5 rats $\pm$ S.E.M. The $17,500 \times$ g rat liver supernatant was utilized as the enzyme and enzyme activity was expressed as nmoles of product formed/mg microsomal protein/hour.

[b] Results are expressed as the mean value obtained with 8 rats after administration of pentobarbital as an intraperitoneal dose of 35 mg/kg.

[c] Significantly different from control values ($p < 0.05$).

Although Mutch and Hurley (1974) found no significant decrease in the total liver zinc levels in rats fed zinc-deficient diets for similar periods of time, it would have made a more definitive study if microsomal levels of zinc, copper, magnesium, etc. had been determined by Becking and Morrison (1970a). Perhaps the copper content of microsomes increased to a level where inhibition of drug metabolism occurred, or microsomal metal levels may have been altered, changing the degree of substrate binding and thus microsomal metabolism.

The relevancy of these zinc depletion studies in rats to man is debatable. All animals exhibiting decreased drug metabolism are in extremely poor clinical condition, having all the visible signs of severe zinc deficiency (kangaroo posture, low body weight, rough fur, etc.). This fact necessitated the use of control animals fed ad libitum and an isocaloric control group in order to eliminate possible changes in drug metabolism caused by the low food intake of the deficient rats. What effect marginal zinc deficiency, a condition more comparable to that found in humans, would have on liver drug metabolism has not been determined.

F. Selenium

Selenium, an essential trace element for experimental and domestic animals (World Health Organization Expert Committee, 1973) has not been proved as an essential element for man. Pathological conditions which resulted from long-term selenium toxicity in humans have not been identified. Selenium has been shown to be toxic to rats at dietary levels 5–10 times higher than optimal dietary levels (Palmer and Olson, 1974). The nutritional status of the animal and the form of selenium present in the diet may dictate the degree of toxicity (World Health Organization Expert Committee, 1973).

Carpenter (1972) reported an impairment in rat hepatic drug metabolism activity during vitamin E depletion. Since then, most studies on the possible effects of selenium on liver microsomal drug metabolism have been carried out to investigate the interrelationship of dietary levels of selenium and vitamin E on microsomal drug metabolism. The effects of Vitamin E and selenium on liver microsomal drug metabolism have been reported by Caygill et al. (1973), Diplock (1974), and Giasuddin et al. (1975).

Studies by Siami et al. (1972) and Burk et al. (1974; Burk and Masters, 1975) have shown that selenium-deficient diets do not cause alterations in rat liver drug metabolism. No alteration in the metabolism of hexobarbital or aminopyrine was noted in selenium-deficient rats. The recent studies by Burk et al. (1974; Burk and Masters, 1975) have confirmed that dietary selenium levels play a minimal role in maintaining optimal levels of hepatic microsomal drug metabolism, but a role for dietary selenium, distinct from Vitamin E, in the synthesis of microsomal components has been discussed (Burk *et al.*, 1974; Burk and Masters, 1975). These results do not refute the hypothesis of Diplock (1974) that there is a vitamin E-dependent role for selenium in the microsomal electron transport system. They suggest a second mechanism by which dietary selenium would alter drug metabolism.

Data from Burk and Masters (1975) are presented in Table XI. Comparing the rate of drug metabolism in rats fed selenium-deficient diets and diets adequate in selenium, it is evident that dietary levels of selenium (up to the nutritionally optimal concentration) do not alter hepatic drug metabolism. It is apparent that the induction of ethylmorpnine demethylase activity by phenobarbital was impaired in selenium-deficient rats. No such impairment was noted in the induction of biphenyl hydroxylase activity or pentobarbital sleeping time. Results published by Burk and Masters (1975), not shown in Table XI, indicated no impairment of the induction of cytochrome c reductase activity or cytochrome b_5 level after phenobarbital administration to selenium-deficient rats. Under similar conditions the induction of cytochrome P-450 was inhibited by 50%.

Although the role of dietary selenium in drug metabolism is unknown at this time, the studies by Burk and Masters (1975) strongly suggest a role for selenium in microsomal drug metabolism distinct from Vitamin

TABLE XI
Effect of Phenobarbital on the Induction of Hepatic Drug Metabolism in Selenium-Deficient and Control Rats[a]

Diet and treatment	Ethylmorphine[b] demethylase	Biphenyl[c] hydroxylase	Pentobarbital sleeping time (minutes)
Se-deficient	2.5 ± 0.6 (10)	0.9 ± 0.11 (3)	139 ± 28 (10)
Se-deficient + Phenobarbital	6.6 ± 1.6 (11[d])	4.72 ± 0.62 (6)	15 ± 4 (10)
Se-0.5 ppm	3.2 ± 1.0 (10)	0.84 ± 0.08 (3)	111 ± 18 (8)
Se-0.5 ppm + Phenobarbital	11.7 ± 1.6 (10)[d]	4.95 ± 1.45 (5)	15 ± 2 (9)

[a] Results are expressed as the mean value ± S.D. Figures in parentheses represent number of animals used. Data represent a summary of that published by Burk and Masters (1975).
[b] Ethylmorphine demethylase activity reported as nmoles formaldehyde/mg protein/minute.
[c] Biphenyl hydroxylase activity reported as nmoles 4-hydroxybiphenyl/mg protein/minute.
[d] Significantly different ($p < 0.001$).

E. Considering known importance of selenium in the nutrition of domestic food producing animals and its probable essentiality to man, it is hoped that researchers will continue to investigate the possible effects of dietary selenium levels on drug metabolism. Possible effects of long-term marginally toxic levels of selenium on microsomal drug metabolism metabolic activity should be studied.

III. NONESSENTIAL MINERALS

In any discussion of the effects of dietary minerals on drug metabolism the possible role of the so-called nonessential, and in most cases toxic, minerals should be considered. The toxicology of trace minerals have been reviewed by many authors and an overview of the field prepared by Bremner (1974). The minerals chosen for review at this time (lead, cadmium, and mercury) represent minerals which are extremely widespread naturally as well as being common, man-added, environmental pollutants. They therefore have the potential of being a component of man's diet.

There is no evidence that lead, cadmium, or mercury are essential to man or animals. Interest in these elements is primarily due to their toxic effects, due in part, to their bioaccumulation. Man's usual exposure (other than occupational) to these toxic minerals arises from low-level, long-term exposures. Most experiments carried out to date do not yield results which are relevant to this form of exposure. Since there is such a dirth of information which can be extrapolated to the long-term low-level type of exposure, it is hoped that this review will stimulate research on the effects of low dietary concentrations of heavy metals.

A. Lead

The alteration of drug metabolism by lead has been reported after acute intravenous administration (Alvares *et al.*, 1972), acute oral administration (Norpath *et al.*, 1974), and low and high dietary levels of lead for long periods of time (Phillips *et al.*, 1971); Alvares *et al.*, 1976; Becking, 1976a). The intravenous chronic administration of high doses of lead will not be discussed in detail. Inhibition of drug metabolism was found by Alvares *et al.* (1972) and the relevance of these studies to man's oral intake of lead has been adequately discussed by Becking (1976a) and Alvares *et al.* (1976). Data presented in Table XII indicate the lack of effect of very high chronic doses of dietary lead on drug metabolism in rats. These data are in essential agreement with those recorded by Al-

ABLE XII

fect of Chronic Administration of Lead on Microsomal Protein and Cytochrome P-450 Content
d Drug Metabolic Activity of Rat Liver[a]

Lead added to diet (ppm)	Enzyme activity[b]			Microsomal	
	Aniline hydroxylase	Aminopyrine demethylase	p-Nitrobenzoic acid reductase	Protein (mg/gm wet liver)	P-450 (nmoles/mg protein)
0	48.8 ± 3.3	53.1 ± 6.4	14.1 + 2.4	28.7 ± 0.7	0.76 ± 0.03
15,000	39.8 ± 3.6	49.8 ± 5.7	11.0 ± 5.7	30.0 ± 0.8	0.94 ± 0.07[c]
30,000	42.0 ± 2.1	54.1 ± 6.2	11.4 ± 1.7	31.4 ± 1.3[c]	0.95 ± 0.05[c]

[a] Dams were given lead in their diet throughout gestation and lactation. After weaning, rats were
the same diet for 10 weeks post-partum. Data taken from Becking (1976a).
[b] Enzyme activity is expressed as nmoles of product formed by the 17,500 × g rat liver super-
tant/mg microsomal protein/hour. Results are expressed as the mean value obtained with 7 rats
S.E.M.
[c] Values significantly different from controls ($p < 0.05$).

vares *et al.* (1976), although the dietary level of lead was lower in the
studies reported by Alvares *et al.* (1976) and the animals were fully
weaned prior to the administration of the lead-containing diet. The
stimulation of microsomal protein and cytochrome P-450 (Table XII)
may be the result of a longer exposure to a higher dietary level of lead.
These findings, using two slightly different dietary regimens, indicate
that the young rat is extremely resistant to high dietary levels of lead.
There is no apparent sensitivity to lead in extremely young rats, similar
to that found in man. Such species variation must be considered in any
experimental animal study where results are to be extrapolated to man.

Drug metabolism in humans exposed to lead has been studied by
Alvares *et al.* (1975, 1976). These subjects, both children and adults,
were exposed to sources of lead other than diet, but considering that
blood leads were determined as a measure of total exposure, one can
extrapolate to the low-level exposure from the diet more easily than
studies in rats, reported by Becking (1976a) and from Alvares *et al.* (1976).
The plasma half-life of antipyrine was prolonged in children suffering
from acute lead poisoning but returned to control values after chelation
therapy (Alvares *et al.*, 1975). Recent studies in eight adult subjects,
exposed at least 3 months to excessively high environmental lead levels,
failed to corroborate the findings in children (Alvares *et al.*, 1976). Although all adult human subjects displayed significant clinical signs of
lead poisoning, only minimal nonsignificant changes were noted in microsomal enzyme activity as measured by the plasma half-life of an-

tipyrine. These findings are similar to those observed in extremely young rats chronically exposed to high dietary lead levels. If the rat experiments were relevant to the situation found in man one would not expect to find lower drug metabolism in children with high blood lead levels. The human studies of Alvares *et al.* (1975, 1976) support the hypothesis that plumbism may have more direct effects on the liver of humans in the prepubertal state then on adults. Although the number of patients studied was relatively small, hopefully similar studies will be carried out to examine drug metabolism in humans under other dietary and/or environmental stresses.

B. Cadmium

The effects of high dietary levels of cadmium on rat liver drug metabolism are shown in Table XIII. Results of lower dietary levels of cadmium given in drinking water for up to 180 days have been summarized by Becking (1976). It was found that after 60 days 200 ppm cadmium in the drinking water did not alter rat liver drug metabolism but a slight stimulation of microsomal protein content was noted. Perhaps the level of cadmium in the liver was approaching the level needed to stimulate drug metabolism as shown by Wagstaff (1973b) and summarized in Table XIII.

From the studies of Wagstaff (1973b) and Becking (1976a) it would appear that low dietary levels of cadmium will have a minimal effect on rat liver microsomal drug metabolism. Although the inhibition of drug metabolism after parenteral administration of cadmium salts has been reported (Unger and Clausen, 1973; Hadley *et al.*, 1974), it is almost impossible to extrapolate these experimental results to man and animals.

TABLE XIII
Effects of High Dietary Cadmium Levels on Rat Liver Microsomal Enzymes[a]

Cadmium added to diet (ppm)	Hexobarbital sleeping time (minutes)	Nitroanisole O-demethylase (μmoles p-nitrophenol/ gm liver/hour)
0	81 ± 5	0.60 ± 0.10
500	46 ± 7[b]	1.27 ± 0.06[b]
1000	53 ± 3[b]	1.27 ± 0.11[b]

[a] Results are expressed as the mean value obtained from 5 rats ± S.E.M.
[b] Significantly different from control values ($p < 0.05$). Data taken from Wagstaff (1973b).

TABLE XIV

Rat Liver Microsomal Drug Metabolism after Acute Exposure to Methyl Mercuric Chloride[a]

	Control	Mercury treated
Ethylmorphine demethylase		
(μmoles formaldehyde/mg protein/hour)	0.33 ± 0.05	0.18 ± 0.03[b]
Aniline Hydroxylase	45.5 ± 2.3	25.9 ± 5.6[b]
(μmoles p-aminophenol/mg protein/hour)		
Hexobarbital sleeping time	40 ± 7	65 ± 6[b]
(minutes)		
Cytochrome P-450	0.54 ± 0.01	0.32 ± 0.04[b]
(μmole/mg protein)		

[a] Results are expressed as the mean value obtained from 5 rats ± S.E.M. Data taken from Alvares *et al.* (1972).

[b] Significantly different from control values ($p<0.05$). Data taken from Wagstaff (1973b).

Man's dietary intake of cadmium should not exceed approximately 1 μg/kg/day (World Health Organization Expert Committee, 1973). Such a dose would give blood and tissue levels of cadmium much lower than those found after chronic intraperitoneal administration of this metal. If it is possible to extrapolate from experiments in rats where the cadmium was administered in water or the diet, it would appear that low doses of dietary cadmium would be without effect on the hepatic drug metabolizing enzymes. What effects these cadmium levels would have on kidney or lung microsomal drug metabolism remains to be determined.

C. Mercury

To date no studies have been conducted on the effect of dietary methyl mercury on hepatic drug metabolism. The less toxic inorganic form of mercury has been fed to rats at excessively high dietary levels (500–2000 ppm) by Wagstaff (1973a). As with cadmium acetate, Wagstaff (1973b) has shown that mercuric acetate stimulates hepatic drug metabolism in adult rats. Whether this is due to the heavy metal or the high level of acetate anion should be investigated.

From the studies of Alvares *et al.* (1972) and Lucier *et al.* (1972, 1973) methyl mercury, after chronic parenteral administration, inhibits hepatic drug metabolism in rats. The extent of such inhibition is shown in Table XIV. No data exist to indicate the effect of methylmercury on drug metabolism in humans exposed to this containment in the fish component of their daily diet.

IV. CONCLUSION AND RESEARCH NEEDS

Dietary minerals do play a role in microsomal drug metabolism in experimental animals, but no data exist to indicate the effect of such minerals on drug metabolism in domestic animals, and only isolated reports are available on their effects on human drug metabolism. Some of the apparent reasons to consider additional research in this area are: the need to maintain adequate human nutrition; to help prevent diseases such as cancer, the incidence of which might be augmented by changes in nutritional status (Clayson, 1975); to understand the mechanism of action of dietary minerals on drug metabolism, thus assisting in the formulation of a standard, nutritionally optimum diet for experimental animals—such a diet might avoid some of the interlaboratory differences found during the toxicity testing of environmental chemicals and drugs, when such differences are due to nutritional factors; to delineate the role of dietary minerals in changing the toxic potential of drugs and environmental chemicals.

All research reported to date has concentrated on the effect of single minerals on drug metabolism. The effects of dietary minerals on drug metabolism in tissues other than liver, especially lung and kidney should be encouraged. The marked decrease in intestinal drug metabolism during iron deficiency must be investigated further. As well, studies should be initiated on the potential effect of marginal deficiencies of more than one dietary mineral acting in concert. It is impossible to discuss the toxicity or deficiency of one element without considering the effects of a deficiency or excess of another interacting element or elements. If all possible mineral interrelationships were considered for experimentation, the task would be impossible to carry out. By careful examination of the nutritional literature, and utilizing the theoretical calculations of Hill and Matrone (1970) priority for future study can be given to many possible combinations of dietary minerals.

The nutritional factors affecting lead toxicity have been reviewed by Mahaffey (1974) and Klauder and Petering (1975). Drug metabolism may indeed be inhibited by dietary lead when animals are marginally deficient in calcium, iron, or copper. Low dietary calcium enhances lead toxicity (Mahaffey et al. (1973) and dietary iron, copper, and zinc alter the absorption of lead in rats. As reviewed in this paper, dietary copper, zinc, and iron, when studied separately, alter drug metabolism in rodents. No studies on the interrelationships of these three minerals have been published. These are only some examples of possible interrelationships, and we must not forget such other important interactions as selenium–vitamin E, protein–selenium, selenium–mercury and the physiologic relationship between magnesium and potassium.

The depletion of microsomal iron content by dietary cadmium reported by Whanger (1973) suggests a possible effect on drug metabolism of low dietary concentrations of cadmium. It remains for future research to determine whether those people marginally deficient in iron are more sensitive to environmental levels of cadmium than those receiving adequate diets.

A major task facing the nutritionist and toxicologist is relating the immense body of experimental animal data to man. Perhaps with an increased data base from animal studies, and a better understanding of the metabolic differences between man and animals, models could be developed to assist in answering questions on the effects of dietary minerals on human drug metabolism. After reviewing the literature in the area of minerals and drug metabolism a disturbing observation is the apparent lack of recent work on the effects of dietary constituents on drug metabolism. Biochemists and pharmacologists appear to be more interested in cytochrone P-450 for its own sake rather than carrying out studies to delineate the role of P-450 in drug metabolism, and factors which may affect its *in vivo* function. Perhaps biochemists and nutritionists could combine their expertise more effectively to elucidate the effect of dietary minerals on drug metabolism.

REFERENCES

Al-Rashid, R. A., and Spangler, J. (1971). Neonatal copper deficiency. *N. Engl. J. Med.* **285,** 841–843.

Alvares, A. P., Leigh, S., Cohn, J., and Kappas, A. (1972). Lead and methyl mercury: Effects of acute exposure on cytochrome P-450 and the mixed-function oxidase system in the liver. *J. Exp. Med.* **135,** 1406–1409.

Alvares, A. P., Kapelner, S., Sassa, S., and Kappas, A. (1975). Drug metabolism in normal children, lead-poisoned children and normal adults. *Clin. Pharmacol.Ther.* **17,** 179–183.

Alvares, A. P., Fischbrin, A., Sassa, S., Anderson, K. E., and Kappas, A. (1976). Lead intoxication: Effects on cytocrhome P-450-mediated hepatic oxidations. *Clin. Pharmacol. Ther.* **19,** 183–190.

Arvela, P., and Karki, N. T. (1971). Effect of cerium on drug metabolizing activity in rat liver. *Experientia* **27,** 1189–1190.

Becking, G. C. (1972). Influence of dietary iron levels on hepatic drug metabolism *in vivo* and *in vitro* in the rat. *Biochem. Pharmacol.* **21,** 1585–1593.

Becking, G. C. (1973). Vitamin A status and hepatic drug metabolism in the rat. *Can. J. Physiol. Pharmacol.* **51,** 6–11.

Becking, G. C. (1974). Comparison of *in vitro* hepatic drug metabolism, plasma half-lives and pentobarbital sleeping times in potassium-deficient rats. *Proc. Can. Fed. Biol. Soc.* **17,** 68.

Becking, G. C. (1976a). Trace elements and drug metabolism. *Med. Clin. North Am.* **60,** 813–830.

Becking, G. C. (1976b). Hepatic drug metabolism in iron-, magnesium- and potassium-deficient rats. *Fed. Proc., Fed. Am. Soc. Exp. Biol.* **35,** 2480–2485.

Becking, G. C., and Morrison, A. B. (1970a). Hepatic drug metabolism in zinc-deficient rats. *Biochem. Pharmacol.* **19,** 895–902.

Becking, G. C., and Morrison, A. B. (1970b). Role of dietary magnesium in the metabolism of drugs by NADPH-dependent rat liver microsomal enzymes. *Biochem. Pharmacol.* **19,** 1639–2644.

Bremner, I. (1974). Heavy metal toxicities. *Q. Rev. Biophys.* **7,** 75–124.

Burk, R. F., and Masters, B. S. S. (1975). Some effects of selenium deficiency on the hepatic microsomal cytochrome *P*-450 system in the rat. *Arch. Biochem. Biophys.* **170,** 124–131.

Burk, R. F., Mackinnon, A. M., and Simon, F. R. (1974). Selenium and hepatic microsomal hemoproteins. *Biochem. Biophys. Res. Commun.* **56,** 431–436.

Carpenter, M. P. (1972). Vitamin E and microsomal drug hydroxylations. *Ann. N.Y. Acad. Sci.* **203,** 81–92.

Catz, C. S., Juchau, M. R., and Yaffe, S. J. (1970). Effects of iron, riboflavin and iodide deficiencies on hepatic drug-metabolizing enzyme systems. *J. Pharmacol. Exp. Ther.* **174,** 197–205.

Caygill, C. P. J., Diplock, A. T., and Jeffery, E. H. (1973). Studies on selenium incorporation into, and electron-transfer function of, liver microsomal fractions from normal and Vitamin E-deficient rats given phenobarbitone. *Biochem. J.* **136,** 851–858.

Clayson, D. B. (1975). Nutrition and experimental carcinogenesis: A review. *Cancer Res.* **35,** 3292–3300.

Coon, M. J., Autor, A. P., and Strobel, H. W. (1971). Role of phospholipid in electron transfer in a reconstituted liver microsomal enzyme system containing cytochrome *P*-450. *Chem. Biol. Interact.* **3,** 248–250.

Crichton, R. R. (1973). A role for ferritin in the regulation of iron metabolism. *FEBS Lett.* **34,** 125–128.

Dingell, J. V., Joiner, P. E., and Hurwitz, L. (1966). Impairment of drug metabolism in calcium deficiency. *Biochem. Pharmacol.* **15,** 971–976.

Diplock, A. T. (1974). A possible role for trace amounts of selenium and Vitamin E in the electron-transfer system of rat liver microsomes. *In* "Trace Element Metabolism in Animals-2" (W. G. Hoekstra *et al.,* eds.), pp. 147–160. Univ. Park Press, Baltimore, Maryland.

Dunlap, W. M., James, W., III, and Hume, D. M. (1974). Anemia and neutropenia caused by copper deficiency. *Ann. Intern. Med.* **80,** 470–476.

Fouts, J. R., and Pohl, R. J. (1971). Further studies on the effects of metal ions on rat liver microsomal reduced nicotinamide adenine dinucleotide phosphate cytochrome *P*-450 reductase. *J. Pharmacol. Exp. Ther.* **179,** 91–100.

Giasuddin, A. S. M., Caygill, C. P. J., Diplock, A. T., and Jeffery, E. H. (1975). The dependence on vitamin E and selenium of drug demethylation in rat liver microsomal fractions. *Biochem. J.* **146,** 339–350.

Gortner, W. A. (1975). Nutrition in the United States, 1900 to 1974. *Cancer Res.* **35,** 3246–3253.

Hadley, W. M., Miya, T. S., and Bousquet, W. F. (1974). Cadmium inhibition of hepatic drug metabolism in the rat. *Toxicol. Appl. Pharmacol.* **28,** 284–291.

Halsted, J. A. (1973). Zinc deficiency in man. *Lancet* **1,** 1447–1448.

Hambridge, K. M., Hambridge, C., Jacob, M., and Baum, J. D. (1972). Low levels of zinc in hair, anorexia, poor growth and hypogensia in children. *Pediatr. Res.* **6,** 868–874.

Hattersley, P. G. (1964). What so innocuous as iron? *Calif. Med.* **101,** 381–382.

Hedges, J. D., and Kornegay, E. T. (1973). Interrelationship of dietary copper and iron as measured by blood parameters, tissues stores and feedlot performance of swine. *J. Anim. Sci.* **37**, 1147-1154.

Hill, C. H., and Matrone, G. (1970). Chemical parameters in the study of *in vivo* and *in vitro* interactions of transition elements. *Fed. Proc., Fed. Am. Soc. Exp. Biol.* **29**, 1474-1481.

Hirsch, G. H. (1974). Effects of potassium depletion in rats on renal organic ion transport. *Can. J. Biochem.* **52**, 90-92.

Hoensch, H., Woo, C. H. and Schmid, R. (1975). Cytochrome *P*-450 and drug metabolism in intestinal villous and crypt cells of rats: Effect of dietary iron. *Biochem, Biophys. Res. Commun.* **65**, 399-406.

Humphrey, H. P., and Heaton, F. W. (1972). Relationship between the thyroid hormone and mineral metabolism in the rat. *J. Endocrinol.* **53**, 113-123.

Jacques, A., and Witschi, R. (1973). Beryllium effects on anylhydrocarbon hydroxylase in rat lung. *Arch. Environ. Health* **27**, 243-247.

Karp, R. J., Haaz, W. S., Starko, K., and Gorman, J. M. (1974). Iron deficiency in families of iron-deficient inner-city school children. *Am. J. Dis. Child.* **128**, 18-20.

Kato, R., and Takahashi, A. (1968). Thyroid hormone and activities of drug metabolizing enzymes and electron transport systems of rat liver microsomes. *Mol. Pharmacol.* **4**, 109-120.

Katsikas, J. K., and Goldsmith, C. (1971). Disorders of potassium metabolism. *Med. Clin. North Am.* **55**, 503-512.

Klauder, D. S., and Petering, H. G. (1975). Protective value of dietary copper and iron against some toxic effects of lead in rats. *Environ. Health Perspect.* **12**, 77-80.

Kubota, J., Lazar, V. A., and Losee, F. L. (1968). Copper, zinc, cadmium and lead in human blood from 19 locations in the United States. *Arch. Environ. Health* **16**, 788-793.

Lucier, G. W., McDaniel, O. S., Brubaker, P. E., and Klein, R. (1972). Effects of methylmercury hydroxide on rat liver microsomal enzymes. *Chem. Biol. Interact.* **4**, 265-280.

Lucier, G. W., Matthews, II. B., Brubaker, P. E., Klein, R., and McDaniel, O. S. (1973). Effects of methylmercury on microsomal mixed-function oxidase components of rodents. *Mol. Pharmacol.* **9**, 237-246.

MacIntyre, I. (1967). Magnesium metabolism. *Adv. Intern. Med.* **13**, 143-154.

Mahaffey, K. R. (1974). Nutritional factors and susceptibility to lead toxicity. *Environ. Health Perspect.* **1**, 107-112.

Mahaffey, K. R., Goyer, R., and Haseman, J. K. (1973). Dose-response to lead ingestion in rats fed low dietary calcium. *J. Lab. Clin. Med.* **82**, 91-100.

Menaker, W. (1954). Influence of protein intake on magnesium requirement during protein synthesis. *Proc. Soc. Exp. Biol. Med.* **85**, 149-151.

Moffitt, A. E., Jr., and Murphy, S. D. (1973a). Effect of excess and deficient copper intake on rat liver microsomal enzyme activity. *Biochem. Pharmacol.* **22**, 1463-1476.

Moffitt, A. E., Jr., and Murphy, S. D. (1973b). Effect of excess and deficient copper intake on hepatic microsomal metabolism and toxicity of foreign chemicals. *Trace Substances Environ. Health—7, Proc. Univ. Mo. Annu. Conf., 7th, 1973* pp. 213-223.

Mutch, P. B., and Hurley, L. S. (1974). Effect of zinc deficiency during lactation on postnatal growth and development of rats. *J. Nutr.* **104**, 828-842.

Norpath, K., Ho, S., and Witting, V. (1974). Indukton mikrosomaler Hämoproteide in der Rattenleber nach oraler Gabe verschiedener Bleisalze. *Int. Arch. Arbeitsmed.* **33**, 139-151.

O'Malley, K., and Stevenson, I. H. (1973). Iron deficiency anaemia and drug metabolism. *J. Pharm. Pharmacol.* **25**, 339-340.

Pal, B. (1974). Zinc in animal and human nutrition. *Indian J. Nutr. Diet.* **11**, 91-109.

Palmer, I. S., and Olson, D. E. (1974). Relative toxicities of selenite and selenate in the drinking water of rats. *J. Nutr.* **104,** 306–314.

Peters, M. A., and Fouts, J. R. (1970). The influence of magnesium and some other divalent cations of hepatic microsomal drug metabolism *in vitro.. Biochem. Pharmacol.* **19,** 533–544.

Phillips, W. E. J., Villeneuve, D. C., and Becking, G. C. (1971). The effects of lead ingestion on the body burden of DDT, liver Vitamin A and microsomal enzyme activity in the rat. *Bill. Environ. Contam. Toxicol.* **6,** 570–575.

Saenger, P., Rifkind, A. B., and New, M. I. (1976). Changes in drug metabolism in children with thyroid disorders. *J. Clin. Endocrinol. Metab.* **42,** 155–159.

Sandstead, H. H., Prasad, A. S., Schulert, A., Farid, Z., Miole, A., Jr., Bassily, S., and Darby, W. J. (1967). Human zinc deficiency, endocrine manifestations and response to treatment. *Am. J. Clin. Nutr.* **20,** 422–442.

Seelig, M. S. (1972). Review: Relationships of copper and molybdenum to iron metabolism. *Am. J. Clin. Nutr.* **25,** 1022–1037.

Sharpless, G. R. (1946). The effects of copper on liver tumor induction by *p*-dimethylaminoazobenzene. *Fed. Proc., Fed. Am. Soc. Exp. Biol.* **5,** 239–240.

Siami, G., Schulert, A. R., and Neal, R. A. (1972). A possible role for the mixed-function oxidase enzyme system in the requirement for selenium in the rat. *J. Nutr.* **102,** 857–861.

Smith, W. O., Baxter, D. J., Linder, A., and Ginn, H. E. (1962). Effect of magnesium depletion on renal function in the rat. *J. Lab. Clin. Med.* **59,** 211–219.

Symes, A. L., Sourkes, T. L., Youdim, M. B. H., Gregoriadis, G., and Birnbaum, H. (1969). Decreased monamine oxidase activity in liver of iron-deficient rats. *Can. J. Biochem.* **47,** 999–1002.

Toback, F. G., Ordonez, N. G., Bortz, S. L., and Spargo, B. H. (1976). Zonal changes in renal structure and phospholipid metabolism in postassium-deficient rats. *Lab. Invest.* **34,** 115–124.

Underwood, E. J. (1971). "Trace Elements in Human and Animal Nutrition," 3rd ed. Academic Press, New York.

Unger, M., and Clausen, J. (1973). Liver cytochrome *P*-450 activity after intraperitoneal administration of cadmium salts in the mouse. *Environ. Physiol. & Biochem.* **3,** 236–242.

Wagstaff, D. (1973a). Enhancement of hepatic detoxification enzyme activity by dietary mercuric acetate. *Bull. Environ. Contamin. Toxicol.* **9,** 10–14.

Wagstaff, D. (1973b). Stimulation of liver detoxification enzymes by dietary cadmium acetate. *Bull. Environ. Contamin. Toxicol.* **10,** 328–332.

Wattenberg, L. W. (1975). Effects of dietary constituents on the metabolism of chemical carcinogens. *Cancer Res.* **35,** 3326–3331.

Welt, L. G. (1964). Experimental magnesium depletion *Yale J. Biol. Med.* **36,** 325–349.

Whanger, P. D. (1973). Effect of dietary cadmium on intracellular distribution of hepatic iron in rats. *Res. Commun. Chem. Pathol. Pharmacol.* **5,** 733–740.

Williams, R. T. (1975). Detoxication mechanisms. *In* "Physiological and Pharmacological Biochemistry" (H. F. K. Blaschko, ed.), pp. 211–266. Butterworth, London.

World Health Organization Expert Committee (1973). Trace elements and human nutrition. *W.H.O. Tech. Rep. Ser.* **532.**

14

Drug Metabolism and Infantile Undernutrition

FERNANDO MONCKEBERG, MARIA BRAVO, and
ONOFRE GONZALEZ

I. INTRODUCTION

Even today, in many countries of the world a high percentage of children suffer from undernutrition. Because of adverse sanitary condition, as well as alterations of the immunological system, they show a high incidence of infectious and parasitic disease (Schlesinger and Stekel, 1974). In severe cases of undernutrition, intercurrent diseases acquire a greater importance, increasing the risk of death (Monckeberg, 1971a). As a consequence, physicians must use a variety of pharmacological agents with the object of treating these secondary diseases. Generally, it is assumed "a priori" that the absorption, metabolism, and excretion of these drugs is similar to that observed in eutrophic children. Nevertheless, this has not been demonstrated, and it is probably not so. Indeed, the reverse may be true.

Diverse data in the literature point out that in severe protein–calorie undernutrition there are numerous alterations of organs and systems that aggravate the undernutrition and make recovery difficult. The mechanism of intestinal absorption (Anderson, 1966; Monckeberg *et al.*, 1958; Platt *et al.*, 1964a; Bowil *et al.*, 1967), liver function (Platt *et al.*, 1964b), endocrine system (Monckeberg, 1971b; Beas *et al.*, 1966; Monckeberg *et al.*, 1964), the central nervous system (Dobbing, 1967; Monckeberg, 1967; Stock and Smith, 1963; Cravioto *et al.*, 1966), the renal function (Gordillo, 1964; Alleyne, 1967; Smith, 1959), the hemato-poietic system (Stekel and Smith, 1969a,b) and the immune system (Schlesinger and Stekel, 1974) are altered. All this leads one to think that many drugs could have a different action in undernutrition, or that their detoxification or excretion processes might be altered.

In recent years it has been observed with increasing frequency that severe undernutrition occurs in the early months of life (Monckeberg, 1970). In Chile, for example, 72% of severe undernourished are under 6 months old. At that age the liver functions as well as the renal functions have not reached total maturity. It is widely recognized that animals of varying maturity exhibit differences in drug metabolism. The fact that severe undernutrition is frequent during the first months of life when the human organism is in early stages of maturation and development, probably indicates a higher risk associated with the administration of certain drugs at that age.

There is very little information about the relation between drug han-dling and protein–calorie malnutrition in humans. It is imperative to know more about this because under different nutritional circumstances the doses or the intervals of drug administration may be different, or some drugs should not be used at all. Unfortunately the results of this research are not easily extrapolated from animal investigations.

II. ANTIPYRETIC DRUG METABOLISM

One of the most widely used drugs in pediatric practice is acetyl-salicylic acid, the toxicity of which differs with age. Thus, for example, in the treatment of rheumatic fever of children or adults the therapeutic concentrations are obtained only with salicylate blood levels of 30 mg/100 ml (Corbun, 1943). However, clinical signs of intoxication ap-pear in infants of a few months of age, with such low blood concen-trations as 10 mg/100 ml (Monckeberg *et al.*, 1960).

Because of these reported findings we studied in our Institute the kinetics of salicylate plasma concentrations in infants with severe under-nutrition (marasmus). With this object, two groups of children were chosen, all under 1 year of age: A control group included nine normal

TABLE I
Summary of Patients Studied

	Age at the time of study (months)	Birth weight (kg)	Weight time of study (kg)	Height (cm)	Percentage deficit weight	Dose acetylsalicylate (mg)
Control						
1	14.1	—[b]	8.970	—	—	108.0
2	12.6	3.150	9.600	78.0	2	116.4
3	12.1	2.500	9.100	74.5	4	110.0
4[a]	11.2	3.000	6.780	71.5	26	81.6
5	10.2	2.540	9.010	73.0	3	108.0
6	6.4	2.630	6.750	70.0	5	81.0
7	6.0	3.200	6.100	63.0	2	73.2
8	6.0	—	5.740	65.0	—	68.4
9	3.9	—	6.400	63.5	—	76.8
Undernourished						
10	11.2	2.800	3.700	60.0	60	44.4
11	9.0	2.680	4.500	63.0	46	55.2
12	5.2	2.550	3.860	60.0	37	45.6
13	5.2	3.000	3.650	59.0	40	46.2
14	5.2	3.000	3.700	60.0	37	45.0
15	5.0	3.050	4.360	59.5	27	52.3
16	4.6	3.200	3.460	56.0	40	41.5
17	4.4	4.000	3.600	60.0	42	43.2
18	4.3	3.600	3.860	58.0	31	45.8

[a] Recovered undernourished child.
[b] No data were obtainable.

TABLE II
Plasma Half-Life (in Hours) of Total, Protein-Bound and Free Salicylate in Normal and
Undernourished Children

Status	Plasma salicylate half-life (hours)[a]		
	Total	Protein-bound	Free
Eutrophic	1.40 ± 0.26	1.68 ± 0.54	1.1 ± 0.2
Undernourished	2.80 ± 0.80	1.40 ± 0.20	7.5 ± 2.0
$p <$	0.50	NS[b]	0.01

[a] Mean ± standard error of the mean.
[b] Probability not significant by the "t" test.

infants, and a test group of nine infants with severe marasmic undernutrition. These children showed no edema, hypoproteinemia, or marked anemia (Table I). Both groups were injected with acetylsalicylic acid intravenously in one dose of 12 mg/kg body weight. The drug used was "Aspegic Roche," which is a lysine acetylsalicylate with glycine buffer. Blood samples were obtained from both groups at times 0, 10, 25, 28, 30, 40, 60, 120, and 480 minutes after the drug administration. In each one of these samples the free plasma and protein bound drug were determined following the method of Potter and Guy (1964). With these data, the plasma elimination constant and the half-life of free and protein-bound salicylate were calculated.

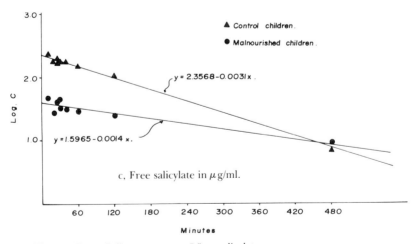

Fig. 1. Rate of disappearance of free salicylate.

TABLE III

Plasma Salicylate Elimination Constants ($K_{min} \times 10^3$) for
Eutrophic and Marasmic Patients Injected Intravenously with
Lysine Acetylsalicylate (Aspegic)

Nutritional status	$K^a_{min} \times 10^3$		
	Total	Protein-bound	Free
Eutrophic	10.9 ± 2.5^b	11.2 ± 2.8	12.3 ± 2.8
Marasmic	5.2 ± 1.0	10.3 ± 2.3	2.3 ± 0.7
$p <$	0.001	NS^c	0.001

[a] The fraction of salicylate eliminated from plasma each minute.
[b] Mean ± standard error of the mean.
[c] Probability not significant by the "t" test.

In normal conditions, salicylates are bound in a high percentage to serum albumins (85–95%) (Gillette, 1972). A smaller fraction remains free. Different reports in the literature (Brodie, 1966) lead one to think that protein-bound salicylates would represent a real drug reserve that would be liberated as free salicylate in the proportion as it is used, metabolized, and eliminated. It has been postulated that the real active fraction of plasma salicylate would be that remaining free.

Table II shows a prolongation of the half-life of total salicylates in severely undernourished compared to eutrophic children ($p < 0.05$). This difference is higher when the half-life of free salicylates is calculated separately. Thus, the latter was 1.1 hours for normal infants and 7.5 hours for undernourished infants ($p < 0.001$). Figure 1 shows the rate of disappearance of free salicylates in both groups of children.

Table III shows the plasma elimination constants of total, protein-bound and free salicylates. The elimination constant of free salicylate was much lower in undernourished than in normal children. While in normal children it was 12.3, in the undernourished it was 2.3 ($p < 0.001$).

These results have an enormous clinical importance because when using salicylates as antipyretics they are prescribed in repeated doses according to the changes of temperature. It is easily understandable that, if the undernourished infant has a prolonged half-life of free salicylates, toxic levels can be reached by the additive action of the successive doses. This is even more serious, since the clinical symptoms of salicylate intoxication in the small child are predominately hyperthermia and acidosis (Monckeberg et al., 1960).

III. METABOLISM OF ANTIBIOTICS

Recently Mehta *et al.* (1975) reported that severe undernourished children also present alterations in the absorption and metabolism of chloramphenicol. The administration of this drug in undernourished children produced the following differences in relation to normal children:

1. Peak plasma levels were generally attained in 4 hours or more in contrast to 2 hours in the normal.

2. The peak plasma levels were higher in children suffering from protein–calorie undernutrition than in controls.

3. The drug took much longer to clear from the plasma of undernourished children.

The longer time taken to achieve the peak level may be due to a slower absorption, because children show many alterations of intestinal absorption (lipids, carbohydrates, vitamin B_{12}) (Mehta *et al.*, 1975), as well as morphological alterations of the intestinal mucosa (Brunser *et al.*, 1966). But, as in the case of salicylates, the delayed clearance of the drug is probably due to a lesser biotransformation velocity, or a slower renal clearance. Alterations in renal plasma flux, glomerular filtration, and renal excretion have been described in undernourished children, but are not so important as to explain by themselves the clearance delay of these drugs.

IV. SUMMARY AND CONCLUSIONS

The most probable explanation is that some processes of biotransformation of these drugs are altered in the liver. In severely undernourished children, diverse alterations of hepatic function as well as histological changes (Platt *et al.*, 1964b) have been described. In electron microscopy studies, changes have been described in the endoplasmic reticulum in humans (Theron and Lienberg, 1963) as well as in animals (Oroy *et al.*, 1966; Svoboda *et al.*, 1966). Most enzymes involved in drug metabolism reside in the endoplasmic reticulum (isolated as microsomes). It is therefore possible that alterations in biotransformation of drugs might be a common factor in children suffering from severe undernutrition.

In general, biotransformation of drugs has two phases of reactions (Gillette, 1966). In the first phase there occur all the reactions changing a nonpolar compound into a polar one which is more rapidly excreted. In the second phase of metabolism there is a synthetic step, so that the compound is conjugated with an endogenous molecule. The products of the second phase, often referred to as conjugated products, are usually water-soluble acids which are readily excreted. The metabolism of most foreign compounds, involves both phases of reactions, but there are some compounds, particularly those that already possess a functional group, that undergo only the second phase.

The enzymes involved in the first phase require oxygen, NADPH, and cytochrome P-450 (Gillette, 1963). It is well documented in the literature that the hepatic microsomal drug metabolism system in rats is affected

TABLE IV

Effect of Protein–Calorie Undernutrition (Marasmus) and Pheno-barbital Induction on Liver Cytochrome P-450 in Male Rats 17 Days Old[a]

Groups	Optical density (450–489 mμ)	Ratio (Phe/saline)
Control + saline (Pool 1)	0.022	
		5.55
Control (Pool 1) + Phe[b]	0.122	
Control + saline (Pool 2)	0.034	
		3.12
Control (Pool 2) + Phe	0.106	
Marasmus (Pool 1) + saline	0.070	
		2.47
Marasmus (Pool 1) + Phe	0.173	
Marasmus + (Pool 2) saline	0.064	
		4.56
Marasmus (Pool 2) + Phe	0.292	

[a] Rats were injected intraperitoneally with 25 mg phenobarbital/kg body weight during 5 days, controls being injected with saline. All values are referred to 3.5 mg microsomal protein/ml. Pools are of 8 animals.

[b] Phe = phenobarbital.

by several specific nutrient deficiencies and low protein diets (Marshall and McLean, 1969; Dickerson *et al.*, 1971; Kato, 1967; Gillette *et al.*, 1969; Kato and Gillette, 1965; Dixon *et al.*, 1960). These studies mostly involve adult animals. In our Institute, the levels of cytochrome *P*-450 were studied in young rats before and after the administration of phenobarbital, and were compared to marasmic rats of the same age. Marasmic rats showed the same degree of induction when phenobarbital was administered (Table IV).

Many other enzymes concerned in the metabolism of foreign compounds are also located in the hepatic endoplastic reticulum, as for example, the glucuronyltransferase enzymes that catalyze the synthesis of glucuronic acid conjugates, a two-phase reaction. Mehta *et al.*, (1975), studying two children suffering severe undernutrition and receiving chloramphenicol, found in their liver biopsies a significant reduction of glucuronyltransferase, using bilirubin as substrate. Although the information gathered is preliminary, it suggests alterations that would interfere with an efficient conjugation of drugs.

Results analyzed here establish the need for further investigation, especially clinical research in order to acquire a better understanding of how the severely undernourished child reacts to different drugs. With the few drugs about which there is some information, evident alterations in their handling can be observed. The severely undernourished child (marasmus) of only a few months of age is very difficult to treat, and even in hospitals they have a 30% mortality rate. This is why one must be extremely careful in the use of drugs, even those that might seem innocuous.

REFERENCES

Alleyne, G. A. (1967). The effect of severe protein calorie malnutrition on the function of Jamaican children. *Pediatrics* **39**, 400.

Anderson, C. (1966). Intestinal malabsorption in childhood. *Arch. Dis. Child.* **41**, 571.

Beas, F., Monckeberg, F., and Horwitz, I. (1966). The response of the thyroid gland to thyroid stimulating hormone in infant malnutrition. *Pediatrics* **38**, 1003.

Bowil, M., Barbezot, G., and Hansen, J. D. L. (1967). Carbohydrates absorption in malnourished children. *Am. J. Clin. Nutr.* **20**, 89.

Brodie, R. R. (1966). Pharmacological and clinical implications of drug transport. *In* "Transport Function of Plasma Proteins" (P. Desgrez and P. de Traverse, eds.), p. 137. Am. Elsevier, New York.

Brunser, O., Reid, W., Monckeberg, F., and Maccioni, A. (1966). Jejunal biopsies in infant malnutrition. *Pediatrics* **38**, 605.

Corbun, A. (1943). Salicylate and rheumatic fever. *Bull. Johns Hopkins Hosp.* **73**, 435.

Cravioto, J., Dilicardie, E., and Birch, H. (1966). Nutrition, growth and neurologic development. *Pediatrics* **38**, 319.

Dickerson, J., Basu, T., and Park, D. (1971). Protein nutrition and drug metabolizing enzymes in the liver of the growing rat. *Proc. Nutr. Soc.* **30,** 5A.

Dixon, R., Shultice, W., and Fouts, J. (1960). Factors affecting drug metabolism by liver microsomes. IV, Starvation. *Proc. Soc. Exp. Biol. Med.* **103,** 333.

Dobbing, J. (1967). Effect of experimental undernutrition on development of the nervous system. *In* "Malnutrition, Learning and Behavior," (Nevin S. Scrimshaw and John S. Gordon, eds.) p. 181. The MIT Press, Cambridge.

Gillette, J. (1963). Metabolism of drugs and other foreign compounds by enzymatic mechanism. *Prog. Drug Res.* **6,** 13.

Gillette, J. (1966). Biochemistry of drug oxidation and reduction by enzymes in hepatic endoplasmic reticulum. *Adv. Pharmacol.* **4,** 219.

Gillette, J. (1972). Overview of protein binding. *Ann. N.Y. Acad. Sci.* **226,** 6.

Gillette, J. R., Conney, A. H., Cosmides, G. J., Estabrook, R. W., Fouts, J. R., and Mannering, G. J., eds. (1969). "Microsomes and Drug Oxidations" p. 547. Academic Press, New York.

Gordillo, G. (1964). Transtornos renales en niños con desnutrición avanzada. *Bol. Med. Hosp. Infant. Mex. (Span. Ed.)* **21,** 699.

Kato, R. (1967). Effects of starvation and refeeding on the oxidation of drugs by liver microsomes. *Biochem. Pharmacol.* **16,** 871.

Kato, R., and Gillette, J. (1965). Effects of starvation on NADPH dependent enzymes in liver microsomes of male and female rats. *J. Pharmacol. Exp. Ther.* **150,** 273.

Marshall, W., and McLean, A. (1969). The effect of oral phenobarbitone on the hepatic microsomal cytochrome *P*-450 and demethylation activity in rats fed normal and low protein diet. *Biochem. Pharmacol.* **18,** 153.

Mehta, S., Kalsi, H., Jayareman, S., and Mathur, V. (1975). Chloramphenicol metabolism in children with protein–calorie malnutrition. *Am. J. Clin. Nutr.* **28,** 977.

Monckeberg, F. (1967). Effects of early malnutrition on subsequent physical and psychological development. *In* "Malnutrition Learning and Behaviour" (N. Scrimshaw, and J. Gordon, eds.) p. 278. The MIT Press, Cambridge.

Monckeberg, F. (1970). Factors Conditioning Malnutrition in Latin America, with Special Reference to Chile. Advices for a volunteers action. *In* "Malnutrition is a problem of Ecology," (P. György and O. L. Kline, eds.) p. 23. S. Karger, Basel.

Monckeberg, F. (1971a). Malnutrition and socioeconomic development. *Bull. Protein Advisory Group* **11,** 9.

Monckeberg, F. (1971b). Endocrine mechanism in nutritional adaptation. *Sci. Publ. Pan. Am. Health Organ.* **222,** 121.

Monckeberg, F., Manzur, F., and Lopez, M. (1958). Algunos factores que incluencian la absorción de grasas en el lactante desnutrido. *Pediatria (Santiago)* **1,** 132.

Monckeberg, F., Jiménez, J., Oxman, S., and Aedo, R. (1960). Intoxicación salicílica en el niño *Pediatria (Santiago)* **3,** 108.

Monckeberg, F., Beas, F., Horwitz, I., Davancens, C. and Figueroa, M. (1964). Oxygen consumption in infant malnutrition. *Pediatrics* **33,** 554.

Oroy, J., Somorajski, T., Zimmermann, R., and Rady, P. (1966). Effects of postnatal protein deficiency on weight gain, serum protein enzymes, cholesterol and liver ultrastructure in subhuman primates. *Am. J. Pathol.* **48,** 796.

Platt, B. S., Heard, C. R. C., and Stewart, R. J. C. (1964a). "Symposium on the Role of Gastro-intestinal Tract in Protein Metabolism." Oxford Univ. Press, London and New York.

Platt, B. S., Heard, C. R. C., Stewart, R. J. C. (1964b). Experimental protein-calorie deficiency. *In* "Mammalian Protein Metabolism" (H. Munro, and J. Allison, eds.) Vol. 2, p. 476. Academic Press, New York.

Potter, C., and Guy, E. (1964). Micromethod for analysis of plasma salicylate. *Proc. Soc. Exp. Biol. Med.* **116,** 658.

Schlesinger, L., and Stekel, A. (1974). Impaired cellular immunity in marasmic infants. *Am. J. Clin. Nutr.* **27,** 615.

Smith, Roger. (1959). Urinary acidification in infantile malnutrition. *Lancet,* 764.

Stekel, A., and Smith, N. (1969a). Hematological studies of severe undernutrition in infancy. *Pediatr. Res.* **3,** 320.

Stekel, A., and Smith, N. (1969b). Hematological studies of severe undernutrition in infancy. *Pediatr. Res.* **3,** 338.

Stock, M., and Smith, P. (1963). Does undernutrition during infancy inhibit brain growth and subsequent intellectual development. *Arch. Dis. Child.* **38,** 546.

Svoboda, D., Grady, H., and Higginson, J. (1966). The effects of chronic protein deficiency in rats. *Lab. Invest.* **14,** 731.

Theron, J., and Lienberg, N. (1963). Some observations in fine cytology of parenchymal liver cells in kwashiorkor. *J. Pathol. Bacteriol.* **86,** 109.

15

Effects of Dietary Protein on Drug Metabolism

T. COLIN CAMPBELL

I. INTRODUCTION

Before we consider what role protein nutrition may play in drug metabolism, let us first consider whether protein intake varies sufficiently to accommodate significant effects on these extremely important reactions. It is generally accepted within the public health and research communities that malnutrition due to protein–calorie insufficiency is one of the four major nutritional problems within the world. Latham (1974) concludes that protein–calorie malnutrition of young children is the world's most important and devastating nutritional problem. The disease symptoms range from kwashiorkor, which is precipitated by a deficiency of protein and certain essential amino acids, to nutritional marasmus, which represents primarily a deficit of calories, but also including protein.

The relative importance of the deficiencies associated with these two nutrients remains somewhat debatable, in part because of the lack of distinction, but extensive overlap, of clinical symptoms. Within the past 25 years, however, considerable emphasis has been placed on the so-called protein gap (Phillips, 1973), although more recently recommendations have been made that more emphasis be placed on an adequate food intake (Latham, 1974; R. W. Engel, personal communication), rather than concentrating on protein-rich foods. Whatever outcome is eventually realized for the relative importance of protein versus calories remains to be established.

On the other hand, what *is* known is that protein intake varies widely in various parts of the world. The median per capita intake of total protein for various countries ranges at least three-fold (Food and Agricultural Organization, 1964–1966), with still greater variation for individuals *within* countries. This wide range in total protein consumption is primarily contributed by a more widely varying range in the consumption of meat protein (Clark and Turner, 1973). For example, the range in the median consumption patterns for meat protein is about twentyfold, ranging from a low of 3.6 gm/person/day for Rwanda to 71.8 gm/person/day for Uruguay. Many ambitious projects have been premised on the assumption that if countries are to improve their overall nutrition, a higher intake of meat protein must be realized (Phillips, 1973).

In addition to the great variation in the intake of dietary protein through traditional dietary patterns, there are also a large number of individuals whose protein status may be impaired by other means. Such a deficiency occurs in the abnormal diets of chronic alcoholics, narcotic and other drug addicts, depressed psychopaths, and food faddists (Boyd, 1969). These brief comments are intended to convey the message that protein intake varies from below the recommended dietary allowances to amounts which are several times these allowances. Within the context of our own experimentation on the effect of protein nutrition on drug metabolism, we would suggest that there is ample room for the intake of this nutrient to influence the activities of the drug-metabolizing enzyme system.

Other information which is fundamental to an understanding of this type of interaction is that concerned with the role of drug metabolism in the resultant pharmacologic and toxicologic activities of the compounds which are metabolized by this enzyme system.

First, we must recognize that substrates of this enzyme system include a wide variety of rather lipophilic substances. Foreign chemicals such as drugs, adventitious food residues, and intentional food additives, together with endogenous steroid hormones, may all be metabolized. Therefore, such events as hormonal balance, pharmacologic activity, acute chemical toxicity, and chemical carcinogenesis may all be influenced by the metabolism of the chemicals which induce these events.

What role, then, does metabolism of these chemicals play in their eventual activities? The respective biological response obtained will depend, as a first approximation, on whether the rate-limiting reaction catalyzes either detoxification or activation of the parent substance. The cytochrome P-450-dependent mixed-function oxidase (MFO) primarily located in the liver is generally considered to be the predominant enzyme involved in these reactions. However, the important reactions, which are catalyzed by various transferases and hydrases and which form products even more water-soluble and excretable, must not be overlooked.

What role does protein nutrition play in the metabolism and biologic activity of these foreign compounds, and can that effect be predicted? For many compounds, the reaction sequences may be exceedingly complex and render an answer difficult to obtain. One reasonably simple approach to an understanding of these reactions is to first ask whether the biological activity of interest is reversible after the compound is cleared from the tissue; expressed another way, is the response dosage-dependent? That is, the interactions of pharmaceutical chemicals with mammalian tissue target sites should be readily reversible, whether these are the pharmacologically desirable end-points or the sometimes unavoidable side-reactions.

If there is a single enzymatic reaction involved in the metabolism of such chemicals, then the relative activity of that enzyme will determine the duration and intensity of response. A good example of this type of mechanism is one demonstrating the effect of dietary protein levels on the response to barbiturates. That is, the activity of the MFO enzyme system is inversely correlated with barbiturate sleeping times in several laboratory animal species (Quinn *et al.*, 1958). The higher the rate of metabolism of pentobarbital by the MFO enzyme system to the less active products, the faster is the plasma clearance and the shorter is the sleeping time. Moreover, Kato *et al.* (1968) demonstrated in rats that the decrease of serum pentobarbital was directly related to dietary protein concentrations ranging from 0–50%.

Whereas protein deficiency *increases* the activity of barbiturates, it *decreases* the toxicities of substances such as heptachlor (Weatherholtz *et al.*, 1969) and octamethylpyrophosphoramide (Kato *et al.*, (1968), since each of these substances are metabolized to more toxic products by the MFO system. All of these observations are consistent with our data which show that low protein intakes depress MFO enzyme activities (Mgbodile and Campbell, 1972; Hayes *et al.*, 1973; Campbell, 1976).

Whereas reversible interactions and single enzymatic reactions simplify the interpretations above, what can be said for those chemicals whose tissue effects are irreversible and whose metabolism includes more than one reaction? These conditions are characteristic of chemical carcinogens and necrogenic agents. Interpretation of this type of event relies on a more complete understanding of the several reactions which are sequenced and perhaps coordinated in the production of a reaction intermediate which is more reactive than the parent compound. Moreover, the toxic event appears to depend on an irreversible reaction between the target site within the cell and the reactive component. Such a reaction may result in the formation of a covalent bond with the resulting irreversible cell damage. Gillette and co-workers (1974) have carried out a series of elegant studies with agents such as the halobenzenes, furosamide and acetaminophen showing that cell necrosis is a function of the amount of reactive intermediate of these chemicals which covalently binds critical molecules. These workers have concluded that the best estimator of toxic response in this type of reaction is the proportion of the dose which forms the reactive intermediate and which covalently binds critical macromolecules within the target tissue (Gillette, 1974a,b).

For this latter type of toxicity, therefore, any of several metabolic events may influence the proportion of the dose which forms this highly reactive intermediate. In other words, there are enzymatic reactions which activate the parent compound and there are enzymatic reactions which deactivate the reactive product; there are requirements for cosubstrates involved in the conjugation of the reactive intermediate that must be met; and there may be alternate noncritical target sites which siphon off important quantities of reactive intermediate. These complexities may be illustrated with the scheme for the metabolism of chemical carcinogens shown in Fig. 1. This type of metabolic scheme should also apply to other irreversibly toxic lesions. That is, the probability for lesion formation, or alternatively, the severity of the lesion, should depend on the proportion of the dose which forms the ultimately toxic metabolite and which covalently binds the most critical target receptor site. As can be seen, there are several reactions and cosubstrate availabilities which may influence the amount of ultimately toxic metabolic formed. In the case of carcinogenesis, reactions which proceed via the hatched arrows eventually lead to neoplasia. Some carcinogens may form the ultimate carcinogen directly via MFO metabolism; others, like benzopyrene, appear to involve a minimum three-step reaction sequence forming an epoxide, then a diol, and finally a second epoxide group on another part of the molecule (Wislocki *et al.*, 1976); still others, like AAF, may form the *N*-hydroxy proximate carcinogen but then require transferase-catalyzed conjugation reactions to form the ultimate carcinogen (De Baun *et al.*, 1970). In each of these cases, the quantity of ultimate carcinogen formed should relate directly to the proportion

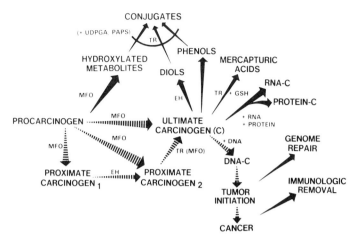

Fig. 1. Metabolism of chemical carcinogens. MFO, mixed function oxidase; TR, transferase(s); EH, epoxide hydrase; GSH, glutathione; UDPGA, uridine diphosphoglucuronic acid; PAPS, (3'-phosphoadenosine 5'-phosphosulfate); DNA-C, DNA-carcinogen adduct.

of the dose which binds or alkylates DNA as well as directly to the tumorigenicity. Opposed to the reaction sequences with the hatched arrows are the various reaction sequences with solid arrows which are intended to show detoxification mechanisms. These involve several steps. First, the original chemical may form less active products; second, the ultimate carcinogen may rearrange or react to be diverted from its reaction with DNA or whatever is the critical macromolecule; third, the covalently-bound DNA may be repaired; and fourth, one last valve may include immunologic removal of the tumor cells.

In theory, there are several mechanisms within this scheme which could regulate the quantity of covalently-bound carcinogen. First, the activity of the rate-limiting enzyme could be involved and that could theoretically be the epoxide hydrase or one of the transferases, as well as the MFO; second, the availability of cosubstrates (such as GSH, UDPGA, PAPS), may be rate-limiting; third, the relative specific MFO activities for detoxification and activation, whatever these are, must be considered; fourth, at least in theory, the availability of alternate reaction sites for the ultimate carcinogen (such as RNA and protein), may be involved; and fifth, there may be specific transport mechanisms, such as with the carcinogen-binding proteins, which deliver either the procarcinogen or its ultimate carcinogen to selected molecular or subcellular sites.

For other "irreversible" toxicities, the terms "ultimately toxic metabolite" and "toxicity" could be used in place of "ultimate carcinogen" and "neoplasia," respectively.

II. EFFECT OF PROTEIN DEFICIENCY ON
MIXED-FUNCTION OXIDASE ENZYME SYSTEM

Much of our initial investigations on the effect of protein deficiency on drug metabolism reactions was concerned with the effect of dietary protein deficiency on the MFO enzyme system.

Throughout out studies we have employed Sprague-Dawley-derived male rats 21 days of age. On procurement, they were housed individually in stainless steel wire-bottom cages, provided tap water ad libitum and fed a 20% casein semi-purified diet for 2 days. They were then divided into three groups and fed either a 5% casein diet (Group I); a 20% casein diet pair-fed to Group I (Group II); or a 20% casein diet fed *ad libitum* (Group III). The basal diet (20% casein) was previously described by Weatherholtz *et al.* (1969), and consisted of the following: (in grams) sucrose 69.6; vitamin-free casein, 20.0; Mazola corn oil, 4.0; Jones Foster salt mixture, 4.0; vitamin mixture, 2.2; and DL-methionine, 0.2. The 5% casein diet was kept isocaloric by replacing the casein with an equivalent amount of sucrose. The ranges of body weight gains for these animals were approximately 5–7 gm (Group I), 35–50 gm (Group II), and 80–110 (Group III). Each group was comprised of 4–7 animals, and each experiment was replicated a minimum of 6 times. Livers from each group were pooled and each assay was replicated 2–3 times.

The methods and materials used for the various assays were published elsewhere (Hayes *et al.*, 1973; Mgbodile *et al.*, 1973; Hayes and Campbell, 1974). Substrates for the MFO enzyme system were chosen to represent the classical type I (ethylmorphine, EM) and type II (aniline, AN) compounds.* Classical inducers of MFO enzyme activity used in these experiments included phenobarbital (PB), which increases cytochrome P-450 content and enzyme activity for a broad spectrum of substrates, and 3-methylcholanthrene (MC), which increases cytochrome P-448 (P_1-450) content and enzyme activity for a more limited spectrum of substrates generally characterized by aromatic hydrocarbons such as benzo(a)pyrene.

The livers of the protein-deficient animals were characterized by cells higher in lipid content and larger in size (relative to body weight) than the livers of the protein-adequate control animals (Table I). Histological examination of tissue slices confirmed the higher content of lipid (Mgbodile, 1973). Feeding the protein-deficient diets for 2 weeks was

---

*Type I ligands produce a difference spectrum characterized by an absorption peak at 385–390 nm and a trough at 419–425 nm, whereas type II substrates produce a different spectrum characterized by an absorption peak at 426–435 nm and a trough at 390–405 nm.

TABLE I
Representative Protein Deficiency Effects on Rat Liver Cell Constituents[a]

Cell parameter	Dietary protein[b]	
	5%	20%
Lipid content (%)	6.64 ± 0.09[c]	2.10 ± 0.02
Cell volume ($\mu^3 \times 10^{-3}$)	4.45 ± 0.17	2.76 ± 0.19
Liver DNA (mg/gm)	1.26 ± 0.09	2.18 ± 0.12
Microsomal protein (mg/gm)	10.5 ± 0.5	18.0 ± 1.5

[a] From Mgbodile and Campbell (1972) and Mgbodile (1973).
[b] Animals were pair-fed.
[c] Data represent means ± S.E., wet tissue basis.

associated with fewer cells per liver weight, as demonstrated with the DNA content; also, there was less microsomal protein per unit weight of liver. These data suggest that the amount of microsomal protein per unit weight of tissue depends, in part, on the number of cells. Apparently consumption of the protein-deficient diets is associated with a lower rate of liver cell proliferation in these growing animals.

Representative data, which demonstrate the effect of protein deficiency on MFO enzyme activities are shown in Table II. There was a 50–65% decrease in the MFO enzyme activities in the 5% casein group compared to the 20% control groups. Cytochrome P-450 content and P-450 reductase activity were decreased approximately the same amount

TABLE II
Representative Protein Deficiency Effects on Rat Liver MFO Enzyme Activities[a]

	Dietary protein		
	5%	20%	20%
Feeding protocol	ad lib	pair-fed[b]	ad lib
Enzyme activities			
P-450, nmoles/mg protein	0.12 ± 0.02	0.48 ± 0.10	0.42 ± 0.04
P-450 reductase[c]	7 ± 1	19 ± 1	16 ± 2
V_{max}, EM[d]	340 ± 50	940 ± 40	900 ± 60
V_{max}, AN[e]	10 ± 1	20 ± 2	20 ± 3

[a] From Hayes and Campbell (1974).
[b] Pair-fed to 5% protein animals.
[c] Nmoles P-450 reduced/mg protein/minute ± range (duplicate assays).
[d] Nmoles HCHO/mg protein/hour ± S.E.
[e] Nmoles p-aminophenol/mg protein/hour ± S.E.

as the EM N-demethylase and AN hydroxylase activities. When these decreases are coupled with the decrease in total microsomal protein content usually observed in the low-protein animals (see Table I), the total MFO decrease per unit body weight may be as great as 75–80%, within the 14 day feeding trial. In other studies, in our laboratory, (unpublished observations), we have found that most of this decrease can be achieved within the first 8 days.

Because there was higher lipid content in the protein-deficient livers and because phosphatidylcholine was known to be required for MFO enzyme activity, we therefore examined various relationships between phosphatidylcholine, cytochrome P-450, and enzyme kinetic parameters. These studies were premised on the observation that when protein-deficient animals were administered either PB or MC in order to induce MFO enzyme activities, the cytochrome component was increased substantially more than the phosphatidylcholine (Table III). The greater abundance of phosphatidylcholine was associated with a substantially greater number of "binding sites" for EM and a lower K_m for metabolism of EM. These data suggested that the induced synthesis of P-450 without a concommittant increase of phosphatidylcholine resulted in a hemoprotein activity characterized by fewer binding sites and a higher K_m. Accordingly, the K_m may represent a diffusion rate for the substrate penetrating into the vicinity of the active site; that is, when an environment about the active site is made more hydrophobic with phosphatidylcholine, the lipophilic substrates of this enzyme approach the catalytic site with greater facility. These data (but not the interpretation) are in accord with those of others who chemically removed the

TABLE III
Effects of *In Vivo* Administration of PB and MC on EM N-Demethylase Kinetics of Rat Liver Microsomes of Protein-Deficient Animals[a]

Parameter	Control	PB[b]	Control[c]	MC[c]
ΔA_{max}/nmole P-450 ($\times 10^3$)	21.0 ± 5.0	6.0 ± 1.2	22.4 ± 4.2	3.2 ± 0.6
K_m, mM	0.12 ± 0.03	0.19 ± 0.04	0.15 ± 0.02	0.24 ± 0.03
PC/P-450[d]	170 ± 30	65.7 ± 9.4	230 ± 45	69.2 ± 9.8

[a] From Hayes *et al.* (1973), Mgbodile *et al.* (1973), and Hayes and Campbell (1974).

[b] Phenobarbital (80 mg/kg) administered ip on days 11–14 in 0.9% saline; control animals administered 0.9% saline only.

[c] 3-Methylcholanthrene (20 mg/kg) administered ip on days 13–14 in corn oil; control animals administered corn oil only.

[d] Mg phosphatidylcholine/nmole P-450 (P-448 for MC-induced microsomes).

TABLE IV

Effects of Protein Deficiency on Kinetic Parameters of EM N-Demethylase of Rat Liver Microsomes[a]

Parameter	Dietary protein		
	5%	20%	20%
Feeding protocol	ad lib	pair-fed[b]	ad lib
ΔA_{max}/nmole P-450 ($\times$ 10³)	21.8 ± 4.4	12.8 ± 1.9	16.2 ± 2.7
K_m, mM	0.13 ± 0.02	0.14 ± 0.02	0.16 ± 0.02
PC/P-450[c]	200.0 ± 40.0	61.0 ± 14.0	57.0 ± 10.0

[a] From Hayes *et al.* (1973), Mgbodile *et al.* (1973), and Hayes and Campbell (1974).
[b] Pair-fed to 5% protein animals.
[c] μg phosphatidylcholine/nmole P-450.

phosphatidylcholine component with isooctane extraction (Leibman and Estabrook, 1971) or phospholipase c treatment (Chaplin and Mannering, 1970). MC-induced microsomes (Table III) show the same trends to an even greater degree. This enhancement is probably due to a replacement of a large proportion of the cytochrome P-450 with cytochrome P-448. When the same parameters were examined as functions of dietary treatment (Table IV), these trends were much less marked. Even though there was a much greater phosphatidylcholine contribution in the microsomes of the protein-deficient animals, there was only a modest increase in EM binding sites and a very slight, but insignificant, decrease in the K_m. We have concluded, therefore, that dietary protein does not alter the phosphatidylcholine involvement in hemoprotein activity, even though there is an accumulation of lipid within these cells.

An analysis of the effect of protein deficiency on MFO enzyme induction is shown in Table V. PB was administered on the last 4 days of the experiment to permit maximum enzyme induction. Protein deficiency decreased not only the basal MFO activities but also the induced activities, compared to the animals fed 20% dietary protein. Although the percentage increases were remarkably similar for all four enzyme activities, the induced activities in the protein-deficient animals were much lower than the induced activities for the control animals. Since enzyme induction of MFO enzyme activities is known to modify toxic and pharmacologic activities (Campbell and Hayes, 1974), it may be important to determine whether protein deficiency alters responses which are dependent on these capacities.

TABLE V

Effect of Protein Deficiency on MFO Enzyme Induction[a]

| | Dietary protein[b] | | | |
| | 5% | | 20% | |
Enzyme activity	Control	Induced[c]	Control	Induced[c]
EM N-demethylase (nmoles HCHO produced/hour/mg protein)	400 ± 48.0	1670 ± 320 (76)	1200 ± 70.0	4730 ± 590 (75)
AN hydroxylase (nmoles p-aminophenol/hour/mg protein)	8.6 ± 1.2	30.3 ± 13.6 (72)	23.8 ± 1.8	75.8 ± 8.9 (69)
Cytochrome P-450 reductase (nmoles P-450/mg protein)	6.1 ± 1.0	37.9 ± 0.8 (84)	17.1 ± 3.3	135 ± 39 (87)
Cytochrome P-450 (nmoles/mg protein)	0.16 ± 0.03	0.54 ± 0.07 (70)	0.41 ± 0.07	1.84 ± 0.12 (78)

[a] From Mgbodile et al. (1973).

[b] Phenobarbital (80 mg/kg) administered ip on days 11–14 in 0.9% saline; control animals injected with 0.9% saline. All animals in both dietary treatment groups were pair-fed to equalize food intake.

[c] Numbers in parentheses show percentage increases.

As previously discussed, the final outcome for the effect of protein deficiency on toxic and pharmacologic responses may be determined by any one of several reactions, particularly those which are rate-limiting. The simplest system is that which involves only one reaction and reversible interaction between the chemical and its tissue target site. Knowing whether that reaction represents either detoxication or activation would enable one to predict the effect of protein deficiency on the biological activity of the chemical. As previously mentioned, for toxicities such as cell necrosis and carcinogenesis, on the other hand, irreversible covalent bonds form between the toxic chemical and the target site. A reactive intermediate is usually produced and is involved in this type of interaction. In turn, reactions involved in both production *and* degradation of the reactive intermediate must be considered, particularly for those reactions which may be rate-limiting.

What effect, then, would protein deficiency have on the metabolism of chemical carcinogens which are metabolized in this manner? The degree of chemical carcinogenesis should depend on the proportion of the dose which forms the ultimate carcinogen and which covalently binds target macromolecules. One of the more interesting carcinogens which has been examined during protein deficiency is aflatoxin, which is the potent hepatocarcinogen produced by *Aspergillus flavus* (Wogan, 1968; Campbell and Stoloff, 1974).

Rats fed protein-deficient diets during the administration of aflatoxin B_1 (AFB$_1$) yielded a dramatically decreased number of tumors after 1 year (Madhavan and Gopalan, 1968). Because the decrease in carcinogenicity should be correlated with a decrease in the amount of covalently bound AFB$_1$ residue, we examined the effect of protein deficiency on the proportion of an ^{3}H-AFB$_1$ dose which binds critical macromolecules in rat liver nuclei (Preston *et al.*, 1976). These data are presented in Table VI. In both control and protein-deficient animals, there was a consistent decrease (70%) in the binding to chromatin, DNA, and chromatin protein. Protein deficiency depressed MFO activity and would suggest that the decrease in binding was due to lower production of the ultimate carcinogen.

However, it may not be possible to draw the simple conclusion that the decreased MFO activity in the protein-deficient animals is responsible for the decreased production of AFB$_1$ product which covalently binds. This is because, as Garner (1975) recently showed, when phenobarbital was administered to rats, less binding of AFB$_1$ to DNA and rRNA occurred, and in his animals, MFO activity should have been induced. Since protein deficiency and phenobarbital administration both depress AFB$_1$ tumorigenicity, the quantity of covalent binding with both of these

TABLE VI
Effect of Protein Deficiency on the Binding of ^{3}-H-AFB$_1$ to Nuclear Macromolecules[a]

AFB$_1$[b] bound to	Dietary protein		
	5%	20%	20%
Feeding protocol	ad lib	pair-fed[c]	ad lib
Chromatin (pmoles/mg DNA)	81.7 ± 16.0	187 ± 8.0	259 ± 36.0
DNA (pmoles/mg)	56.4 ± 9.6	141 ± 14	202 ± 21
Protein (pmoles/mg)	11.9 ± 3.2	21.8 ± 8.3	35.2 ± 21

[a] From Preston *et al.* (1976).
[b] Animals fed for 15 days, then injected on day 16 ip with ^{3}-H-AFB$_1$ (1.90 mg/kg) 6 hours prior to sacrifice.
[c] Pair-fed to 5% protein animals.

treatments would be a satisfactory carcinogenic index, whereas the MFO activity is not. Clearly, then, other reactions involved in AFB$_1$ metabolism might also be modified by treatments such as feeding protein-deficient diets and injecting phenobarbital. The finding that protein deficiency increases hepatic glucuronyltransferase activity in rats (Woodcock and Wood, 1971) certainly indicates that all reactions—both activation and degradation types—must be evaluated in any assessment of protein status on the metabolism of chemical carcinogens.

III. CONCLUSIONS

In conclusion, I wish to emphasize that reasonably modest protein deprivation can alter the metabolism of foreign compounds rather dramatically. Moreover, since protein intakes in man vary widely, it is reasonable to assume that protein nutrition may exert a major influence on our susceptibilities to the toxicities and carcinogenicities of foreign chemicals, as well as on our responsiveness to pharmaceutical preparations. However, before information of this type becomes useful to the clinician or public health scientist, we will need to learn considerably more about the metabolism of the chemicals under investigation, as well as the specific effects of protein deficiency on each of the various reactions involved in the metabolism of these substances.

ACKNOWLEDGMENT

Supported by grants from Hoffman LaRoche Research Foundation, Research Corporation, and National Institutes of Health (RO1 ES 00336, RO1 CA 20079)

REFERENCES

Boyd, E. M. (1969). Diet and drug toxicity. *Clin. Toxicol.* **2,** 423–433.

Campbell, T. C. (1976). The effect of quantity and quality of dietary protein on drug metabolism. *Fed. Proc.* **35,** 2470–2474.

Campbell, T. C., and Hayes, J. R. (1974). Role of nutrition in the drug-metabolizing enzyme system. *Pharmacol. Rev.* **26,** 171–197.

Campbell, T. C., and Stoloff, L. (1974). Implication of mycotoxins for human health. *J. Agric. Food Chem.* **22,** 1006–1015.

Chaplin, M. D., and Mannering, G. J. (1970). Role of phospholipids in the hepatic microsomal drug-metabolizing system. *Mol. Pharmacol.* **6,** 631–640.

Clark, C., and Turner, J. B. (1973). World population growth and future food trends. *In* "Man, Food and Nutrition" (M. Rechcigl, Jr., ed.), pp. 55–77. Chem. Rubber Publ. Co., Cleveland, Ohio.

De Baun, J. R., Miller, E. C., and Miller, J. A. (1970). Reactivity *in vivo* of the carcinogen N-hydroxy-2-acetylaminofluorene. *Science,* **167,** 184–186.

Food and Agriculture Organization. (1964–1966). "Food Balance Sheets." FAO, Rome.

Garner, R. C. (1975). Reduction in binding of (^{14}C) aflatoxin B_1 to rat liver macromolecules by phenobarbitone pretreatment. *Biochem. Pharmacol.* **24,** 1553–1556.

Gillette, J. R. (1974a). A perspective on the role of chemically reactive metabolites of foreign compounds in toxicity. I. Correlation of changes in covalent binding of reactivite metabolites with changes in the incidence and severity of toxicity. *Biochem. Pharmacol.* **23,** 2785–2794.

Gillette, J. R. (1974b). A perspective on the role of chemically reactive metabolites of foreign compounds in toxicity. II. Alterations in the kinetics of covalent binding. *Biochem. Pharmacol.* **23,** 2927–2938.

Gillette, J. R., Mitchell, J. R., and Brodie, B. B. (1974). Biochemical mechanisms of drug toxicity. *Annu. Rev. Pharmacol.* **14,** 271–288.

Hayes, J. R., and Campbell, T. C. (1974). Effect of protein deficiency on the inducibility of the hepatic microsomal drug-metabolizing enzyme system. III. Effect of 3-methyl-cholanthrene induction on activity and binding kinetics. *Biochem. Pharmacol.* **23,** 1721–1731.

Hayes, J. R., Mgbodile, M. U. K., and Campbell, T. C. (1973). Effect of protein deficiency on the inducibility of the hepatic microsomal drug-metabolizing enzyme system. I. Effect on substrate interaction with cytochrome *P*-450. *Biochem. Pharmacol.* **22,** 1005–1014.

Kato, R., Oshima, T., and Tomizawa, S. (1968). Toxicity and metabolism of drugs in relation to dietary protein. *Jpn. J. Pharmacol.* **18,** 356–366.

Latham, M. C. (1974). Protein–calorie malnutrition in children and its relation to psychological development and behavior. *Physiol. Rev.* **54,** 541–565.

Leibman, K. C., and Estabrook, R. W. (1971). Effects of extraction with isooctane upon the properties of liver microsomes. *Mol. Pharmacol.* **7,** 26–32.

Madhavan, T. V., and Gopalan, C. (1968). The effect of dietary protein on carcinogenesis of alfatoxin. *Arch. Pathol.* **85,** 133–137.

Mgbodile, M. U. K. (1973). Microsomal mixed function oxidation mechanisms associated with dietary protein insufficiency. Ph.D. Dissertation, Virginia Polytechnic Institute and State University, Blacksburg.

Mgbodile, M. U. K., and Campbell, T. C. (1972). Effect of protein deprivation of male weanling rats on the kinetics of hepatic microsomal enzyme activity. *J. Nutr.* **102,** 53–60.

Mgbodile, M. U. K., Hayes, J. R., and Campbell, T. C. (1973). Effect of protein deficiency on the inducibility of the hepatic microsomal drug-metabolizing enzyme system. II.

422   T. Colin Campbell

Effect on enzyme kinetics and electron transport system. *Biochem. Pharmacol.* **22**, 1125-1132.

Phillips, R. W. (1973). Increasing output of animal production relative potential of specific meat-producing animals. *In* "Man, Food and Nutrition" (M. Rechcigl, Jr., ed.), pp. 147-162. Chem. Rubber Publ. Co., Cleveland, Ohio.

Preston, R. S., Hayes, J. R., and Campbell, T. C. (1976). The effect of protein deficiency on the *in vivo* binding of aflatoxin B_1 to rat liver macromolecules. *Life Sci.* **19**, 1191-1198.

Quinn, G. P., Axelrod, J., and Brodie, B. B. (1958). Species, strain, and sex differences in metabolism of hexobarbitone, amidopyrine, antipyrine, and aniline. *Biochem. Pharmacol.* **1**, 152-159.

Weatherholtz, W. M., Campbell, T. C., and Webb, R. E. (1969). Effect of dietary protein levels on the toxicity and metabolism of heptachlor. *J. Nutr.* **98**, 90-94.

Wislocki, P. G., Wood, A. W., Chang, R. L., Levin, W., Yagi, H., Hernandez, O., Dansette, P. M., Jerina, D. M., and Conney, A. H. (1976). Mutagenicity and cytotoxicity of benzo-(a)pyrene arene oxides, phenols, quinones, and dihydrodiols in bacterial and mammalian cells. *Cancer Res.* **36**, 3350-3357.

Wogan. G. N. (1968). Biochemical responses to aflatoxins. *Cancer Res.* **28**, 2282-2287.

Woodcock, B. G., and Wood, G. C. (1971). Effect of protein-free diet on UDP-glucuronyltransferase and sulfotransferase activities in rat liver. *Biochem. Pharmacol.* **20**, 2703-2713.

16

Effect of Amino Acid Intake on Ethanol Toxicity

CHARLES O. WARD and MICHAEL A DORATO

I. INTRODUCTION

Ethanol is one of the most ubiquitous of human foodstuffs, having been discovered by mankind before the onset of recorded history. It has been used by every major civilization discovered to date. Despite the fact that its food value is limited to its caloric content and that its principal effects on the human body are central nervous system depression and gastric irritation, it is an integral part of each major meal in many parts of the world and has been for centuries.

In addition to its use as a food, ethanol is also the most widely used psychoactive substance in the world. The United States has the unfortunate distinction of being the nation with the highest incidence of alcoholism in the world (Gable, 1974). Ethanol is in fact the most widely abused substance in the world today.

II. ETHANOL ABSORPTION AND METABOLISM

Ethanol is rapidly absorbed through the small intestine, some absorption also occurring from the stomach (Mendelson, 1970). The rate of ethanol absorption increases with ethanol concentration to a maximum at 40% (Mendelson, 1970). The CNS depression of ethanol does not vary in concentrations ranging from 30 to 90% (Aston and Stolman, 1966).

The liver plays an important role in the metabolism of ethanol (Fig. 1; Goth, 1974). Hepatic metabolism of ethanol to acetaldehyde, via the alcohol dehydrogenase system, is associated with the generation of excess reducing equivalents, such as NADH (Lieber et al., 1975). The increase in reducing equivalents can partially explain the hepatotoxic effects of ethanol (Mendelson, 1970; Leevy and Baker, 1963; Lieber et al., 1975) and de-emphasize the role of dietary deficiency (Lieber et al., 1975).

At tissue levels associated with central effects, ethanol is metabolized at a relatively constant rate (Gessner, 1973). Only at low tissue levels of ethanol does metabolism occur at a rate proportional to the ethanol

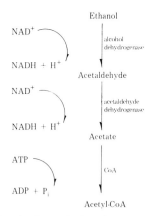

Fig. 1. Ethanol metabolism in liver (Goth 1974). NAD (NADH), nicotine adenine dinucleotide (reduced form); ATP, adenosine triphosphate; ADP, adenosine diphosphate; CoA, coenzyme A.

concentration (Gessner, 1973; Marshall and Fritz, 1953; Owens and Marshall, 1955). The constant rate of ethanol metabolism has been ascribed to the saturation of ethanol clearance mechanisms (Gessner, 1973; Marshall and Fritz, 1953; Makar and Mannering, 1970). In the rat, the rate of ethanol oxidation was independent of blood ethanol levels following the administration of 1–2.5 gm/kg of ethanol (Owens and Marshall, 1955).

In mice, a linear elimination of ethanol during the first 3 hours following ethanol administration was reported (Nelson et al., 1957). The possibility that the rate-limiting factors of ethanol metabolism (Goldstein, 1970; Frosander, 1970; Smith et al., 1957) might not operate during the first hour following ethanol administration was indicated by Owens and Marshall (1955). Nelson et al. (1957), however, reported no difference in metabolic rate during the first or subsequent hours following ethanol administration.

A variety of conditions have been found to alter the rate of ethanol metabolism, for example, weight (Nelson et al., 1957), route of administration, pyruvate, and nicotinamide adenine dinucleotide (Owens and Marshall, 1955). Maintenance of rats on a protein-free diet was found to decrease the rate of ethanol metabolism (Owens and Marshall, 1955; Kerner and Westerfield, 1953). Fasting was reported to decrease the rate of ethanol metabolism by one-third (Owens and Marshall, 1955) to one-half (Smith and Newman, 1959). In vitro studies utilizing the livers of fasting rats have shown that agents which promote the reoxidation of reduced nicotinamide adenine dinucleotide also increased the rate of ethanol metabolism (Smith and Newman, 1959). The livers of well-fed rats did not respond in the same way.

Whether chronic ethanol administration results in an adaptive increase in ethanol elimination has been a matter of considerable disagreement (Pieper and Sheen, 1973). Recently, it has been agreed that metabolic tolerance is a factor in ethanol elimination (Hawkins and Kalant, 1972). Pieper and Sheen (1973) reported metabolic tolerance in ethanol-dependent nonhuman primates. Majchrowicz et al. (1968) and Greenberger et al. (1965) found no metabolic tolerance in rodents, however. There is a dose dependency in elevated ethanol elimination rates; moderate amounts of ethanol can be consumed for extended periods of time without the production of metabolic tolerance (Pieper and Sheen, 1973).

Alcohol dehydrogenase is the most important enzyme for the oxidation of ethanol (Hawkins and Kalant, 1972). Since acetaldehyde is the primary ethanol metabolite produced by the alcohol dehydrogenase system (Hawkins and Kalant, 1972; Stotz et al., 1944; Holtzman and

Schneider, 1974), some of the actions of ethanol have been attributed to acetaldehyde (Truitt and Doritz, 1966; Cohen and Collins, 1970; Feldstein *et al.*, 1964).

Whether acetaldehyde makes an important contribution to ethanol toxicity is still a matter of some debate. High blood concentrations of acetaldehyde, 4–6 mg/ml, have been reported to occur without causing obvious signs of intoxication (Macleod, 1950). It has alternately been reported that acetaldehyde is from 30 to 35 times more potent than ethanol as a central nervous system depressant (Holtzman and Schneider, 1974).

III. ACUTE AND CHRONIC TOXICITY OF ETHANOL

Briefly, the acute effect of ethanol in laboratory rodents has the following dose-related response: ataxia, decreased muscle tone, dyspnea, hypomotility, hind leg paralysis, loss of righting reflex, tremors, and death. The chronic effects are related to dependence, target organ histopathology, and death after prolonged ethanol intake.

A. Effects of Acute Amino Acid Administration

Schiller *et al.* (1959) investigated the effect of amino acids as a solution of protein hydrolyzates on ethanol blood levels and elimination. The amino acids were administered iv and ethanol po to chronic alcoholics free of liver impairment. Ethanol utilization curves have shown amino acids to decrease blood ethanol levels and accelerate the rate of disappearance of ethanol from the blood (Schiller *et al.*, 1959). The specific active amino acids in the mixture used by Schiller *et al.* were not determined. Widmark (1933a) also reported selected amino acids to be effective in decreasing blood ethanol levels in dogs, when administered simultaneously with ethanol. Certain amino acids may form a stable complex with ethanol when administered orally, thus impeding its absorption (Widmark, 1933b).

Others (Prigot *et al.*, 1962; Ancona and Caloza, 1963) have reported successful use of amino acid mixtures in managing delerium tremens. Specific amino acids have been indicated in altering the course of ethanol toxicity (Table I).

1. L-*Glutamine and* L-*Glutamate*

It has been postulated that a block in glutamine synthetase exists in alcoholics. Ravel *et al.* (1955) isolated a liver factor which prevents the

TABLE I
Effect of Various Amino Acids on the Toxicity
of Ethanol

Antagonistic	Synergistic
Glutamine	Glycine
Arginine	Serine
Arginine–glutamate	Tryptophan
Lysine	Asparagine
Ornithine	
Glycine	
Asparagine	

toxicity of alcohol for *Streptococcus fecalis*, and identified it as glutamine. Rogers *et al.* (1955) reported orally administered glutamine to be relatively effective in decreasing the voluntary consumption of alcohol by rats. Glutamic acid, a close relative of glutamine, in combination with arginine has been found useful in managing delerium tremors (Ancona and Caloza, 1963). Glutamine supplementation trials in ten alcoholics indicated glutamine as an important addition to other nutritional supplements in decreasing the desire for alcohol in humans (Rogers and Pelton, 1957). Good nutrition was reported to be necessary for success (Rogers and Pelton, 1957). In contrast, however, it has been reported that glutamine is no more effective than a placebo in altering acute alcohol intoxication or in the treatment of alcoholism (Stolt, 1965).

Ethanol has been reported to adversely affect amino acid transport and utilization by various tissues (Chambers and Piccirillo, 1973; Israel *et al.*, 1968). It has also been reported to affect cerebral protein synthesis in mice (Tewari and Noble, 1971). During chronic ethanol intoxication, an increase in γ-aminobutyric acid, glutamate, and aspartate and a decrease in brain glutamine have been reported (Hakkinen and Kulonen, 1961). The brain damage following chronic ethanol administration may be related to an impairment of protein synthesis (Tewari and Noble, 1971). The effect of ethanol on brain amino acids appears to be suppressed by the oral administration of glutamine (Hakkinen and Kulonen, 1961).

2. L-*Arginine*

Arginine has been reported to be of value in the therapy of delerium tremens (Ancona and Caloza, 1963). The use of a combination of malic acid and arginine was successful in treating alcoholic hepatitis and advanced cirrhosis of the liver (Tissot-Fovre and Brette, 1970). Arginine has been reported to decrease some of the toxic effects of ethanol in rats

(Breglia *et al.*, 1973), and to offer some protection against the hepatotoxic effect of ethanol–carbon tetrachloride treatment (Raja, 1973).

3. Glycine

Glycine represents a particular area of controversy in the effects of amino acids on ethanol toxicity. Blum *et al.* (1972) report that both glycine and serine synergize the action of ethanol. They are supported by reports that glycine may act as an inhibitory transmitter in brain and spinal cord (Shark and Aprison, 1971), and serine decreases the firing of spinal neurons (Curtis and Watkins, 1960). Glycine is a strong inhibitor of glutamine synthetase (Lehninger, 1970). The effects of ethanol have been reported to be related to decreased brain glutamine levels and are reversible by the oral administration of glutamine (Hakkinen and Kulonen, 1961). Glycine, however, does not alter blood ethanol levels (Liebhardt and Gastomzyx, 1968). Conversely, Widmark (1933a) and Haggard and Greenberg (1940) reported increased rates of ethanol disappearance from blood, and reduced blood ethanol levels after alanine or

TABLE II

Effect of Oral Pretreatment with Amino Acids on Ataxia and Sleeping Time Following Serial Administration of Ethanol PO

Amino acid	Dose (gm/kg)	Protection[a] factor	Percentage reduction of sleeping time
Lysine-HCl	0.120	2.03	N.S.
Lysine-HCl	2.50	2.95	55.38
Lysine-HCl[b]	0.120	3.26	11.08
Arginine-HCl	0.140	2.17	N.S.
Arginine-HCl	2.88	3.47	56.17
Arginine HCl[b]	0.140	4.39	39.22
Ornithine-HCl	0.111	1.54	N.S.
Ornithine-HCl	2.31	3.01	61.15
Ornithine-HCl[b]	0.111	2.02	N.S.
Glycine-HCl	0.073	2.81	N.S.
Glycine-HCl	1.53	4.70	64.57
Glycine-HCl[b]	0.073	N.S.	N.S.

[a] Protection factor is the number of times onset of ataxia time for test group is greater than onset of ataxia for control group.
[b] Simultaneous administration.

TABLE III
**Effect of Oral Pretreatment with Amino Acids on Ataxia and
Sleeping Time Following Single Dose Administration of Ethanol PO**

Amino acid	Dose (gm/kg)	Protection[a] factor	Percentage reduction of sleeping time
Lysine-HCl	0.120	N.S.	N.S.
Lysine-HCl	2.50	11.55	60.05
Lysine-HCl[b]	0.120	N.S.	N.S.
Arginine-HCl	0.140	N.S.	58.27
Arginine-HCl	2.88	4.79	43.72
Arginine-HCl[b]	0.140	7.26	N.S.
Ornithine-HCl	0.111	N.S.	N.S.
Ornithine-HCl	2.31	3.63	51.51
Ornithine-HCl[b]	0.111	N.S.	N.S.
Glycine-HCl	0.073	N.S.	N.S.
Glycine-HCl	1.53	10.62	98.96
Glycine-HCl	0.0	N.S.	N.S.

[a] Protection factor is the number of times onset of ataxia time for test group is greater than onset of ataxia for control group.
[b] Simultaneous administration.

glycine administration. The formation of a stable amino acid-ethanol complex was reported to reduce ethanol absorption and ethanol blood levels (Widmark, 1933b). Breglia et al. (1973) reported that glycine and other amino acids reduced sleeping time, prolonged the onset of ataxia, and decreased the intensity of loss of righting reflex following po ethanol administration in rats (Tables II and III).

4. L-*Tryptophan*

Olson et al. (1960) have given evidence for a defect in tryptophan metabolism in chronic alcoholics. Jarowski and Ward (1971) reported that the administration of tryptophan does not reverse the central nervous system toxicity and depressant effects of ethanol. The central effects were in fact enhanced, while the LD_{50} was reduced (Jarowski et al., 1971).

5. L-*Lysine*

Ward et al. (1972) reported a slight increase in the po and ip LD_{50} of ethanol followed the administration of lysine in rats. Pretreatment of

430 Charles O. Ward and Michael A. Dorato

TABLE IV
Composition of Various Amino Acid Solutions

Treatment	Composition	Dose
Lysine I	Lysine-HCl, 4.0 gm	1 gm/kg
	Protein hydrolyzate qs	
	20.0 ml	
Lysine II	Lysine-HCl, 4.0 gm	1 gm/kg
	Water qs 20.0 ml	twice daily
Protein hydrolyzate	Aminosol solution	9 ml/kg
	(Abbott Laboratories, Inc.)	

rats with lysine prolonged the onset of ethanol-induced sleeping time and reduced its duration (Ward *et al.*, 1972). Dorato *et al.* (1977) reported an increase in the po LD_{50} of ethanol in mice following a pretreatment with various lysine solutions (Tables IV and V). Doses of lysine, both ip and po, up to 2.5 gm/kg, have been reported to be without pharmacologic effect in rats (Ward *et al.*, 1972). The po LD_{50} of lysine in rats has been reported to be 10.13 ± 0.97 gm/kg, while the LD_{50} of lysine in mice has been reported as 8.021 ± 0.72 gm/kg (Dorato, 1976). Also in mice, the 72-hour po LD_{50} of ethanol has been reported to be $7.48 + 0.47$ gm/kg (Dorato *et al.*, 1977). After treatment with lysine, the LD_{50} of ethanol was increased to 8.99 ± 0.58 gm/kg (Dorato *et al.*, 1977; Table V).

It has also been shown that lysine will decrease ethanol blood levels on simultaneous oral administration and with a 4-day pretreatment

TABLE V
Effect of Lysine on the 72-Hour Oral LD_{50} of Ethanol

Treatment	LD_{50} (mg/kg $\pm$ SD)	Confidence limits	p-Level
Lysine I	8986 ±592.61	8539.57 9432.43	<0.05
Lysine II	8746 ±204.76	8591.75 8900.25	<0.05
Protein[a] hydrolyzate	8127 ±414.26	7814.92 8439.08	NS
Control	7484 ±472.29	7128.21 7839.79	—

[a] Significant at 24 hours.

TABLE VI
Effect of Lysine on Ethanol Blood Levels

| | Blood ethanol levels (mg/ml ± SD) | | | | | |
| | Pretreatment[a] | | | | Simultaneous | |
Treatment	Intraperitoneal[b]	p-Level	Oral[c]	p-Level	Oral[d]	p-Level
Lysine I	4.16 ± 0.57	NS	6.35 ± 1.03	<0.05	3.60 ± 0 58	<0.001
Control	4.06 ± 0.43	—	7.39 ± 0.42	—	6.98 ± 0.29	—
Lysine II	4.67 ± 0.55	NS	6.93 ± 0.66	<0.02	5.20 ± 0.82	<0.02
Control	4.82 ± 0.48	—	7.63 ± 0.26	—	7.35 ± 1.56	—
Protein hydrolyzate	3.70 ± 0.51	NS	5.25 ± 0.59	NS	5.98 ± 0.90	NS
Control	3.98 ± 0.48	—	5.82 ± 0.41	—	5.86 ± 0.38	—

[a] Four-day pretreatment according to Table IV.
[b] Ethanol 3 gm/kg 1 hour after last amino acid dose.
[c] Ethanol 6 gm/kg 1 hour after last amino acid dose.
[d] Ethanol 6 gm/kg simultaneously with last amino acid dose.

TABLE VII
Effect of Lysine on Rate of Ethanol Elimination
from the Blood

Treatment	Elimination (mg/ml/hour ± SD)	p-Level
Lysine I	0.80 ± 0.12	<0.05
Lysine II	0.81 ± 0.09	<0.05
Protein hydrolyzate	0.70 ± 0.08	NS
Control	0.64	—

TABLE VIII
Effect of Lysine on Mean Time on Rotating Roller during Ethanol Inhalation

Treatment	Mean time (minutes ± SD)	p-Level
Lysine I	0.69 ± 0.15	<0.05
Lysine II	0.63 ± 0.16	NS
Control	0.37 ± 0.18	—

(Dorato, 1976; Table VI). In addition, lysine has been shown to increase the rate of disappearance of ethanol from the blood of mice (Dorato, 1976; Table VII).

Using selected amino acids, Breglia *et al.* (1973) showed the greatest prolongation of ethanol ataxia to be produced by lysine. Lysine has also been shown to offer more protection than arginine against induced hepatotoxicity of ethanol–carbon tetrachloride mixtures (Raja, 1973).

In experiments involving the inhalation of ethanol vapors (Dorato, 1976; Dorato *et al.*, 1977), treatment with lysine prolonged the mean time mice were able to maintain their balance on a rotating roller (Table VIII) and decreased the ataxia accompanying ethanol inhalation (Table IX). The mean blood ethanol levels after 4 days of ethanol inhalation were also decreased by treatment with lysine (Table X). When the withdrawal syndrome was evaluated by a convulsion on handling technique lysine was again found to provide protection (Table XI).

6. L-*Ornithine*

Pretreatment of rats with ornithine (2.31 gm/kg) was reported to reduce sleeping time, prolong the onset of ataxia, and decrease the number of animals losing the righting reflex (Breglia *et al.*, 1973).

TABLE IX
Effect of Lysine on Daily Percent Ataxia Seen in Groups Exposed to Ethanol Vapors for 4 D

Treatment	Day-2	p-Level	Day-3	p-Level	Day-4	p-Level	Day-5	p-Level
Lysine I	30	<0.01	40	<0.01	40	NS	30	<0.001
Lysine II	30	<0.01	20	<0.001	20	<0.01	30	<0.001
Control	60	—	70	—	50	—	70	—

TABLE X
Effect of Lysine on Mean Blood Ethanol Level Produced
by the Inhalation of Ethanol Vapors for 4 Days

Treatment	Mean blood ethanol[a] (mg/ml ± SD)	p-Level
Lysine I	1.46 ± 0.18	<0.05
Lysine II	1.58 ± 0.33	NS
Control	2.28 ± 0.52	—

[a] Chamber concentration of 11–15 mg/liter.

B.   Feeding Studies

Dubroff (1973) found that diets supplemented with either lysine or lysine-tryptophan slightly elevated the LD_{50} of ethanol in rats (Table XII). When phenobarbital was tested against supplemental diets, significant decreases in sleeping time and loss of righting reflex occurred only in the lysine–tryptophan supplemented group (Dubroff, 1973).

It was observed that animals maintained on a lysine-supplemented diet showed significantly greater growth rates consistently (Table XIII). This was not true for those maintained on diets supplemented with lysine–tryptophan (Dubroff, 1973). A possible explanation was offered—the lysine–tryptophan diet contained excess lysine which could cause a repression of plasma arginine and lead to decreased

TABLE XI
Effect of Lysine on Ethanol Withdrawal Scores after 4-Day Exposure to Ethanol Vapors[a]

Treatment	Mean ± SD	p-Level	Peak[b] ± SD	p-Level	Mean[c] development ± SD	p-Level
Lysine I	0.73 ±0.27	<0.0005	0.95 ±0.09	<0.001	0.72 ±0.31	<0.02
Lysine II	0.94 ±0.36	NS	1.32 ±0.12	<0.001	0.98 ±0.44	NS
Control	1.38 ±0.58	—	1.94 ±0.05	—	1.39 ±0.68	—

[a] Chamber concentration, 11–15 mg/liter.
[b] Mean of the three highest consecutive scores.
[c] Mean of all scores up to and including the highest mean score.

TABLE XII

Effect of Lysine and Tryptophan Diets on Ethanol Toxicity in Rats

Diet	Sleeping time (minutes)	Loss righting reflex (minutes)	LD_{50} (mg/kg)
Lysine	227.5[a]	6.3[a]	9.0
Lysine–tryptophan	185.0	7.3	9.8[a]
Control	279.2	4.3	8.2

[a] Significant at $p < 0.05$.

weight gain (Kerner and Westerfield, 1953; Smith and Newman, 1959; Pieper and Sheen, 1973).

C. Fasting Plasma Profile Equivalents

Knowledge of limiting essential amino acids will enable one to choose the most appropriate amino acid supplementation to improve the biological value of the protein (Feldstein et al., 1964). The method chosen to determine the limiting amino acid is important. The chemical score technique is based on assumptions which are frequently incorrect (Feldstein et al., 1964). Supplementation with the improper amino acid can lead to amino acid imbalance (Feldstein et al., 1964).

Jarowski et al. (1971) have reported on the utility of the fasting essential amino acid plasma profile in formulating synthetic diets. The Fasting Plasma Profile Equivalent (F.P.P.E.) calculated only once, at a fasted level, and based on a specific diet allows for the determination of the

TABLE XIII

Effect of Lysine and Tryptophan Diets on Body Weight Gain in Rats

Diet	Weight (gm)		Mean weight gain	Percentage increase weight
	Start	End		
Lysine	101.1	212.0	112.9	119.7
Lysine–tryptophan	104.9	210.9	106.2	113.7
Control	107.1	203.1	96.5	93.4

[a] All data are means for 3 separate trials.

exact quantity of an amino acid (A.A.) to be added to a diet. The F.P.P.E. can be determined as follows (Dubroff, 1973; Macleod, 1950):

F.P.P.E. = mM of A.A. in 1 mg of diet/mM of A.A. in liter of plasma of fasted animal

This method has been used to determine the most appropriate amino acid with which to supplement diets of rats (Dubroff, 1973). The animals maintained on these improved diets were then tested for their reaction to stress, such as the administration of ethanol, as described above.

IV. METHODS OF DETERMINING ETHANOL TOXICITY

Various methods are available for the evaluation of ethanol toxicity and the effects of various other drugs upon it. The LD$_{50}$, of course, is useful for determination of acute effects. It is also desirable to have a standardized test with which the extent of behavioral impairment can be measured accurately (Gibbins et al., 1968). A practical test for ethanol intoxication should: (1) permit distinction of several intoxication levels; (2) be reproducible; (3) require a minimum of apparatus and animal training; and (4) be able to express results in exact values (Arvola et al., 1958).

A. Observational Methods

A simple apparatus for detecting neurological deficit in rats and mice consists of a rotating roller (Dunham and Miya, 1957). This test is useful in evaluating the degree of motor impairment produced by ethanol (Walsh, 1973). The ability of mice to walk on a lattice floor without slipping was impaired by ethanol (Arvola, 1961). The effect was quantitated by use of a specially constructed slipping cage (Arvola, 1961). The slipping test provides an objective measure of impaired motor coordination, as related to spontaneous activity, produced by ethanol (Arvola, 1961). Slipping was not found to be related to blood ethanol.

Gibbins et al. (1968) describe a treadmill test whereby an animal is forced to walk a nylon belt which moves continuously over an electrified grid. Falling off the belt elicits a shock and activates a timer to record off-belt time. The total time off the belt has been reported to be linearly related to blood ethanol levels in the range of 150–300 mg/100 ml (Gibbins et al., 1968). The rotating roller test resembles this method, but is more sensitive for mice than for rats (Gibbins *et al.*, 1968). The treadmill test is reportedly equally useful for both mice and rats.

B. Behavioral Methods

Arvola *et al.* (1958) describe a tilted plane test. This test measures a complex of functions composed of vestibular and grasping reflexes, including a strong cortical component. Sliding is measured by placing an animal on the rough surface of a hard board or on 80 mesh wire matting, facing upwards. The board or wire is then tilted through 90° in 5 seconds and the angle at which the animal slides down is recorded (Arvola *et al.*, 1958). The surface of the board used is critical; smooth surfaces are unsuitable (Friedman and Ingalls, 1960). Changes in the sliding angle can be used to characterize the effects of other drugs on ethanol intoxication (Kora, 1964).

Patel and Ward (1976) used a shuttle box similar to that described by Wallgren and Savolainens (1962) to evaluate the effects of lysine on preventing ethanol disruption of the conditioned avoidance response. Lysine was reported to antagonize ethanol-induced decreases in avoidance response (Fig. 2).

C. Blood Ethanol Levels

The motor impairment and behavioral responses produced by ethanol are dose-related; they increase with increasing blood ethanol levels. The methods for determination of blood ethanol levels are many and varied. They have been adequately reviewed by Jain and Cravey (1972a,b). The determination of blood ethanol levels is useful in further understanding how substances, such as lysine, which modify ethanol responses produce their effects.

D. Histopathology of Target Organs

The liver is a well-known target organ of ethanol. The accumulation of lipid and fat in the liver after an alcohol bout had been regarded as subclinical and reversible (Lundquist *et al.*, 1973; Lieber, 1972). Kullen *et al.* (1969) have described a syndrome of sudden fatty liver deaths.

Ethanol has a stimulating effect on the pituitary adrenal axis in the rat and guinea pig (Forbes and Duncan, 1953). This stimulation is characterized by reduction in ascorbic acid and cholesterol levels.

The observation of the effects of ethanol on the above systems and the modification of these effects by amino acids can yield valuable data as to

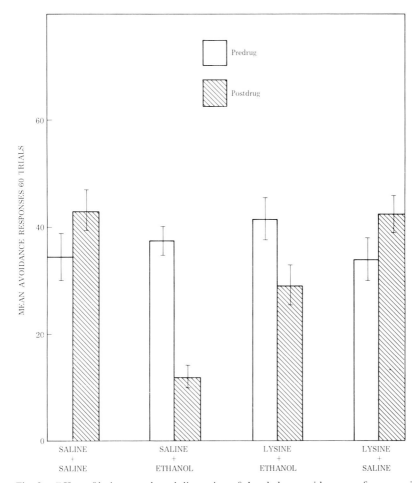

Fig. 2. Effect of lysine on ethanol disruption of shuttle box avoidance performance in trained mice.

the utility of amino acids in the management of chronic alcohol intoxication. Laboratory rodents fed a diet deficient in lysine showed decreased pituitary-adrenal responses to challenging doses of ethanol (Forbes and Duncan, 1958).

Carbon tetrachloride in combination with ethanol has been used as a tool to simulate chronic ethanol hepatotoxicity. It has been found that lysine afforded significant protection against the liver necrolytic effect of ethanol-carbon tetrachloride (Raja, 1973). Arginine showed similar effects, but its index of protection was not as high as that of lysine.

Similar results were also reported for groups tested with amino acids and isopropanol. In inhalation experiments involving the exposure of mice to 11 mg/liter of ethanol vapors for 4 days, the use of lysine afforded protection against liver congestion, focal necrosis,pericentral and panacinar fatty changes (Dorato, 1976).

V.   ROLE OF ACETALDEHYDE IN ALCOHOL TOXICITY

The physiologic and pharmacologic effects of acetaldehyde may be fundamental to the various effects of ethanol (Sheppard *et al.*, 1970). Duritz and Truitt (1966) have suggested that acetaldehyde rather than ethanol may be responsible for the psychopathology of alcoholism. If acetaldehyde accumulation is fundamental to the behavioral changes seen in alcoholism, then slight changes in the aldehyde dehydrogenase system may be the ultimate cause of the behavioral response (Sheppard *et al.*, 1970).

The interaction of ethanol or acetaldehyde, its major metabolite, with various biogenic amines has been indicated as a possible cause of dependence following chronic ethanol administration (Davis *et al.*, 1970; Davis and Walsh, 1970; Cohen and Collins, 1970). It has been postulated that

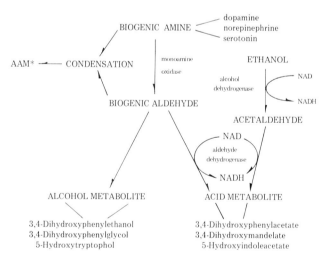

Fig. 3.   Formation of alcohol addictive metabolites (Sprince *et al.*, 1972a, and Deitrich and Erwin, 1975). *Alcohol addictive metabolites: tetrahydropapaveroline, tetrahydro-isoquinoline, tetrahydro-beta-carboline.

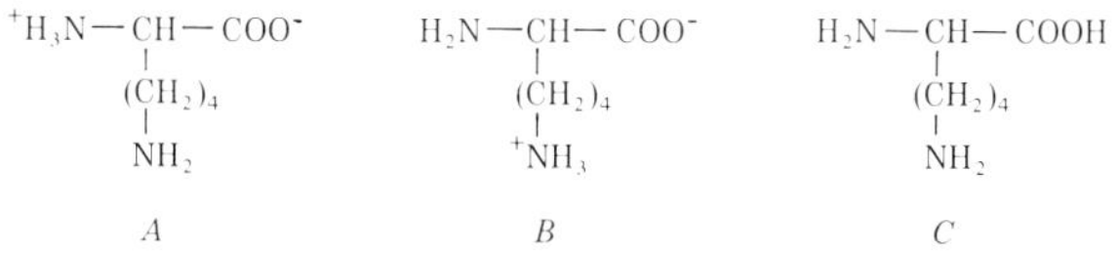

$$^+H_3N—CH—COO^- \qquad H_2N—CH—COO^- \qquad H_2N—CH—COOH$$
$$\underset{NH_2}{\overset{(CH_2)_4}{|}} \qquad \underset{^+NH_3}{\overset{(CH_2)_4}{|}} \qquad \underset{NH_2}{\overset{(CH_2)_4}{|}}$$

A   B   C

Fig. 4. Ionic species of lysine in aqueous solution. Ratio of A to B to C = 320,000 to 1,800,000 to 1

the presence of acetaldehyde leads to localized increases in the concentration of aromatic aldehydes, in tissues rich in biogenic amines (Davis *et al.*, 1970). Further, these highly reactive aldehydes condense with their respective parent amine to yield morphine-like alkaloids (Fig. 3; Davis *et al.*, 1970.

Ortiz *et al.* (1974) reported similar withdrawal, cross dependence, behavioral changes and effects on brain monoamine levels in mice after chronic exposure to ethanol or acetaldehyde vapors.

Effect of Amino Acids on Acetaldehyde Toxicity

Ward *et al.* (1972) have suggested that the co-administration of an excess reactive alpha amino acid such as lysine (Fig. 4) and ethanol might lead to a decrease in ethanol toxicity, the decreased toxicity being due to the condensation of acetaldehyde with the amino acid (Fig. 5).

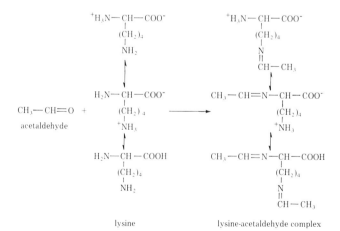

Fig. 5. Reaction of lysine with acetaldehyde (Greenstein and Winitz, 1961).

TABLE XIV
Effect of Lysine on the Toxicity of Acetaldehyde in Rats

Treatment	$LD_{50} \pm 94\%$ limits (gm/kg)	p-Value
Acetaldehyde-lysine mixture	1.2 ± 0.14	N.S.
60-minute Lysine pretreatment	1.8 ± 0.18	<0.05
5-day Lysine pretreatment	1.8 ± 0.18	<0.05
Acetladehyde	1.1 ± 0.15	—

Such an interaction would be expected to: (1) reduce the acute toxicity of ethanol; (2) decrease or prevent alkaloid accumulation; and (3) eliminate the pharmacologic effects of acetaldehyde (Ward *et al.*, 1972).

Lower aldehydes combine rapidly with amino groups (Robert and Penandra, 1954). Sunaga *et al.* (1970) support the lysine–acetaldehyde interaction with the formation of a Schiff base. In rabbits, the products of amino acids and acetaldehyde are reported to be cortical stimulants (Beck *et al.*, 1968). Dorato *et al.* (1977) report that the use of lysine decreases the central nervous system depression and withdrawal syndrome in mice exposed to ethanol vapors for four days. In rats, lysine as a 60-minute or 5-day pretreatment increases the LD_{50} of acetaldehyde (Pfeiffer *et al.*, 1972; Table XIV). Sprince *et al.* (1972b, 1974) reported that cysteine, alone and in combination with thiamine increased survival rates following lethal doses of acetaldehyde.

VI. SUMMARY

Amino acids have been shown, in several investigations, to be capable of reducing the acute and subacute toxic effects of ethanol administration. The LD_{50} of ethanol is increased, blood levels are decreased, and behavioral effects of this psychoactive foodstuff have been modified. It should be noted, also, that these effects of the amino acids are produced at nontoxic doses. It still remains, however, to investigate the potential clinical applications of these findings, and to assess their usefulness in the treatment of acute and chronic alcohol intoxication.

REFERENCES

Ancona, C. V., and Caloza, D. (1963). Observations on the effectiveness of arginine and glutamate therapy in delerium tremens. *J. Neuropsychiatry* **4,** 369.

Arvola, A. (1961). A slipping test for measuring level of alcohol intoxication in the mouse. *Q. J. Stud. Alcohol* **22,** 575.

Arvola, A., Sammalisto, L. and Wallgren, H. (1958). A test for level of alcohol intoxication in the rat. *Q. J. Stud. Alcohol* **19,** 563.

Aston, R., and Stolman, S. (1966). Influence of route and concentration of ethanol upon the central depressant effect in the mouse. *Proc. Soc. Exp. Biol. Med.* **123,** 496.

Beck, R. A., Pfeiffer, C. C., Iliev, U., and Goldstein, L. (1968). Cortical EEG stimulant effect in the rabbit of acetaldehyde—biogenic amine reaction product. *Proc. Soc. Exp. Biol. Med.* **128,** 823.

Blum, K., Wallace, J. E., and Geller, I. (1972). Synergy of ethanol and putative neurotransmitters: Glycine and serine. *Science* **176,** 292.

Breglia, R. J., Ward, C. O., and Jarowski, C. I. (1973). Effect of selected amino acids on ethanol toxicity in rats. *J. Pharm. Sci.* **62,** 49.

Chambers, J. W., and Piccirillo, V. J. (1973). Effects of ethanol on amino acid uptake and utilization by the liver and other organs of rats. *Q. J. Stud. Alcohol, Part A* **34,** 707.

Cohen, G., and Collins, M. (1970). Alkaloids from catecholamines in adrenal tissue: Possible role in alcoholism. *Science* **167,** 1949.

Curtis, D., and Watkins, J. C. (1960). The excitation and depression of spinal neurones by structurally related amino acids. *J. Neurochem.* **6,** 117.

Davis, V. E., and Walsh, M. J. (1970). Alcohol, amines and alkaloids: A possible biochemical basis of alcohol addiction. *Science* **167,** 1005.

Davis, V. E., Walsh, M. J., and Yamanaka, Y. (1970). Augmentation of alkaloid formation from dopamine by alcohol and acetaldehyde, *in vitro. J. Pharmacol. Exp. Ther.* **174,** 401.

Deitrich, R. A., and Erwin, G. (1975). Involvement of biogenic amine metabolism in ethanol addiction. *Fed. Proc., Fed. Am. Soc. Exp. Biol.* **34,** 1962.

Dorato, M. A. (1976). The value of lysine and diethanolamine in reducing the intoxication, dependence and the withdrawal syndrome induced in mice by the inhalation of ethanol. Ph.D. Thesis, St. John's University, Jamaica, New York.

Dorato, M. A., Lynch, V. D., and Ward, C. O. (1977). The effect of lysine and diethanolamine on the blood levels, withdrawal and acute toxicity of ethanol in mice. *J. Pharm. Sci.* **66,** 35.

Dubroff, L. (1973). The effects of lysine and tryptophan on the rate of growth and on the toxicity of barbiturates and ethanol in Sprague-Dawley rats. M. S. Thesis, St. John's University, Jamaica, New York.

Dunham, N. W., and Miya, T. S. (1957). A note on a simple apparatus for detecting neurological deficit in rats and mice. *J. Am. Pharm. Assoc.* **46,** 208.

Duritz, G., and Truitt, E. B. (1966). Importance of acetaldehyde in the action of ethanol on brain norepinephrine and 5-hydroxytryptamine. *Biochem. Pharmacol.* **15,** 711.

Feldstein, A., Hoagland, H., Wong, K., and Freeman, H. (1964). Biogenic amines, biogenic aldehydes and alcohol. *Q. J. Stud. Alcohol* **25,** 218.

Forbes, J. C., and Duncan, G. M. (1953). Effect of intraperitoneal administration of alcohol on the adrenal levels of cholesterol and ascorbic acid in rats and guinea pigs. *Q. J. Stud. Alcohol* **14,** 19.

Forbes, J. C., and Duncan, G. M. (1958). The adrenal response to alcohol intoxication in rats maintained with diets deficient in tryptophan, niacin and lysine. *Q. J. Stud. Alcohol* **19,** 555.

Friedman, S. L., and Ingalls, J. W. (1960). A note on the tilting plane technique for measuring the performance of rats in relation to the degree of their alcohol intoxication. *Q. J. Stud. Alcohol* **21,** 217.

Frosander, O. (1970). Influence of ethanol on the redox state of the liver. *Q. J. Stud. Alcohol, Part A* **31,** 550.

Gable, F. B. (1974). "Psychosocial Pharmacy: The Synthetic Society," p. 61. Lea & Febiger, Philadelphia, Pennsylvania.

Gessner, P. K. (1973). *In vivo* ethanol metabolism: Kinetics of inhibition. *Proc. Annu. Alcohol Conf., 1st NIAAA.* p. 79.

Gibbins, R. J., Kalant, H., and LeBlanc, A. E. (1968). A technique for accurate measurement of moderate degress of alcohol intoxification in small animals. *J. Pharmacol. Exp. Ther.* **159,** 236.

Goldstein, A. (1970). Saturation of alcohol dehydrogenese by ethanol. *N. Engl. J. Med.* **283,** 875.

Goth, A. (1974). "Medical Pharmacology Principles and Concepts," p. 263. C. V. Mosby Co., St. Louis.

Greenberger, N. J., Cohen, R. B., and Isselbacher, K. J. (1965). The effect of chronic ethanol administration on liver alcohol dehydrogenese activity in the rat. *Lab. Invest.* **14,** 264.

Greenstein, J. P., and Winitz, M. (1961). "Chemistry of Amino Acids," p. 448. Wiley, New York.

Haggard, H. W., and Greenberg, L. A. (1940). Studies in the absorption, distribution and elimination of alcohol. V. The influence of glycol upon the absorption of alcohol. *J. Pharmacol. Exp. Ther.* **68,** 482.

Hakkinen, H. M., and Kulonen, E. (1961). Effect of ethanol on the amino acids of the rat brain with reference to the administration of glutamine. *Biochem. J.* **78,** 588.

Hawkins, R. D., and Kalant, H. (1972). The metabolism of ethanol and its metabolic effect. *Pharmacol. Rev.* **24,** 67.

Holtzman, S. G., and Schneider, F. H. (1974). Comparison of acetaldehyde and ethanol depression on motor activity in mice. *Life Sci.* **14,** 1243.

Israel, Y., Salazar, I., and Rosenmann, E. (1968). Inhibitory effects of alcohol on intestinal amino acid transport *in vivo* and *in vitro. J. Nutr.* **96,** 499.

Jain, N. C., and Cravey, R. H. (1972a). Analysis of alcohol. I. A review of chemical and infrared methods. *J. Chromatogr. Sci.* **10,** 257.

Jain, N. C., and Cravey, R. H. (1972b). Analysis of alcohol. II. A review of gas chromatographic methods. *J. Chromatogr. Sci.* **10,** 263.

Jarowski, C. I., and Ward, C. O. (1971). Effect of tryptophan on toxicity and depressant effect of barbiturates and ethanol in rats. *Toxicol. Appl. Pharmacol.* **18,** 603.

Jarowski, C. I., Poccini, A. V., Winitz, M., and Otez, M. C. (1971). The utility of fasting essential amino acid plasma levels in the formulation of nutritionally adequate diets. *Agric. Biol. Chem.* **35**, 1007.

Kerner, E., and Westerfield, W. W. (1953). Effect of diet on rats of alcohol oxidation by liver. *Proc. Soc. Exp. Biol. Med.* **83**, 530.

Kora, F. (1964). Data on the degree of alcohol intoxication in rats examined with the tilting-plane method. *Q. J. Stud. Alcohol* **25**, 253.

Kullen, L. H., Kramer, L., and Fisher, R. (1969). Changing trends in cirrhosis and fatty liver mortality. *Am. J. Public Health* **59**, 1124.

Leevy, C. M., and Baker, H. (1963). Metabolic and nutritional effect of alcoholism. *Arch. Environ. Health* **7**, 453.

Lehninger, A. L. (1970). "Biochemistry," p. 557. Worth, New York.

Lieber, C. S. (1972). Alcohol and the liver. *Med. World News, Gastroenterol. Ed.* p. 25.

Lieber, C. S., Freschke, R., Hasumura, Y., and DeCarli, L. M. (1975). Differences in hepatic and metabolic changes after acute and chronic alcohol consumption. *Fed. Proc., Fed. Am. Soc. Exp. Biol.* **34**, 2060.

Liebhardt, E., and Gastomzyx, J. G. (1968). Bestimmung von Glucose und freien Fettsäuren in Serum nach Gabe von Alkohol und Glycin. *Z. Klin. Chem. Klin. Biochem.* **5**, 377.

Lundquist, A., Wiebe, T., and Belfraje, P. (1973). Liver liquid content in alcoholics. *Acta Med. Scand.* **194**, 555.

Macleod, L. D. (1950). Acetaldehyde in relation to intoxication by ethyl alcohol. *Q. J. Stud. Alcohol* **11**, 385.

Majchrowicz, E., Lipton, M. A., Meek, J. L., and Hall, L. (1968). Effect of chronic ethanol consumption on the clearance of acutely administered ethanol and acetaldehyde from blood in rats. *Q. J. Stud. Alcohol* **29**, 553.

Makar, A. B., and Mannering, G. J. (1970). Kinetics of ethanol metabolism in the intact rat and monkey. *Biochem. Pharmacol.* **19**, 2017.

Marshall, E. K., and Fritz, W. F. (1953). The metabolism of ethyl alcohol. *J. Pharmacol. Exp. Ther.* **109**, 431.

Marshall, E. K., and Owens, A. H. (1955). Rate of metabolism of ethyl alcohol in the mouse. *Proc. Soc. Exp. Biol. Med.* **89**, 573.

Mendelson, J. H. (1970). Alcohol. *In* "Principles of Psychopharmacology" (W. G. Clark and J. Del Giudice, eds.), p. 513. Academic Press, New York.

Nelson, G. H., Kinnard, F. W., and Hay, M. G. (1957). Rate of metabolism of ethanol in the mouse. *Am. J. Physiol.* **190**, 169.

Olson, R. E., Gursey, D., and Vesten, J. W. (1960). Evidence for a defect in tryptophan metabolism in chronic alcoholism. *N. Engl. J. Med.* **263**, 1169.

Ortiz, A., Griffith, P. J., and Littleton, J. M. (1974). A comparison of the effects of chronic administration of ethanol and acetaldehyde to mice: Evidence for a role of acetaldehyde in ethanol dependence. *J. Pharm. Pharmacol.* **26**, 249.

Owens, A. H. and Marshall, E. K. (1955). The metabolism of ethyl alcohol in the Rat. *J. Pharmacol. Exp. Ther.* **115**, 360.

Patel, J., and Ward, C. O. (1976). Evaluation of selected antagonists on the neuropharmacological effects of ethanol in rodents. Unpublished observations.

Pfeiffer, H., Dorato, M. A., and Ward, C. O. (1972). The effect of L-lysine on the toxicity of acetaldehyde in the rat. Unpublished observations.

Pieper, W. A., and Sheen, M. J. (1973). Changes in rate of ethanol elimination associated with chronic administration of ethanol to chimpanzees and rhesus monkeys. *Drug Metab. Dispos.* **1**, 634.

Prigot, A., Cohen, E., Maynard, A., Roden, T. P., and Hjelt-Harvey, I. (1962). The treatment of delerium tremens with amino acids. *Q. J. Stud. Alcohol* **23**, 390.

Raja, P. K. (1973). Effect of amino acid pretreatment on alcohol–carbon tetrachloride toxicity in rats. Personal communication.

Ravel, J. M., Felsig, B., Lansferd, E. M., Trubey, R. H., and Shive, W. (1955). Reversal of alcohol toxicity by glutamine. *J. Biol. Chem.* **214**, 497.

Robert, L., and Penandra, F. S. (1954). Studies on aldehyde–protein interactions. I. Reaction of amino acids with lower aldehydes. *J. Polym. Sci.* **12**, 337.

Rogers, L. L., and Pelton, R. B. (1957). Glutamine in the treatment of alcoholism, a preliminary report. *Q. J. Stud. Alcohol* **18**, 581.

Rogers, L. L., Pelton, R. B., and Williams, R. J. (1955). Voluntary alcohol consumption by rats following administration of glutamine. *J. Biol. Chem.* **214**, 503.

Schiller, J., Peck, R. E., and Goldberg, M. E. (1959). Effect of amino acids on the rate of disappearance of alcohol from the blood. *AMA Arch. Neurol. (Chicago)* **1**, 127.

Shark, R. P., and Aprison, M. H. (1971). The metabolism *in vivo* of glycine and serine in eight areas of the rat central nervous system. *J. Neurochem.* **17**, 1461.

Sheppard, J. R., Alberstein, P., and McClean, G. (1970). Aldehyde dehydrogenase and ethanol preference in mice. *J. Biol. Chem.* **245**, 2876.

Smith, H. E., and Newman, H. W. (1959). The rate of ethanol metabolism in fed and fasting animals. *J. Biol. Chem.* **234**, 1544.

Smith, H. E., Newman, E. J., and Newman, H. W. (1957). Effect of increased diphosphopyridine nucleotide levels on rate of ethanol metabolism in the mouse. *Proc. Soc. Exp. Biol. Med.* **95**, 541.

Sprince, H., Parker, C. M., Smith, G. C., and Gonzales, L. J. (1972a). Alcoholism: Biochemical and nutritional aspects of brain amines, aldehydes and amino acids. *Nutr. Rep. Int.* **5**, 185.

Sprince, H., Parker, C. M., Smith, G. G., and Gonzales, L. J. (1972b). Protection against acetaldehyde toxicity and lethality by L-cysteine plus thiamine. *Fed. Proc., Fed. Am. Soc. Exp. Biol.* **00**, 574.

Sprince, H., Parker, C. M., Smith, G. G., and Gonzales, L. J., (1974). Protection against acetaldehyde toxicity in the rat by L-cysteine, thiamine and L-2-methylthiazalidine 4-carboxylic acid. *Agents Actions* **4**, 125.

Stolt, G. (1965). Glutamin vid Alkoholintoxikation. *Nord. Psykiatr. Tidsskr.* **22**, 39.

Stotz, E., Westerfield, W. W., and Berg, R. O. (1944). The metabolism of acetaldehyde with acetoin formation. *J. Biol. Chem.* **152**, 1944.

Sunaga, K., Imamura, J., and Koide, S. S. (1970). Interaction of 21-dehydroprednisolone with amino acids. *Biochim. Biophys. Acta* **210**, 164.

Tewari, S., and Noble, E. P. (1971). Ethanol and brain protein synthesis. *Brain Res.* **26**, 469.

Tissot-Fovre, A., and Brette, R. (1970). Effects thérapeutiques du malate D-arginine dans le cirrhoses alcooliques. *Therapie* **25**, 629.

Truitt, E. B., and Doritz, G. (1966). The role of acetaldehyde in the actions of ethanol. *In* "Biochemical Factors in Alcoholism" (R. J. Maickel, ed.), p. 66. Pergamon, Oxford.

Wallgren, H., and Savolainens, S. (1962). The effect of ethyl alcohol on a conditioned avoidance response in rats. *Acta Pharmacol Toxicol.* **19**, 59.

Walsh, M. J. (1973). The biochemical aspects of alcoholism. *In* "Alcoholism: Progress in Research and Treatment" (P. G. Bourne and R. Fox, eds.), p. 43. Academic Press, New York.

Ward, C. O., Lau Cam, C. A., Tang, A., Breglia, R. J., and Jarowski, C. I. (1972). Effects of lysine on toxicity and depressant effects of ethanol in rats. *Toxicol. Appl. Pharmacol.* **22,** 422.

Widmark, E. M. P. (1933a). The action of amino acids on blood alcohol. *Biochem. Z.* **265,** 237.

Widmark, E. M. P. (1933b). The influence of the constituents of food stuffs on the alcohol content of the blood. *Biochem. Z.* **267,** 135.

17

Nutritional Effects on Drug–Protein Binding

ARTHUR A. SPECTOR and JOHN E. FLETCHER

I. INTRODUCTION

Many drugs are present in the blood in the form of a complex with plasma proteins. A partial listing of drugs that bind to plasma proteins is presented in Table I. For the most part, drugs that bind to plasma proteins are poorly soluble in aqueous solutions such as plasma and require a carrier to facilitate their movement through the circulation. Albumin, the most abundant protein in blood plasma, is the main trans-

447

TABLE I
A Partial List of Drugs that Bind to Plasma Proteins

Drug	Reference
Acetylsalicylic acid	Pinckard *et al.*, 1973; Sykes, 1970
Bupivacaine	Ghoneim and Pandya, 1974
Camptothecin	Chignell, 1973
Carbenoxolone	Parke and Lindup, 1973
Clofibrate	Spector *et al.*, 1973
Dapsone	Reidenberg and Affrime, 1973
Diazoxide	Sellers and Koch-Weser, 1973
Dicoumarol	Chignell, 1973; O'Reilly, 1973; Levy, 1973
Digitoxin and related cardenolides	Lukas and DeMartino, 1969
Diphenylhydantoin	Borondy *et al.*, 1973; Shoeman *et al.*, 1973
Flufenamic acid	Chignell, 1973
Halofenate	Fletcher *et al.*, 1973; Spector *et al.*, 1973
Methadone	Olsen, 1972
Penicillin and derivatives	Kunin *et al.*, 1973
Phenobarbital	Welch, 1973
Phenylbutazone	Chignell, 1973; Dayton *et al.*, 1973
Probenecid	Dayton *et al.*, 1973
Quinidine	Reidenberg and Affrime, 1973
Salicylate	Krasner *et al.*, 1973
Sulfonamide and derivatives	Anton, 1973
Tetracycline and derivatives	Chignell, 1973; Kunin *et al.*, 1973
Thiopental	Dayton *et al.*, 1973
Tolbutamide	Welch, 1973
Triamterene	Reidenberg and Affrime, 1973
Warfarin	Chignell, 1973; O'Reilly, 1973

port vehicle for drugs. The binding process occurs through physical interactions, not covalent linkage. In most cases, the attachment is stabilized by a combination of nonpolar interactions between the hydrocarbon structures of the drug and hydrophobic amino acid side chains of the protein, plus electrostatic interactions between oppositely charged groups of the drug and the protein.

The binding of a drug to albumin is represented by Eq (1),

$$PA \rightleftharpoons P + A \tag{1}$$

where PA is the concentration of drug–protein complexes, P is the concentration of protein binding sites that do not contain drug, and A is the concentration of unbound drug in the solution.* The unbound concentration, A, regulates the pharmacologic effectiveness of the drug; that is, its potency, distribution, rate of metabolism, and glomerular filtration (Sellers and Koch-Weser, 1973). In effect, the unbound concentration is the therapeutic plasma concentration (Reidenberg and Affrime, 1973). The unbound concentration is determined by the total concentration of drug in the plasma, the availability of albumin binding sites and the affinity of these sites for the drug.

There are two ways in which nutrition can influence drug binding and, hence, transport in the plasma. One is protein–calorie malnutrition, particularly kwashiorkor, where the plasma albumin concentration is reduced considerably. In this situation, there is a lack of available protein binding sites to transport a drug through the plasma. Therefore, at a given plasma concentration, more of the drug is unbound than under normal circumstances. The effective drug concentration is higher, more enters the tissues, and it is excreted more rapidly. Fortunately, this problem is rare, at least in Western civilization. By far the more common way that nutrition might alter drug binding is through a modulating effect of various metabolites on the interaction between the drug and albumin.

In addition to drugs, albumin binds and facilitates the transport of a number of physiologic substances through the plasma. Among these are bilirubin (Jacobsen, 1972; Odell, 1973), bile acids (Green *et al.*, 1971), nonpolar amino acids such as tryptophan (Cunningham *et al.*, 1975; Curzon *et al.*, 1973; Lipsett *et al.*, 1973; McMenamy and Oncley, 1958), lysolecithin (Rutenberg *et al.*, 1973) and free fatty acid (FFA)† (Spector, 1975). Hormones such as thyroxine (Braverman *et al.*, 1969; Tabachnick, 1964; Steiner *et al.*, 1966) and the steroids (Westphal, 1964) also can bind to albumin, but they are transported in the plasma primarily by specific globulins and bind to albumin in appreciable amounts only when they are present in excessive concentrations. Some of these physiological metabolites may modulate the binding of drugs to albumin, by either competing with the drug for common binding sites or producing conformational changes in the structure of the drug binding sites. Although changes in the concentration of any of these metabolic products could result from nutritional influences, the one that appears to be most likely to affect drug binding is FFA.

---

*Formally, the correct parameter is the activity, not the concentration. In practice, however, concentrations almost always are substituted for activities.

†The abbreviations used are: FFA, free fatty acid or acids; ANS, 1-anilino-8-naphthalenesulfonate; HABA, 2-(4'-hydroxyphenylazo)benzoic acid.

II. BINDING TO PLASMA ALBUMIN

Albumin, the most abundant protein in the blood plasma, is present normally at a concentration of 3.5–4.5 gm/dl. Human albumin consists of a single polypeptide chain and has a molecular weight of 66,300 (Finlayson, 1975). It contains either 584 (Behrens *et al.*, 1975) or 585 amino acids (Meloun *et al.*, 1975). Bovine albumin, which is used more often in experimental work because it is more readily available and costs much less, is structurally similar to the human protein and contains 581 amino acids (Brown, 1975). Therefore, most of the binding data obtained with bovine albumin probably is applicable to the human protein. Both albumins are made up of three homologous repeating units called domains. In human albumin, the three domains consist of amino acid residues 1–191, 192–348, and 385–584, respectively (Behrens *et al.*, 1975). The distribution of the three domains is almost identical in bovine albumin, involving amino acid residues 1–190, 191–382, and 383–581 (Brown, 1975). Each of the domains is thought to have the tertiary structure of a cylinder composed of five parallel helices (Brown, 1975). According to this model, the primary binding sites for drugs and metabolites such as fatty acids are holes or pockets within the three cylindrical structures.

Support for this model has come from recent studies of binding to fragments of bovine albumin (Peters and Feldhoff, 1975; Reed *et al.*, 1975; Feldhoff *et al.*, 1975; King, 1973). In this work, bovine albumin was cleaved by pepsin into two fragments; B, which contains amino acid residues 1–306 and A, which contains residues 307–581. Thus, B contains the first cylindrical domain and A the third, while the second domain is cleaved apart by the enzymatic digestion. Each of the two fragments is able to bind organic anions such as octanoate (King, 1973), palmitate, bilirubin, 1-anilino-8-naphthalenesulfonate (ANS), and bromocresol green (Reed *et al.*, 1975). This supports the suggestion that binding sites for large organic compounds are contained on the two outside domains. When the binding exhibited by the two fragments is summed, however, the total is less than that exhibited by the intact albumin molecule. This suggests that a binding region is destroyed when the molecule is cleaved by pepsin. When the two fragments are mixed together in a solution, they form a structure that is similar to the intact albumin molecule, even though there is no covalent bond between amino acid residues 306 and 307. Except for palmitate, these fragments bind more of an organic compound when they are present together in solution than when each is tested separately and their individual binding is summed. This suggests that additional binding sites form when the two fragments combine. One explanation is that the combination causes the second (center) domain to reform and that this central cylinder, like the two outside ones, contains one or more binding sites for certain organic compounds.

Each of the cylinders does not exhibit an equal affinity for a given compound. For example, the strongest long-chain fatty acid binding site is in the carboxyl-terminal region of the molecule, between amino acid residues 377 and 503 and, therefore, probably associated with the third domain (Reed *et al.*, 1975). Although the amino-terminal fragment also binds long-chain fatty acids, the strength of binding is considerably weaker. The same is true for the medium-chain fatty acids, for the domain located in the carboxyl-terminal region of the protein binds octanoate much more tightly than the one located in the amino-terminal region (King, 1973).

A second model for the binding of organic compounds to albumin has been derived from studies with ANS, a fluorescent model compound. As predicted from the cylindrical model deduced from the amino acid sequence data, physical measurements indicate that albumin is folded in the form of three spherical regions which are adjacent to one another (Bloomfield, 1966). The ANS studies suggest that four high affinity binding sites for organic compounds are located in hydrophobic crevices formed by the juncture of the central and two outside spheres, each juncture giving rise to two binding sites (Anderson and Weber, 1969). This binding model differs to some extent with that postulated by Brown (1975) in that the sites are between two adjacent cylindrical regions, not within the cylindrical domain itself.

It is not possible to distinguish between the two models at this time. Both are consistant with the evidence that much of the energy involved in the binding of organic compounds to albumin is due to nonpolar interactions (Klotz *et al.* 1946; Karush and Sonnenberg, 1949; Ray *et al.*, 1966). In the case of the Brown model, the hydrophobic regions are located within the domains, whereas in the Anderson and Weber model they are between the domains. The fragment data is consistent with the Brown model in that the central domain appears to provide the albumin molecule with additional binding capacity. Yet, one could just as easily envision greater binding capacity at the intraspherical clefts due to the presence of the intact central sphere, an interpretation that would make the fragment data also consistant with the Anderson and Weber model. Furthermore, it is possible that structurally different organic compounds bind to albumin in different ways, so that each model may apply only to certain compounds. For example, the main tryptophan binding site appears to be located in the first domain, while the primary bilirubin

452   Arthur A. Spector and John E. Fletcher

binding site involves a region that includes parts of both the first and second domain (Peters, 1975).

III. FREE FATTY ACIDS

Most of the fatty acid contained in the blood plasma is present as a component of complex lipids, i.e., phospholipids, glycerides, and cholesteryl esters. These complex lipids are carried in the plasma as components of lipoproteins. A small quantity of fatty acid, however, is present in the plasma in unesterified form. This fraction of the plasma fatty acid is commonly known as free fatty acid (FFA), the term free being used to indicate that it is in the unesterified form. Actually, more than 99% of the plasma FFA is bound to albumin and, therefore, is not free in the sense of being unbound. From 86–95% of the fatty acids present in the FFA fraction of human plasma contains 16- or 18-carbon atoms (Spector, 1971). FFA interact with albumin through physical binding and, like most drugs, are modeled by Eq (1). Although there is still some debate concerning the ionization of long-chain FFA in aqueous solutions, most investigators believe that FFA are almost totally dissociated at plasma pH and are present predominantly as fatty acid anions (Spector, 1975). In binding to albumin, both electrostatic and nonpolar forces are involved, but the major attractive force is nonpolar (Spector, 1975). Therefore, binding is thought to occur primarily through an insertion of the long fatty acid hydrocarbon chain into nonpolar pockets of the albumin structure (Spector, 1975), either within the cylindrical domains (Brown, 1975) or in crevices between the spherical regions (Anderson and Weber, 1969). The binding of the 16- and 18-carbon atom FFA to albumin is extremely tight, the association constants for binding of the first mole ranging from 6.1×10^7 to $2.6 \times 10^8 M^{-1}$ for human albumin (Ashbrook et al., 1975).* These constants are 150 to 500,000 times larger than those for the binding of the first mole of various drug, where values ranging from 5×10^2 to $4 \times 10^5 M^{-1}$ have been reported (Peters, 1975). Table II compares the first four stepwise equilibrium binding constants for palmitate and oleate, the two most abundant FFA, with those for clofibrate and halofenate, commonly used hypolipidemic drugs. The values for the fatty acids are 100 to 2000 times larger than those for the drugs.

*These calculations do not take into account the possibility of fatty acid dimerization in aqueous solution. If dimerization or other forms of fatty acid association are included in the calculation, the association constants increase to the range of 2.6×10^8 to $9.1 \times 10^8 M^{-1}$ (Ashbrook et al., 1975).

TABLE II
Multiple Equilibrium Binding Constants

K_i	Palmitate[a] (M^{-1})	Oleate[a] (M^{-1})	Clofibrate (M^{-1})	Halofenate (M^{-1})
K_1	6.2×10^7	2.6×10^8	1.5×10^5	5.1×10^5
K_2	2.3×10^7	9.4×10^7	2.4×10^4	1.8×10^5
K_3	1.2×10^7	2.9×10^7	1.2×10^4	7.0×10^4
K_4	3.1×10^6	2.1×10^7	4.7×10^3	2.1×10^4

[a] The constants for the fatty acids assume that there is no association of the unbound fatty acid in the aqueous solution (Spector, 1975).

A. Origin of the Plasma Free Fatty Acids

The plasma FFA arise from two separate sources, each in a different nutritional state. One is the adipose tissue, where fatty acid is stored in the form of triglycerides (Steinberg, 1967). Fatty acid is either synthesized within the adipocytes from precursors derived from glucose (Vrána and Fábry, 1973) or taken up from the triglycerides contained in circulating lipoproteins. The major triglyceride-rich plasma lipoproteins are chylomicrons that are synthesized in the intestinal mucosa and very low density lipoproteins that are synthesized predominantly in the liver (Morrisett et al., 1975). Dietary fat is the source of the fatty acids contained in the triglycerides of chylomicrons, whereas much of the fatty acid contained in the triglycerides of the very low density lipoproteins is synthesized in the liver. Lipoprotein lipase, an enzyme that is produced within the adipocyte but apparently acts at the surface of the capillary endothelium, hydrolyzes the plasma lipoprotein triglycerides during the process of removal from the plasma (Cryer et al., 1975; Higgins and Fielding, 1975; Stewart and Schotz, 1974; Fielding et al., 1974; Blanchette-Mackie and Scow, 1971). The fatty acids released during hydrolysis enter the adipocytes where they are incorporated into triglycerides.

Triglyceride synthesis in adipose tissue is facilitated when the plasma concentrations of glucose and insulin are high, such as in the fed state (Steinberg, 1967). By contrast, fatty acid is released from the adipose tissue in the form of FFA when the circulating levels of glucose and insulin are low, such as during fasting or starvation. The presence of certain fat mobilizing hormones, such as epinephrine, norepinephrine and glucagon, stimulate lipolysis and the release of fatty acid in the form of FFA from the adipose tissue (Steinberg, 1967). Release of norepinephrine from the sympathetic nerve endings in the adipose tissue also stimulates FFA release into the plasma. In summary, net amounts of FFA are released from adipose tissue primarily in the fasting state or at times of stress when the availability of circulating substrate is either low or insufficient to meet metabolic needs (Owen and Reichard, 1971).

A second source of plasma FFA is the triglycerides contained in chylomicrons and very low density lipoproteins (Heimberg *et al.*, 1974). During hydrolysis of the lipoprotein triglycerides, some of the fatty acid that is produced is released into the plasma as FFA, although the bulk is deposited in the tissues. Kinetic measurement with isotopic labels indicate that about 50% of the triglyceride fatty acids are converted to plasma FFA and that plasma FFA is an intermediate in the movement of triglyceride fatty acid to the tissues (Eaton *et al.*, 1969). This is the source of much of the FFA present in the plasma in the fed state. Through this mechanism, the plasma FFA composition can change considerably after a meal, depending on the type of fat that is eaten. For example, linoleic acid composition of the plasma FFA increased from 15 to 45% within 6 to 8 hours after safflower oil was fed to humans (Heimberg *et al.*, 1974). A similar increase in the linoleic acid content in triglycerides occurred during this period, increasing from 20 to 50% of the plasma triglyceride fatty acids. These results support the view that appreciable amounts of the plasma FFA in the postprandial state are derived from plasma triglyceride hydrolysis and, moreover, indicate that the ingestion of a single fat meal is sufficient to change the fatty acid composition of both lipoprotein triglycerides and FFA. This may be important in terms of drug binding in the plasma. If drug binding to albumin can indeed be modulated by FFA, it is possible that the modulation may vary depending on the composition of the fatty acids that comprise the plasma FFA fraction. In turn, this may vary considerably, depending on the type of fat that is consumed at a given meal.

B. Oscillations in Plasma Free Fatty Acid Concentration

The half-life of the plasma FFA is only 1 to 2 minutes (Fredrickson and Gordon, 1958). Release of FFA from the adipose tissue is initiated and terminated rapidly. Likewise, the plasma triglyceride half-life is only 1.5 to 5 hours (Eaton *et al.*, 1969). Based upon these findings, one can predict that the plasma FFA concentration can vary considerably over a short period of time. Some nutritionally-induced modifications in the plasma FFA concentration are listed in Table III. After administration of glucose orally, 1 gm/kg body weight following an overnight fast, the plasma FFA concentration was observed to decrease from 60 to 75% within 1 hour (Shafrir and Gutman, 1965). Even at only 30 minutes after

TABLE III
Effect of Nutrition on Plasma Free Fatty Acid Concentration

Nutritional state	Time[a] (hours)	FFA (μEq/ml)	FFA/Albumin[b] $\bar{\nu}$[c]	Reference
Basal	—	0.30–0.50	0.67	[d]
Glucose load	1	0.09–0.17	0.22	Shafrir and Gutman, 1965
Carbohydrate fed	—[e]	0.09–0.16	0.21	Fredrickson and Gordon, 1958
Fat load	8	0.65–0.08	1.08	Heimberg et al., 1974
Sugarless coffee	4	0.83 ± 0.07[f]	1.38	Bellet et al., 1968
Fasting	16	0.79	1.32	Fredrickson and Gordon, 1958
Fasting	39	1.20 ± 0.08[f]	2.00	Sawin and Willard, 1970

[a] Time that blood was taken following the nutritional perturbation.
[b] Assumes an albumin concentration of 4 gm/dl.
[c] Molar ratio based on the mean FFA value.
[d] Mean range of the basal values reported by all of these references.
[e] Carbohydrate feeding was begun 2 hours before sampling and continued to the time of measurement.
[f] Mean ± S.E.

glucose administration, the plasma FFA concentrations were decreased by about 50%. In a similar study, it was observed that the mean plasma FFA decrease following an oral glucose load was 45%, that the decrease continued for the first 2 hours, and that the rate of decrease was $1.19 \pm 0.06 \mu$ Eq/liter/minute (Gola *et al.*, 1972). On the other hand, ingestion of a fatty meal produces a rise in the plasma FFA concentration (Heimberg *et al.*, 1974). For example, ingestion of safflower oil caused the plasma FFA to increase from 0.32 to 0.66 μ Eq/ml over 12 hours, and a similar coconut oil feeding produced an increase from 0.36 to 0.73 μ Eq/ml over the same period. Unsweetened coffee produced an increase from 0.43 to 0.82 μ Eq/ml over a 3-hour period, apparently because of its caffeine content (Bellet *et al.*, 1968). Fasting for 39 hours caused the plasma FFA to increase from about 0.4 to 1.2 μ Eq/ml in a group of normal patients (Sawin and Willard, 1970). These findings indicate that nutritional factors can have an appreciable influence on the plasma FFA concentration and, as noted in the previous section, even on the plasma FFA composition.

C. Molar Ratio of Free Fatty Acid to Albumin

The molecular weight of albumin is about 66,000 daltons (Peters, 1975). Since normal plasma contains 3.5 to 4.5 gm/dl, there are between 0.53 and 0.68 μmoles/ml of albumin present. In resting subjects, the plasma FFA concentration has been observed to vary from about 0.33 to 0.68 μ Eq/ml (Bellet *et al.*, 1968; Goodman and Gordon, 1958; Sawin and Willard, 1970; Shafrir and Gutman, 1965). In our laboratory, we find the resting venous plasma FFA concentration in samples obtained after the insertion of an indwelling venous catheter to be between 0.31 and 0.93 μ Eq/ml, with a mean value of 0.57 μ Eq/ml in 24 determinations. Based upon these values, we calculate that the molar ratio of FFA to albumin in normal, venous plasma at rest is about 0.94, with a range of 0.46–1.75. Therefore, the molar ratio of FFA to albumin is usually less than 2 under normal, resting conditions. With fasting, plasma FFA values as high as 1.2 μ Eq/ml and 1.7 μ Eq/ml have been obtained (Fredrickson and Gordon, 1958; Sawin and Willard, 1970). After prolonged physical exercise, FFA values as high as 2.5 μ Eq/ml were noted (Havel *et al.*, 1967). We have produced plasma FFA concentrations of 2.2–2.4 μ Eq/ml by administering heparin intravenously to hypertriglyceridemic subjects. However, we have only achieved values of 1.0–1.2 μ Eq/ml in subjects having normal plasma triglyceride concentrations with this method. Assuming that the average plasma albumin concentration is about $0.6\,\mu$ moles/ml, molar ratios of 1.67 to 2.83 have been observed in fasting subjects, and values as high as 3.67 to 4.17 can occur after exercise or heparin administration. Therefore, it is entirely possible in the human to achieve FFA to albumin molar ratios in excess of 2, although this is not a common occurrence. When the molar ratio does exceed 2, FFA begin to bind to other substances in the plasma, such as lipoproteins and erythrocytes (Goodman, 1958b; Goodman and Shafrir, 1959.)

IV. EFFECTS OF FREE FATTY ACIDS ON DRUG BINDING TO PLASMA ALBUMIN

It was recognized more than 20 years ago that fatty acids and many of the drugs that bind to plasma albumin have structural similarities. Both have hydrocarbon groups that can interact with nonpolar regions of the protein and, like FFA, many of the drugs also exist predominantly as anions. Therefore, it was reasonable to assume that both FFA and drugs may compete for the same protein binding sites. The initial tests of this question were made with an organic dye, methyl orange, the dye being employed instead of a drug because it could be measured spectrophotometrically. Displacement of methyl orange was observed when large amounts of FFA were added to bovine albumin, but there was no displacement when less than 2 moles of FFA were added (Cogin and Davis, 1951). Identical results were obtained with human albumin, no displacement being observed when up to 2 moles of FFA were added (Goodman, 1958a). It was noted that the strength of binding of the first 2 moles of fatty acid to the albumin was at least 100 times greater than that of methyl orange and, furthermore, that the association constant for methyl orange was in the same range as that for many of the drugs and other organic compounds that bind to albumin (Goodman, 1958a). Based on these observations, a model was suggested in which albumin was presumed to contain three classes of binding sites. The first class of sites was accessible only to long-chain fatty acids such as the 16- and 18-carbon atom varieties that comprise the bulk of the plasma FFA. Apparently, the long, relatively straight hydrocarbon chain of these FFA enabled them to penetrate into the high energy binding sites, whereas compounds with bulky ring groups, such as methyl orange and many drugs, cannot reach these sites. On the other hand, a secondary group of four or five sites which bind FFA with an association constant in the range of 1×10^4 to $5 \times 10^5\,M^{-1}$, was considered to be accessible to fatty acids as well as other organic compounds such as drugs (Goodman,

1958a). This model accounted for the observation that methyl orange was displaced by the more strongly binding FFA only when more than 2 moles of fatty acid were bound to albumin.

We have confirmed these findings using several other optically active organic model compounds that lend themselves to either spectrophotometric or fluorescence measurements. For example, 2-(4'-hydroxyphenylazo)benzoic acid (HABA) was displaced from human albumin only when 3 moles of either palmitate or oleate were added (Spector and Imig, 1971). These measurements were made by equilibrium dialysis, and the displacement produced by 3 moles of palmitate was about 15–20%. Similar equilibrium dialysis measurements revealed that ANS also was displaced from bovine and human albumins only when 3 or more moles of fatty acids were present (Santos and Spector, 1972, 1974). Again, the displacements were only about 15–20%. HABA, ANS, and methyl orange are considered to be experimental model compounds that structurally are representative of drugs that bind to albumin. Therefore, the results obtained with these model compounds suggested that many drugs also would not be displaced until the molar ratio of FFA to albumin exceeded 2. As noted in Section III, C, there are situations in which the molar ratio does exceed 2 in the human, but these are uncommon occurrences. For the most part, the FFA to albumin molar ratio varies between 0.5 and 2.0 in normal individuals, a range where drug binding should not be affected according to the predictions made from the work with the model compounds.

A. Binding Studies with Radioactive Drugs

The conclusions of the dye studies were confirmed using a number of labeled drugs. Addition of either 3.5 or 7 moles of palmitate appreciably reduced the binding of salicylate, diphenylhydantoin, phenylbutazone, bromosulphthalein, sulfadiazine, thiopental and bishydroxycoumarin to albumin as measured by equilibrium dialysis (Rudman et al., 1971). Significant differences were not observed, however, when less than 3.5 moles of palmitate were added.

As shown in Fig. 1, we have obtained a similar result by equilibrium dialysis when we tested the binding of a hypolipidemic drug, halofenate, to human serum albumin. When the molar ratio of palmitate to albumin was 3.0, we were able to demonstrate a decrease in halofenate binding of between 15 and 30%. As in evident from Fig. 1, however, there is considerable scattering in these binding data in spite of the fact that this is a straightforward physicochemical measurement. Because of this scattering, we were not able to distinguish any consistent effect on halofenate

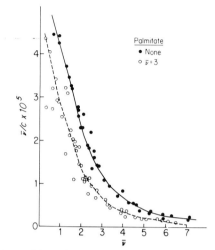

Fig. 1. Effect of fatty acid on the binding of halofenate to human plasma albumin. These data were obtained by equilibrium dialysis at 37°C in a calcium-free Krebs Ringer phosphate buffer, pH 7.4. The human plasma albumin concentration was 0.15 mM, and where present, the palmitate concentration was 0.45 mM. ^{14}C-labeled halofenate was employed for these assays. ●, No palmitate; ○, $\bar{v} = 3$.

binding when the molar ratio of palmitate to albumin was less than 3.0 (Spector *et al.*, 1973), although there was a suggestion from the data that the points obtained at intermediate FFA concentrations might actually lie between the control isotherm and that obtained when 3 moles of palmitate were present. At most, however, these reduction in binding can be only 5–10%. Differences in binding on the order of 5–10% might still have some effect *in vivo*. For these reasons, we again turned to the dye and fluorescent compounds in order to make much more sensitive measurements of the possible effects of 0.5–2.0 moles of FFA on the binding of a second organic compound.

B. Fluorescence Studies

Our initial studies were done with ANS and bovine albumin, a system in which there is no measurable displacement of the dye by equilibrium dialysis until the molar ratio of FFA to albumin reaches 3.0 (Santos and Spector, 1972). Yet, when ANS fluorescence was measured, a definite reduction in fluorescence was noted in the FFA to albumin molar ratio range of 0 to 3 (Santos and Spector, 1972). At molar ratio 3, there was a 15–28% reduction in ANS fluorescence, values that were in agreement with the decrease in ANS binding as measured by equilibrium dialysis.

At molar ratio 1, however, there also was a 3–10% reduction in ANS fluorescence. Likewise, at molar ratio 2, there was a 7–21% reduction in ANS fluorescence. Similar reductions in ANS fluorescence were produced by fatty acids containing 12–18 carbon atoms. The reductions were not accompanied by any shift in the wavelength of maximum fluorescence. These findings indicated that the very sensitive and reproducible fluorescence assay was able to detect changes in ANS binding over the usual range of FFA to albumin molar ratios even though they could not be detected by the more cumbersome equilibrium dialysis method.

Much more complex data were obtained when ANS was tested with human albumin (Santos and Spector, 1974). Again, no significant differences in ANS binding could be detected when the FFA to albumin molar ratio was less than 3. Yet, changes in fluorescence were noted at FFA–albumin molar ratios of 1 and 2. Unlike the finding with bovine albumin, however, the fluorescence of ANS was greater at molar ratios 1 and 2 as compared with fatty acid-poor human albumin. As in the case of bovine albumin, there was no modification in the wavelength of maximum ANS fluorescence. This finding suggested that in the lower concentration range, FFA might actually increase ANS binding by about 10%, not cause displacement. Although indirect, these results with ANS also provide some support for the view that changes in FFA concentration within the usual physiologic range might influence to a small extent the binding of a second organic compound to plasma albumin.

C.   2-(4′-Hydroxyphenylazo)benzoic Acid

HABA is an organic dye that readily binds to plasma albumin. When it binds, there is a marked shift in its absorption spectrum (Baxter, 1964). In the absence of albumin, HABA has a maximum absorbance at 348 nm. When it binds to albumin, however, an absorption maximum develops in the region of 480 nm (Baxter, 1963). The absorbance at 480 nm is correlated with the quantity of HABA bound to albumin.

When the effect of FFA on HABA binding to albumin was tested by equilibrium dialysis, results similar to those observed with halofenate (Fig. 1), ANS (Santos and Spector, 1972), and a number of commonly used drugs (Rudman *et al.*, 1971) were noted (Spector and Imig, 1971). No reduction in HABA binding could be demonstrated until the molar ratio of FFA to albumin reached 3.0. As shown in Fig. 2, however, a decrease in HABA absorbance at 480 nm occurred as the FFA concentration was raised, and small reductions were observed even when the FFA–albumin molar ratio was varied between 0 and 2. When the palmi-

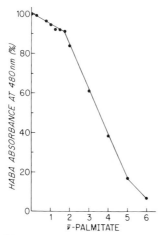

Fig. 2. Effect of fatty acid concentration on 2-(4'-hydroxyphenylazo)benzoic acid binding to bovine plasma albumin. Binding is measured as absorbance of the dye at 480 nm. The fatty acid added was palmitate, and the symbol, $\bar{\nu}$, denotes the molar ratio of palmitate to albumin present in the solution.

tate to albumin molar ratio was 3.0, HABA absorbance was decreased by 38% as compared with fatty acid-poor bovine albumin. This corresponded to a 15–25% reduction in binding as measured by equilibrium dialysis (Spector and Imig, 1971). A 16% reduction in absorbance occurred when the palmitate molar ratio was raised from 0 to 2. As in the case of the fluorescence results with ANS, these HABA data suggest that a small decrease in binding occurs within the range of FFA–albumin molar ratios that can be produced by nutritional variations, on the order of 5–15%. This must be considered as speculative, however, for the absorbance changes cannot be equated rigorously to changes in the amount of HABA that is bound.

Another spectrophotometric observation made with HABA suggests that the molecular interactions between this organic compound and its binding sites are altered when the FFA–albumin molar ratio varies. As shown in Fig. 3, there is a small but progressive red shift in the wavelength of maximum absorbance when the molar ratio of palmitate to human albumin is raised from 0 to 7.4. With fatty acid-poor albumin, the actual wavelength of maximum absorbance was 481 nm. There was no change when one mole of palmitate was added, but the maximum then increased gradually to 490 nm until the molar ratio reached 6.5. The maximum occurred at 482 nm when the molar ratio was 1 and 483 nm when it was 2.5. Therefore, the red shift began to occur within the lower range of palmitate–albumin molar ratios, in this case beginning at

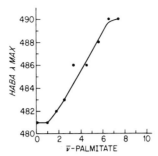

Fig. 3. Effect of fatty acid concentration on the wavelength of maximum absorbance of the 2-(4'-hydroxyphenylazo)benzoic acid–human plasma albumin complex. The fatty acid added was palmitate, and the symbol, $\bar{\nu}$, denotes the molar ratio of palmitate to albumin present in the solution.

1.0. Again, this cannot be equated with a binding change in a strict sense. The finding does suggest, however, that there is a progressive modification in the interaction between HABA and its binding sites as the FFA content of the albumin increases. Although it is reasonable to suggest that this might be associated with or mirror a change in the strength of binding, such an interpretation remains conjectural.

In summary, our spectroscopic data suggest that small changes in the plasma FFA concentration may alter the binding of an organic ligand to albumin. Proof that this actually occurs, however, has not as yet been obtained with drugs. Based upon our results, we would predict that the binding changes are on the order of only 5–15%. In our hands, equilibrium dialysis data usually are too scattered to conclusively demonstrate such small differences. Therefore, definitive information with drugs will have to await the development of more accurate and reproducible binding methods.

V. MECHANISM OF FATTY ACID-INDUCED ALBUMIN BINDING CHANGES

As seen in Fig. 1, plasma albumin can bind more than 7 moles/mole of halofenate. Large binding capacities also have been noted for other drugs (Rudman *et al.*, 1971), indicating that multiple binding to a single albumin molecule can occur. Similarly, albumin has a large capacity to bind FFA (Goodman, 1958a; Spector *et al.*, 1969). Using Eq (2),

$$\bar{\nu} = \frac{K_1 A + 2K_1 K_2 A^2 + \ldots n K_1 \ldots K_n A^n}{1 + K_1 A + K_1 K_2 A^2 + \ldots K_1 \ldots K_n A^n} \tag{2}$$

one can calculate the association constants for the multiple binding of a compound to albumin (Fletcher *et al.*, 1973). The first four binding constants for palmitate and oleate, the most prevalent acids comprising the plasma FFA, and for clofibrate and halofenate, two hypolipidemic drugs, are listed in Table II. The values for the fatty acids are 100 to 2000 times larger than those for the drugs. From the binding data available in the literature for many other drugs, it can be estimated that their binding constants also are very much smaller than those for the long-chain FFA. Therefore, if FFA and drugs were to compete for the same albumin sites, the drug should be displaced as long as FFA were available to occupy the binding site. Since the succeeding K_i for multiple binding are smaller than K_1 (see Table II), displacement of some drug from the protein should occur when the drug moves to a weaker site. As noted in Section IV, however, we have not been able to measure any consistent decrease in drug binding by equilibrium dialysis when either 1 or 2 moles of FFA are added to albumin. Others have had the same experience (Cogin and Davis, 1951; Goodman, 1958a; Rudman *et al.*, 1971). Therefore, it is generally agreed that albumin is able to carry up to 2 moles of FFA without having any serious impediment in its ability to bind a second organic compound. The simplest explanation, which was first put forward by Goodman (1958a), is that albumin contains two binding sites that are accessible only to long-chain FFA.

A. Separation of Binding Sites

This separation of FFA and drug binding sites is illustrated schematically in Fig. 4. In the upper panel, two types of binding sites are depicted. The N_1 sites, shown on the left side, are the class that is specific for FFA. Either because they possess a long, straight hydrocarbon chain or they have such a high energy of binding, FFA are able to penetrate into these sites. Because of their more bulky structure or lesser binding energy, drugs and other organic compounds such as ANS, HABA, or methyl orange cannot reach these sites. There appear to be two N_1 sites. In addition, there is a second class of albumin binding sites that are available to all types of organic compounds, including drugs and FFA. These are denoted as the N_2 class and are shown on the right side of the model. The general symbol A^- is used to indicate that many types of organic anions can bind to the N_2 sites. Each albumin molecule contains four or five N_2 sites (Goodman, 1958a). When the FFA concentration is high and the N_1 sites approach saturation, the excess FFA spills over and begins to fill the N_2 sites. This leads to competition between FFA and other compounds for the N_2 sites, accounting for the displacement of

HSA BINDING; FUNCTIONAL MODEL

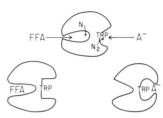

Fig. 4.   Schematic representation of fatty acid and drug binding to plasma albumin; the conformational model. N_1 is used to represent the class of two binding sites that are specific for long-chain fatty acids. N_2 represents the secondary or general organic anion binding sites, the anions being abbreviated as A^-. The tryptophan residue, abbreviated as TRP, is shown as being located in the region of one of the main N_2 sites. The bottom left-hand panel indicates that binding of FFA to the N_1 sites may influence the conformation of the N_2 sites. Likewise, the bottom right-hand panel indicates that anion binding to the N_2 sites may alter the conformation of the N_1 sites. This model was constructed from data obtained with human albumin, but the available evidence suggests that it also applies to bovine albumin.

halofenate (Fig. 1) and HABA (Fig. 2) when the albumin solution contains more than 2 moles of palmitate. As shown in Fig. 4, the single tryptophan residue of human albumin is present at one of these N_2 binding sites (Swaney and Klotz, 1970; Gambhir *et al.*, 1975).

Assuming that this model involving separation of the N_1 and N_2 binding sites is correct, one must develop an explanation for our HABA and ANS data which suggest that some organic anion displacement occurs even when the molar ratio of FFA to albumin is in the range of 0–2. Two explanations are possible. One involves conformational changes in the binding sites, whereas the other involves competitive binding. It is possible that both processes occur simultaneously.

B.   Conformational Change

This concept is illustrated schematically in the lower panels of Fig. 4. According to this hypothesis, FFA binding to the N_1 sites causes a change in the three-dimensional structure of the N_2 sites. This is shown in Fig. 4 as a change in shape of the N_2 sites from a circular to a square shape when FFA occupy the N_1 sites. The extent of the conformational change depends on the amount of FFA present at the N_1 sites, accounting for the progressive decrease in HABA absorbance seen in Fig. 2 when the palmitate concentration was raised from 0 to 2. According to this interpretation, the strength of binding changes as the conformational change increases. The red shift in HABA absorbance that occurs as the palmitate concentration is raised (Fig. 3) is consistent with the occurrence of conformational changes. This could account for a progressively different molecular interaction between the site and the chromaphor, producing the spectral red shift. The types of conformational changes that are envisioned are not gross disorganizations in the albumin tertiary structure. Rather, the concept is one of subtle changes in the regions of the N_2 sites. There is some experimental evidence for small conformational changes in bovine albumin when relatively little FFA is bound (Glazer and Sanger, 1963; Soetewey *et al.*, 1972).

If binding at the N_1 sites can produce conformational changes in the N_2 sites, there is reason to suspect that the reverse also could occur; namely, that organic anion binding at the N_2 sites might alter the conformation of the N_1 sites. This is depicted in the lower right-hand panel of Fig. 4. Such a mechanism could explain how small amounts of a drug such as clofibrate, which is bound much less tightly (Table II), can displace some FFA from plasma albumin (Thorp, 1963; Spector and Soboroff, 1971; Meisner, 1975).

C. Competitive Binding

It is also possible to account for the displacement of an organic compound by competitive binding even if there are separate N_1 and N_2 sites. This follows from a fractional analysis of FFA binding to plasma albumin.

Distribution Analysis of Fatty Acid Binding

Since the multiple equilibrium constants for FFA binding are available as is shown in Table II, one can calculate the distribution of FFA in an albumin solution using Eq (3),

$$FP_i = \frac{[PA_i]}{[P_T]} = \frac{iK_1K_2\ldots K_i[A]^i}{1 + K_1[A] + \ldots K_1\ldots K_n[A]^n} \tag{3}$$

where FP_i is the fraction of the *total albumin* that binds a given amount of FFA. In this way, the percentage of albumin molecules in a solution that contain $0, 1, 2, 3 \ldots n$ moles of FFA at a given total FFA and albumin concentration can be estimated. Rather than being widely separated, the K_i values for FFA binding are fairly close in magnitude (see Table II). Therefore, FFA would tend to spread over several sites of roughly similar strength rather than be completely localized to one specific site. Using different approaches, similar conclusions were reached by Cun-

TABLE IV
Oleate–Albumin Species Calculated by Distribution
Analysis

Molar ratio[a]	Albumin molecules (%)[b]						
	0[c]	1	2	3	4	5	6
0.5	58	34	7	1	0	0	0
1.0	31	43	22	4	0	0	0
2.0	6	26	40	20	7	1	0
3.0	1	8	27	29	24	10	1

[a] Total moles oleate/mole albumin in solution.
[b] Assumes an albumin concentration of 0.58 mM.
[c] Number of oleate molecules per albumin molecule.

ningham et $al.$ (1975), Wosilait and Soler-Argilaga (1975), and Wosilait et $al.$ (1976).

As shown in Table IV, this prediction was borne out by the actual calculations. For example, when the molar ratio of $total$ oleate to albumin is one, the largest percentage of the albumin molecules, 43%, also contains 1 mole of FFA. However, 31% of the albumin molecules contain no FFA, 22% contain 2 moles and 4% contain 3 moles of FFA. Similarly, when the solution contains 2 moles of oleate, 40% of the albumin molecules contain 2 moles of FFA. Yet, 6% contain no FFA, 26% contain 1 mole, 20% contain 3 moles, 7% contain 4 moles, and 1% contain 5 moles of FFA. Therefore, 28% of the albumin molecules contain more than 2 moles of FFA even though the total number of moles of oleate per mole of albumin is only 2. Intermediate distributions occur when the molar ratio of $total$ oleate to albumin is between 1 and 2.

Possible Relationship to Drug Binding. Independently of the model that is selected for the grouping of the albumin binding sites, one would predict that albumin molecules are less well suited to bind a second compound as their FFA content increases. Before the results of the distribution analysis were known, one might argue that all of the drug binding sites were unfilled when the albumin solution contained less than 2 moles/mole of FFA. This, of course, assumes the existence of two N_1 sites specific for FFA. The distribution analysis indicates that this is incorrect; that is, all of the FFA under these conditions would not be segregated to only two binding sites even if there are two specific N_1 sites. It is likely that albumin molecules containing 3 or more moles of FFA have at least some of their drug binding sites occupied by fatty acid molecules.* This should lead to competitive binding between these FFA molecules and drug molecules that, on a statistical basis, might happen to interact with the site. The net result would be some decrease in the strength of drug binding due to competition with these FFA for the sites. Therefore, on the basis of competition alone, one can account for a 5–15% decrease in binding when the molar ratio of FFA to albumin is between 0 and 2. According to this interpretation, the red shift in the HABA binding spectrum (Fig. 3) is due to interactions between the dye and the hydrocarbon tails of fatty acids present at the drug binding sites, not to conformational changes as postulated in Fig. 4. Furthermore, the greater drug displacement that occurs when the molar ratio of FFA to albumin exceeds 2 can be explained as an extension of the process whereby more of the albumin molecules contain larger numbers of FFA molecules, and no new or separate mechanism needs to be postulated.

VI. SUMMARY AND CONCLUSIONS

Drug binding takes place in the blood plasma. It involves the combination of a drug with a plasma protein, usually albumin, to enhance its solubility and to facilitate its transport through the circulation. Binding is important because it influences the pharmacologic potency, metabolism, and excretion of a drug.

Nutrition can influence drug binding in two ways. One is to reduce the amount of available albumin. This can occur in severe protein–calorie malnutrition. In Western civilization, however, this is a relatively rare occurrence. Nutrition also can influence drug binding by producing variations in the concentration of metabolites that are transported by albumin. These include nonpolar amino acids such as tryptophan, bile salts, bilirubin, lysolecithin, and FFA. All of these substances in theory should influence drug binding. The concentrations of amino acids and FFA are especially prone to nutritional influences.

Competitive binding between drugs and the nonpolar amino acids has not been studied in enough detail to determine whether nutritional var-

---

*The multiple equilibrium constants used for the distribution binding calculations deal with complexes of FFA and albumin, not specific binding sites on the albumin molecule. Therefore, no information about specific binding sites can be derived from the distribution analysis. On a statistical basis, one might predict that there would be a greater tendency for a fatty acid molecule to approach the unfilled site having the highest binding energy. Although such a prediction seems reasonable, any assignment of FFA molecules to specific albumin sites on the basis of the multiple equilbrium and distribution analyses is entirely speculative.

iations play any role. Since tryptophan probably binds to the same albumin site as some drugs (Gambhir *et al.,* 1975) and tryptophan binding varies with the nutritional state (Lipsett *et al.,* 1973), it probably would be worthwhile to examine this possibility in some detail.

A considerable amount of detailed information already is available concerning FFA. Although there appears to be a separation of some FFA and drug binding sites, displacement of drugs will occur when the FFA–albumin molar ratio exceeds 2. This results predominantly from competitive binding at the secondary albumin binding sites. Nutritional effects, however, usually cause the FFA–albumin molar ratio to vary only between 0 and 2, and there is debate as to whether FFA variation within this range has any influence on drug binding. No conclusive effect can be demonstrated by classical binding studies. Using model compounds and spectroscopic assays, however, we have demonstrated changes that may indicate binding differences on the order of 5–15% over the molar ratio range of 0–2. We suggest that such changes result from either a conformational change in the drug binding sites produced by the binding of FFA to other regions of the albumin molecule, or competitive binding. Distribution analyses calculated from the multiple equilibrium binding constants for the long-chain FFA suggests that there is some spill-over of fatty acids to the drug binding sites in some of the albumin molecules in the solution, even when the FFA–albumin molar ratio is only 1–2. This could lead to competitive binding between the FFA and the drug in these more heavily loaded albumin complexes.

VII. RESEARCH NEEDS

Three lines of investigation would contribute useful information to the subject of nutrition and drug binding. One is competitive binding studies between drugs and nonpolar amino acids such as tryptophan, especially over the range of amino acid concentrations that can occur in different nutritional states. This would indicate whether the variations in plasma amino acid concentration that can be produced nutritionally might have any real influence on drug binding. The other two types of investigation deal with the FFA studies described in this report. First, pharmacologic data are needed to determine whether binding changes on the order of 5–15% are important in terms of drug transport and effectiveness. It may be that even if such differences occur, they are too small to have pharmacologic significance. If so, further work on the role of FFA could be terminated. Conversely, if small changes in drug binding are important pharmacologically, it would be important to document that the types of changes predicted by our spectroscopic studies occur with actual drugs. This probably will require the application of newer binding methods or, alternatively, technical improvements in the currently used equilibrium dialysis method.

ACKNOWLEDGMENTS

We wish to thank Merck Sharp and Dohme Research Laboratories, West Point, Pennsylvania, for supplying halofenate and ^{14}C-labeled halofenate; Ayerst Laboratories, New York, New York, for providing clofibrate; and Imperial Chemical Industries Limited, Macclesfield, Cheshire, England, for supplying ^{14}C-labeled clofibrate.

These studies were supported in part by research grants from the National Heart and Lung Institute (HL 14,230 and HL 14,781) and the American and Iowa Heart Association (74-689)

REFERENCES

Anderson, S. R., and Weber, G. (1969). Fluorescence polarization of the complexes of 1-anilino-8-naphthalenesulfonate with bovine serum albumin. Evidence for preferential orientation of the ligand. *Biochemistry* **8**, 371–377.

Anton, A. H. (1973). Increasing activity of sulfonamides with displacing agents: A review. *Ann. N.Y. Acad. Sci.* **226**, 273–292.

Ashbrook, J. D., Spector, A. A., Santos, E. C., and Fletcher, J. E. (1975). Long-chain fatty acid binding to human plasma albumin. *J. Biol. Chem.* **250**, 2333–2338.

Baxter, J. H. (1963). Dissimilarity of changes induced in absorption spectrum of 2-(4'-hydroxyphenylazo)benzoic acid by different serum albumins. *Proc. Soc. Exp. Biol. Med.* **113**, 197–202.

Baxter, J. H. (1964). Differences in serum albumins reflected in absorption spectra of a bound dye. *Arch. Biochem. Biophys.* **108**, 375–383.

Behrens, P. O., Spiekerman, A. M., and Brown, J. R. (1975). Structure of human serum albumin. *Fed. Proc., Fed. Am. Soc. Exp. Biol.* **34**, 591 (2106).

Bellet, S., Kershbaum, A., and Finck, E. M. (1968). Response of free fatty acids to coffee and caffeine. *Metab. Clin. Exp.* **17**, 702–707.

Blanchette-Mackie, E. J., and Scow, R. O. (1971). Sites of lipoprotein lipase activity in adipose tissue perfused with chylomicrons. Electron microscopic cytochemical study. *J. Cell Biol.* **51**, 1–25.

Bloomfield, V. (1966). The structure of bovine serum albumin at low pH. *Biochemistry* **5**, 684–689.

Borondy, P., Dill, W. A., Chang, T., Buchanan, R. A., and Glazko, A. J. (1973). Effect of protein binding on the distribution of 5,5-diphenylhydantoin between plasma and red cells. *Ann. N.Y. Acad. Sci.* **226**, 82–87.

Braverman, L. E., Arky, R. A., Foster, A. E., and Ingbar, S. H. (1969). Effect of physiological variations in free fatty acid concentration on the binding of thyroxine in the serum of euthyroid and thyrotoxic subjects. *J. Clin. Invest.* **48**, 878–884.

Brown, J. R. (1975). Structure of bovine serum albumin. *Fed. Proc., Fed. Am. Soc. Exp. Biol.* **34**, 591 (2105).

Chignell, C. F. (1973). Recent advances in methodology: Spectroscopic techniques. *Ann. N.Y. Acad. Sci.* **226,** 44–59.

Cogin, G. E., and Davis, B. D. (1951). Competition in the binding of long-chain fatty acids and methyl orange to bovine serum albumin. *J. Am. Chem. Soc.* **73,** 3135–3138.

Cryer, A., Davies, P., Williams, E. R., and Robinson, D. S. (1975). The clearing factor lipase activity of isolated fat cells. *Biochem. J.* **146,** 481–488.

Cunningham, V. J., Hay, L., and Stoner, H. B. (1975). The binding of L-tryptophan to serum albumins in the presence of nonesterified fatty acids. *Biochem. J.* **146,** 653–658.

Curzon, G., Friedel, J., and Knott, P. J. (1973). The effect of fatty acids on the binding of tryptophan to plasma protein. *Nature (London)* **242,** 198–200.

Dayton, P. G., Israili, Z. H., and Perel, J. M. (1973). Influence of binding on drug metabolism and distribution. *Ann. N.Y. Acad. Sci.* **226,** 172–194.

Eaton, R. P., Berman, M., and Steinberg, D. (1969). Kinetic studies of plasma free fatty acid and triglyceride metabolism in man. *J. Clin. Invest.* **48,** 1560–1579.

Feldhoff, R. C., Reed, R. G., and Peters, T., Jr. (1975). Structural features and ligand-binding properties of two halves of bovine albumin. *Fed. Proc., Fed. Am. Soc. Exp. Biol.* **34,** 591.

Fielding, P. E., Shore, B. G., and Fielding, C. J. (1974). Lipoprotein lipase: Properties of the enzyme isolated from post-heparin plasma. *Biochemistry* **13,** 4318–4323.

Finlayson, J. S. (1975). Physical and biochemical properties of human albumin. *In* "Proceedings of the Workshop in Albumin" (J. T. Sgouris and A. René, eds.), pp. 31–56. Nat. Inst. Health, Bethesda, Maryland.

Fletcher, J. E., Ashbrook, J. D., and Spector, A. A. (1973). Computer analysis of drug–protein binding data. *Ann. N.Y. Acad. Sci.* **226,** 69–81.

Fredrickson, D. S., and Gordon, R. S., Jr. (1958). The metabolism of albumin-bound C^{14}-labeled unesterified fatty acids in normal human subjects. *J. Clin. Invest.* **37,** 1504–1515.

Gambhir, K. K., McMenamy, R. H., and Watson, F. (1975). Positions in human serum albumin which involve the indole binding site. *J. Biol. Chem.* **250,** 6711–6719.

Ghoneim, M. M., and Pandya, H. (1974). Plasma protein binding of bipivacaine and its interaction with other drugs in man. *Br. J. Anaesth.* **46,** 435–438.

Glazer, A. N., and Sanger, F. (1963). Effect of fatty acid on the iodination of bovine serum albumin. *J. Mol. Biol.* **7,** 452–453.

Gola, A., Frydecka, I., and Słónczewski, B. (1972). Free fatty acids curve in normals during the oral glucose tolerance test. *Clin. Chim. Acta* **38,** 127–130.

Goodman, D. S. (1958a). The interaction of human serum albumin with long-chain fatty acid anions. *J. Am. Chem. Soc.* **80,** 3892–3898.

Goodman, D. S. (1958b). The interaction of human erythrocytes with sodium palmitate. *J. Clin. Invest.* **37,** 1729–1735.

Goodman, D. S., and Gordon, R. S., Jr. (1958). The metabolism of plasma unesterified fatty acid. *Am. J. Clin. Nutr.* **6,** 669–680.

Goodman, D. S., and Shafrir, E. (1959). The interaction of human low density lipoproteins with long-chain fatty acid anions. *J. Am. Chem. Soc.* **81,** 364–370.

Green, H. O., Mortiz, J., and Lack, L. (1971). Binding of sodium taurocholate by bovine serum albumin. *Biochim. Biophys. Acta* **231,** 550–552.

Havel, R. J., Ekelund, L.-G., and Holmgren, A. (1967). Kinetic analysis of the oxidation of palmitate-1-^{14}C in man during prolonged heavy muscular exercise. *J. Lipid Res.* **8,** 366–373.

Heimberg, M., Dunn, G. D., and Wilcox, H. G. (1974). The derivation of plasma free fatty acids from dietary neutral fat in man. *J. Lab. Clin. Med.* **83,** 393–402.

Higgins, J. M., and Fielding, C. J. (1975). Lipoprotein lipase. Mechanism of formation of triglyceride-rich remnant particles from very low density lipoproteins and chylomicrons. *Biochemistry* **14**, 2288-2293.

Jacobsen, C. (1972). Chemical modification of the high-affinity bilirubin binding site of human serum albumin. *Eur. J. Biochem.* **27**, 513-519.

Karush, F., and Sonnenberg, M. (1949). Interaction of homologous alkyl sulfates with bovine serum albumin. *J. Am. Chem. Soc.* **71**, 1369-1376.

King, T. P. (1973). On the location of the primary organic ligand binding site of bovine plasma albumin. *Ann. N.Y. Acad. Sci.* **226**, 94-100.

Klotz, I. M., Walker, F. M., and Pivan, R. B. (1946). The binding of organic ions by proteins. *J. Am. Chem. Soc.* **68**, 1486-1490.

Krasner, J., Giacoia, G. P., and Yaffe, S. J. (1973). Drug–protein binding in the newborn infant. *Ann. N.Y. Acad. Sci.* **226**, 101-114.

Kunin, C. M., Craig, W. A., Kornguth, M., and Monson, R. (1973). Influence of binding on the pharmacologic activity of antibiotics. *Ann. N.Y. Acad. Sci.* **226**, 214-224.

Levy, G. (1973). Relationship between plasma protein binding, distribution, and anticoagulant action of dicoumarol. *Ann. N.Y. Acad. Sci.* **226**, 195-199.

Lipsett, D., Madras, B. K., Wurtman, R. J., and Munro, H. N. (1973). Serum tryptophan level after carbohydrate ingestion: Selective decline in nonalbumin-bound tryptophan coincident with reduction in serum free fatty acids. *Life Sci.* **12**, Part II, 57-64.

Lukas, D. S., and DeMartino, A. G. (1969). Binding of digitoxin and some related cardenolides to human plasma proteins. *J. Clin. Invest.* **48**, 1041-1053.

McMenamy, R. H., and Oncley, J. L. (1958). The specific binding of L-tryptophan to serum albumin. *J. Biol. Chem.* **233**, 1436-1447.

Meisner, H. (1975). Displacement of palmitate from albumin by chlorophenoxyisobutyrate. *Biochem. Biophys. Res. Commun.* **66**, 1134-1140.

Meloun, B., Morávek, L., and Kostka, V. (1975). Complete amino acid sequence of human serum albumin. *FEBS Lett.* **58**, 134-137.

Morrisett, J. D., Jackson, R. L., and Gotto, A. M., Jr. (1975). Lipoproteins: Structure and function. *Annu. Rev. Biochem.* **44**, 183-207.

Odell, G. B. (1973). Influence of binding on the toxicity of bilirubin. *Ann. N.Y. Acad. Sci.* **226**, 225-237.

Olsen, G. D. (1972). Methadone binding to human plasma albumin. *Science* **176**, 525-526.

O'Reilly, R. A. (1973). The binding of sodium warfarin to plasma albumin and its displacement by phenylbutazone. *Ann. N.Y. Acad. Sci.* **226**, 293-308.

Owen, O. E., and Reichard, G. A., Jr. (1971). Fuels consumed by man: The interplay between carbohydrates and fatty acids. *Prog. Biochem. Pharmacol.* **6**, 177-213.

Parke, D. V., and Lindup, W. E. (1975). Quantitative and qualitative aspects of the plasma protein binding of carbenoxolone, an ulcer-healing drug. *Ann. N.Y. Acad. Sci.* **226**, 200-213.

Peters, T., Jr. (1975). Serum albumin. *In* "The Plasma Proteins: Structure, Function, and Genetic Control" (F. W. Putnam, ed.), 2nd ed., Vol. 1, pp. 133-181. Academic Press, New York.

Peters, T., Jr., and Feldhoff, R. C. (1975). Fragments of bovine serum albumin produced by limited proteolysis. Isolation and characterization of tryptic fragments. *Biochemistry* **14**, 3384-3388.

Pinckard, R. N., Hawkins, D., and Fan, R. S. (1973). The influence of acetylsalicylic acid on the binding of acetrizoate to human albumin. *Ann. N.Y. Acad. Sci.* **226**, 341-354.

Ray, A., Reynolds, J. A., Polet, H., and Steinhardt, J. (1966). Binding of large organic anions and neutral molecules by native bovine serum albumin. *Biochemistry* **5**, 2606-2616.

Reed, R. G., Feldhoff, R. C., Clute, O. L., and Peters, T., Jr. (1975). Fragments of bovine serum albumin produced by limited proteolysis. Conformation and ligand binding. *Biochemistry* **14**, 4578–4583.

Reidenberg, M. M., and Affrime, M. (1973). Influence of disease on binding of drugs to plasma proteins. *Ann. N.Y. Acad. Sci.* **226**, 115–126.

Rudman, D., Bixler, T. J., II, and Del Rio, A. E. (1971). Effect of free fatty acids on binding of drugs by bovine serum albumin, by human serum albumin and by rabbit serum. *J. Pharmacol. Exp. Ther.* **176**, 261–272.

Rutenberg, H. L., Lacko, A. G., and Soloff, L. A. (1973). Inhibition of lecithin:cholesterol acyltransferase following intravenous administration of heparin in man. *Biochim. Biophys. Acta* **326**, 419–427.

Santos, E. C., and Spector, A. A. (1972). Effect of fatty acids on the binding of 1-anilino-8-naphthalenesulfonate to bovine serum albumin. *Biochemistry* **11**, 2299–2302.

Santos, E. C., and Spector, A. A. (1974). Effects of fatty acids on the interaction of 1-anilino-8-naphthalenesulfonate with human plasma albumin. *Mol. Pharmacol.* **10**, 519–528.

Sawin, C. T., and Willard, D. A. (1970). Normal rise in plasma free fatty acids during fasting in patients with hypopituitarism. *J. Clin. Endocrinol. Metab.* **31**, 233–234.

Sellers, E. M., and Koch-Weser, J. (1973). Influence of intravenous injection rate on protein binding and vascular activity of diazoxide. *Ann. N.Y. Acad. Sci.* **226**, 319–332.

Shafrir, E., and Gutman, A. (1965). Patterns of decrease of free fatty acids during glucose tolerance tests. *Diabetes* **14**, 77–83.

Shoeman, D. W., Benjamin, D. M., and Azarnoff, D. L. (1973). The alteration of plasma proteins in uremia as reflected in the ability to bind diphenylhydantoin. *Ann. N.Y. Acad. Sci.* **226**, 127–130.

Soetewey, F., Rosseneu-Motreff, M., Lamote, R., and Peeters, H. (1972). Size and shape determination of native and defatted bovine serum albumin monomers. II. Influences of the fatty acid content on the conformation of bovine serum albumin monomers. *J. Biochem. (Tokyo)* **71**, 705–710.

Spector, A. A. (1971). Metabolism of free fatty acids. *Prog. Biochem. Pharmacol.* **6**, 130–176.

Spector, A. A. (1975). Fatty acid binding to plasma albumin. *J. Lipid Res.* **16**, 165–179.

Spector, A. A., and Imig, B. (1971). Effect of free fatty acid concentration on the transport and utilization of other albumin-bound compounds: Hydroxyphenylazobenzoic acid. *Mol. Pharmacol.* **7**, 511–518.

Spector, A. A., and Soboroff, J. M. (1971). Effect of chlorophenoxyisobutyrate on free fatty acid utilization by mammalian cells. *Proc. Soc. Exp. Biol. Med.* **137**, 945–947.

Spector, A. A., John, K., and Fletcher, J. E. (1969). Binding of long-chain fatty acids to bovine serum albumin. *J. Lipid Res.* **10**, 56–67.

Spector, A. A., Santos, E. C., Ashbrook, J. D., and Fletcher, J. E. (1973). Influence of free fatty acid concentration on drug binding to plasma albumin. *Ann. N.Y. Acad. Sci.* **226**, 247–258.

Steinberg, D. (1967). The dynamics of FFA mobilization and utilization. *Prog. Biochem. Pharmacol.* **3**, 139–150.

Steiner, R. F., Roth, J., and Robbins, J. (1966). The binding of thyroxine by serum albumin as measured by fluorescence quenching. *J. Biol. Chem.* **241**, 560–567.

Stewart, J. E., and Schotz, M. C. (1974). Release of lipoprotein lipase activity from isolated fat cells. II. Effect of heparin. *J. Biol. Chem.* **249**, 904–907.

Swaney, J. B., and Klotz, I. M. (1970). Amino acid sequence adjoining the lone tryptophan of human serum albumin. A binding site of the protein. *Biochemistry* **9**, 2570–2574.

Sykes, B. D. (1970). A nuclear magnetic resonance study of the binding of acetylsalicylic acid to human serum albumin. *Biochem. Biophys. Res. Commun.* **39**, 508–515.

Tabachnick, M. (1964). Thyroxine–protein interactions. I. Binding of thyroxine to human serum albumin and modified albumins. *J. Biol. Chem.* **239**, 1242–1249.

Thorp, J. M. (1963). An experimental approach to the problem of disordered lipid metabolism. *J. Atheroscler. Res.* **3**, 351–360.

Vrána, A., and Fábry, P. (1973). Dietary carbohydrates and adipose tissue metabolism. *Prog. Biochem. Pharmacol.* **8**, 189–215.

Welch, R. M. (1973). A method for studying the interactions of drugs with bishydroxy-coumarin (dicoumarol) in dogs. *Ann. N.Y. Acad. Sci.* **226**, 259–266.

Westphal, U. (1964). Binding of steroids to proteins. *J. Am. Oil Chem. Soc.* **41**, 481–490.

Wosilait, W. D., and Soler-Argilaga, C. (1975). A theoretical analysis of the multiple binding of palmitate by bovine serum albumin: The relationship to uptake of free fatty acids by tissues. *Life Sci.* **17**, 159–166.

Wosilait, W. D., Soler-Argilaga, C., and Nagy, P. (1976). A theoretical analysis of the binding of palmitate by human serum albumin. *Biochem. Biophys. Res. Commun.* **71**, 419–426.

18

Lipids in Drug Detoxication

ADELBERT E. WADE, WILLIAM P. NORRED, and JENET
S. EVANS

I. INTRODUCTION

Many tissues of the body have the capacity to metabolize drugs and other foreign compounds. Although enzymes associated with the endoplasmic reticulum of mammalian hepatocytes are quantitatively the most important in this respect the influence of drug-metabolizing enzymes associated with tissues at other portals of entry (i.e., lungs and intestine) should not be overlooked. Alteration in the activity of these so-called microsomal enzymes affects the duration and intensity of action of such agents as drugs, hormones, and environmental contaminants. The consequences of unrecognized alterations in the function of these mixed-function oxidases range from the acquisition of unreliable data during drug testing to dangerous overdosage toxicity in man resulting from impaired metabolism of therapeutic agents (Campbell and Hayes, 1974; Conney, 1967). Purposeful manipulation of these enzymes, on the other hand, may have far reaching consequences in enhancing or preventing chemical carcinogenesis (Czygan et al., 1974; Miller and Miller, 1965; Rogers and Newberne, 1971; Wattenberg et al., 1976; Wynder, 1976, Hopkins and West, 1976), in modifying chronic medication, or in treating drug and chemically induced toxicities (Chadwick et al., 1977).

II. FUNCTION OF LIPOPROTEIN IN THE DRUG-METABOLIZING ENZYME SYSTEM

Enzymes responsible for oxidative and some reductive reactions of drugs are associated with the lipoprotein membranes of endoplasmic reticulum. When microsomes are solubilized and the components purified it may be demonstrated that three components of the endoplasmic reticulum are essential for drug metabolism: The hemochromogen, cytochrome P-450, NADPH cytochrome P-450 reductase, and lipid. This lipid accounts for about 30–40% of the dry weight of hepatic endoplasmic reticulum (Glaumann and Dallner, 1968; Siekevitz, 1963). It is well established that lipids are essential for proper function of enzymes bound to these membranes. For example, (1) Removal of the phospholipid with detergents or phospholipases or subjecting microsomes to peroxidation diminishes drug metabolizing activity (Kamataki and Kitagawa, 1973; Omura and Sato, 1964; Wills, 1971). (2) Hydrolysis of phospholipids to the corresponding α, β-diglycerides or phosphatidic acid with phospholipase C or D, or extraction with isooctane or l-butanol and acetone, alters substrate binding to cytochrome P-450 and inhibits Type I substrate metabolism (Chaplin and Mannering, 1970; Eling and DiAugustine, 1971; Leibman and Estabrook, 1971; Vore et al., 1974a,b). (3) Phosphatidylcholine restores metabolic activity to a solubilized cytochrome P-450-NADPH cytochrome P-450 reductase system and also restores activity to microsomes treated with phospholipases or extracted with isoctane or 1-butanol and acetone (Coon *et al.*, 1971; Lu *et al.*, 1969a; Strobel *et al.*, 1970; Vore *et al.*, 1974a). (4) During enzyme induction with phenobarbital, phospholipid, cholesterol, and triglyceride concentrations of microsomes increase as proteins increase (Cooper and Feuer, 1972); Glaumann and Dallner, 1968; Infante *et al.*, 1971; Orrenius *et al.*, 1965, 1969; Young *et al.*, 1971). (5) Phenobarbital or 3-methylcholanthrene induction increases the incorporation of linoleate into phospholipid at almost the exact time that the concentration of other components of the drug hydroxylation system increase (Davison and Wills, 1974). (6) The sex differences in phospholipid content of rat hepatic microsomes may be related to their sex differences in drug-metabolizing activity, since the elevated phospholipid fractions seen in males are the same ones that increase during induction of drug-metabolizing enzymes (Belina *et al.*, 1975). (7) Phospholipid appears to be essential for the NADPH-dependent reduction of cytochrome P-450 since electron transfer from NADPH to cytochrome P-450 occurs at a rate sufficient to support substrate hydroxylation only when phosphatidylcholine is present (Coon *et al.*, 1971; Strobel *et al.*, 1970).

Addition of unsaturated fatty acids to an incubation mixture of substrate with microsomal enzymes inhibits metabolism of the drug substrate (DiAugustine and Fouts, 1969). Thus it appears that fatty acids must be incorporated into phospholipids of the membrane to be functional. In solubilized preparations of cytochrome P-450 and NADPH cytochrome P-450 reductase, the phospholipid phosphatidylcholine appears to form a dissociable complex with the cytochrome and its reductase. Whether this is responsible for the enhanced electron transfer is unknown; more information is needed about the nature of this complexation and whether similar complexations occur *in vivo*.

III. EFFECT OF DIETARY LIPID ON COMPOSITION OF HEPATIC ENDOPLASMIC RETICULUM

Phosphatidylcholine, a phospholipid essential for optimal drug-metabolizing enzyme activity appears to be synthesized by the methylation of phosphatidylethanolamine by the action of S-adenosylmethionine-dependent methyltransferase in smooth endoplasmic reticulum (Natori, 1963) rather than by direct incorporation of choline. The long-chain fatty acids esterified to the alpha (No. 1) carbon of glycerol is usually saturated whereas an unsaturated fatty acid is usually attached to the beta (No. 2) carbon.

Increasing amounts of dietary corn oil (0,3%, 10%) produced decreasing concentrations of palmitoleic (16:1) and oleic (18:1) acids of phospholipids of washed hepatic microsomes whereas linoleic (18:2) and arachidonic (20:4) acid contents were increased. Measurable quantities of eicosatrienoic acid (20:3) were found in microsomes from rats fed the fat-free diet but not in microsomes recovered from rats fed diets containing corn oil. Docosapentaenoic acid (22:5) was highest in microsomes from rats fed the diet containing 3% corn oil (Norred and Wade, 1972).

Others (Mohrhauer and Holman, 1963; Century, 1973; Kaschnitz, 1970; Trewhella and Collins, 1973; Agradi *et al.*, 1975) have reported similar changes in fatty acid composition of microsomes or whole liver resulting from feeding fat-free diets or diets containing saturated or unsaturated fatty acids. An interesting observation was that eicosatrienoic acid appeared to replace arachidonic acid in the synthesis of phosphatidylcholine in rats fed fat-free or saturated fat diets. For example, concentration of arachidonoyl phosphatidylcholine dropped from a normal of 49.3% to 1.7% in fat-deficient rats and eicosatrienoyl phosphatidylcholine increased from undetectable levels in the normal rat to 39.9% in the deficient rat (Trewhella and Collins, 1973). In our experience (Norred and Wade, 1972) the total eicosatrienoic plus arachidonic acids of phospholipids of microsomes from animals fed fat-free diet is equal to the arachidonic acid level in those fed diets containing 3% corn oil. This appears to be true also when comparing those fatty acids in microsomes from rats fed saturated fat or various unsaturated fats (Agradi *et al.*, 1975). Dietary fats that are not normally found in liver microsomes apparently do not accumulate in lipids of the endoplasmic reticulum: Erucic acid (22:1) does not accumulate in liver microsomes of animals fed a diet rich in erucate from rapeseed oil (Agradi *et al.*, 1975).

IV. ROLE OF DIETARY LIPID IN HEPATIC MICROSOMAL DRUG METABOLISM

A. Effect of Saturated Fatty Acids on Rate of Drug Metabolism

Caster *et al.* (1970a) fed varying concentrations of eight saturated fatty acids (4:0 to 18:0) to male rats. All diets contained 1.8% safflower oil to provide optimal levels of essential fatty acids. The major effect upon drug-metabolizing activity of rat liver was associated with the absolute amount of fat in the diet and was independent of chain length. An increase in saturated fatty acid content of the diet from 15% to 35% doubled the rate of aniline hydroxylase while producing no effect on hexobarbital oxidase. Century (1969) reported that rats fed 7% beef fat metabolized hexobarbital and aminopyrine more slowly than rats fed unsaturated fatty acids. Agradi *et al.* (1975) reported that rats fed a diet containing 10% saturated fat to age 3 or 4 months exhibited decreased concentration of hepatic cytochrome *P*-450, and decreased activities of benzpyrene hydroxylase but not aniline hydroxylase when compared to rats fed diets containing various unsaturated fats. Marshall and McLean (1971a) reported that the concentration of cytochrome *P*-450 achieved following induction with phenobarbital is determined by the nature of the dietary fat with the greatest level of induction occurring in rats fed the more highly unsaturated fat. Norred and Wade (1973) reported that a diet containing 3% coconut oil (largely saturated fatty acids) failed to support phenobarbital induction of hexobarbital oxidase or aniline hydroxylase to the extent afforded by a diet containing corn oil. Hietanen *et al.* (1975) reported that rats fed cocoa butter or cocoa butter plus cholesterol in concentrations such that total fat was 24–34% w/w resulted in hepatic microsomes having only 10% of the activity of those recovered from rats fed a standard diet or a diet containing an equivalent concentration of cholesterol. On the other hand, neither cocoa butter nor olive oil affected the activity of *p*-nitroanisole *O*-demethylase whereas feeding high levels of cholesterol enhanced this activity about twofold.

The effects of dietary saturated fat on aniline metabolism reported by Caster *et al.* (1970a) may have been secondary to the supply or availability of NADPH or other cofactors. Thus it appears from this and other work that treatments which promote fatty acid synthesis (carbohydrate feeding) increases utilization of NADPH or other cofactors for this in preference to the drug-metabolizing function. On the other hand, those factors depressing fatty acid synthesis (fat ingestion, starvation) may free more NADPH for utilization in drug-catabolizing reactions. The reason all substrates are not affected by the same concentration of fat to the same degree may reflect differing quantitative requirements for NADPH since various substrates are metabolized at vastly different maximal rates. (e.g., The apparent V_{max} for aniline hydroxylase in male rat liver microsomes is about 20–50 nmoles/mg protein. Ethylmorphine demethylase V_{max} is about 300–400 nmole/mg protein/hour). On the other hand, certain fats may accumulate in liver or other tissues and act as competitive inhibitors of selective drug-metabolizing enzymes (e.g., unsaturated fatty acids added to incubation mixtures inhibited metabolism of Type I substrates without affecting Type II substrate metabolism).

B. Effect of Polyunsaturated and Essential Fatty Acids on Rate of Drug Metabolism

Dietary or intubated polyunsaturated or essential fatty acids appear to induce greater mixed-function oxidase (MFO) activity than observed in microsomes recovered from rats fed fat-free diets or diets containing saturated fats. Male rats fed diets containing 3 or 10% corn oil as a source of linoleate for 21 days have greater hepatic MFO activity associated with aniline, heptachlor, or hexobarbital metabolism than those fed a fat-free diet. Using a single saturating substrate concentration in incubation mixtures containing 9000 g supernatant of male rat liver homogenates, aniline hydroxylation was increased an average of 31%, hexobarbital oxidation was increased an average of 80% and heptachlor epoxidase was increased 160% in male rats fed 3% corn oil over animals fed the fat-free diet (Caster et al., 1968; Norred and Wade, 1972; Wade et al., 1969). A diet containing 10% corn oil resulted in a 39% increase of aniline hydroxylase, 28% increase in hexobarbital oxidase, and 148% increase in heptachlor epoxidase activity (Table I). In experiments where dietary intake of corn oil furnished zero, 0.27, 0.54, 1.3, 3.8 and 11.7% of calories, half maximal changes in metabolism of aniline occurred at about 0.1% of calories and for hexobarbital and ethylmorphine, it occurred in male rats receiving corn oil at 1–1.5% of calories (Caster et al., 1970b).

In other experiments arachidonate in doses of 0.3–100 μl per day for 21 days was administered to male rats by oral intubation. Maximum rates of aniline hydroxylation and hexobarbital oxidation were achieved by liver 9000 g supernatant fractions from rats fed 1.0 and 10 μl (0.8 or 8 mg) of arachidonate per day (Wade et al., 1972). Although direct comparison of these dietary effects may not be valid, these data suggest that approximately 32 mg corn oil ingested each day providing maximal aniline metabolism is equivalent to 0.8 mg arachidonate, and 420 mg corn oil per day is equivalent to 8 mg arachidonate in providing maximum hexobarbital oxidation. Menhaden oil appeared to support aniline and hexobarbital metabolic reactions at doses of 0.001 μl per day at levels significantly higher than those from rats fed a fat-free diet

TABLE I

Effect of Corn Oil Consumption on Drug Metabolism by 9000 g Supernatant Fraction of Male Rat Liver Homogenates

Diet	Aniline hydroxylase[a]	Hexobarbital oxidase[a]	Heptachlor epoxidase[a]
Fat-free	0.88 ± 0.08[b]	3.44 ± 0.54[b]	2.45 ± 0.36
3% Corn oil	1.15 ± 0.07[b]	6.19 ± 0.56[b]	6.37 ± 0.50
10% Corn oil	1.22 ± 0.13	4.40 ± 0.35	6.07 ± 0.3

[a] μmole/gm liver/hours.
[b] Mean of three experiments.

(Wade *et al.*, 1972). Marshall and McLean (1971b) reported that aniline hydroxylation was approximately 30% higher in rats fed 10 days on diets containing 15% herring oil than in rats fed fat-free diet. Although Century (1969, 1973) could detect no change in hexobarbital or aminopyrine metabolism by 9000 *g* supernatant of rat liver homogenates as a result of increasing concentrations of corn oil in the diet from 0.5 to 10%, menhaden oil incorporated in the diet (7%) enhanced hexobarbital metabolism approximately 40% and aminopyrine about 30% when compared to rats fed beef fat. Patel and Pawar (1972) reported an increase in ethylmorphine and aniline metabolism by 9000 *g* supernatant fractions of liver homogenate from rats fed a synthetic diet containing 6% groundnut oil ad libitum for 6 weeks compared to rats fed fat-free diet. Béraud *et al.* (1975) reported that diets containing 30% lipid resulted in microsomal enzyme aniline hydroxylase, aminopyrene demethylase, *p*-nitroanisole demethylase, and *N*-methylaniline demethylase activities 1.5–1.8 times greater than those from rats fed 1% lipid containing diets with no change in cytochrome *P*-450 content. Kaschnitz (1970) reported a decrease in aniline hydroxylation in microsomes from rats fed fat-free diet for 7 weeks. Rats fed saturated fat (10% w/w) until 3–4 months of age yielded microsomes having 33–53% as much benzpyrene hydroxylase activity as microsomes from rats fed 10% rapeseed oil, olive oil or safflower oil (Agradi *et al.*, 1975). However only the diet containing 10% safflower oil enhanced aniline hydroxylase activity. The apparent discrepancy between this finding and those from our laboratory may lie in the assay systems used since the aniline hydroxylase activity reported by Agradi *et al.* (1975) is about one-tenth that reported by us.

We attempted to evaluate the mixed-function oxidase system by measuring the apparent kinetics of substrate metabolism by washed hepatic microsomes from rat liver (Norred and Wade, 1972) (Tables II and III). In these experiments the apparent V_{max} for aniline hydroxylase, hexobarbital oxidase, and ethylmorphine demethylase in male rats were enhanced 56%, 53%, and 47% respectively by diets containing 3% corn oil. Male rats ingesting diet containing 10% corn oil yielded microsomes having V_{max} 8, 118 and 45% greater for aniline, hexobarbital, and ethylmorphine than those ingesting the fat-free diet (Norred and Wade, 1972). Thus a diet containing 3% corn oil may afford maximal drug-metabolizing activity for aniline and ethylmorphine, whereas hexobarbital oxidase may require up to or more than 10% corn oil for maximal activity.

In the female rat V_{max} for aniline hydroxylation was unchanged by diet containing 3% corn oil but increased 40% by the diet containing

TABLE II
Effect of Corn Oil Consumption on the Apparent Kinetics of Drug Metabolism by Hepatic Microsomes from Male Rats

Diets	Substrate	V_{max} (nmoles/mg protein/hour)	K_m(mM)
Fat-free	Aniline	57.3 ± 4.6[a]	0.065 ± 0.014[a]
	Hexobarbital	386.1 ± 47.0[b]	0.188 ± 0.058[b]
	Ethylmorphine	400.7 ± 28.6[c]	0.290 ± 0.126[c]
3% Corn oil	Aniline	89.4 ± 6.7[a]	0.101 ± 0.018[a]
	Hexobarbital	591.4 ± 60.6[b]	0.265 ± 0.087[b]
	Ethylmorphine	588.4 ± 21.9[c]	0.284 ± 0.054[c]

[a] Mean of six experiments.
[b] Mean of four experiments.
[c] Mean of two experiments.

10% corn oil (Table III). The apparent V_{max} for hexobarbital oxidation was increased twofold by both corn oil containing diets. Feeding female rats diet containing 3 and 10% corn oil enhanced ethylmorphine demethylase 50–60%.

The apparent K_m's for aniline, hexobarbital, or ethylmorphine were statistically similar in male and female rats regardless of whether the diet

TABLE III
Effect of Corn Oil Consumption on Apparent Kinetics of Drug Metabolism by Hepatic Microsomes from Female Rats

Diet	Substrate	V_{max} (nmoles/mg protein/hour)	K_m(mM)
Fat-free	Aniline[a]	21.2 ± 0.8[c]	0.080 ± 0.009
	Hexobarbital	50.1 ± 13.7[b]	0.064 ± 0.033
	Ethylmorphine	53.3 ± 6.8[b,c]	1.132 ± 0.297
3% Corn oil	Aniline[a]	24.3 ± 1.3	0.082 ± 0.087
	Hexobarbital	100.2 ± 15.3	0.130 ± 0.040
	Ethylmorphine	81.0 ± 3.6	0.995 ± 0.046
10% Corn oil	Aniline[a]	28.9 ± 2.5	0.103 ± 0.063
	Hexobarbital	93.9 ± 14.8	0.093 ± 0.035
	Ethylmorphine	86.7 ± 5.5	0.956 ± 0.147

[a] Mean of four experiments.
[b] Significantly different from rats fed 3% corn oil.
[c] Significantly different from rats fed 10% corn oil.

was fat-free or supplemented with 3% corn oil. A diet containing 10% corn oil significantly elevated the K_m for hexobarbital in male rats (Norred and Wade, 1972).

The evidence derived from these studies indicates that increases in microsomal enzyme activity induced by dietary lipid ingestion were due primarily to increases in enzyme concentration. The lack of changes in apparent K_m for these substrates suggest that dietary corn oil does not induce qualitative differences in the components of this drug-metabolizing enzyme system.

In vitro metabolic changes induced by dietary lipid do not always correlate with changes in in vivo activity. The scanty in vivo data (dealing primarily with hexobarbital sleeping time) is conflicting, with investigators reporting no alterations to slight increases in hexobarbital sleep time exhibited by rats fed various levels of fat (Caster et al., 1970b; Century, 1973; Kaschnitz, 1970). Shakman (1974) implied that the toxicity of the chlorinated hydrocarbon, dieldrin, is increased in states of essential fatty acid deficiency but correlations with drug-metabolizing activity was lacking. We determined hexobarbital sleeping times in male and female rats fed fat-free diet or diet supplemented with 3% corn oil. Narcosis from the intraperitoneal injection of hexobarbital sodium (100 mg/kg body weight) was the same in female rats fed fat-free diet or diet supplemented with 3% corn oil (Table IV). In male rats fed fat-free diet, hexobarbital-induced narcosis was 52% longer than in rats fed the diet supplemented with 3% corn oil. In a time course study we found that no change in sleep time of male rats was evident after feeding fat-free or corn oil supplemented diet for 10 days but that a significant reduction in sleep time was evident in those fed 3% corn oil diet for 21 days (W. P. Norred and A. E. Wade, unpublished results). In a similar experiment using Wistar strain mice we found no significant change in sleep time after 5 days on diet but a significant reduction was evident in male mice fed 3% corn oil diet for 10, 15, 20 or 25 days (Fig. 1).

TABLE IV
Effect of Corn Oil Consumption on Hexobarbital Sleeping Time

Diet	Number	Male (minutes)	Number	Female (minutes)
Fat-free	18	35.2 ± 2.9[a]	17	97.9 ± 4.8
3% Corn oil	15	23.1 ± 1.8	17	89.1 ± 3.8

[a] Significantly different from rats fed 3% corn oil ($p < 0.05$).

HEXOBARBITAL SLEEPING TIME

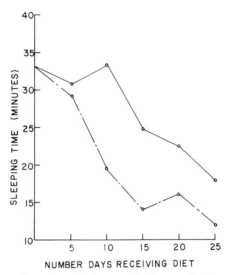

Fig. 1. The effect of number of days on fat-free or lipid supplemented diet on hexobarbital sleeping time in mice. (————), 0% corn oil; (– – –), 3% corn oil.

V. ROLE OF DIETARY LIPID ON COMPONENT ENZYMES OF DRUG-METABOLIZING SYSTEM

A. Quantity and Quality of Cytochrome P-450

Feeding a synthetic fat-free diet to male and female rats results in significant reduction in cytochrome P-450 (Norred and Wade, 1972). Male rats fed a diet containing 3% corn oil had cytochrome P-450 levels approximately 38% higher than those fed the same diet but devoid of corn oil. A diet with 10% corn oil fed to male rats yielded microsomes having 42% more cytochrome P-450. In female rats fed 3 and 10% corn oil diet, the cytochrome P-450 concentration of liver microsomes was respectively 57 and 70% higher than that of rats fed the fat-free diet (Table V).

Kaschnitz (1970) found only 73% as much cytochrome P-450 in liver microsomes of rats fed hydrogenated coconut oil as their sole fat source compared to rats fed a standard laboratory chow while Agradi *et al.* (1975) reported 38–47% as much P-450 in microsomes of rats fed a diet containing 10% saturated fat compared to those fed diet containing 10% lipids with unsaturation indexes of 93 to 147. Oral administration of

TABLE V

Effect of Corn Oil Consumption on Cytochrome P-450 Content and NADPH Cytochrome c Reductase Activity of Hepatic Microsomes

Diet	Sex	Cytochrome P-450[a]	NADPH cytochrome c reductase[b]
Fat-free	M	0.589 ± 0.047[c]	111.6 ± 9.4
	F	0.371 ± 0.031[d]	101.6 ± 8.5[e]
3% Corn oil	M	0.810 ± 0.050[c]	110.6 ± 6.3
	F	0.581 ± 0.053[d]	125.4 ± 4.1[e]
10% Corn oil	M	0.836 ± 0.067	—
	F	0.632 ± 0.063[d]	146.3 ± 13.9[e]

[a] nmoles/mg microsomal protein.
[b] nmoles cytochrome c reduced/mg protein/minute.
[c] Mean of six experiments.
[d] Mean of three experiments.
[e] Mean of two experiments.

arachidonic acid ($0.3-100 \mu$l/day) or menhaden oil ($0.001-100.0 \mu$l/day) to male rats for 21 days did not significantly alter cytochrome P-450 content (Wade *et al.*, 1972).

B. Activity of NADPH-Cytochrome c Reductase and Glucose-6-Phosphate Dehydrogenase

The activity of NADPH cytochrome c reductase was significantly elevated in female rats fed diets containing 3% or 10% corn oil for 21 days (Table V). However this enzyme was not significantly altered by dietary corn oil or by arachidonate or menhaden oil administration to male rats (Wade *et al.*, 1972). Dietary lipid appears to play only a minor role in the overall synthesis or activity of this enzyme. Since 80–90% of NADPH cytochrome c reductase activity remained in microsomes following extensive removal of neutral fat, phospholipid, and cholesterol by 1-butanol-acetone extraction, this finding was not unexpected (Vore *et al.*, 1974a).

Glucose-6-phosphate dehydrogenase activity in hepatic soluble fraction is markedly reduced in rats fed high levels of linseed oil, menhaden oil, or arachidonate (Century, 1972, 1973; Wade *et al.*, 1972) and moderately reduced in male rats fed 3% corn oil (Wade *et al.*, 1972). Since adequate amounts of glucose-6-phosphate dehydrogenase activity are found even in starved or thiamine-deficient rats this reduction in activity would not be expected to influence drug-metabolizing activity.

VI. EFFECT OF DIETARY LIPID ON SUBSTRATE INTERACTION WITH CYTOCHROME P-450

The formation of a complex between substrate and the oxidized form of cytochrome P-450 is an obligatory step in the oxidation of drugs and other xenobiotics (Orrenius et al., 1972). Various drugs added to oxidized washed microsomes or purified preparations of cytochrome P-450 produce characteristic absorbance changes in difference spectrum which probably reflects the interaction of the drug with the terminal oxidase. Most drugs evaluated produce one of only three types of absorbance changes in the visible spectrum (Type I, II, and modified Type II) and the magnitude of this change is related to the concentration of cytochrome P-450. Upon addition of increasing concentrations of substrate to cytochrome P-450, a series of absorbance curves are obtained from which an apparent dissociation constant (K_s) may be calculated. Pretreatment of animals with many drugs, hormones, or environmental toxicants may selectively increase the concentration of one or more of the several forms of cytochrome P-450 thought to exist in hepatic endoplasmic reticulum. These alterations which affect the overall response of the animal to administered drugs or xenobiotics, may be detected by measuring the spectral changes induced by the addition of several ligands to the cytochrome P-450 preparation.

The apparent spectral dissociation constant (K_s) for hexobarbital and aniline binding to microsomes from male and female rats was unaltered by the addition of corn oil to the diet. This provides strong evidence that the binding sites on the enzyme or the form of cytochrome P-450 present were not qualitatively changed by these diets. Maximal spectral absorbance changes (A_{max}) were observed in microsomes prepared from rats fed diets containing 3% corn oil. When calculated on the basis of cytochrome P-450 content, however, these changes in absorbance were minimized. Thus it appears from these data and from the unchanged K_m for substrate metabolism that binding of substrate to microsomal cytochrome P-450 is only minimally affected by diets which alter membrane lipid composition, the quantity of cytochrome P-450 and/or the rate of drug metabolism (Norred and Wade, 1972).

Two accepted methods for detecting qualitative alterations in cytochrome P-450 induced by diet or drugs are the determination of the extinction coefficient for the cytochrome or the determination of difference absorbance spectra using ethylisocyanide as the ligand. Extinction coefficients of cytochrome P-450 were unchanged by the level of fat in the diet.

Ethylisocyanide, when added to dithionite reduced microsomes, produces a characteristic absorption spectrum with absorbance peaks occurring at 430 and 455 nm. The relative heights of these absorbance peaks is indicative of the type of cytochrome P-450 which exists in the microsomes (Sladek and Mannering, 1966). Induction with the hydrocarbon 3-methylcholanthrene (3-MC) alters the relative peak heights of this absorption spectrum as the concentration of a species of cytochrome P-450 termed cytochrome P_1-450 (P-448) increases.

The ethylisocyanide difference spectra of microsomes from male or female rats fed diet containing 3 or 10% corn oil were not consistently altered, again indicating that significant qualitative changes in cytochrome P-450 had not occurred. It appears that several species of cytochrome P-450 exist in microsomes of control animals (Jefcoate et al., 1970) and only two forms have been examined in these dietary studies. Whether other species of P-450 are affected by dietary fat awaits further study.

VII. EFFECT OF DIETARY LIPID ON INTESTINAL MIXED-FUNCTION OXIDASE ACTIVITY

Hietanen et al. (1975) reported that intestinal benzpyrene hydroxylase activity was highest in rats fed standard diet and that rats fed diets containing high levels of cholesterol plus cocoa butter, olive oil, or olive oil plus cholesterol exhibited benzpyrene hydroxylase activities 30–80% of this. Wattenberg (1972) reported finding little or no benzpyrene hydroxylase activity in rats fed fat-free or fat-supplemented diets and deduced that intestinal aryl hydrocarbon hydroxylase (AHH) activity, when present, was the result of induction by compounds in the diet. He further demonstrated that these inducers were found in various vegetable compounds of commercial diets being particularly high in those from the Brassecacaea family.

VIII. EFFECT OF DIETARY LIPID ON THE INDUCTION OF HEPATIC DRUG-METABOLIZING ENZYMES

A. Phenobarbital Induction

Marshall and McLean (1971b) reported that polyunsaturated fatty acids in the diet, but not saturated fatty acids, permit maximum induction of cytochrome P-450 by drugs. The increase in cytochrome P-450 in response to phenobarbital induction in rats fed coconut oil, olive oil, or fat-free diet was only half that obtained in rats fed linoleic acid or herring oil. Aniline hydroxylase was induced 12% more in rats fed 15% herring oil diet than in rats fed fat-free diet.

Century (1969, 1973) reported that phenobarbital induction of hexobarbital oxidase and aminopyrine demethylase was more pronounced in rats provided a diet with 7% corn oil, 7% linseed oil, or 7% menhaden oil than in those fed beef fat. Increased hexobarbital metabolism was reflected in shorter hexobarbital sleep times. Low levels of corn oil (0.3–0.8%) did not significantly alter induction patterns in microsomes compared with rats fed beef fat. In mice, however, enhancement of phenobarbital induction was evident only with diets containing 7% menhaden oil.

In our experiments, feeding fat-free or corn oil-supplemented diets did not significantly alter food consumption or weight gains in male or female Sprague Dawley rats over the 3 week feeding period (Table VI). The injection of phenobarbital (80 mg/ kg body weight/ day) during the last 4 days of these experiments did not significantly alter food consumption or weight gain; however, the intraperitoneal injection of 3-methylcholanthrene (20 mg/kg body weight/ day) generally reduced food consumption.

Concentrations of cytochrome P-450 per mg microsomal protein were 26 and 29% higher in female rats fed 3 or 10% corn oil following phenobarbital induction and 64% higher ($p < 0.05$) in males fed 3% corn oil diet (Tables VII and VIII). These increases in concentration were accompanied by increased liver weight (as proportion of body weight)and/or increased microsomal protein content, thus when calculated on the basis of body weight, cytochrome P-450 was increased 110% in males fed 3% corn oil diet and 67 and 29% in females fed 3 and 10% corn oil diet.

The apparent V_{max} for aniline hydroxylase was induced to higher levels by phenobarbital in male and female rats fed corn oil diets than in those fed the fat-free diet. However K_m was altered significantly only in females fed the diet containing 3% corn oil. V_{max} for ethylmorphine demethylation in females was increased by the administration of phenobarbital equally in fat-free and corn oil-fed rats with K_m for ethylmorphine altered only by 3% corn oil (Tables IX and X). The administration of phenobarbital during the last 4 days of the feeding experiment increased the apparent V_{max} for hexobarbital oxidase 35 and 52% more in male rats fed 3% corn oil than in their controls fed fat-free diet (Tables IX and XI). Feeding the same diet supplemented with 3% coconut oil,

TABLE VI

Accumulative Weight Gain in Grams of Female and Male Rats Fed Fat-Free Diet and Diet Supplemented with 3% Corn Oil Using 3-Methylcholanthrene as Inducer 4 Days before Decapitation

Diet	Sex	Control			3-Methylcholanthrene		
		Week-1	Week-2	Week-3	Week-1	Week-2	Week-3
Fat-free	F	22.1 ± 1.0^a	51.3 ± 1.5	70.5 ± 1.9	22.1 ± 2.0	51.7 ± 2.8	69.1 ± 2.8
3% Corn oil	F	26.6 ± 1.4	54.9 ± 2.5	76.2 ± 2.7	26.9 ± 0.9	55.8 ± 2.8	71.4 ± 3.5
Fat-free	M	34.7 ± 1.4	68.3 ± 3.8	103.0 ± 5.6	34.3 ± 1.6	70.7 ± 3.0	102.3 ± 3.9
3% Corn oil	M	36.3 ± 2.5	76.3 ± 4.0	115.7 ± 4.9	38.1 ± 1.2	77.5 ± 2.5	108.5 ± 3.5

[a] Significantly different from rats fed 3% corn oil diet ($p < 0.05$).

TABLE VII
Effect of Corn Oil Consumption and Phenobarbital Pretreatment of Female Rats on Parameters of Microsomal Drug-Metabolizing System

Diet	Pretreatment	Liver wt. (gm/100 gm body wt.)	Microsomal protein (mg/gm liver)	Cytochrome P-450 (nmole/mg)	NADPH Cytochrome c reductase (nmole reduced/mg protein/minute)
Fat-free	Control	4.74 ± 0.09	22.4 ± 0.9	0.271 ± 0.015[b,c]	105.9
	Phenobarbital	5.72 ± 0.19[a]	24.6 ± 1.1[b]	0.659 ± 0.036[a]	173.3
3% Corn oil	Control	4.67 ± 0.19	24.1 ± 1.0	0.438 ± 0.049	131.4
	Phenobarbital	5.88 ± 0.17[a]	31.0 ± 0.5[a,c]	0.829 ± 0.045[a]	187.7
10% Corn oil	Control	4.50 ± 0.20	22.8 ± 1.8	0.423 ± 0.026	112.2
	Phenobarbital	5.35 ± 0.26[a]	26.1 ± 2.1	0.850 ± 0.075[a]	178.1

[a] Significantly different from control rats fed same diet.
[b] Significantly different from rats fed 3% corn oil given the same pretreatment.
[c] Significantly different from rats fed 10% corn oil given the same pretreatment.

TABLE VIII

Effect of Corn Oil Consumption and Phenobarbital Pretreatment on Some Hepatic Microsomal Parameters of Male Rats

Diet	Pretreatment	Liver wt. (gm/ 100 gm body wt.)	Microsomal protein (mg/gm liver)	Cytochrome P-450 (nmole/mg)	Ethylisocyanide difference spectra (Δ A455nm/Δ A430nm)
Fat-free	Control	5.10 ± 0.13	19.3 ± 1.6	0.985 ± 0.124	0.858 ± 0.087
	Phenobarbital	5.93 ± 0.09[a,b]	25.4 ± 2.3[a]	1.618 ± 0.090[a,b]	1.213 ± 0.043[a,b]
3% Corn oil	Control	5.02 ± 0.13	21.2 ± 1.8	1.241 ± 0.126	0.897 ± 0.032
	Phenobarbital	6.72 ± 0.09[a]	28.6 ± 1.1[a]	2.660 ± 0.153[a]	1.467 ± 0.056[a]

[a] Significantly different from control rats fed same diet.
[b] Significantly different from rats fed 3% corn oil given same pretreatment.

TABLE IX
Effect of Dietary Lipid Consumption and Phenobarbital Pretreatment on Kinetics of Substrate Metabolism in Male Rats

Diet	Pretreatment	Hexobarbital		Aniline	
		V_{max} (nmoles met./mg protein/hour)	K_m (mM)	V_{max} (nmoles met./mg protein/hour)	K_m (mM)
Fat-free	Control	331.2 ± 43.1	0.270 ± 0.079	40.05 ± 5.1[b]	0.014 ± 0.008
	Phenobarbital	621.2 ± 34.9[a]	0.222 ± 0.035	75.5 ± 11.2[a,b]	0.049 ± 0.020
3% Corn oil	Control	386.2 ± 73.0	0.211 ± 0.118	85.6 ± 11.5	0.051 ± 0.018
	Phenobarbital	839.4 ± 90.2[a]	0.248 ± 0.072	160.8 ± 14.3[a]	0.085 ± 0.019

[a] Significantly different from control rats fed same diet.
[b] Significantly different from rats fed 3% corn oil given same pretreatment.

TABLE X

Effect of Dietary Lipid Consumption and Phenobarbital Pretreatment on Kinetics[a] of Substrate Metabolism in Female Rats

Diet	Pretreatment	Ethylmorphine		Aniline	
		V_{max} (nmoles met./mg protein/hour)	K_m (mM)	V_{max} (nmoles met./mg protein/hour)	K_m (mM)
Fat-free	Control	53.3 ± 6.8[c,d]	1.132 ± 0.297	8.6 ± 0.2[c,d]	0.045 ± 0.004[c]
	Phenobarbital	337.3 ± 11.9[b]	0.744 ± 0.074	25.2 ± 2.7[b,c,d]	0.013 ± 0.014[c]
3% Corn oil	Control	81.0 ± 3.6	0.955 ± 0.046	16.7 ± 0.7	0.008 ± 0.009[d]
	Phenobarbital	333.4 ± 6.6[b]	0.823 ± 0.042[b]	34.3 ± 1.9[b]	0.065 ± 0.017[b]
10% Corn oil	Control	86.7 ± 5.5	0.956 ± 0.147	16.9 ± 0.9	0.039 ± 0.010[c]
	Phenobarbital	358.5 ± 20.2[b]	0.971 ± 0.135	42.2 ± 3.5[b]	0.067 ± 0.023

[a] Apparent kinetics derived from 6 substrate concentrations spanning the K_m.

[b] Significantly different from control rats fed same diet.

[c] Significantly different from rats fed 3% corn oil given same pretreatment.

[d] Significantly different from rats fed 10% corn oil given same pretreatment.

TABLE XI
Effect of Dietary Lipid Consumption on Kinetics of Substrate Metabolism by Hepatic Microsome from Phenobarbital Pretreated Male Rats

Diet	Hexobarbital		Aniline	
	V_{max} (nmoles met./mg protein/hour)	K_m (mM)	V_{max} (nmoles met./mg protein/hour)	K_m (mM)
Fat-free	563.2 ± 73.9	0.101 ± 0.063	117.1 ± 13.1	0.089 ± 0.023
3% Coconut oil	629.1 ± 57.2	0.122 ± 0.047	154.1 ± 16.0	0.100 ± 0.023
3% Corn oil	857.0 ± 29.9[a]	0.193 ± 0.020	205.2 ± 17.7[a]	0.172 ± 0.030

[a] Significantly different from rats fed fat-free diet.

which is high in saturated fat, was no more effective than fat-free diet in allowing full expression of phenobarbital induction (Table XI).

Microsomal enzyme induction by phenobarbital also increased the ratio of the peak heights of the ethylisocyanide binding spectrum in male rats fed the synthetic diets in a manner similar to that induced by the polycyclic hydrocarbon, 3-methylcholanthrene (Table VIII). The increase in the ratio was greater in corn oil-fed rats than in those fed fat-free diet. Induction with phenobarbital of rats fed lab chow does not alter the ratio of ethylisocyanide absorption peaks, while induction with 3-methylcholanthrene increases the magnitude of absorbance at 455 nm relative to that at 430 nm (Sladek and Mannering, 1966). It is conceivable that the synthetic diet produces a particular pattern of cytochrome P-450 species and that phenobarbital administration alters this pattern. Davison and Wills (1974) reported that the administration of phenobarbital increased the proportion of linoleic acid in phosphatidylcholine and phosphatidylethanolamine while decreasing the proportion of oleic, arachidonic, and docosahexaenoic acids. The finding that phenobarbital increases the ethylisocyanide absorbance ratio more in rats fed the corn oil diet than in rats fed a fat-free diet indicates a role of essential fatty acid in determining the reactivity of various cytochrome P-450 species to chemical inducers.

B. 3-Methylcholanthrene (3-MC) Induction

The injection of 3-MC (20 mg/kg, ip for 4 days) increased microsomal cytochrome P-450 approximately twofold in male rats fed fat-free or 3% corn oil diet. NADPH cytochrome c reductase activity (which is the same in male rats fed corn oil or fat-free diet) is induced about 30% by 3-MC in rats fed 3% corn oil ($p < 0.05$) but is not increased significantly in those fed fat-free diets. The ratio of the ethylisocyanide difference spectrum ($\Delta A_{455nm}/\Delta A_{430\ nm}$) was increased about threefold in male and females fed the fat free and fat-supplemented diets (Tables XII and XIII).

In female rats, 3-MC increased cytochrome P-450 threefold in animals fed fat-free diet and about twofold in those fed 3% or 10% corn oil diets. NADPH cytochrome c reductase was increased 20 and 40% respectively in rats fed 3 or 10% corn oil diet; however, injection of 3-MC decreased cytochrome c reductase levels in those fed 10% corn oil diet. Although the concentration of cytochrome P-450 was lower in control rats fed the fat-free diet than in those fed 3 or 10% corn oil diet, following induction with 3-MC, hepatic microsomal cytochrome P-450 concentrations were 35% greater in males fed 3% corn oil ($p < 0.05$) and 19 and 41% higher in females fed 3 and 10% corn oil respectively ($p < 0.05$) (Table XIII).

The administration of 3-MC enhanced the apparent V_{max} of aniline hydroxylation (Type II) to significantly higher levels in male and female rats fed diets containing corn oil than in rats fed fat-free diet. The apparent K_m for this reaction was significantly higher in male rats fed fat-free diet than in controls or 3-MC induced male rats fed 3% corn oil. No changes in K_m were observed in females (Tables XIV and XV). Ethylmorphine demethylase and hexobarbital oxidase activities (Type I) were either unchanged or decreased by the administration of 3-MC in male and female rats with no change in K_m being observed. Since Davison and Wills (1974) found that 3-MC administration failed to increase

TABLE XII

Effect of Dietary Corn Oil Consumption and 3-Methylcholanthrene (3-MC) Pretreatment of Male Rats on Content of Cytochrome P-450[b] and NADPH Cytochrome c Reductase in Hepatic Microsomes

Diet	Pretreatment	N	NADPH cytochrome c reductase[a]	Cytochrome P-450 (nmole/mg protein)	Ethylisocyanide difference spectra ($\Delta A_{455nm}/\Delta A_{430nm}$)
Fat-free	Methocel	5	111.6 ± 9.4	0.526 ± 0.015^e	0.84 ± 0.05
	3-MC[c]	5	122.0 ± 9.5	$1.097 \pm 0.099^{d,e}$	$2.46 \pm 0.06^{d,e}$
3% Corn oil	Methocel	4	110.6 ± 6.3	0.794 ± 0.021	0.97 ± 0.02
	3-MC[c]	6	140.7 ± 4.7^d	1.480 ± 0.088^d	2.81 ± 0.08^d

[a] nmoles reduced/mg protein/minute.
[b] Cytochrome induced by 3-MC has λ max at 448 nm.
[c] 3-MC suspended in 0.5% Methocel solution.
[d] Significantly different from control rats fed same diet.
[e] Significantly different from rats fed 3% corn oil given same pretreatment.

TABLE XIII

Effect of Dietary Corn Oil Consumption and 3-Methylcholanthrene Pretreatment of Female Rats on Content of Cytochrome P-450 and NADPH Cytochrome c Reductase in Hepatic Microsomes[a]

Diet	Pretreatment[b]	N	NADPH cytochrome c reductase[c]	Cytochrome P-450 (nmole/mg protein)	Ethylisocyanide difference spectra ($\Delta A_{455nm}/\Delta A_{430nm}$)
Fat-free	Methocel	9	101.6 ± 8.5[e,f]	0.237 ± 0.023[e,f]	0.64 ± 0.04
	3-MC	11	115.2 ± 6.3	0.732 ± 0.044[d,e,f]	2.10 ± 0.16[d]
3% Corn oil	Methocel	8	125.4 ± 4.1	0.459 ± 0.028	0.70 ± 0.04
	3-MC	12	111.9 ± 4.7[d]	0.868 ± 0.036[d,f]	1.87 ± 0.21[d]
10% Corn oil	Methocel	4	146.3 ± 14.0	0.466 ± 0.020	0.72 ± 0.05
	3-MC	5	89.9 ± 14.7[d]	1.035 ± 0.057[d,e]	1.98 ± 0.12[d]

[a] Mean of two experiments.

[b] 3-MC administered on last four days of experiment (20 mg/kg, ip) suspended in methocel.

[c] nmoles reduced/mg protein/minute.

[d] Significantly different from control rats fed same diet.

[e] Significantly different from rats fed 3% corn oil given same pretreatment.

[f] Significantly different from rats fed 10% corn oil given same pretreatment.

the incorporation of linoleic acid into phosphatidylcholine, they postulated that linoleic acid in the β position of this phospholipid is necessary for the electron transfer from NADPH to cytochrome P-450 and that this is the limiting step in side chain oxidation or demethylation reactions.

The injection of 3-MC for 4 days prior to testing did not alter hexobarbital sleeping times of female rats but apparently prolonged narcosis in male rats fed 3% corn oil. On the other hand phenobarbital (80 mg/kg, ip for 4 days) reduced sleeping time of hexobarbital to 36% of control in female rats fed fat-free diet and to 20% of control in female rats fed 3% corn oil diet. Century (1973) also observed greater induction in male rats fed corn oil diet (Table XVI).

In order to explain the "permissive effect" of dietary unsaturated fatty acids on enzyme induction by phenobarbital, Marshall and McLean (1971b) proposed a mechanism whereby an endogenous factor serves as a "mediator" between inducing agents and increased content of cytochrome P-450. If normal metabolic inactivation of this endogenous factor is blocked by phenobarbital, the inductive process is initiated. Unsaturated fatty acids are suggested to enhance phenobarbital's ability to block hydroxylation of the endogenous factor and thus to enhance enzyme

TABLE XIV

Effect of Corn Oil Consumption and 3-Methylcholanthrene Pretreatment of Female Rats on Apparent Kinetics of Aniline Hydroxylase and Ethylmorphine Demethylase Activities in Hepatic Microsomes

Diet	Aniline Hydroxylase		Ethylmorphine Demethylase	
	V_{max}[a]	K_m (mM)	V_{max}[a]	K_m (mM)
Fat-free				
Control	15.8 ± 0.3[c,d]	0.036 ± 0.004	73.7 ± 4.4[d]	0.359 ± 0.072
3-MC	19.8 ± 0.5[b,c,d]	0.038 ± 0.007	63.5 ± 6.9	0.400 ± 0.136
3% Corn oil				
Control	20.4 ± 0.6	0.027 ± 0.010	88.8 ± 7.4	0.455 ± 0.114
3-MC	22.8 ± 0.6[b,d]	0.039 ± 0.007	70.4 ± 3.5	0.381 ± 0.064
10% Corn oil				
Control	19.3 ± 0.3	0.030 ± 0.003	89.5 ± 4.2	0.475 ± 0.067
3-MC	27.4 ± 0.6[b,c]	0.045 ± 0.005	69.9 ± 3.0[b]	0.421 ± 0.059

[a] nmoles metabolized/mg protein/hour.
[b] Significantly different from control rats fed same diet.
[c] Significantly different from rats fed 3% corn oil given same pretreatment.
[d] Significantly different from rats fed 10% corn oil given same pretreatment.

TABLE XV

Effect of Corn Oil Consumption on Apparent Kinetics of Drug Metabolism by Hepatic Microsomes from Male Rats Pretreated with 3-Methylcholanthrene (3-MC)

Diet	Aniline Hydroxylase		Ethylmorphine Demethylase		Hexobarbital Oxidase	
	$V_{max}{}^c$	K_m (mM)	$V_{max}{}^c$	K_m (mM)	$V_{max}{}^c$	K_m (mM)
Fat-free						
Control	24.3 ± 0.2^b	0.034 ± 0.002^b	281.6 ± 48.8	0.417 ± 0.241	280.6 ± 17.3	0.198 ± 0.035
3-MC	$29.8 \pm 0.3^{a,b}$	0.028 ± 0.002	481.7 ± 170.0	1.469 ± 0.966	247.4 ± 37.0^b	0.092 ± 0.036
3% Corn oil						
Control	32.5 ± 0.4	0.022 ± 0.002	360.7 ± 29.6	0.334 ± 0.092	450.3 ± 83.3	0.329 ± 0.149
3-MC	39.8 ± 0.5^a	0.021 ± 0.002	272.9 ± 11.3^a	0.240 ± 0.039	462.6 ± 79.8	0.289 ± 0.128

[a] Significantly different from control rats fed same diet.

[b] Significantly different from rats fed 3% corn oil given same pretreatment.

[c] nmoles metabolized/mg protein/hour.

TABLE XVI

Effect of Corn Oil Consumption and 3-Methylcholanthrene or Phenobarbital Induction on Hexobarbital Sleeping Time

Diet	Pretreatment	N	Male (minutes)	N	Female (minutes)
Fat-free	Control	18	35.2 ± 2.9^c	9	94.7 ± 9.8
	3-MC	8	37.1 ± 4.3	8	100.2 ± 8.7
	Control		44.4^a	9	94.2 ± 6.6
	Phenobarbital		$32.2^{a,b,c}$	11	$34.8 \pm 3.0^{b,c}$
3% Corn Oil	Control	15	23.1 ± 1.8	8	86.1 ± 9.3
	3-MC	8	29.5 ± 1.6^b	9	83.3 ± 6.7
	Control		43.7^d	10	86.1 ± 4.7
	Phenobarbital		$26.7^{d,b}$	11	17.2 ± 1.5^b

[a] Diet contained 6.3% beef fat and 0.7% corn oil (Century, B. 1973).
[b] Significantly different from control rats fed same diet.
[c] Significantly different from rats fed corn oil given same pretreatment.
[d] Diet contained 7% corn oil (Century, B. 1973).

induction. This theory may be an oversimplification. The possible role of dietary fat in altering the conformation of microsomal membranes (and consequently the properties of cytochrome P-450) was not considered in this model. Nor does the theory explain the observation that rats fed a fat-free diet have less cytochrome P-450 than rats fed corn oil even in the absence of phenobarbital induction. However, the theory may explain the lower degree of induction observed when phenobarbital is administered to rats fed a fat-free or coconut oil-supplemented diet when compared to rats fed corn oil.

The fact that 3-MC induces Type II substrate (aniline) metabolism to higher levels in animals fed a source of polyenoic acids also suggests that fatty acids are involved in allowing full expression of this interaction. Why 3-MC is a limited substrate inducer has been explained on the basis of its selected induction of cytochrome P_1-450 (P-448) which appears to be involved in the metabolism of the polycyclic hydrocarbons such as benzpyrene and Type II substrates such as aniline. From the kinetics of Type I substrate metabolism it appears that this selective enhancement of cytochrome P_1-450 is accompanied with decreases in P-450 associated with corresponding decreases in the V_{max} for ethylmorphine demethylation. Findings to date indicate that a source of polyenoic fatty acids is necessary for optimal activity of the microsomal drug metabolizing system. Deprivation of dietary lipids results in changes in relative content of microsomal phospholipid fatty acids, and associated with these changes are decreased metabolism of hexobarbital, aniline, and ethylmorphine, decreased content of cytochrome P-450, and decreased binding of aniline and hexobarbital to microsomes. These quantitative alterations may be associated with qualitative alteration of some microsomal constituents as evidenced by a shift in the ethylisocyanide difference spectrum during induction with phenobarbital. In addition to their role in facilitating electron transport from NADPH cytochrome P-450 reductase to the P-450 drug complex, polyenoic acids may be necessary in synthesizing hepatic endoplasmic reticulum capable of maintaining a full complement of cytochrome P-450, holding this hemoprotein in its optimum conformation or influencing the coupling and decoupling of the cytochrome P-450 and cytochrome P-450 reductase systems (Stier, 1976).

REFERENCES

Agradi, E., Spagnuolo, C., and Galli, C. (1975). Dietary lipids and aniline and benzpyrene hydroxylations in liver microsomes. *Pharmacol. Res. Commun.* **7,** 469–480.

Belina, H., Cooper, S. D., Farkas, R., and Feuer, G. (1975). Sex difference in the phospholipid composition of rat liver microsomes. *Biochem. Pharmacol.* **24,** 301–303.

Béraud, M., Gaillard, D., and Derache, R. (1975). Influence des regimes alimentaires sur la stimulation des monoxygenases microsomales du foie de rat induite par la dimethyl-2,3 quinoxaline. *Eur. J. Toxicol.* **8,** 212–219.

Campbell, T. C., and Hayes, J. R. (1974). Role of nutrition in the drug-metabolizing enzyme system. *Pharmacol. Rev.* **25,** 171–197.

Caster, W. O., Wade, A. E., Greene, F. E., and Meadows, J. S. (1968). Effect of small changes in dietary thiamine or essential fatty acid in altering the rate of drug detoxication in the liver of the rat. *Fed. Proc., Fed. Am. Soc. Exp. Biol.* **27,** 549.

Caster, W. O., Wade, A. E., Norred, W. P., and Bargmann, R. E. (1970a). A differential effect of dietary saturated fat on the metabolism of aniline and hexobarbital by the rat liver. *Pharmacology* **3,** 177–186.

Caster, W. O., Wade, A. E., Greene, F. E., and Meadows, J. S. (1970b). Effect of different levels of corn oil in the diet upon the rate of hexobarbital, heptachlor and aniline metabolism in the liver of the male white rat. *Life Sci.* **9,** 181–190.

Century, B. (1969). Lipids affecting drug metabolism and cellular functions. *In* "Drugs Affecting Lipid Metabolism," (W. L. Holmes, ed.) pp. 629–638. Plenum, New York.

Century, B. (1972). Effect of dietary lipid on various liver enzymes and on *in vivo* removal of 3,4-dimethoxyphenylethylamine, 3,4-dihydroxyphenylalanine and 5-hydroxytryptophan in rats. *J. Nutr.* **102,** 1067–1077.

Century, B. (1973). A role of the dietary lipid in the ability of phenobarbital to stimulate drug detoxification. *J. Pharmacol. Exp. Ther.* **185,** 185–194.

Chadwick, R. W., Simmons, W. S., Bryden, C. C., Chuang, L. T., Key, L. M., and Chadwick, C. J. (1977). Effect of dietary lipid and dimethyl sulfoxide on lindane metabolism. *Tox. and Appl. Pharmac.* **30,** 391–410.

Chaplin, M. D., and Mannering, G. J. (1970). Role of phospholipids in the hepatic microsomal drug-metabolizing system. *Mol. Pharmacol.* **6,** 631–640.

Conney, A. H. (1967). Pharmacological implications of microsomal enzyme induction. *Pharmacol. Rev.* **19**, 317–366.

Coon, M. J., Strobel, H. W., Autor, A. P., Heidema, J., and Duppel, W. (1971). Functional components of the liver microsomal enzyme system catalyzing fatty acid, hydrocarbon and drug hydroxylation. *Proc. Biochem. Soc.* **125**, 2–3.

Cooper, S. D., and Feuer, G. (1972). Relation Between drug-metabolizing activity and phospholipids in hepatic microsomes. I. Effects of phenobarbital, carbon tetrachloride and actinomycin D. *Can. J. Physiol. Pharmacol.* **50**, 568–575.

Czygan, P., Greim, H., Garro, A., Schaffner, F., and Popper, H. (1974). The effect of dietary protein deficiency on the ability of isolated hepatic microsomes to alter the mutagenicity of a primary and a secondary carcinogen. *Cancer Res.* **34**, 119–123.

Davison, S. C., and Wills, E. D. (1974). Studies on the lipid composition of the rat liver endoplasmic reticulum after induction with phenobarbitone and 20-methylcholanthrene. *Biochem. J.* **140**, 461–468.

DiAugustine, R. P., and Fouts, J. R. (1969). The effects of unsaturated fatty acids on hepatic microsomal drug metabolism and cytochrome *P*-450. *Biochem. J.* **115**, 547–554.

Eling, T. E., and DiAugustine, R. P. (1971). A role for phospholipids in the binding and metabolism of drugs by hepatic microsomes. *Biochem. J.* **123**, 539–549.

Glaumann, H., and Dallner, G. (1968). Lipid composition and turnover of rough and smooth microsomal membranes in rat liver. *J. Lipid Res.* **9**, 720–729.

Hietanen, E., Laitinen, M., Vainio, H., and Hänninen, O. (1975). Dietary fats and properties of endoplasmic reticulum. II. Dietary lipid induced changes in activities of drug-metabolizing enzymes in liver and duodenum of rat. *Lipids* **10**, 467–472.

Hopkins, G. J., and West, C. E., (1976). Possible roles of dietary fats in carcinogenesis. *Life Sciences.* **19**, 1103–1116.

Infante, R., Petit, D., Polonski, J., and Caroli, J. (1971). Microsomal phospholipid biosynthesis after phenobarbital administration. *Experientia* **27**, 640–642.

Jefcoate, C. R. E., Calabrese, R. L., and Gaylor, J. L. (1970). Ligand interaction with hemoprotein *P*-450. III. The use of *n*-octylamine and ethylisocyanide difference spectroscopy in the quantitative determination of high- and low-spin *P*-450. *Mol. Pharmacol.* **6**, 390–401.

Kamataki, T., and Kitagawa, H. (1973). Effects of lipid peroxidation on activities of drug-metabolizing enzymes in liver microsomes of rats. *Biochem. Pharmacol.* **22**, 3199–3207.

Kaschnitz, R. (1970). Aryl 4-hydroxylase, cytochrome *P*-450 and microsomal lipids in essential fatty acid deficiency. *Hoppe-Seyler's Z. Physiol. Chem.* **351**, 771–774.

Leibman, K. C., and Estabrook, R. W. (1971). Effects of extraction with isooctane upon the properties of liver microsomes. *Mol. Pharmacol.* **7**, 26–32.

Lu, A. Y. H., Junk, K. W., and Coon, M. J. (1969a). Resolution of the cytochrome *P*-450 containing w-hydroxylation system of liver microsomes into three components. *J. Biol. Chem.* **244**, 3714–3721.

Lu, A. Y. H., Strobel, H. W., and Coon, M. J. (1969b). Hydroxylation of benzphetamine and other drugs by a solubilized form of cytochrome *P*-450 from liver microsomes: lipid requirement for drug demethylation. *Biochem. Biophys. Res. Commun.* **36**, 545–551.

Marshall, W. J., and McLean, A. E. M. (1971a). Dietary lipid requirements for hepatic microsomal enzyme induction in the rat. *Proc. Nutr. Soc.* **30**, 66A.

Marshall, W. J., and McLean, A. E. M. (1971b). A requirement for dietary lipids for induction of cytochrome *P*-450 by phenobarbital in rat liver microsomal fraction. *Biochem. J.* **122**, 569–573.

Miller, J. A., and Miller, E. C. (1965). Metabolism of drugs in relation to carcinogenicity. *Ann. N.Y. Acad. Sci.* **123**, 125–140.

Mohrrauer, H., and Holman, R. T. (1963). The effect of dose level of essential fatty acids upon fatty acid composition of the rat liver. *J. Lipid Res.* **4**, 151–159.

Natori, Y. (1963). Studies on ethionine. *J. Biol. Chem.* **238**, 2075–2080.

Norred, W. P., and Wade, A. E. (1972). Dietary fatty acid-induced alterations of hepatic microsomal drug metabolism. *Biochem. Pharmacol.* **21**, 2887–2897.

Norred, W. P., and Wade, A. E. (1973). Effect of dietary lipid ingestion on the induction of drug-metabolizing enzymes by phenobarbital. *Biochem. Pharmacol.* **22**, 432–436.

Omura, T., and Sato, R. (1964). The carbon monoxide-binding pigment of liver microsomes. *J. Biol. Chem.* **239**, 2370–2378.

Orrenius, S., Ericsson, J. L. E., and Ernster, L. (1965). Phenobarbital-induced synthesis of the microsomal drug-metabolizing enzyme system and its relationship to the proliferation of endoplasmic membranes. *J. Cell Biol.* **25**, 627.

Orrenius, S., Das, M., and Gnosspelius, Y. (1969). Overall biochemical effects of drug induction of liver microsomes. In "Microsomes and Drug Oxidations" (J. R. Gillette, et al., eds.), p. 251. Academic Press, New York.

Orrenius, S., Wilson, B. J., von Bahr, C., and Schenkman, J. B. (1972). On the significance of drug-induced spectral changes in liver microsomes. In "Biological Hydroxylation Mechanisms" (G. S. Boyd and R. M. S. Smellie, eds.), pp. 55–77. Academic Press, New York.

Patel, J. M., and Pawar, S. S. (1972). Activities of phenobarbital induced liver microsomal enzymes in rats fed protein- and fat-free diets. *Indian J. Biochem. Biophys.* **9**, 277–278.

Rogers, A. E., and Newberne, P. M. (1971). Nutrition and aflatoxin carcinogenesis. *Nature (London)* **229**, 62–63.

Shakman, R. A. (1974). Nutritional influences on the toxicity of environmental pollutants. *Arch. Environ. Health* **28**, 105–113.

Siekevitz, P. (1963). *Protoplasm: Endoplasmic reticulum and microsomes and their properties.* *Annu. Rev. Physiol.* **25**, 15–40.

Sladek, N. E., and Mannering, G. J. (1966). Evidence for a new P-450 hemoprotein in hepatic microsomes from methylcholanthrene-treated rats. *Biochem. Biophys. Res. Commun.* **24**, 668–674.

Stier, A. (1976). Lipid structure and drug-metabolizing enzymes. *Biochem. Pharmacol.* **25**, 109–113.

Strobel, H. W., Lu, A. Y. H., Heidema, J., and Coon, M. J. (1970). Phosphatidylcholine requirement in the enzymatic reduction of hemoprotein P-450 and in fatty acid, hydrocarbon and drug hydroxylation. *J. Biol. Chem.* **245**, 4851–4854.

Trewhella, M. A., and Collins, F. D. (1973). A comparison of the relative turnover of individual molecular species of phospholipids in normal rats and in rats deficient in essential fatty acids. *Biochim. Biophys. Acta* **296**, 34–50.

Vore, M., Hamilton, J. G., and Lu, A. Y. H. (1974a). Organic solvent extraction of liver microsomal lipid. *Biochem. Biophys. Res. Commun.* **56**, 1038–1044.

Vore, M., Lu, A. Y. H., Kuntzman, R., and Conney, A. H. (1974b). Organic solvent extraction of liver microsomal lipid II. *Mol. Pharmacol.* **10**, 963–974.

Wade, A. E., Caster, W. O., Greene, F. E., and Meadows, J. S. (1969). Effect of thiamine and dietary linoleate levels on hepatic drug metabolism in the male rat. *Arch. Int. Pharmacodyn. Ther.* **181**, 466–473.

Wade, A. E., Wu, B., and Caster, W. O. (1972). Relationship of dietary essential fatty acid consumption to hepatic drug hydroxylation. *Pharmacology* **7**, 305–314.

Wattenberg, L. W. (1972). Dietary modification of intestinal and pulmonary aryl hydrocarbon hydroxylase activity. *Toxicol. Appl. Pharmacol.* **23**, 741–748.

Wattenberg, L. W., Loub, W. D., Lam, L. K., and Speier, J. L. (1976). Dietary constituents altering the responses to chemical carcinogens. *Fed. Proc., Fed. Am. Soc. Exp. Biol.* **35,** 1327–1331.

Wills, E. D. (1971). Effects of lipid peroxidation on membrane-bound enzymes of the endoplasmic reticulum. *Biochem. J.* **123,** 983–991.

Wynder, E. L. (1976). Nutrition and cancer. *Federation Proc.* **35,** 1309–1315.

Young, D. L., Powell, G., and McMillan, W. O. (1971). Phenobarbital-induced alteration in phosphatidylcholine and triglyceride synthesis in hepatic endoplasmic reticulum. *J. Lipid Res.* **12,** 1–8.

19

Dietary Effects on Carcinogenicity of Drugs and Related Compounds

ADRIANNE E. ROGERS

I. INTRODUCTION

Diet influences the induction of tumors by carcinogens of many different chemical classes. Both nutrient and nonnutrient dietary components can affect the incidence, number, size, site, latent period, and histologic type of tumors induced in experimental animals and may be responsible for the epidemiologic characteristics of many human tumors. Prevention or retardation of tumor development by dietary alterations is one of the major goals of research programs in nutrition and cancer which have been developed and are now being expanded by the National Institutes of Health and other public and private agencies which support biomedical research. People are exposed to carcinogenic chemicals inadvertently by inhalation of contaminated air, ingestion of contaminated food or water, or by skin contact with contaminated surfaces; they can be exposed intentionally to carcinogenic chemicals or irradiation for therapeutic purposes or by their own choice in smoking tobacco or sunbathing. Some exposures can be decreased or eliminated, but reduction to zero exposure often is not possible even when the carcinogen is known, and at present most are not known. For these reasons, definition of general principles which govern biological responses to carcinogens is important since such definition offers the hope of modifying the responses. Nutritional condition of animals and their specific dietary intake are significant modifiers of response to carcinogens as are immunologic status, endocrine status, and age. The interactions of these modifiers of carcinogenesis with each other and with carcinogen-exposed tissues contribute to the outcome of carcinogen exposure.

Among environmental exposures to carcinogens which may not be reducible but may, on the contrary, increase are exposures to therapeutic agents which are carcinogenic. The list of such agents is small, but it includes X-irradiation and many agents used in chemotherapy of cancer, a group of drugs which is expanding rapidly in size and use. Nutritional modification of carcinogenic effects of therapeutic compounds is a goal toward which research should be directed. Exploitation of the special case of interactions between antifolate drugs and citrovorum factor in reducing toxicity of the drugs is an example of nutrient manipulation to influence drug effects. (Bertino and Nixon, 1969). There are indications from experimental studies that carcinogenicity of therapeutic agents or compounds which are chemically similar to them can be modified by dietary alterations. These studies are reviewed in the sections which follow.

II. REVIEW

Therapeutic agents which are or may be carcinogenic in humans or experimental animals are listed in Table I. Solar irradiation and X-irradiation are listed and will be discussed briefly, but discussion will be devoted primarily to chemical agents which are both therapeutic and carcinogenic or potentially carcinogenic. In each section the evidence for carcinogenicity of each drug or group of drugs is discussed first and is followed by discussion of evidence for nutrient or dietary effects on carcinogenicity by the drugs or related compounds. These sections are followed by general discussion of dietary effects on chemical carcinogenesis. Insofar as possible, references have been chosen for citation which are recent and review older references. In the literature on drugs

TABLE I
Therapeutic Agents which Are or May Be Carcinogenic in Humans and Experimental Animals

Agent	Carcinogenic in		References
	Species	Organ	
Antitumor agents			
Adriamycin	Rat	Mammary gland	Bertazzoli et al., 1971; Marquardt et al., 1976
Azothiaprine	Human	Hematopoietic	
		Lymphoreticular	Sieber, 1975; Silvergleid and Schrier, 1974
	Rat	Zymbal's gland	Frankel et al., 1970
Chlorambucil	Human	Hematopoietic	Steigbigel et al., 1974
	Rat	Lymphoreticular	Weisburger et al., 1975a
	Mouse	Lymphoreticular	Weisburger et al., 1975a
		Lung	Weisburger et al., 1975a
		Ovary	Weisburger et al., 1975a
Cyclophosphamide	Human	Urinary bladder	Bachur et al., 1975; Rosner and Grünwald, 1974;
		Lymphoreticular	Tannenbaum and Schur, 1974; Wall and
		Hematopoietic	Clausen, 1975
		Müllerian duct	
	Rat	Mammary gland	Weisburger et al., 1975a
	Mouse	Lymphoreticular	Walker and Bole, 1973
Daunomycin	Rat	Mammary gland	Bertazzoli et al., 1971; Marquardt et al., 1976
5-(3,3-Dimethyl-1-	Rat	Lymphoreticular	Beal et al., 1975
triazene)-imidazole-		Uterus	
4-carboxamide (DTIC)		Mammary gland	
Melphalan	Human	Hematopoietic	Karchmer et al., 1974; Kyle et al., 1974; Rosner
			and Grünwald, 1974; Sieber, 1975
	Rat	Connective tissue	Weisburger et al., 1975a
	Mouse	Lymphoreticular	Weisburger et al., 1975a
		Lung	

(continued)

TABLE I, *continued*

Agent	Carcinogenic in		References
	Species	Organ	
Procarbazine	Nonhuman primate	Hematopoietic	O'Gara et al., 1971
	Rat	Hematopoietic	Lemon, 1975; Weisburger, 1969; Weisburger et al., 1975a
		Lymphoreticular	
		Mammary gland	
	Mouse	Hematopoietic	Kelly et al., 1969; Weisburger et al., 1975a
		Lung	
		Kidney	
		Uterus	
Streptozotocin	Rat	Kidney	Mauer et al., 1974; Rakieten et al., 1971
		Liver	Schoental, 1975
		Pancreas	Weisburger et al., 1975a
		Muscle	
	Mouse	Lung	Weisburger et al., 1975a
		Kidney	
		Uterus	
Thiotepa	Human	Hematopoietic	Greenspan and Tung, 1974; Rosner and Grünwald, 1974
X-irradiation	Human	Lymphoreticular	Arsenau et al., 1972; Jablon, 1975; Rosner and Grünwald, 1974, 1975
		Hematopoietic	Selinger and Koff, 1975
		Thyroid	
		Vascular	
		Bone	
		Other sites irradiated	

	Species	Site	References
	Mouse	Lymphoreticular, Uterus, Lung, Harderian gland, Gastrointestinal tract, Thyroid, Meninges	Ershoff et al., 1969
Steroid hormones			
Estrogens	Human	Uterus, Vagina, Liver	Cutler et al., 1972; Edmonson et al., 1976; Herbst et al., 1971; Mack et al., 1976; D. C. Smith et al., 1975; Ziel and Finkle, 1975
	Rat	Mammary gland, Uterus, Pituitary	Ershoff, 1964; Leonard, 1973
	Mouse	Mammary gland, Uterus, Cervix, Testis, Pituitary, Lymphoreticular	Dunn and Green, 1963; Leonard, 1973; Pullinger, 1961
Androgens	Hamster	Kidney	Hamilton et al., 1975
	Human	Liver	Farrell et al., 1975, Meadows et al., 1974
	Mouse	Liver	Andervont, 1950
Agents active in nervous system			
Amphetamine (?)[a]	Human	Lymphoreticular	Newell et al., 1973 (Boston Collaborative Drug Surveillance Program, 1974a)[b]
Dibenamine	Rat	Connective tissue, Gastrointestinal tract	Weisburger et al., 1974
Diphenylhydantoin (?)	Human	Lymphoreticular	Anthony, 1970; Li et al., 1975 (Clemmesen, et al., 1974)
L-Dopa (?)	Mouse	Lymphoreticular	Kruger and Harris, 1972
Phenacetin (?)	Human	Melanocyte	Lieberman and Shupack, 1974
	Human	Kidney	Johansson et al., 1974 (Editorial, 1969)

(continued)

TABLE I, *continued*

Agent	Carcinogenic in		References
	Species	Organ	
Phenobarbital	Mouse	Liver	Jones and Butler, 1975; Thorpe and Walker, 1973
Reserpine (?)	Human	Mammary gland	Armstrong et al., 1974; Boston Collaborative Drug Surveillance Program, 1974b; Heinonen et al., 1974 (Laska et al., 1975 Mack et al., 1975; O'Fallon et al., 1975)
Antibacterial, antiparasitic agents			
Chloramphenicol (?)	Human	Hematopoietic	H. J. Cohen and Huang, 1973; Fraumeni, 1967
Isonicotonic acid hydrazide (?)	Human	Bladder	Miller, 1974 (Hammond et al., 1967)
	Rat	Anus	Peacock and Peacock, 1966
	Mouse	Lung	Peacock and Peacock, 1966; Severi and Biancifiori, 1968
Nitrofurans	Rat	Urinary bladder	Cohen et al., 1975
		Kidney	Erturk et al., 1969
		Mammary gland	
		Forestomach	
		Lung	
		Lymphoreticular	
		Vasculature	

Agent	Species	Site	References
	Mouse	Urinary bladder Forestomach Lymphoreticular	S. M. Cohen et al., 1973
	Hamster	Urinary bladder Kidney Forestomach Adrenal	Croft and Bryan, 1973
5-Nitroimidazole	Mouse	Lymphoreticular Lung	Rustia and Shubik, 1972
For treatment of dermatologic diseases			
Arsenic	Human	Skin Vascular Lung	Cole and Goldman, 1975 Lander et al., 1975 Lee and Fraumeni, 1969 Morris et al., 1974
Coal tar ointments (?)	Human	Skin Gastrointestinal tract	Boyd and Doll, 1954 Rook et al., 1956 (Higginson, 1966); Swanbeck and Hellström, 1971)
Solar irradiation	Human Mouse	Skin Skin	Emmett, 1973; Jablon, 1975; Mason et al., 1975 Blum, 1959; Freeman et al., 1970; Winkelmann et al., 1963

[a] Agents followed by (?) are subjects of both positive and negative reports with respect to carcinogenicity in humans. References to the negative reports are given in parentheses.

which are or may be carcinogenic, the initial publications often are reports of one or a few cases; later publications review these and add more data. The later publications have been cited for convenience of readers who are reminded that credit for the initial observation is due to the earlier investigators cited in those publications.

Identification of chemicals carcinogenic for humans is difficult, and much of the evidence used is derived from studies in experimental animals or from human industrial exposures. In Table I the only compounds listed without question marks as human carcinogens are drugs used in chemotherapy of cancer, steroid sex hormones, and arsenic.

The antitumor drugs are used in situations in which the benefit outweighs the risk of inducing a second cancer; studies of dietary influences on their activity may yield methods of decreasing risks attendant on their use. Sex hormones are used in many different situations. The risks of tumor induction increase with duration of exposure; manipulation of dosage schedules and possibly dietary alterations may reduce the risks. Prolonged use of these compounds must be regarded as unsafe and should be restricted to conditions for which no other treatment is available. Arsenicals may pose a problem in industrial pollution but are no longer significant in therapeutics.

Drugs listed as questionably or possibly carcinogenic for people and as carcinogenic in experimental animals include widely-used compounds whose possible risks are of great concern. Determination of their carcinogenicity should be made as rapidly as possible and methods sought to reduce the risks associated with their use.

A few therapeutic agents in addition to those listed in Table I may be cocarcinogenic under certain conditions. Immunosuppressive agents such as antilymphocyte globulin (ALG), the folate antimetabolite, methotrexate, and corticosteroids probably contribute to the increased cancer incidence in recipients of organ grafts (Hoover and Fraumeni, 1975a). ALG increased hepatic vascular tumors in rats treated with azoxymethane (Kroes et al., 1975) and enhanced metastasis of transplanted tumors (James and Salsbury, 1974). There are conflicting data on its effect on development of spontaneous lymphoreticular tumors in mice (Burstein and Allison, 1970; Ben-Yaakov et al., 1975). Methotrexate enhanced tumor induction by 7, 10-dimethylbenzanthracene (DMBA) in hamsters and has been associated with appearance of tumors at several organ sites in humans, but the evidence is not extensive (Bailin et al., 1974; Shklar et al., 1966). Allopurinol, a drug used in treatment of gout and neoplasia was carcinogenic in rat urinary bladder (Wang et al., 1976).

In experimental animals, sex determines both potency and site of action of many carcinogenic chemicals, e.g., N-2-fluorenylacetamide (AAF) and aflatoxin B_1 (AFB_1). Ovarian hormones and prolactin are required for induction of mammary tumors in rats by DMBA, but exogenous ovarian hormones also can be anticarcinogenic (Lemon, 1975; Newberne and Williams, 1969; Shellabarger and Soo, 1973). Since phenothiazines, which are used intensively as tranquilizers, stimulate prolactin release they may be of some significance in breast cancer (Hoover and Fraumeni, 1975a).

A third category of therapeutic agents which may be of concern in carcinogenesis is composed of amines which can be nitrosated in the stomach or other tissues to form carcinogenic nitrosamines (Hoover and Fraumeni, 1975a; Wogan et al., 1975). Agents in this group have varied and extensive use and include chlorpromazine, oxytetracycline, and ephedrine.

III. ANTITUMOR AGENTS

The carcinogenicity of antitumor agents, as of other chemical carcinogens, may depend upon one or more tissue reactions, e.g., damage to macromolecules or other nucleophiles, immunosuppression, and viral activation. Their cytotoxicity, and therefore their therapeutic effect, is strongly but not entirely dependent upon proliferation of target cells (Valeriote and van Putten, 1975). Their carcinogenicity also may be dependent on proliferation of target cells since the majority induce tumors of the rapidly dividing cells of the hematopoietic and/or lymphoreticular systems, but several other tissues with a smaller population of proliferating cells such as mammary gland, kidney, and urinary bladder are susceptible to them as well. The relationships between DNA synthesis, mitosis, and chemical carcinogenesis are not established and are undoubtedly complicated by factors such as carcinogen delivery, uptake and metabolism, and DNA repair.

Evidence for carcinogenicity of antitumor drugs in humans is composed largely of reports of patients treated for lymphoreticular tumors who subsequently developed myelocytic or lymphocytic leukemia. There has been discussion of the possibility that development of the second tumors is part of the natural course of lymphoreticular malignancy in people whose life span is lengthened by chemotherapy, but azathioprine, cyclophosphamide, melphalan, thiotepa and X-irradiation have been associated with tumor induction also in people treated for nonmalignant diseases or tumors at sites other than the lymphoreticular system. In addition, the compounds have induced tumors at sites other than the lymphoreticular or hematopoietic systems (Greenspan and Tung, 1974; Kyle et al., 1974; McAdam et al., 1974; Rosner and Grünwald, 1974, 1975; Sieber, 1975; Silvergleid and Schrier, 1974; Tannenbaum and Schur, 1974; Wall and Clausen, 1975). Animal studies support the evidence for carcinogenicity of this group of agents (Table I).

There are several points of interest with respect to dietary interactions with carcinogenesis by chemotherapeutic agents. The probable relationship between cell proliferation and susceptibility to carcinogens is probably important with these agents since their cytotoxicity is related to cell proliferation. Growth and cell division of normal tissues and tumors are decreased in animals chronically underfed an adequate diet, and cell division in normal tissues can be virtually abolished temporarily by starvation (MacDonald et al., 1963; Tannenbaum, 1959). Tumor induction and growth may be either enhanced or decreased in animals fed diets inadequate or excessive in specific nutrients. Such diets may induce cell division in normal tissues and thereby enhance their susceptibility to chemical carcinogenesis.

We have found an example in rats fed a high fat diet marginally deficient in lipotropes (choline, methionine, and folic acid) and certain amino acids. The deficient rats grow normally, except for a small lag in the first 4–6 weeks after weaning, and often weigh more than rats fed an adequate diet. They are, however, more susceptible to both chronic toxicity and carcinogenicity of many different chemicals, particularly AFB_1 and other chemicals carcinogenic for the liver (Rogers et al., 1974; Rogers and Newberne, 1975; Rogers, 1975). The deficiency stimulates DNA synthesis and cell division in hepatocytes (Rogers and Newberne, 1971) which in itself enhances carcinogenesis by azobenzenes and nitroso compounds but not by AFB_1 (Craddock and Frei, 1974; Rogers et al., 1971; Warwick, 1967). Another example is hypervitaminosis A which increases cell division in hamster cheek pouch epithelium and increases tumor induction by DMBA at that site (Polliack and Levij, 1967, 1969).

Increasing dietary protein stimulates body and tumor growth up to the point at which the protein reaches toxic levels; it may also alter tumor site (Ross and Bras, 1973; Shay et al., 1964).

Another point of interest with respect to dietary interactions with this and other groups of carcinogens is the dietary effect on metabolic activation or excretion. Many nutrients influence activity of hepatic and other tissue enzymes responsible for metabolism of foreign chemicals (Campbell and Hayes, 1974). Nonnutrient food components can induce activity of the enzymes (Wattenberg, 1975). Because of the complexity of metabolic pathways and, in most cases, lack of knowledge of the active forms of drugs and other chemicals, the effect on carcinogenesis of dietary manipulation of enzyme activity cannot be predicted (Gillette, 1976). If cytotoxic and carcinogenic metabolites are different, dietary manipulation might be useful in favoring formation of the former; with compounds such as 5-(3,3-Dimethyl-1-triazene)-imidazole-4-carboxamide (DTIC) and streptozotocin which undergo extensive metabolism to several different metabolites (Beal et al., 1975; Gunnarsson et al., 1974; Schein et al., 1967) this is a possible approach to reduction of carcinogenic hazard.

Streptozotocin is naturally occurring nitrosourea antibiotic and antitumor agent which is toxic to pancreatic B cells in several species and carcinogenic in rodents (Rakieten et al., 1971; Weisburger et al., 1975a). Because it depletes tissues of NAD, several studies of interactions between nicotinamide and streptozotocin have been performed. Toxicity of the compound can be blocked by simultaneous administration of the vitamin, but carcinogenicity may be increased, decreased, or unchanged (Table II).

The effect of nicotinamide apparently is exerted through repletion of tissue NAD–NADP (Gunnarsson et al., 1974; Schein et al., 1967). The coenzymes are required for respiration and many reactions of intermediary metabolism and also for functioning of the microsomal oxidases which metabolize streptozotocin. Elucidation of the effects of niacin supplementation on streptozotocin metabolism, carcinogenicity, and antitumor activity should be of great interest and may increase its usefulness by decreasing the carcinogenic and toxic hazards of its use. A second antitumor antibiotic, adriamycin, is metabolized to several compounds which vary in toxicity (Bachur, 1975). Its potential usefulness is great and might be enhanced by dietary manipulation of metabolism.

Most of the antitumor compounds listed are direct or indirect alkylating agents; probably nucleic acid alkylation is responsible for both their antitumor effect and their carcinogenicity. Therefore dietary or other alterations aimed at decreasing carcinogenicity without decreasing tumor cytotoxicity would have to exploit differences in susceptibility of tumor and normal tissue to the alterations. The ability to block toxicity of methotrexate in normal tissues by administration of folate without blocking completely its toxicity to tumors gives hope that other tissue-tumor differences can be found and used.

Nitrosamine and hydrazine carcinogens are alkylating agents which may be considered as models for exploration of dietary effects on alkylating chemotherapeutic agents. Procarbazine is a hydrazine, and the alkylating species of the nitrogen mustards may be similar or identical to compounds derived from nitrosamines and hydrazines (Druckrey, 1970;

TABLE II
Effect of Nicotinamide on Streptozotocin Carcinogenesis in Rats

		Tumor incidence		
Reference	Nicotinamide	Pancreas (%)	Liver (%)	Kidney (%)
Rakieten et al., 1971[a]	0	4	—	—
	+	64	—	—
Weisburger et al., 1975a[b]	0	8	0 (Males) 41 (Females)	40
	+	12	18 (Males) 10 (Females)	48

[a] Streptozotocin 50 mg/kg iv; nicotinamide 350 mg/kg ip 10 minutes before and 180 minutes after streptozotocin.
[b] Streptozotocin 6 or 12 mg/kg ip, three times/week for 6 months; nicotinamide 250 mg/kg ip by same schedule.

Magee and Barnes, 1967). Nitrosamine carcinogenesis is enhanced in liver by lipotrope deficiency and in kidney by protein deficiency, but tumor induction in other organs, e.g., lung and urinary bladder, is not affected (Hard and Butler, 1970; McLean and Magee, 1970; Rogers *et al.,* 1974; Rogers, 1975). Both N-nitrosodiethylamine (DENA) and N-nitrosodibutylamine (DBN) are significantly more hepatocarcinogenic in lipotrope-deficient rats; DENA is more carcinogenic for the esophagus as well if given in high but not low dosage. The dietary effect on DENA hepatocarcinogenesis is consistently repeatable and is being used to measure the effects of diet supplements on susceptibility to carcinogenesis (Fig. 1). DBN induces a high incidence of tumors in lung and bladder of both control and deficient rats despite the enhancement of hepatocarcinoma induction in deficient rats. If the carcinogens are activated and deactivated locally in each case there must be a difference in susceptibility of the enzymes of different tissues to lipotrope deficiency. Liver cells are highly sensitive to the deficiency, and the decreased microsomal oxidase activity it induces may be responsible for alteration of carcinogenesis at that site (Rogers and Newberne, 1971).

The demonstration that DENA induces tissue folate deficiency in the presence of adequate dietary folate (Poirier and Whitehead, 1973) suggests that specific cellular defects in 1-carbon metabolism may contribute to the dietary effect. Hematopoietic and lymphoreticular tissues, and tumors arising from them, are sensitive to alterations of supply of folate, vitamin B_{12}, and methyl groups which is the basis of antimetabolite chemotherapy of tumors of these tissues. Their rapid cell turnover, which creates the need for methyl groups, is responsible also for their susceptibility to alkylating agents. Further research into basic lipotrope interactions in the two tissues, and tumors arising from them, and into interactions between lipotropes and carcinogenesis, may demonstrate mechanisms which can be used to reduce carcinogenicity of the alkylating agents without reducing their tumor cytotoxicity.

The complexity of such studies is great. In examining lipotropic and other dietary effects on DENA carcinogenesis in liver, we have found that supplementation of the diet with a single lipotrope, choline, has no effect, but supplementation with the three major lipotropes, choline, methionine, and folic acid, or with the amino acids in which the diet is deficient, which include methionine, reduces tumor induction (Fig. 1) (Rogers, 1977b). A pivotal role for methionine is suggested by this result and by the observation that dietary methionine but not folate itself prevents induction of tissue folate deficiency by DENA (Poirier and Whitehead, 1973).

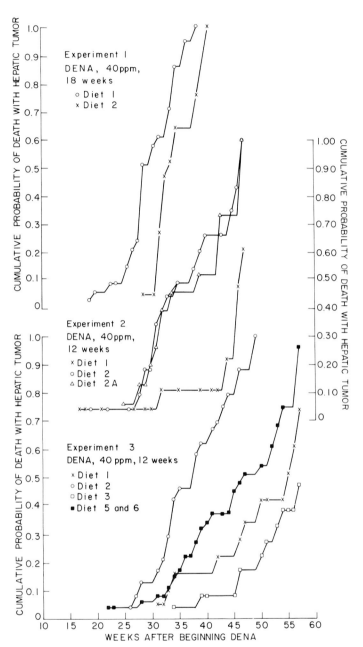

Fig. 1. Cumulative probability of death with hepatocarcinoma in rats fed DENA in: diet 1, Adequate in all known respects for rats; diet 2, marginally deficient in lipotropes and amino acids, high in beef fat; diet 2A, diet 2 + choline; diet 3, diet 1 + beef fat to equal amount in diet 2; diets 5 and 6, diet 2 supplemented with lipotropes (diet 5) or amino acids (diet 6).

A hydrazine [1, 2-dimethylhydrazine (DMH)] is a more effective colon carcinogen in lipotrope-deficient rats than in normal rats (Rogers and Newberne, 1973). The observation offers a model for investigating lipotrope–carcinogen interactions in a tissue with rapid cell turnover and perhaps less metabolic complexity than liver. Interaction between dietary lipid and hydrazine carcinogenesis was reported in DMH-treated rats fed either 5 or 20% corn oil or lard. Rats fed 20% fat had a higher incidence of colon tumors and a greater number of tumors per rat than rats fed 5% fat. (Reddy *et al.*, 1975). High fat diets do not consistently enhance DMH carcinogenesis (Rogers and Newberne, 1975; Wilson *et al.*, 1977).

In other studies of nutrient effects on DMH carcinogenesis, both vitamin A-deficient and hypervitaminotic A rats were exposed to the carcinogen. Vitamin A deficiency induces abnormalities of intestinal mucosa and increases induction of colon tumors by AFB_1 (Newberne and Rogers, 1973). However, DMH colon carcinogenesis is not altered by increased dietary vitamin A and is only slightly, if at all, enhanced by deficiency of the vitamin (Rogers *et al.*, 1973). Two hydrazine drugs are listed in Table 1: procarbazine and isonicotinic acid hydrazide (INH). Procarbazine is unquestionably carcinogenic in rodents, and studies of dietary effects on its activity are indicated. Patients treated for tuberculosis with INH over long periods do not have increased tumor incidence (Hammond *et al.*, 1967;) although there is an informal report in the form of a letter that bladder cancer may be increased in such patients (Miller, 1974). Studies of INH in rodents have been negative except for increased incidence of pulmonary ademonas in strains of mice in which the tumors occur spontaneously (Peacock and Peacock, 1966; Severi and Biancifiore, 1968; Toth and Shubik, 1966).

Effects of several diet components on tumor induction in mice by X-irradiation have been found, and certain specific results require further study. A general result can be stated, i.e., that ingestion of a natural ingredient diet protects mice against X-ray carcinogenesis in the lymphoreticular system and uterus compared to ingestion of any of several purified diets (Ershoff *et al.*, 1969). A protective effect of natural ingredient diets compared to purified diets has been observed also in studies of chemical or spontaneous carcinogenesis in rats, mice, and hamsters (Rogers, 1977a; Smith *et al.*, 1975b).

IV. STEROID HORMONES

The hormones of significance in this group are the sex steroids. The major adrenocortical hormones may contribute to increased tumor inci-

dence in immunosuppressed patients, but no significant primary carcinogenic activity has been demonstrated for them. Natural and synthetic estrogens are carcinogenic in experimental animals, and there is
strong epidemiologic evidence that estrogens are carcinogenic in
women. Evidence was reported for transplacental carcinogenesis in the
vagina by diethylstilbestrol (Herbst *et al.*, 1971) and for endometrial
carcinogenesis in patients with gonadal dysgenesis treated with the same
compound (Cutler *et al.*, 1972). There have been several reports in the
past year of increased endometrial carcinoma in women exposed during
menopause to one or more estrogen preparations (Mack *et al.*, 1975,
1976; Smith *et al.*, 1975; Ziel and Finkle, 1975). The evidence has promoted publication of several cautionary notes regarding therapeutic use
of estrogens (Federal Drug Administration, 1976; Ryan, 1975; Weiss,
1975). Contraceptive estrogen usage by young women has been associated with development of hepatoma in a few cases, an association
considered significant because of the rarity of the tumor (Edmondson *et
al.*, 1976; Nissen *et al.*, 1975). There have been several studies of breast
cancer incidence in users and nonusers of estrogens, but no significant
association has been found (Boston Collaborative Drug Surveillance
Program, 1974c; Vessey *et al.*, 1975).

In rodents, several different forms of estrogen are carcinogenic for
mammary gland, uterus, ovary, and pituitary (Ershoff, 1964; Lemon,
1975; Leonard, 1973). Diethylstilbestrol induces renal carcinoma in male
hamsters (Hamilton *et al.*, 1975). Interactions with pituitary prolactin
secretion may be prominent (Hamilton *et al.*, 1975; Leonard, 1973).
Both prolactin and endogenous estrogens are major conditioning factors
for growth and development of mammary tumors, either chemically
induced or occurring spontaneously in rodents (Meites, 1972; Quadri *et
al.*, 1974; Sinha *et al.*, 1973). Estrogens can be anticarcinogenic in female
rodents treated with other chemicals carcinogenic for mammary gland
(Lemon, 1975; Shellabarger and Soo, 1973) and in males treated with
AFB_1 to induce liver tumors (Newberne and Williams, 1969).

The complexity of interactions between hormones or between hormones and chemical carcinogens in tumor induction and the further
complexities added by nutritional effects on hormone secretion combine
to discourage experimental studies in this area. Epidemiologic studies
indicate a role for diet in etiology of breast, uterine and ovarian cancer
and point to a need for increased understanding of nutritional effects on
hormone secretion, metabolism, and activity, particularly the gonadal
and pituitary hormones. Geographic variations in breast cancer have
been linked to estrogen metabolism, age at menarche, age at first birth,
and body size (Berg, 1975a; deWaard, 1975; Lipsett, 1975; MacMahon,

1975; Zumoff et al., 1975). To some extent endometrial and ovarian cancer follow the same epidemiologic patterns (Berg, 1975a). Nutrition in childhood and perhaps even during gestation influences both age at menarche and body size and is probably a major factor in development of the endocrine-dependent cancers (Frisch and McArthur, 1974).

Breast cancer is influenced by nutritional and endocrine events relatively early in life. This may be the reason that as yet no significant effect of contraceptive hormone therapy on breast cancer incidence has been found and suggests that no conclusions as to safety can be reached until cohorts of women exposed early in life have been followed for their life span (Vessey et al., 1975). Endometrial susceptibility to carcinogenesis may be determined later in life as is suggested by the increased incidence in diabetics and women treated with estrogens for menopausal symptoms (Mack et al., 1976). Hormonal and morphologic correlates in the menstrual cycle are established, but nutritional effects on them are not known except under conditions of virtual starvation and extreme weight loss (Frisch and McArthur, 1974; Owen, 1975). Studies of effects of dietary changes, such as those conjectured to be the basis of geographic differences in cancer incidence, on hormone metabolism in women have not been reported and should be performed.

In experimental animals there is considerable evidence that diet influences mammary tumor induction by chemical carcinogens, e.g., DMBA and AAF, but experimental studies of dietary effects on hormonal induction of mammary or other endocrine-dependent tumors or on hormone secretion, metabolism, and activity are lacking. Ershoff (1964) presented evidence which suggested that natural ingredient diets are protective against estrogen-induced ovarian and uterine tumors in rats when compared to purified diets. Natural ingredient diets protect rats against AAF or DMBA induction of mammary tumors (Carroll, 1975; Commoner et al., 1970; Engel and Copeland, 1952a). Increasing dietary fat increases the incidence and decreases the latent period for spontaneous mammary tumors in C_3H and DBA mice, and obesity in C_3H mice overcomes the inhibitory effect on tumor development of castration (Silverstone and Tannenbaum, 1950; Waxler and Leef, 1966). Severe caloric or protein restriction decreases mammary tumor development in rats and mice and is associated with decreased secretion of estrogen and pituitary hormones. In rats, DMBA mammary carcinogenesis is significantly enhanced by diets high in vegetable fat (Carroll, 1975).

Although dietary fat content has been correlated positively with mammary tumor induction by chemical carcinogens in several studies, effects of dietary protein have not been consistent, probably because of variable effects of protein on body growth (Carroll, 1975; Shay et al.,

1964). The quality of protein fed could influence tumor growth and explain differences between natural ingredient diets based on vegetable protein and purified diets based on casein; however no significant difference is found in the induction of mammary tumors by DMBA between rats fed soy protein and rats fed casein (Carroll, 1975). Dietary supplementation with a single amino acid, arginine, decreases DMBA mammary carcinogenesis in rats without affecting body weight gain. Arginine decreases tumor induction or growth in other model systems as well (Takeda *et al.*, 1975).

Interactions of dietary protein and lipid, lipid metabolism, and chemical mammary carcinogenesis have been demonstrated in protein- and lipotrope-deficient rats in which DMBA tumor induction is markedly inhibited despite a high level of dietary fat (Tanaka and Dao, 1965). The effect is opposite to the effect of feeding an adequate diet high in fat as reported and reviewed by Carroll (1975), probably because of abnormalities of carcinogen metabolism and hormone metabolism induced by the combined dietary deficiencies. In our studies of rats fed the marginally lipotrope-deficient, high fat diet, DMBA carcinogenesis is inhibited; there is no significant effect of the diet on body weight or weight or morphology of ovaries and pituitary.

The dietary effect on AAF mammary carcinogenesis is less consistent but some retardation of tumor induction occurs in deficient rats. Addition of beef fat to the control adequate diet to equal the fat content of the deficient diet also retards mammary tumor induction although it increases body weight gain (Rogers, 1977c; Table III). This suggests that the kind as well as the level of dietary fat may be important. Carroll's

TABLE III
Tumors Induced in Rats Fed Adequate (Diet 1) or Marginally Lipotrope-Deficient (Diet 2) Diets Containing AAF

| | | Percentage of rats with carcinoma of | | |
Diet	Number of rats	Mammary gland	Liver	Zymbal's gland
Sprague-Dawley female rats				
1	31	65	0	6
2	32	41	0	6
Fischer female rats				
1	25	0	36	8
2	25	8	72	0
Sprague-Dawley male rats				
1	21	0	19	5
2	27	0	41	11

studies and most studies cited in his review (1975) utilized vegetable oils although in some experiments lard or hydrogenated vegetable fats were studied. In a recent study, tumor induction by DMBA was significantly increased in rats fed 20% corn oil compared to rats fed 5% corn oil. Administration of either antiestrogenic or antiprolactin compounds decreased tumor incidence, and the antiprolactin compound abolished the dietary effect (Chan and Cohen, 1974). The authors suggest that high fat diets stimulate tumor induction by stimulating prolactin secretion.

In summary, extreme dietary changes which markedly modify body weight gain and sexual maturation alter induction of mammary tumors in rodents by chemical carcinogens; the direction of the change in tumor incidence generally parallels the change in body weight. The relationship can be shown by altering either caloric or protein intake. Effects of less drastic dietary changes are variable but may be more pertinent to human disease. Dietary protein, specific amino acids, or lipotropes can influence tumor induction or development. Investigation of interactions of the nutrient changes with hormonal secretion and metabolism may clarify some of the effects. Interactions between diet and induction of mammary and other tumors by estrogens have not been studied but may be of great significance. Estrogen carcinogenesis in the endometrium of rodents has been demonstrated but not intensively studied. Epidemiologic evidence in people makes it imperative to do so and to investigate dietary effects in animal models for endometrial tumors.

Association between occurrence of liver tumors and either androgen or estrogen treatment has been reported in humans (Edmondson et al., 1976; Farrell et al., 1975; Meadows et al., 1974; Nissen et al., 1975). The estrogen-induced tumors reported to date have been histologically benign, but several have bled massively; some androgen-induced tumors have been malignant. Because of the liver's central role in hormone metabolism and its sensitivity to dietary changes, investigation of effects of hormonal carcinogens on liver under different dietary conditions will be of interest.

One further source of concern with respect to carcinogenicity of estrogens is the report from the Boston Collaborative Drug Surveillance Program (1974c) of increased cholelithiasis in patients exposed to exogenous estrogens. Gall stones are the major risk factor associated with biliary tract cancer and are associated also with increased caloric intake and obesity (Fraumeni, 1975). Endometrial cancer is associated with a history of gallbladder disease (Mack et al., 1976). Thus a combination of factors already implicated in endometrial cancer, i.e., exposure to exogenous estrogens, excessive caloric intake, and obesity (MacMahon, 1974) may result also in increased biliary tract cancer.

V. AGENTS ACTIVE IN THE NERVOUS SYSTEM

This group of drugs has been implicated in induction of lymphoreticular, renal, and mammary tumors, and in stimulation of growth of malignant melanoma in humans. In the cases of amphetamine, diphenylhydantoin, and reserpine, positive epidemiologic studies have been countered by comparable negative studies; in the case of phenacetin, epidemiologic evidence is derived primarily from one geographic area in which special conditions of exposure exist, and there is no report of its carcinogenicity in general therapeutic usage.

A significant relationship between recent amphetamine use and onset of Hodgkin's disease was found by Newell *et al.* (1973) but not by the Boston Collaborative Drug Surveillance Program (1974a). The two studies were performed in different areas and populations and differed somewhat in methodology. A major difference is that amphetamine use by both patients and controls was much greater in Newell's study than in the Boston study. Exposure history was evaluated only for 2 years or less prior to onset of disease which is probably a relatively brief period for carcinogenesis in humans, and its significance must be questioned. A positive history for the period covered may be considered to indicate a longer duration of exposure.

There are conflicting reports on carcinogenicity of diphenylhydantoin, in many cases combined with phenobarbital, in patients with epilepsy. Autopsy and clinical studies of patients with lymphoma have demonstrated a significant association with diphenylhydantoin exposure (Anthony, 1970; Li *et al.*, 1975). There are in addition several published case reports (reviewed in Li *et al.*, 1975). However in 9136 epileptic patients treated for many years with diphenylhydantoin and phenobarbital, there was no increase in lymphoreticular tumors (Clemmesen *et al.*, 1974). There was a small increase in liver tumors, but it was not statistically significant (Clemmesen, 1975; Schneiderman, 1974).

Diphenylhydantoin induces lymphoreticular tumors in mice (Kruger and Harris, 1972); phenobarbital induces hepatic tumors in mice (Thorpe and Walker, 1973; Jones and Butler, 1975). Phenobarbital has interesting properties as a cocarcinogen in rat liver. When given simultaneously with either AAF or DENA, it decreases the effective carcinogenicity of both compounds, but if it is given after carcinogen treatment it increases induction of liver tumors (Peraino *et al.*, 1971, 1975; Weisburger *et al.*, 1975b). Diphenylhydantoin given after AAF treatment does not affect induction of liver tumors (Peraino *et al.*, 1975).

Reserpine usage was associated with increased breast cancer incidence in women in three studies published in 1974 (Armstrong *et al.*, 1974;

Boston Collaborative Drug Surveillance Program, 1974b; Heinonen *et al.*, 1974), but subsequent studies demonstrated no association (Laska *et al.*, 1975; Mack *et al.*, 1975; O'Fallon *et al.*, 1975). A recent evaluation of all the evidence led to the conclusion that the association was unproved and probably not of significance (Editorial, 1975).

Phenacetin is an aromatic amine chemically related to the known carcinogens β-naphthylamine and certain fluorenes including AAF. It has been associated with tumors of the renal pelvis or urinary bladder in patients who had chronically taken overdoses of compounds which contained caffeine and phenazone in addition to phenacetin (Johansson *et al.*, 1974). Most of the cases have been reported from Sweden but there are case reports from other areas as well (reviewed in Johansson *et al.*, 1974). The question has been raised of the contribution of caffeine and phenazone to carcinogenicity of phenacetin-containing compounds (Editorial, 1969); further epidemiologic and experimental studies are required to established the carcinogenicity of the analgesic compounds. Urinary tract tumors associated with phenacetin-containing compounds have occurred in people who had renal damage and malfunction. An effect of dose on phenacetin metabolism has been reported (Raaflaub and Dubach, 1969). The patients may have been exposed to metabolites which do not appear in significant quantities in normal humans or have smoked or used other drugs. Cocarcinogenic effects of tobacco smoke or caffeine may be significant (Schmauz and Cole, 1974). At this time definite assessment of the carcinogenic risk to normal humans of therapeutic phenacetin use cannot be made.

Aromatic amines are carcinogenic for humans (Fraumeni, 1975) and experimental animals, and dietary effects on their carcinogenicity and metabolism have been studied using AAF as the model compound. AAF is hydroxylated and sulfated in the liver; the sulfate ester of N-OH-AAF is thought to be the ultimate hepatic carcinogen; other derivatives may be active in mammary gland and other tissues (De Baun *et al.*, 1970; Weisburger *et al.*, 1972; Gutman *et al.*, 1972). Rats fed natural ingredient diets are protected against AAF carcinogenesis compared to rats fed purified diets (Commoner *et al.*, 1970; Engel and Copeland, 1952a). Varying casein levels in the diet do not have a consistent effect; extremely high levels (60%) decrease mammary and hepatic tumor induction in most experiments in female rats. Supplementation of the 60% casein diet with vitamin B_{12} and folate probably enhances mammary tumor induction, which is further evidence for a role of 1-carbon metabolism in carcinogenesis (Engel and Copeland, 1952b). As discussed above, the interactions between dietary lipotropes and AAF carcinogenesis are complex; diets deficient in lipotropes depress mammary tumor induction by AAF in female rats. In contrast, induction of hepatic tumors in male or female rats is enhanced by lipotrope deficiency and depressed by addition of lipotropes to an adequate diet (Miller and Miller, 1972; Rogers, 1975). Lipotrope deficiency alters AAF metabolism as indicated by excretion of metabolites in the urine, and this may be the mechanism for alterating its carcinogenicity (Poirier *et al.*, 1977).

Urinary tract carcinogenesis by aromatic amines is susceptible to dietary influence. Induction of bladder tumors is increased by addition of tryptophan or indole to the diet of rats, or addition of indole but not trypotophan to the diet of hamsters (Dunning *et al.*, 1950; Oyasu *et al.*, 1972). Deficiency of vitamin B_6 may enhance bladder tumor induction in rats (Miyakawa *et al.*, 1973). The dietary alteration depressed food and AAF intake, decreased induction of hepatic tumors, and prolonged life span. Increased bladder tumor incidence may have been due to these effects rather than to specific cocarcinogenic effects. However bladder tumors are rarely found in rats fed AAF in adequate and balanced diets.

Dibenamine, an α-adrenergic blocking agent, has not been related to tumors in humans but is both carcinogenic and anticarcinogenic in rats. It decreases hepatocarcinoma induction by DENA but induces tumors at the injection site or in the intestine (Weisburger *et al.*, 1974).

L-Dopa has been associated temporally with activation of malignant melanoma in several patients, and the question has been raised of its stimulatory effects on the tumor because it is incorporated into melanin (Lieberman and Shupack, 1974). It has not been associated with induction of tumors.

The agents discussed in this section are all amines active in the nervous system. Although in most cases their carcinogenicity is not established, evidence suggests that some, at least, are weak carcinogens in humans or experimental animals. The possibility of nitrosation of amines with formation of carcinogenic nitrosamines has been raised by several investigators particularly with respect to drugs (Berg, 1975b; Wogan *et al.*, 1975). The nitrosation product of ephedrine, which is pharmacologically and chemically related to amphetamine, is carcinogenic for mice (Wogan *et al.*, 1975). Nitrosation of many compounds by dietary nitrite has been demonstrated *in vivo* with formation of toxic and/or carcinogenic substances (Mirvish, 1975; Newberne and Shank, 1973). Dietary alterations which reduce nitrosation as well as reduction of dietary nitrite may be useful in reducing carcinogenic risks of these compounds. Ascorbic acid reduces nitrosation *in vitro* and *in vivo* (Mirvish, 1975). Effects of other dietary components have not been demonstrated.

VI.   ANTIBACTERIAL AND ANTIPARASITIC AGENTS

Chloramphenicol, like the antitumor agents, is toxic to hematopoietic cells and may be carcinogenic for them (H. J. Cohen and Huang, 1973; Fraumeni 1967). The number of cases of leukemia reported in chloramphenicol-treated patients is small, but their association with prior drug-induced aplastic anemia suggests that they are significant.

The nitrofurans are a large group of antibiotic compounds whose use has been prohibited or severely restricted because of their carcinogenicity in several organs and several animal species. Human tumors have not been associated with them. The compounds are useful experimentally in investigation of structure–activity relationships in carcinogenesis and in studies of nutrient effects on bladder carcinogenesis. Vitamin A deficiency enhances tumor induction by a nitrofuran in rats but hypervitaminosis A is no more protective than adequate dietary vitamin A (S. M. Cohen *et al.*, 1974). Lipotrope deficiency has no effect (Rogers, 1975). Studies of the effect of dietary protein and other nutrients discussed above which influence AAF induction of bladder tumor on nitrofuran carcinogenesis may be helpful in elucidation of general nutrient effects on bladder and other urinary tract cancer.

Isonicotinic acid hydrazide, which is listed in this group, was discussed above.

5-Nitroimidazoles are carcinogenic in mice and mutagenic for bacteria (Rustia and Shubik, 1972; Speck *et al.*, 1976; Voogd *et al.*, 1974). No human tumors have been associated with their use, but they are of concern because they or their mutagenic metabolites appear in urine of treated humans (Speck *et al.*, 1976). The significance of mutagenicity thus demonstrated is not known, but its observation raises questions of safety. Dietary effects on activity of this group of compounds have not been described.

VII.   AGENTS FOR TREATMENT OF DERMATOLOGIC
DISEASES

Carcinogenicity of arsenic, which has been used in the past in human and veterinary medicine for treatment of dermatologic and systemic diseases and as a nonspecific tonic, has been strongly suggested in humans by association of tumors with agricultural or industrial exposure; carcinogenicity has not been demonstrated in experimental animals (Cole and Goldman, 1975; Lee and Fraumeni, 1969). Development of skin tumors in patients treated with arsenic was reported in 1888, and case reports have continued to appear up to the present (Morris et al., 1974). Chronic liver disease and hepatic angiosarcomas were found in patients exposed occupationally to arsenic; rare cases of angiosarcoma have been reported in association with its medicinal use (Lander et al., 1975). As with vinyl chloride-induced hepatic angiosarcomas, there may be an enhancement of susceptibility to arsenical carcinogenesis by alcohol intake, but dietary studies have not been reported.

Known carcinogens in coal tar preparations are the polycyclic aromatic hydrocarbons which are carcinogenic for skin, respiratory tract, gastrointestinal tract and mammary gland in experimental animals. Their importance in industrial, tobacco, and urban air carcinogenesis is great and has been reviewed (Pike et al., 1975). The hydrocarbons are used extensively in experimental carcinogenesis. Therapeutic use of hydrocarbons occurs in coal tar preparations applied directly to the skin, a route by which the compounds are carcinogenic in experimental animals and have been reported to be carcinogenic in humans (Rook et al., 1956), but other studies have demonstrated no association (Higginson, 1966; Swanbeck and Hellström 1971). Relationships between structure, carcinogenicity, and mutagenicity have been reviewed (Fahmy and Fahmy, 1973).

Dietary influences on hydrocarbon carcinogenesis at several sites including skin have been extensively studied. In the absence of dietary lipotrope deficiency, high fat diets enhance hydrocarbon carcinogenesis in skin and mammary gland (Carroll, 1975). Vitamin A inhibits hydrocarbon tumor induction in the upper gastrointestinal tract of hamsters and may influence respiratory tract carcinogenesis but the effects are not consistent. (Chu and Malmgren, 1965; Saffiotti et al., 1967; Smith et al., 1975a,b). Riboflavin-deficient mice are more susceptible to hydrocarbon induction of skin tumors than mice fed diets adequate or excessive in riboflavin (Wynder and Chan, 1970).

Solar irradiation is strongly associated with squamous carcinoma of the skin in humans and less strongly with basal cell tumors and malignant melanoma (Emmett, 1973). Tumor induction in experimental animals can be increased or decreased by administration of photoactive compounds (Emmett, 1973; O'Neal and Griffin, 1957; Joseph-Bravo et al., 1976). These include polycyclic aromatic hydrocarbons, discussed above, and vitamin A and riboflavin. The effect of the hydrocarbons is dose-dependent (Emmett, 1973; Clark, 1964). Utilization of vitamin A or other carotenoid absorption of UV light may be useful in modifying carcinogenic risks of actinic radiation to the skin or even in enhancing UV breakdown of circulating carcinogens (Newberne et al., 1974;

Joseph-Bravo *et al.*, 1976). Careful assessment is required because there is some evidence that vitamin A may enhance tumor induction in squamous epithelium (Polliack and Levij, 1967, 1969). Serum riboflavin drops rapidly in animals exposed to UV irradiation; increased riboflavin intake decreases AFB_1 carcinogenicity for the liver in light-exposed but not normal rats (Joseph-Bravo *et al.*, 1976). Investigation of riboflavin effects on UV carcinogenesis is needed.

VIII. DISCUSSION

Dietary effects on chemical carcinogenesis are often subtle, may be inconsistent, and are in most cases poorly understood. They do however offer promise in prevention of tumor induction in people for whom carcinogen exposure cannot be reduced or eliminated because the carcinogens are not known, cannot be eliminated from the environment, or offer benefits which may outweigh the risk of tumor development. Several useful drugs fall into the last category and have been specifically discussed.

There are some generalizations which can be made with respect to dietary effects on chemical carcinogenesis in experimental animals which may be useful even if an effect on tumor induction by a particular drug has not been demonstrated. They are listed below.

1. Deficiency of certain specific nutrients, e.g., vitamin A, riboflavin, lipotropes (methionine, choline, folate) tends to increase tumor induction provided the deficiency is not so severe that weight gain is greatly reduced.

2. Increased antioxidant content of the diet tends to decrease tumor induction.

3. Diets composed of natural ingredients, tend to decrease tumor induction compared to purified diets composed of refined ingredients.

4. Increased caloric intake leading to increased growth and body weight tends to increase tumor induction and development.

5. Increase in the relative amount of fat in the diet tends to increase tumor induction.

The extent to which these points apply to chemical carcinogenesis varies and exceptions to each one can be found. Nutritional effects on metabolism of carcinogens, hormones, and other chemicals are extensive and undoubtedly contribute to dietary alterations of tumor induction as do nutritional effects on target organ susceptibility arising from alteration of cell division, differentiation, DNA repair, and carcinogen uptake.

There are recent reviews of the nutrient effects listed (Apffel, 1976; Bollag, 1970; Carroll, 1975; Maugh, 1974; Rogers, 1977a; Ross and Bras, 1973; Rogers and Newberne, 1975; Rivlin, 1973; Wattenberg, 1975). While general dietary changes, such as decreasing caloric and fat intake, may be recommended appropriately for many population groups as a measure to alter the epidemiology of occurrence of certain tumors and other diseases, elucidation of specific nutrient interactions with specific chemicals or drugs may allow more effective measures in cases of unavoidable exposure.

Vitamin A in doses far in excess of the nutritional requirement reduces tumor induction by polycyclic aromatic hydrocarbons in the upper gastrointestinal tract or skin of hamsters (Chu and Malmgren, 1965; Saffiotti et al., 1967; Smith et al., 1975a,b). Therefore it is effective under conditions in which it can be applied directly in large amounts to carcinogen-treated squamous epithelium and is anticarcinogenic even if applied after carcinogen treatment. Although it has been reported to be effective also in the respiratory tract (Saffiotti et al., 1967), results have not been consistent, and enhancement of tumor development has been found in some experiments (Smith et al., 1975a,b). Enhancement of tumor induction was found also in hamster cheek pouch (Polliack and Levij, 1967, 1969). Vitamin A deficiency enhances colon tumor induction by AFB_1 and perhaps by DMH but not by N-methyl, N-nitronitroso guanidine (MNNG) (Narisawa et al., 1976; Newberne and Rogers, 1973; Rogers, 1975; Rogers and Newberne, 1975; Rogers et al., 1973). Hypervitaminosis A has no effect.

Riboflavin deficiency enhances cutaneous carcinogenesis in mice and induction of hepatic tumors by azo dyes in rats. The protective effect probably is the result of maintenance of normal tissue levels of the flavin coenzymes (Rivlin, 1973). In its interactions with UV irradiation and chemical carcinogenesis, riboflavin may form a complex with the carcinogen and enhance its photochemical breakdown (Joseph-Bravo et al., 1976).

Lipotropes have long been known to influence hepatic carcinogenesis by chemically different compounds, and one of the lipotropes, methionine, may be responsible for some of the effects on carcinogenesis of dietary protein level. Supplementation of the marginally lipotrope-deficient diet referred to above has yielded complex and sometimes surprising results (Rogers, 1977b). When DENA carcinogenesis is compared in rats fed an adequate, casein-based diet or the marginally lipotrope-deficient diet based on peanut meal, deficient rats invariably develop a higher incidence of hepatocarcinoma than adequately fed rats. If the lipotrope deficiency is corrected using choline alone, the dietary effect on tumor induction is not corrected. If all three lipotropes, choline, methionine, and folate, or six amino acids including methionine, in which peanut meal is deficient, are added to the diet, hepatocarcinoma induction decreases almost to the level in rats fed the adequate diet; life span increases, but rats develop a high incidence of hepatic hemangiosarcoma.

Antioxidant inhibition of carcinogenesis may be one of mechanisms by which natural ingredient diets decrease chemical carcinogenesis. The food antioxidants BHA and BHT reduce tumor induction by polycyclic aromatic hydrocarbons in the gastrointestinal tract or mammary gland of rats and mice and also reduce induction of hepatocarcinoma by AAF in rats (Ulland, *et al.* 1973; Wattenberg, 1972, Table IV). A mixture of antioxidants fed to mice reduced UV skin carcinogenesis (Black, 1974). Sulfhydryl compounds counteract the toxicity and carcinogenicity of chemicals and of X-irradiation through their antioxidant or nucleophilic reactions, directly or via glutathione (GSH), and possibly also through a controlling or permissive effect on cell division (Harington, 1967; Apffel, 1976; Wattenberg, 1974). Tissue GSH levels tend to increase during carcinogen treatment (Harington, 1967; Poirier *et al.*, 1977). Sulfhydryl compounds vary in their ability to block toxicity and carcinogenicity of chemicals and may not block both effects. Several sulfhydryl compounds blocked induction of mammary tumors and adrenal necrosis by DMBA in rats, but cysteamine blocked only tumor induction (Marquardt *et al.*, 1974; Wattenberg, 1974).

TABLE IV

Inhibition of Chemical Carcinogenesis in Rats Given BHT

Carcinogen	Reference	Target organ	Percentage of rats with tumor	
			BHT	0
Sprague-Dawley female rats				
DMBA	Wattenberg, 1972	Mammary gland	28	80
N-OH-AAF	Ulland *et al.*, 1973	Mammary gland	40	80
AAF		Mammary gland	35	20
Sprague-Dawley male rats				
AAF		Liver	20	70
N-OH-AAF		Liver	15	60
Fischer male rats				
AAF		Liver	13	90
N-OH-AAF		Liver	50	64

Enhancement of tumor induction has been reported in rats treated with sulfate. Since AAF must be hydroxylated and sulfated to be active, increased availability of sulfate might be expected to enhance its carcinogenicity and has been shown to do so (Weisburger *et al.*, 1972). Azo dye carcinogenesis is enhanced by dietary sulfate (Blunck and Crowther, 1975). Manipulation of dietary and tissue antioxidant and sulfur content may alter the carcinogenicity of some of the drugs discussed and should be investigated.

The other general nutrient effects listed have been discussed above.

There are many questions in this area on which further studies are needed. The carcinogenicity of drugs is a potentially serious hazard which must be defined in experimental animals as carefully as possible and followed up by studies in people exposed for therapeutic reasons. Establishment of nutrient effects on carcinogenesis and elucidation of responsible mechanisms are major research needs in development of measures for protection of humans from unavoidable carcinogenic hazards. The two groups of carcinogenic drugs from which protection is most urgently needed are antitumor agents and steroid sex hormones. Studies of dietary effects on their carcinogenicity and also on cell division and hormone secretion and metabolism may provide information on which protective dietary measures can be based.

ACKNOWLEDGMENT

The author's studies discussed in this chapter were supported in part by NIH-NCI contract NO1-CP-33238.

REFERENCES

Andervont, H. B. (1950). Studies on occurrence of spontaneous hepatomas in mice of strains C3H and CBA. *J. Natl. Cancer Inst.* **11**, 581–592.

Anthony, J. J. (1970). Malignant lymphoma associated with hydantoin drugs. *Arch. Neurol. (Chicago)* **22**, 450–454.

Apffel, C. A. (1976). Nonimmunological host defenses: A review. *Cancer Res.* **36**, 1527–1537.

Armstrong, B., Stevens, N., and Doll, R. (1974). Retrospective study of the association between use of Rauwolfia derivatives and breast cancer in English women. *Lancet* **2**, 672–675.

Arsenau, J. C., Sponzo, R. W., Levin, D. L., Schnipper, L. E., Bonner, H., Young, R. C., Canellos, G. P., Johnson, R. E., DeVita, V. T., 1972. Non-lymphomatons malignant tumors complicating Hodgkin's Disease. Possible association with intensive therapy. *N. Engl. J. Med.* **287**: 1119–1122.

Bachur, N. R. (1975). Adriamycin (NSC-123127) pharmacology. *Cancer Chemother. Rep., Part 3* **6**, 153–158.

Bailin, P. L., Jindale, J. P., Roenigk, H. H., and Hogan, M. D. (1974). Is methotrerate therapy for psoriasis carcinogenic? *J. Am. Med. Assoc.* **232**, 359–362.

Beal, D. D., Skibba, J. C., Croft, W. A., Cohen, S. M., and Bryan, G. T. (1975). Carcinogenicity of the antineoplastic agent, 5-(3,3-dimethyltriazene)-imidazole-4-carboxamide, and its metabolites in rats. *J. Natl. Cancer Inst.* **54**, 951–957.

Ben-Yaakor, M., Meshorer, A., and Haran-Ghera, N. (1975). Enhancement and retardation of spontaneous reticulum cell neoplasm development in SJL/J mice. *J. Natl. Cancer. Inst.* **54**, 443–448.

Berg, J. W. (1975a). Can nutrition explain the pattern of international epidemilogy of hormone-dependent cancers? *Cancer Res.* **35**, 3345–3350.

Berg, J. W. (1975b). Diet. *In* "Persons at High Risk of Cancer; An Approach to Cancer Etiology and Control", (J. F. Fraumeni, Jr., ed.), Chapter 13, pp. 201–224. Academic Press, New York.

Bertazzoli, C., Chieli, T., and Solcia, E. (1971). Different incidence of breats carcinomas or fibroadenomas in daunomycin or adriamycin treated rats. *Experientia* **27**, 1209–1210.

Bertino, J. R., and Nixon, P. F. (1969). Nutritional Factors in the design of more selective anti-tumor agents. *Cancer Res.* **29**, 2417–2421.

Black, H. S. (1974). Effects of dietary antioxidants on actinic tumor induction. *Res. Commun Chem. Pathol. Pharmacol.* **7**, 783–786.

Blum, H. F. (1959). "Carcinogenesis by Ultraviolet Light." Princeton Univ. Press, Princeton, New Jersey.

Blunck, J. M., and Crowther, C. E. (1975). Enhancement of azo dye carcinogenesis by dietary sodium sulphate. *Eur. J. Cancer* **11**, 23–31.

Bollag, W. (1970). Vitamin A and vitamin A acid in the prophylaxis and therapy of epithelial tumours. *Int. J. Vitam. Nutr. Res.* **40**, 300–314.

Boston Collaborative Drug Surveillance Program (1974a). Amphetamines and malignant lymphoma. *J. Am. Med. Assoc.* **229**, 1462–1463.

Boston Collaborative Drug Surveillance Program. (1974b). Reserpine and breast cancer. *Lancet* **2**, 669–671.

Boston Collaborative Drug Surveillance Program. (1974c). Surgically confirmed gallbladder disease, venous thromboembolism, and breast tumors in relation to postmenopausal estrogen therapy. *N. Engl. J. Med.* **290**, 15–19.

Boyd, J. T., and Doll, R. (1954). Gastro-intestinal cancer and the use of liquid paraffin. *Br. J. Cancer* **8**, 231–237.

Burstein, N. A., and Allison, A. C. (1970). Effect of antilymphocytic serum on the appearance of reticular neoplasma in SJL/J mice. *Nature* **225**: 1139–1140.

Campbell, T. C., and Hayes, J. R. (1974). Role of nutrition in the drug-metabolizing enzyme system. *Pharmacol. Rev.* **26**, 171–197.

Carroll, K. K. (1975). Experimental evidence of dietary factors and hormone-dependent cancers. *Cancer Res.* **35**, 3374–3383.

Chan, P. C., and Cohen, L. A. (1974). Effect of dietary fat; antiestrogen, and antiprolactin on the development of mammary tumors in rats. *J. Natl. Cancer Inst.* **52**, 25–30.

Chu, E. W., and Malmgren, R. A. (1965). An inhibitory effect of vitamin A on the induction of tumors of forestomach and cervix in the Syrian hamster by carcinogenic polycyclic hydrocarbons. *Cancer Res.* **25**, 884–895.

Clark, J. H. (1964). The effect of long ultraviolet radiation on the development of tumors induced by 20-methycholanthrene. *Cancer Res.* **24**, 207–210.

Clemmesen, J., Fuglsang-Fredericksen, V. and Plum, C. M. (1974). Are anticonvulsants oncogenic? *Lancet* **1**, 705–707.

Clemmesen, J. (1975). Phenobarbitone, liver tumors and thorotrast. *Lancet* **1**, 37–38.

Cohen, H. J., Huang, A. T.-F., (1973). A marker chromosome abnormality. *Arch. Intern. Med.* **132**, 440–443.

Cohen, S. M., Lower, G. M., Jr., Erturk, E., and Bryan, G. T. (1973). Comparative carcinogenicity in Swiss mice of N-[4-(5-nitro-2-furyl) - 2 thiazolyl] acetamide and structurally related 5-nitrofurans and 4-nitrobenzenes. *Cancer Res.* **33**, 1593–1597.

Cohen, S. M., Wittenburg, J. F., and Bryan, G. T. (1974). *Fed. Proc., Fed. Am. Soc. Exp. Biol.* **33**, 2208.

Cohen, S. M., Erturk, E., von Esch, A. M., Cronetti, A. J., and Bryan, G. T. (1975). Carcinogenicity of 5-nitrofurans and related compounds with amino-heterocyclic substituents. *J. Natl. Cancer Inst.* **54**, 841–850.

Cole, P., and Goldman, M. B. (1975). Occupation. *In* "Persons at High Risk of Cancer: An Approach to Cancer Etiology and Control" (J. F. Fraumeni, Jr., ed.), Chapter 11, pp. 167–184. Academic Press, New York.

Commoner, B., Moolum, J. C., Senturia, B. H., Jr., and Jernberg, J. L. (1970). The effects of 2-acetylaminofluorene and nitrite on free radicals and carcinogenesis in rat liver. *Cancer Res.* **30**, 2091–2097.

Craddock, V. M., and Frei, J. V. (1974). Induction of liver cell adenomata in the rat by a single treatment with N-methyl-N-nitrosourea given at various times after partial hepatectomy. *Br. J. Cancer* **30**, 503–511.

Croft, W. A., and Bryan, G. T. (1973). Production of urinary bladder carcinomas in male hamsters by N-(4-(5-Nitro-2furyl) -2thiazolyl) formamide, N-(4-(5-nitro-2-furyl)-2 thiazolyl)-acetamide, or formic acid 2-(4-5-nitro-2-furyl)-2 thiazolyl) hydrazide. *J. Natl. Cancer Inst.* **51**, 941–949.

Cutler, B. S., Forbes, A. P., Ingersoll, F. M., and Scully, R. E. (1972). Endometrial carcinoma after stilbestrol therapy in gonadal dysgenesis. *N. Engl. J. Med.* **287**, 628–630.

De Baun, J. R., Miller, E. C., and Miller, J. A. (1970). N-Hydroxy-2-acetylaminofluorene Sulfotransferase: Its probable role in carcinogenesis and in protein-(methion-S-yl) binding in rat liver. *Cancer Res.* **30**, 577–595.

de Waard, F. (1975). Breast cancer incidence and nutritional status with particular reference to body weight and height. *Cancer Res.* **35**, 3351–3356.

Druckrey, H. (1970). Production of colonic carcinomas by 1,2-dialkylhydrazines and azoxyalkanes. *In* "Carcinoma of the Colon and Antecedent Epithelium," ed. Burdette, W. J., Chap. 20, 267–279. Chas C. Thomas Springfield.

Dunn, T. B., and Green, A. W. (1963). Cysts of the epididymis, cancer of the cervix, granular cell myoblastoma, and other lesions after estrogen injection in newborn mice. *J. Natl. Cancer Inst.* **31**, 425–455.

Dunning, W. F., Curtis, M. R., and Maun, M. E. (1950). The effect of added dietary tryptophan on the occurrence of 2-acetylaminofluorene-induced liver and bladder cancer in rats. *Cancer Res.* **10**, 454–459.

Editorial. (1969). Analgesic Abuse and Tumors of the renal pelvis. *Lancet* **2**, 1233–1234.

Editorial. (1975). Rauwolfia and breast cancer. *Lancet* **2**, 312–313.

Edmondson, H. A., Henderson, B. E., and Benton, B. (1976). Liver-cell adenomas associated with use of oral contraceptives. *N. Engl. J. Med.* **294**, 470–472.

Emmett, E. A. (1973). Ultraviolet radiation as a cause of skin tumors. *Crit. Rev. Toxicol.* 211–255.

Engel, R. W., and Copeland, D. H. (1952a). Protective action of stock diets against the cancer-inducing action of 2-acetylaminofluorene in rats. *Cancer Res.* **12**, 211–215.

Engel, R. W., and Copeland, D. H. (1952b). The influence of dietary casein level on tumor induction with 2-acetylaminofluorene. *Cancer Res.* **12**, 905–908.

Ershoff, B. H. (1964). Effects of diet on pituitary tumor induction by estrogens. *Exp. Med. Surg.* **22**, 28–32.

Ershoff, B. H., Bajawa, G. S., Field, J. B., and Bavetta, L. A. (1969). Comparative effects of purified diets and a natural food stock ration on the tumor incidence of mice exposed to multiple sublethal doses of total body X-irradiation. *Cancer Res.* **29**, 780–788.

Erturk, E., Cohen, S. M., Price, J. M., and Bryan, G. T. (1969). Pathogenesis, histology, and transplantability of urinary bladder carcinomas induced in albino rats by oral administration of N-(4-(5-nitro-2-furyl)-2-thiazolyl) formamide. *Cancer Res.* **29**, 2219–2228.

Fahmy, O. G., and Fahmy, M. J. (1973). Oxidative activation of benz(2)anthracene and methylated derivatives in mutagenesis and carcinogenesis. *Cancer Res.* **33**, 2354–2361.

Farrell, G. C., Uren, R. F., Perkins, K.W., Joshua, D. E., Baird, P. J., and Kronenburg, H. (1975). Androgen-induced hepatoma. *Lancet* **1**, 430–432.

Federal Drug Administration. (1976). Estrogens and endometrial cancer. *FDA Drug Bull.* **6**, 18–19.

Frankel, H. H., Yamamoto, R. S., Weisburger, E. K., and Weisburger, J. H. (1970). Chronic toxicity of azathioprine and the effect of this immunosuppressant on liver tumor induction by the carcinogen N-hydroxy-N-2-fluorenylacetamide. *Toxicol. Appl. Pharmacol.* **17**, 462–480.

Fraumeni, J. F., Jr. (1975). Respiratory carcinogenesis: An epidemiologic appraisal. *J. Natl. Cancer Inst.* **55**, 1039–1046.

Fraumeni, J. F., Jr. (1967). Bone marrow depression induced by chloramphenicol or phenylbutazone. Leukemia and other sequelae. *J. Am. Med. Assoc.* **201**, 828–834.

Freeman, R. G., Hudson, H. T., and Carnes, M. A. (1970). Ultraviolet wavelength factors in solar radiation and skin cancer. *Int. J. Dermatol.* **9**, 232–236.

Frisch, R. E., and McArthur, J. W. (1974). Menstrual cycles: Fatness as a determinant of minimum weight for height necessary for their maintenance and onset. *Science* **185**, 949–951.

Gillette, J. R. (1976). Environmental factors in drug metabolism. *Fed. Proc., Fed. Am. Soc. Exp. Biol.* **35**, 1142–1147.

Greenspan, E. M., Tung, B. G. (1974). Acute myeloblastic leukemia after cure of ovarian cancer. *J. Am. Med. Assoc.* **230**, 418–423.

Gunnarsson, R., Berne, C., and Hellerström, C. (1974). Cytotoxic effects of streptozotocin and N-nitrosomethylurea on the pancreatic B cells with special regard to the role of nicotinamide-adenine dinucleotide. *Biochem. J.* **140**, 487–494.

Gutmann, H. R., Malejka-Giganti, D., Barry, E. J., and Rydell, R. E. (1972). On the correlation between the hepatocarcinogenicity of the carcinogen, N-2-fluorenylacetamide, and its metabolic activation by the rat. *Cancer Res.* **32**, 1554–1561.

Hamilton, J. M., Flake, A., Saluja, P. G., and Maguire, S. (1975). Hormonally induced renal neoplasia in the male Syrian hamster and the inhibitory effect of 2-bromo-2-ergocryptine methanesulfonate. *J. Natl. Cancer Inst.* **54**, 1385–1400.

Hammond, E. C., Selikoff, I. J., and Robitzek, E. H. (1967). Isoniazid therapy in relation to later occurrence of cancer in adults and in infants. *Br. Med. J.* **2**, 792–795.

Hard, G. C., and Butler, W. H. (1970). Cellular analysis of renal neoplasia: Light microscope study of the development of interstitial lesions induced in the rat kidney by a single carcinogenic dose of DMN. *Cancer Res.* **30**, 2806–2815.

Harington, J. S. (1967). The sulfhydryl group and carcinogenesis. *Adv. Cancer Res.* **10**, 247–309.

Heinonen, O. P., Shapiro, S., Tuonimen, L., and Monson, R. R. (1974). Reserpine use in relation to breast cancer. *Lancet* **2**, 675-677.

Herbst, A., Ulfelder, H., and Poskanzer, D. C. (1971). Adenocarcinoma of the vagina: Association of maternal stillbestrol therapy with tumor appearance in young women. *N. Engl. J. Med.* **284**, 878-881.

Higginson, J. (1966). Etiological factors in gastrointestional cancer in man. *J. Natl. Cancer Inst.* **37**, 527-545.

Hoover, R., and Fraumeni, J. F., Jr. (1975a). Drugs. *In* "Persons at High Risk of Cancer: An Approach to Cancer Etiology and Control" (J. F. Fraumeni, Jr., ed.), Chapter 12, pp. 185-199. Academic Press, New York.

Hoover, R., and Fraumeni, J. F., Jr. (1975b). Drugs in clinical use which cause cancer. *J. Clin. Pharmacol.* **2**, 16-23.

Jablon, S. (1975). Radiation. *In* "Persons at High Risk of Cancer: An Approach to Cancer Etiology and Control" (J. F. Fraumeni, Jr., ed.), Chapter 10, pp. 151-165. Academic Press, New York.

James, S. E., and Salsbury, A. J. (1974). Facilitation of metastasis by antithymocyte globulin. *Cancer Res.* **34** 367-370.

Johansson, S., Angervall, L., Bengtsson, V., and Wahlgvist, L. (1974). Uroepithelial tumors of the renal pelvis associated with abuse of phenacetin-containing analgesics. *Cancer* **33**, 743-753.

Jones, G., and Butler, W. H. (1975). Morphology of spontaneous and induced neoplasia. *In* "Mouse Hepatic Neoplasia" (W. H. Butler and P. M. Newberne, eds.), Chap. 3, pp. 21-59. Elsevier Amsterdam.

Joseph-Bravo, P. I., Findley, M., and Newberne, P. M. (1976). Some interactions of light, riboflavin, and aflatoxin B_1 *in vivo* and *in vitro*. *J. Toxicol. Environ. Health* **1**, 353-376.

Karchmer, R. K., Amare, M., Larsen, W. E., Mallouk, A. G., and Caldwell, G. G. (1974). Alkylating agents as leukemogens in multiple myeloma. *Cancer* **33**, 1103-1107.

Kelly, M. G., O'Gara, R. W., Yancey, S. F., Kumidini, G., Botkins, C., and Oleverio, V. T. (1969). Comparative carcinogenicity of N-isopropylα (2-methylhydrazino)-P-toluamide. HCl (procarbazine hydrochloride), its degradation products, other hydrazines, and isonicotinic acid hydrazide. *J. Natl. Cancer Inst.* **42**, 337-344.

Kroes, R., Berkrens, J. M., and Weisburger, J. H. (1975). Immunosuppression in primary liver and colon tumor induction with N-hydroxy-N-2-fluorenylacetamide and azoxymethane. *Cancer Res.* **35**, 2651-2656.

Kruger, G. R. F., and Harris, D. (1972). Is phenytoin carcinogenic? *Lancet* **2**, 323.

Kyle, R. A., Pierre, R. V., and Bayrd, E. D. (1974). Primary amyloidosis and acute leukemia associated with melphalan therapy. *Blood* **44**, 333-337.

Lander, J. J., Stanley, R. J., Summer, H. W., Boswell, D. C., and Aach, R. D. (1975). Angiosarcoma of the liver associated with Fowler's solution (potassium arsenite). *Gastroenterology* **68**, 1582-1586.

Laska, E. M., Meisner, M., Siegel, C., Fischer, S., and Wanderling, J. (1975). Matched-pairs study of reserpine use and breast cancer. *Lancet* **2**, 296-300.

Lee, A. M., and Fraumeni, J. F., Jr. (1969). Arsenic and respiratory cancer in man: An occupational study. *J. Natl. Cancer Inst.* **42**, 1045-1052.

Lemon, H. M. (1975). Estriol prevention of mammary carcinoma induced by 7, 12-dimethylbenzanthracene and procarbazine. *Cancer Res.* **35**, 1341-1353.

Leonard, B. J. (1973). The use of rodents for studies of toxicity in contraceptive research. *Meet. Pharmacol. Models Assess Toxicity Side Effects Fertil. Regul. Agents* pp. 34-73.

Li, F. P., Willard, D. R., Goodman, R., and Vawter, G. (1975). Malignant lymphoma after diphenylhydantoin (Dilantin) therapy. *Cancer* **36**, 1359-1362.

Lieberman, A. N., and Shupack, J. L. (1974). Levodopa and melanoma. *Neurology* **24**, 340-343.

Lipsett, M. B. (1975). Hormones, nutrition and cancer. *Cancer Res.* **35**, 3359-3361.

McAdam, L., Paulers, H. E., and Peter, J. B. (1974). Adenocarcinomia of the lung during azathioprine therapy. *Arthritis Rheum.* **17**, 92-94.

MacDonald, R. A., Rogers, A. E., and Pechet, G. S. (1963). Growth and regeneration of the liver. *Ann. N. Y. Acad. Sci.* **3**, 70-84.

Mack, T. M., Henderson, B. E., Gerkins, V. R., Arthur, M., Baptista, J., and Pike, M. C., (1975). Reserpine and breast cancer in a retirement community. *N. Engl. J. Med.* **292**, 1366-1367.

Mack, T. M., Pike, M. C., Henderson, B. E., Pfeffer, R. I., Gerkins, V. R., Arthur M., Brown, S. E. (1976). Estrogen and endometral cancer in a retirement community. *N. Engl. J. Med.* **294**, 1262-1267.

McLean, A. E. M., and Magee, P. N. (1970). Increased renal carcinogenesis by dimethylnitrosamine in protein deficient rats. *Br. J. Exp. Pathol.* **51**, 587-590.

MacMahon, B. (1974). Risk factors for endometrial cancer. *Gynecol. Oncol.* **2**, 122-129.

MacMahon, B. (1975). Formal discussion of "breast cancer incidence and nutritional status with particular reference to body weight and height." *Cancer Res.* **35**, 3357-3358.

Magee, P. N., and Barnes, J. M. (1967). Carcinogenic nitroso compounds. *Adv. Cancer Res.* **10**, 163-246.

Marquardt, H., Sapozink, M. D., and Zedeck, M. S. (1974). Inhibition by cysteamine-HC of oncogenesis induced by 7, 12-dimethylbenz(a)anthracene without affecting toxic ity. *Cancer Res.* **34**, 3387-3390.

Marquardt, H., Philips, F. S., and Sternberg, S. S. (1976). Tumorigenicity *in vivo* and induction of malignant transformation and mutagenesis in cell cultures by adriamycin and daunomycin. *Cancer Res.* **36**, 2065-2069.

Mason, T. J., McKay, F. W., Hoover, R., Blot, W. J., and Fraumeni, J. F. Jr. (1975). "Atlas of Cancer Mortality for U.S. Counties: 1950-1969." Publ. No. (NIH) 75-780. U.S. Department of Health, Education and Welfare, Washington, D.C.

Mauer, S. M., Lee, C. S., Najarian, J. S., and Brown, D. M. (1974). Induction of malignant kidney tumors in rats with streptozotocin. *Cancer Res.* **34**, 158-160.

Maugh, T. H. (1974). Vitamin A; potential protection from carcinogens. *Science* **186**, 1198.

Meadows, A. T., Naiman, J. L., and Valdes-Dapena, M. (1974). Hepatoma associated with androgen therapy for aplastic anemia. *J. Pediat.* **84**, 109-111.

Meites, J. (1972). Relation of prolactin and estrogen to mammary tumorigenesis in the rat. *J. Natl. Cancer Inst.* **48**, 1217-1224.

Miller, C. T. (1974). Isoniazid and cancer risks. JAMA 230: 1254.

Miller, E. C., and Miller, J. A. (1972). Approaches to the mechanisms and control of chemical carcinogenesis. Bertner Foundation Award Lecture. *In* "Environment and Cancer, 24th Annual Symposium," pp. 5-39. M. D. Anderson Hospital, Williams, & Wilkins, Baltimore, Maryland.

Mirvish, S. S. (1975). Formation of N-nitroso compounds: chemistry, kinetics and *in vivo* occurence. Toxicol. Appl. Pharmacol. 31:325-351.

Miyakawa, M., Yoshida, O., Harada, T., and Kato, T. (1973). The effect of urinary B-glucuronidase inhibition on the induction of bladder tumors with 2-acetylaminofluorene in rats. *Invest. Urol.* **10**, 256-261.

Morris, J. S., Schmid, M., Newman, S., Scheuer, P. J., Path, M. R. C., and Sherlock, S. (1974). Arsenic and noncirrhotic portal hypertension. *Gastroenterology* **64**, 86-94.

Narisawa, T., Reddy, B. S., Wong, C. Q., and Weisburger, J. H. (1976). Effect of Vitamin A deficiency in rat colon carcinogenesis by N-methyl-N'-nitro-N-nitrosoguanidine. *Cancer Res.* **36,** 1379–1383.

Newberne, P. M., and Rogers, A. E. (1973). Rat colon carcinomas associated with aflatoxin and marginal vitamin A. *J. Natl. Cancer Inst.* **50,** 439–448.

Newberne, P. M., and Shank, R. C. (1973). Induction of liver and lung tumors in rats by the simultaneous administration of sodium nitrite and morpholine. *Food Cosmet. Toxicol.* **11,** 819–825.

Newberne, P. M., and Williams, G. (1969). Inhibition of aflatoxin carcinogenesis by diethystilbestrol in male rats. *Arch. Environ. Health* **19,** 489–497.

Newberne, P. M., Chan, W. C. M., and Rogers, A. E. (1974). Influence of light, riboflavin and carotene on the response of rats to the acute toxicity of aflatoxin and monocrotaline. *Toxicol. Appl. Pharmacol.* **28,** 200–208.

Newell, G. R., Rawlings, W., Kinnean, B. K., and Correa, P. (1973). Case control study of Hodgkin's disease. 1. Results of the interview questionnaire. *J. Natl. Cancer Inst.* **51,** 1437–1441.

Nissen, E. D., Kent, F., and Kent, D. R. (1975). Liver tumors and oral contraceptives. *Obstet. Gynecol.* **46,** 460–467.

O'Fallon, M. W., Labarthe, D. R., and Kurland, L. T. (1975). Rauwolfia derivatives and breast cancer. *Lancet* **2,** 292–296.

O'Gara, R. W., Adamson, R. H., Kelly, M. G., and Dalgard, D. W. (1971). Neoplasms of the hematopoietic system in nonhuman primates: Report of one spontaneous tumor and two leukemias induced by procarbazine. *J. Natl. Cancer Inst.* **46,** 1121–1130.

O'Neal, M. A., and Griffin, A. C. (1957). The effect of oxypsoralen upon ultraviolet carcinogenesis in albino mice. *Cancer Res.* **17,** 911–914.

Owen, J. A., Jr. (1975). Physiology of the menstrual cycle. *Am. J. Clin. Nutr.* **28,** 333–338.

Oyasu, R., Kitajima, T., Hopp, M. L., and Sumie, H. (1972). Enhancement of urinary bladder tumorigenesis in hamsters by coadministration of 2-acetylaminofluorene and indole. *Cancer Res.* **32,** 2027–2033.

Peacock, A., and Peacock, P. R. (1966). The results of prolonged administration of isoniazid to mice, rats and hamsters. *Br. J. Cancer* **20,** 307–325.

Peraino, C., Fry, R. J. M., and Staffeldt, E. (1971). Reduction and enhancement by phenobarbital of hepatocarcinogenesis induced in the rat by 2-acetylaminofluorene. *Cancer Res.* **31,** 1506–1512.

Peraino, C., Fry, R. J. M., Staffeldt, E., and Christopher, J. P. (1975). Comparative enhancing effects of phenobarbital amobarbital, diphenylhydantoin, and dichlorodiphenyltrichloroethane on 2-acetylaminofluorene-induced hepatic tumorigenesis in the rat. *Cancer Res.* **35,** 2884–2890.

Pike, M. C., Gordon, R. J., Henderson, B. E., Menck, H. R., and Soo Hoo, I. (1975). Air pollution. *In* "Persons at High Risk of Cancer. An Approach to Cancer Etiology and Control" (J. F. Fraumeni, Jr., ed.). Chapter 14, pp. 225–239. Academic Press, New York.

Poirier, L. A., and Whitehead, V. M. (1973). Folate deficiency and formiminoglutamic acid excretion during chronic diethylnitrosamine administration to rats. *Cancer Res.* **33,** 383–388.

Poirier, L. A., Grantham, P. H., and Rogers, A. E. (1977). The effects of marginal lipotrope-deficient diet on the hepatic levels of S-adenosylmethionine and on the urinary metabolites of 2-acetylaminofluorene in rats. *Cancer Res.* **37,** 744–748.

Polliack, A., and Levij, I. S. (1967). Increased incidence of carcinoma induced by DMBA in the hamster cheek pouch in response to vitamin A. *Nature (London)* **216,** 187–188.

Polliack, A., and Levij, I. S. (1969). The effect of topical vitamin A on papillomas and intraepithelial carcinomas induced in hamsters cheek pouches with 9, 10-dimethyl-1, 2, benzanthracene. *Cancer Res.* **29**, 327–332.

Pullinger, B. (1961). Increase in mammary carcinoma and adenoma incidence and incidence of other tumors in C3HF virgin females after ovariectomy and high dosage with some estrogens. *Br. J. Cancer* **15**, 574–578.

Quadri, S. K., Keadzik, G. S., and Meites, J. (1974). Counteraction by prolactin of androgen-induced inhibition of mammary tumor growth in rats. *J. Natl. Cancer Inst.* **52**, 875–878.

Raaflaub, J., and Dubach, V. C. (1969). Dose-dependent change in the pattern of phenacetin metabolism in men and its possible significance in analgesic nephropathy. *Klin. Wochenschr.* **47**, 1286–1287.

Rakieten, N., Gordon, B. S., Beatty, A., Cooney, D. A., Davis, R. D., and Schein, P. S. (1971). Pancreatic islet cell tumors produced by the combined action of streptozotocin and nicotinamide. *Proc. Soc. Exp. Biol. Med.* **137**, 280–283.

Reddy, B. S., Mastromarino, A., and Wynder, E. L. (1975). Further leads on metabolic epidemiology of large bowel cancer. *Cancer Res.* **35**, 3403–3406.

Rivlin, R. S. (1973). Riboflavin and cancer: A review. *Cancer Res.* **33**, 1977–1986.

Rogers, A. E. (1975). Variable effects of a lipotrope-deficient, high-fat diet on chemical carcinogenesis in rats. *Cancer Res.* **35**, 2469–2474.

Rogers, A. E. (1977a). Dietary effects on chemical carcinogenesis in the livers of rats. *In* "Proceedings of Conference on Hepatoma in Rats" (W. Butler and P. M. Newberne, eds.). M.I.T. Press, Cambridge, Mass. (in press).

Rogers, A. E. (1977b). Reduction of N-nitrosodiethylamine carcinogenesis in rats by lipotrope or amino acid supplementation of a marginally deficient diet. *Cancer Res.* **37**, 194–199.

Rogers, A. E., and Newberne, P. M. (1971). Diet and aflatoxin B toxicity in rats. *Toxicol. Appl. Pharmacol.* **20**, 113–121.

Rogers, A. E., and Newberne, P. M. (1973). Dietary enhancement of intestinal carcinogenesis by dimethylhydrazine in rats. *Nature (London)* **246**, 491–492.

Rogers, A. E., and Newberne, P. M. (1975). Dietary effects on chemical carcinogenesis in animal models for colon and liver tumors. *Cancer Res.* **35**, 3427–3431.

Rogers, A. E., Kula, N. S., and Newberne, P. M. (1971). Absence of an effect of partial hepatectomy on aflatoxin B carcinogenesis. *Cancer Res.* **31**, 491–495.

Rogers, A. E., Herndon, B. J., and Newberne, P. M. (1973). Induction by dimethylhydrazine of intestinal carcinoma in normal rats fed high or low levels of vitamin A. *Cancer Res.* **33**, 1003–1009.

Rogers, A. E., Sanchez, O., Feinsod, F. M., and Newberne, P. M. (1974). Dietary enhancement of nitrosamine carcinogenesis. *Cancer Res.* **34**, 96–99.

Rogers, A. E. (1977c). In preparation.

Rook, A. J., Gresham, G. A., and Davis, R. A. (1956). Squamous epithelioma possibly induced by the therapeutic application of tar. *Br. J. Cancer.* **10**, 17–23.

Rosner, F., and Grünwald, H. (1974). Multiple myeloma terminating in acute leukemia. *Am. J. Med.* **37**, 927–939.

Rosner, F., and Grünwald, H. (1975). Hodgkins Disease and Acute Leukemia, *Am. J. Med.* **58**, 339–353.

Ross, M. H., and Bras, G. (1973). Influence of protein under- and over- nutrition on spontaneous tumor prevalence in the rat. *J. Nutr.* **103**, 944–963.

Rustia, M., and Shubik, P. (1972). Induction of lung tumors and malignant lymphomas in mice by metronidazole. *J. Natl. Cancer Inst.* **48**, 721–729.

Ryan, K. J. (1975). Cancer risk and estrogen use in the menopause. *N. Engl. J. Med.* **293,** 1199–1200.

Saffiotti, V., Montesano, R., Sellakumar, A. R., and Borg, S. A. (1967). Experimental cancer of the lung. Inhibition by vitamin A of the induction of tracheobronchial squamous metaplasia and squamous cell tumors. *Cancer* **20,** 857–864.

Schein, P. S., Cooney, D. A., and Vernon, M. L. (1967). The use of nicotinamide to modify the toxicity of streptozotocin diabetes without loss of antitumor activity. *Cancer Res.* **27,** 2324–2332.

Schmauz, R., and Cole, P. (1974). Epidemiology of cancer of the renal pelvis and ureter. *J. Natl. Cancer Inst.* **52,** 1431.

Schneiderman, M. A. (1974). Phenobarbitone and liver tumours. *Lancet* **2,** 1085.

Schoental, R. (1975). Pancreatic islet cell and other tumors in rats given heliotrine, a monoester pyrrolizidine alkaloid, and nicotinamide. *Cancer Res.* **35,** 2020–2024.

Selinger, M., and Koff, R. S. (1975). Thorotrast and the liver. A reminder. *Gastroenterology* **68,** 799–803.

Severi, L., and Biancifiori, C. (1968). Hepatic carcinogenesis in CBA/Cb/Se mice and Cb/Se rats by isonicotinic acid hydrazide and hydrazine sulfate. *J. Natl. Cancer Inst.* **41,** 331–349.

Shay, H., Gruenstein, M., and Shimkin, M. B. (1964). Effect of casein, lactalbumin, and ovalbumin on 3-methylcholanthrene-induced mammary carcinoma in rats. *J. Natl. Cancer Inst.* **33,** 243–253.

Shellabarger, C. J., and Soo, V. A. (1973). Effects of neonatally administered sex steroids on 7, 12-Dimethylbenz(a) anthracene-induced mammary neoplasia in rats. *Cancer Res.* **33,** 1567–1569.

Shklar, G., Cataldo, E., and Fitzgerald, A. L. (1966). The effect of methotrexon on chemical carcinogensis of hamster buccal pouch. *Cancer Res.* **26,** 2218–2224.

Sieber, S. M. (1975). Cancer chemotherapeutic agents and carcinogenesis. *Cancer Chemother. Rep.* **59,** 915–918.

Silvergleid, A. J., and Schrier, S. L. (1974). Acute myelogenous leukemia in two patients treated with azathioprine for nonmalignant diseases. *Am. J. Med.* **57,** 885–888.

Silverstone, H., and Tannenbaum, A. (1950). The effect of the proportion of dietary fat on the rate of formation of mammary carcinoma in mice. *Cancer Res.* **10,** 448–453.

Sinha, D., Cooper, D., and Dao, T. L. (1973). The nature of estrogen and prolactin effect on mammary tumorigensis. *Cancer Res.* **33,** 411–414.

Smith, D. C., Prentice, R., Thompson, D. J., and Herrmann, W. L. (1975). Association of exogenous estrogen and endometrial carcinoma. *N. Engl. J. Med.* **293,** 1164–1167.

Smith, D. M., Rogers, A. E., Herndon, B. J., and Newberne, P. M. (1975a). Vitamin A (retinyl acetate) and benzo(a)pyrene-induced respiratory tract carcinogenesis in hamsters fed a commercial diet. *Cancer Res.* **35,** 11–16.

Smith, D. M., Rogers, A. E., and Newberne, P. M. (1975b). Vitamin A and benzo(a)pyrene carcinogenesis in the respiratory tract of hamsters fed a semisynthetic diet. *Cancer Res.* **35,** 1485–1488.

Speck, W. T., Stein, A. B., and Rosenkranz, H. S. (1976). Mutagenicity of metronidazole: Presence of several active metabolites in human urine. *J. Natl. Cancer Inst.* **56,** 283–284.

Steigbigel, R. T., Kim, H., Potolsky, A., and Schrier, S. L. (1974). Acute myeloproliferative disorder following long-term chlorambucil therapy. *Arch. Intern. Med.* **134,** 728–731.

Swanbeck, G., and Hellström, L. (1971). Analysis of etiological factors in squamous cell skin cancer of different locations. 4. Concluding remarks. *Acta Derm.-Venereol.* **57,** 151–155.

Takeda, Y., Tominaga, T., Tei, N., Kitamura, M., Taga, S., Murase, J., Jaguchi, T., and Miwatani, T. (1975). Inhibitory effect of L-arginine on growth of rat mammary tumors induced by 7, 12-Dimethylbenz(a)anthracene. *Cancer Res.* **35**, 2390-2393.

Tanaka, Y., and Dao, T. L. (1965). Effect of hepatic injury on induction of adrenal necrosis and mammary cancer by 7, 12-dimethylbenz(a)anthracene in rats. *J. Natl. Cancer Inst.* **35**, 631-640.

Tannenbaum, A. (1959). Nutrition and cancer. In "The Physiopathology of Cancer" (F. Hamburger, ed.), (Hoeber), New York. Vol. 2, pp. 517-562. Harper.

Tannenbaum, H., and Schur, P. H. (1974). Development of reticulum cell sarcoma during cyclophosphamide therapy. *Arthritis Rheum.* **17**, 15-18.

Thorpe, E., and Walker, A. I. T. (1973). The toxicology of dieldrin (HEOD*) II. Comparative long-term oral toxicity studies in mice with dieldrin, DDT, phenobarbitone, β BHC and γ BHC. *Food Cosmet. Toxicol* II 433-442.

Toth, B., and Shubik, P. (1966). Carcinogenesis in Swiss mice by isonicotinic acid hydrazide. *Cancer Res.* **26**, 1473-1475.

Ulland, B. M., Weisberger, J. H., Yamamoto, R. S., and Weisburger, E. K. (1973). Antioxidants and carcinogenesis, butylated hydroxytoluene, but not diphenyl-p-phenylenediamine, inhibits cancer induction by N-2-fluorenylacetamide and by N-hydroxy-N2-fluorenylacetamide in rats. *Food Cosmet. Toxicol.* **11**, 199-207.

Valeriote, F., and van Putten, L. (1975). Proliferation-dependent cytotoxicity of anticancer agents: A review. *Cancer Res.* **35**, 2619-2630.

Vessey, M. P., Doll, R., and Jones, K. (1975). Oral contraceptives and breast cancer. *Lancet* **1**, 941-943.

Voogd, C. E., Van Der Stel, J. J., and Jacobs, J. J.J. A. A. (1974). The mutagenic action of nitroimidazoles. *Mutat. Res.* **26**, 483-490.

Walker, S. E., and Bole, G. G., Jr. (1973). Augmented incidence of neoplasia in NZB/NZW mice treated with long term cyclophosphamide. *J. Lab. Clin. Med.* **82**, 619-633.

Wall, R. L., and Clausen, K. P. (1975). Carcinoma of the urinary bladder in patients receiving cyclophosphamide. *N. Engl. J. Med.* **293**, 271-273.

Wang, C. Y., Hayashida, S., Pamukcu, A. M., and Bryan, G. T. (1976). Enhancing effect of allopurinol on the induction of bladder cancer in rats by N-(4-(5-nitro-2-furyl)-2-thiazolyl) formamide. *Cancer Res.* **36**, 1551-1555.

Warwick, G. P. (1967). The covalent binding of metabolites of tritiated 2-methyl-4-dimethylaminoazobenzene to rat liver nucleic acids and proteins, and the carcinogenicity of the unlabeled compound in partially hepatectomized rats. *Eur. J. Cancer* **3**, 227-233.

Wattenberg, L. W. (1972). Inhibition of carcinogenic and toxic effects of polycyclic hydrocarbons by phenolic antioxidants and ethoxyquin. *J. Natl. Cancer Inst.* **48**, 1425-1430.

Wattenberg, L. W. (1974). Inhibition of carciogenic and toxic effects of polycyclic hydrocarbons by several sulfur-containing compounds. *J. Natl. Cancer Inst.* **52**, 1583-1587.

Wattenberg, L. W. (1975). Effects of dietary constituents on the metabolism of chemical carcinogens. *Cancer Res.* **35**, 3326-3331.

Waxler, S. H., and Leef, M. F. (1966). Augmentation of mammary tumors in castrated obese C3H mice. *Cancer Res.* **26**, 860-862.

Weisburger, E. K., Ward, J. M., and Brown, C. A. (1974). Dibenamine: Selective protection against diethylnitrosamine-induced hepatic carcinogenesis but not oral, pharyngeal and esophageal carcinogenesis. *Toxicol. Appl. Pharmacol.* **28**, 477-484.

Weisburger, J. H. (1969). Procarbazine: Chemical immunosuppressant also powerful carcinogen. *Science* **165**, 517.

Weisburger, J. H., Yamamoto, R. S., Williams, G. M., Grantham, P. H., Matsushima, T., and Weisburger, E. K. (1972). On the sulfate ester of N-hydroxy-N-2-fluorenylacetamide as a key ultimate hepatocarcinogen in the rat. *Cancer Res.* **32**, 491–500.

Weisburger, J. H., Griswold, D. P., Prejean, J. P., Casey, A. E., Wood, H. B., and Weisburger, E. K. (1975a). The carcinogenic properties of some of the principal drugs used in clinical cancer chemotherapy. *Recent Results Cancer Res.* **52**, 1–17.

Weisburger, J. H., Madison, R. M., Ward, J. M., Viguera, C., and Weisburger, E. K. (1975b). Modification of diethylnitrosamine liver carcinogenesis with phenobarbital but not with immunosuppression. *J. Natl. Cancer Inst.* **54**, 1185–1188.

Weiss, N. S. (1975). *Risks and benefits of estrogen use. N. Engl. J. Med.* **293** 1200–1202.

Wilson, R. B., Hutcheson, D. P., and Wideman, L. (1977). Dimethylhydrazine-induced colon tumors in rats fed diets containing beef fat or corn oil with or without wheat bran. *Am. J. Clin. Nutr.* **30**, 176–181.

Winklemann, R. K., Zollman, P. E., and Baldis, E. J. (1963). Squamous cell carcinoma produced by ultraviolet light in hairless mice. *J. Invest. Dermatol.* **40**, 217–220.

Wogan, G. N., Paglialunga, S., Archer, M. C., and Tannenbaum, S. R. (1975). Carcinogenicity of nitrosation products of ephedrine, sarcosine, folic acid, and creatinine. *Cancer Res.* **35**, 1981–1984.

Wynder, E. L., and Chan, P. C. (1970). The possible role of riboflavin deficiency in epithelial neoplasia. II. Effect on skin tumor development. *Cancer* **26**, 1221–1224.

Ziel, H. K., and Finkle, W. D. (1975). Increased risk of endometrial carcinoma among users of conjugated estrogens. *N. Engl. J. Med.* **293**, 1167–1170.

Zumoff, B., Fishman, J., Bradlow, H. L., and Hellman, L. (1975). Hormone profiles in hormone-dependent cancers. *Cancer Res.* **35**, 3365–3373.

Section III

USE OF DRUGS IN ANIMAL FEEDS

20

The Role of Antibiotics in Efficient Livestock Production

VIRGIL W. HAYS

I. INTRODUCTION

Antibiotic feed supplements have been extensively used in every major livestock-producing country for more than 25 years. In the United States alone, more than 1.0 million kg are used annually as diet supplements. The total amounts sold for nonmedical uses vary from year to year; but, according to United States Tariff reports (1949–1973), the amounts sold since 1963 have averaged 1.05 million kg annually (Fig. 1). Such wide acceptance of antibiotics is attributed to their established benefits of increasing growth rate, improving feed conversion, and reducing mortality and morbidity from clinical or subclinical infections.

Antibiotics commonly used in livestock production as dietary additives include bacitracin, chlortetracycline, neomycin, oxytetracycline, oleandomycin, penicillin, streptomycin, and tylosin. Recently flavomycin and

PRICE AND SALES VOLUME OF ANTIBIOTICS FOR NONMEDICAL USES

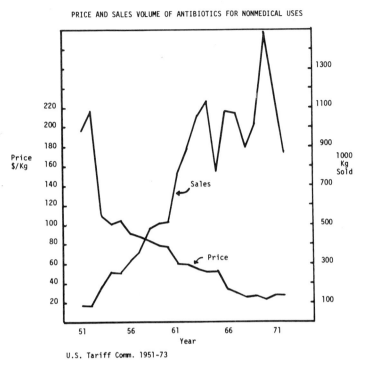

U.S. Tariff Comm. 1951-73

Fig. 1. Average price and total sales of antibiotics for nonmedical uses for the years 1951 to 1972.

virginiamycin have been added to the approved list. Among those presently used, some are more effective as growth promotants than others. Other antibiotics have been used experimentally and show promise as effective additives, and several not approved as feed additives are used as therapeutic agents.

The number of antibiotics approved for use in livestock and poultry production, either as feed additives or for therapeutic usage, totals about thirteen. This is a substantial number; however, Raper (1952) reported that some 300 antibiotics had been described and partially evaluated by 1952. Since that time numerous others have been discovered and evaluated. Thus, only a small percentage has been found to have major application. The large majority are unsuitable for one or more reasons, including low activity, toxicity to the host animal, and resulting residues in animal tissues. Of course, some antibiotics may be quite effective but offer no particular biological advantage over those presently used, thus their development cannot be justified on a cost basis. Though the quantity produced and sold varies from year to year, about 40% of the antibiotics sold are for nonmedical uses and the majority would be for feed additives (Fig. 2).

performance of animals have one thing in common, their ability to suppress or inhibit the growth of certain microorganisms. Their chemical composition and bacterial spectrum differ widely. Some of the effective antibiotics are readily absorbed into the vascular system of the host animal, whereas others are hardly absorbed at all. Their chemical composition, bacterial spectrum, and absorption and excretion patterns certainly influence bactericidal and bacteriostatic properties and effectiveness against specific systemic infections; however, these characteristics are less readily associated with effectiveness as a routine growth promotant.

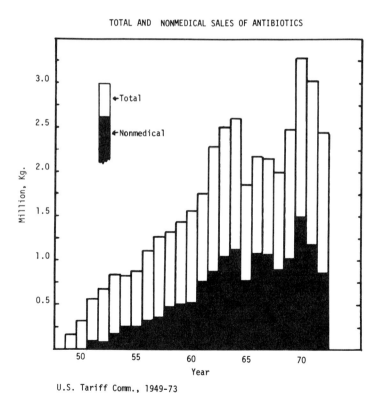

Fig. 2. Sales of antibiotics for medical and nonmedical uses for the years 1949 to 1973.

II. MODE OF ACTION

For the growth-promoting activity of antibiotics, at least three modes of action have been postulated, and each has varying degrees of support: (a) *a metabolic effect,* in that the antibiotics directly affect the rate or pattern of the metabolic processes in the host animal; (b) *a nutrient-sparing effect* in which the antibiotics may reduce the dietary requirement for certain nutrients by stimulating the growth of desirable organisms that synthesize vitamins or amino acids, by depressing the organisms that compete with the host animal for nutrients, by increasing the availability of nutrients via chelation mechanisms, or by improving the absorptive capacity of the intestinal tract; (c) *a disease-control effect,* through suppression of organisms causing clinical or subclinical manifestations of disease, by inhibition of multiplication of organisms that produce toxins, or by limiting their capacity to produce toxins which reduce performance but result in no obvious symptoms of disease.

A. Metabolic Effect

The first of these, the metabolic effect, has the type of support that could also be attributed to a disease-control effect, as the rate of metabolism may certainly be influenced by systemic infections. There is evidence that metabolic reactions in the host animal are influenced by antibiotics. Braude and Johnson (1953) reported that the feeding of chlortetracycline affected water and nitrogen excretion and suggested that it may influence the metabolic rate of pigs. Brody *et al.* (1954), using rat liver homogenates, found that tetracyclines inhibit fatty acid oxidation by the mitochondria. Weinberg (1957) likewise showed that, in bacteria, phosphorylation and oxidation reactions requiring magnesium ions were inhibited by tetracyclines. Hash *et al.* (1964) demonstrated that the tetracyclines inhibited protein synthesis.

Numerous reports illustrate that antibiotics do have metabolic implications, and their bacteriostatic or bactericidal properties can be largely explained on the basis of metabolic effects. However, in view of the nature of the animal responses, the normal tissue levels of the antibiotics when added to the diet at growth-promoting levels and the levels necessary to mediate such biochemical responses, the metabolic effects could hardly account for the growth promotion in animals fed diets supplemented with moderate levels of antibiotics.

B. Nutrient-Sparing Effect

The nutrient-sparing effect has considerable research support. It is well recognized that certain intestinal organisms synthesize vitamins and amino acids that are essential to animals and that other bacteria require and compete with the host animal for these dietary essential nutrients.

Moore *et al.* (1946) reported that streptomycin stimulated the growth or permitted rapid growth of some yeasts; and, Anderson *et al.* (1952a) found that feeding diets containing penicillin increased the numbers of intestinal coliforms other than *Escherichia coli*. Such organisms synthesize nutrients that are dietary essentials for the animals; thus, if a diet is deficient in certain vitamins, this deficiency could be partly corrected by the microbial synthesis.

Other reports show a depression in growth of organisms that are considered competitive with the host animals for dietary needs. March and Biely (1952) indicated that the bacteria most affected by chlortetracycline were the lactobacilli. Anderson *et al.* (1952b) and Johansson and Sarles (1949) also reported that antibiotics caused a reduction in the numbers of lactobacilli. Anderson *et al.* (1952b) reported that penicillin decreased the number of enterococci in the cecum of the chick. The lactobacilli require amino acids in relatively similar proportional amounts as does the pig; studies have shown that levels and sources of proteins that support maximum growth in pigs are also near optimum for the multiplication of lactobacilli in the intestinal tract (Kellogg *et al.*, 1964). It has also been observed that those antibiotics most effective in reducing the number of these organisms in the intestinal tract are also the most effective as routine growth promotants (Kellogg *et al.*, 1966). A reduction in populations of organisms that compete with the host animal for the dietary essential nutrients would be beneficial, especially if the levels of critical nutrients were critically low. This may partially explain the unusually large responses reported for some experiments in the early 1950's, a time when much was to be learned about the optimum levels of many of the essential amino acids and vitamins.

Catron *et al.* (1953) reported an increase rate of glucose absorption in animals fed rations fortified with antibiotics, thus providing additional evidence for the improved nutrient utilization resulting from feeding antibiotics. Braude *et al.* (1955) demonstrated that the gut wall was thinner in pigs fed rations containing an antibiotic than the intestinal wall of pigs fed diets not containing antibiotics. Rusoff *et al.* (1954) and Coates (1953) observed similar effects in calves and chicks, respectively. Coates also noted that feeding chicks the intestinal contents of infected chicks resulted in a thickening of the intestinal wall. Similar effects of antibiotics on the thickness of the intestinal wall have been reported by others (Coates *et al.*, 1955; Gordon, 1952, 1955; Gordon *et al.*, 1957–1958; Hill *et al.*, 1957; Taylor and Harrington, 1955). The thinner intestinal wall implies a potential for improved absorption (Taylor, 1957) and is assumed to be a result of the inhibition of the organisms which damage or produce toxins which in turn damage intestinal tissue. This proposed mode of action, that is, improved utilization of nutrients because of a more healthy intestinal wall, could actually be classed as a reduction in subclinical diseases or an inhibition of toxin production.

Catron *et al.* (1952), Burnside *et al.* (1954), and Beacom (1959a,b) report research which suggests that the level of protein required by pigs for maximum performance is less in the presence of dietary supplements of antibiotics. Table I summarizes the response of pigs to varying protein levels in the presence or absence of antibiotics and shows that the level of protein required for maximum gains was less in the presence of antibiotics. Rate of gain was depressed by low protein in the absence but not in the presence of the antibiotic. Also, Hogue *et al.* (1957) reported

TABLE I

Effect of Chlortetracycline on Weight Gains of Pigs Fed Protein at Four Levels[a]

Weight of pigs (kg)	Protein level fed (%)	Average daily gain (gm)		Feed efficiency[b]	
		Control	Fed chlor-tetracycline	Control	Fed chlor-tetracycline
To 34 34 to 68 68 to 91	20 17 14	690	760	3.90	3.54
To 34 34 to 68 68 to 91	18 15 12	708	754	3.83	3.60
To 34 34 to 68 68 to 91	16 13 10	740	760	3.72	3.55
To 34 34 to 68 68 to 91	14 11 8	681	754	3.74	3.59

[a] Catron *et al.* (1952).
[b] Units of feed per unit of gain.

TABLE II

Effect of Chlortetracycline on Growth of Calves Fed Milk
at Two Levels[a]

	Daily gain	
Level of milk fed	Average (gm)	Improvement (%)
Low		
Control	481	
Fed chlortetracycline	534	11.3
High		
Control	527	
Fed chlortetracycline	554	5.1

[a] Hogue et al. (1957).

that the amount of milk, which reflects quality of protein, in the diet of
young dairy calves influenced their response to antibiotics. Though the
growth rate of the calves was higher on the higher levels of milk, the
response to chlortetracycline was greater (11.3% versus 5.1%) on the
poorer quality diet (Table II). In a comprehensive summary of the effects of antibiotics on the performance of beef cattle, Burroughs et al.
(1959) also noted that animals on the diets that resulted in less rapid and
efficient gains showed a greater percentage response to chlortetracycline
(Table III).

Lucas (1957), Braude et al. (1953a,b), Stokstad (1954), Burnside et al.
(1949), and others present evidence of an association between diet and

TABLE III

Effect of Chlortetracycline on Weight Gains of Beef Cattle Fed Higher and Lower Gaining Diets[a]

Diet and number of comparisons	Daily gain		Feed efficiency[b]	
	Average (kg)	Improvement (%)	Average	Improvement (%)
Higher gaining diets (34 comparisons)				
Control	1.057		10.34	
Fed chlortetracycline	1.103	4.3	9.96	3.7
Lower gaining diets (31 comparisons)				
Control	0.645		12.31	
Fed chlortetracycline	0.681	5.6	11.45	7.0

[a] Burroughs et al. (1959).
[b] Units of feed per unit of gain.

antibiotic response. The response to antibiotics is generally greater if the antibiotics are included in an inadequate diet. This response suggests an improved utilization of nutrients at critical or suboptimal levels and could be attributed to nutrient synthesis by intestinal organisms, reduced competition from bacteria for critical nutrients or improved absorption.

Though there is substantial evidence that antibiotics will markedly enhance the performance of animals fed a diet low in protein or inadequate in other nutrients, there is evidence that the effect on nutrient utilization is other than direct. Meade and Forbes (1956), Wallace *et al.* (1954), and Bush *et al.* (1959) present evidence suggesting that enhancement in growth is largely a result of increased food intake, and though total nitrogen, calcium or other nutrients retained is greater, the percentages retained by the two groups of animals (those fed antibiotics and those not fed antibiotics) are similar. However, environmental conditions existing in most balance studies (extreme cleanliness, one animal per pen, and controlled temperature) are not conducive to dramatic antibiotic responses.

The increased response to antibiotics in the presence of nutritional stresses is of economic importance to livestock producers, since it is often economically desirable or pragmatically convenient for the producer to feed nutrient sources or levels that will not promote maximum rate of gain. In livestock-feeding programs, antibiotics may partially bridge the gap between optimum and economically practical diets for animals.

C. Disease-Control Effect

Though there is rather extensive evidence of nutrition and antibiotic response relationships, such effects appear secondary to the disease-control effect. Numerous studies support the conclusion that the major benefits derived from the inclusion of antibiotics as routine feed additives result from their suppression or control of subclinical or nonspecific diseases. Early in the history of antibiotics as supplements to animal feeds, it was noted that the degree of response to antibiotics was inversely related to the general well being of the experimental animals. Speer *et al.* (1950) observed that healthy, well-nourished pigs did not respond to antibiotic supplements when the pigs were housed in carefully cleaned and disinfected pens that had not previously housed other pigs. These findings have been confirmed by other workers and with other species (Catron *et al.*, 1951; Coates *et al.*, 1951; Hill *et al.*, 1952).

Studies involving clean and contaminated environments illustrate that the response is greater in contaminated environments. Bowland (1956) presented results of pig tests involving a new and an old barn. His data,

TABLE IV

Effect of Chlortetracycline on Weight Gains of Pigs in Different Environments[a]

Environment and chlortetracycline fed	Daily gain		Feed efficiency[b]	
	Average (gm)	Improvement (%)	Average	Improvement (%)
New barn				
Control	604		4.15	
Chlortetracycline (9 gm/ton)	649	7.5	3.92	5.5
Old barn				
Control	604		4.21	
Chlortetracycline (9 gm/ton)	690	14.2	3.78	10.2

[a] Bowland (1956).
[b] Units of feed per unit of gain.

TABLE V

Response to Tylosin by Pigs Housed in Two Environments—New Barn versus Dirt Lots[a]

Environment and tylosin level[c]	New house			Dirt lots[b]		
	0	+	Improvement (%)	0	+	Improvement (%)
Average daily daily gain (kg)						
Starter	0.55	0.63	14.6	0.42	0.50	19.0
Grower	0.84	0.82	2.4	0.58	0.68	17.2
Finisher	0.95	0.99	4.2	0.73	0.80	9.6
Feed/gain						
Starter	2.48	2.29	7.7	2.74	2.53	7.6
Grower	2.53	2.56	4.2	3.19	2.94	8.0
Finisher	3.16	3.15	0.3	3.70	3.52	4.9

[a] Wachholz and Heidenreich (1970).
[b] Area had been used several years for rearing pigs.
[c] 110, 44 and 11 mg/kg, respectively for starter, grower, and finisher diets.

summarized in Table IV, show that antibiotics resulted in a 14.3% increase in growth rate of pigs housed in the old barn, whereas in the new
barn, antibiotics resulted in only a 7.5% increase in growth rate. Similar
differences were noted for improvements in feed conversion for the new
and old barn environments.

Wachholz and Heidenreich (1970) provide additional data that the
cleanliness of the environment affects the magnitude of the response to
antibiotics (Table V). They tested the growth promoting effects of tylosin in a new barn and in a dirt lot facility that had been used for pigs for
several years. The increased rate of gain from supplementing the diet
with tylosin averaged 2.4–14.6% in the new barn as compared with 9.6–
19% in the less desirable environment.

Hays and Speer (1960) conducted two field tests comparing the effectiveness of different levels of the antibiotic spiramycin (Table VI). In one
test, the building was emptied, thoroughly cleaned and disinfected be-

TABLE VI
**Effect of Spiramycin and Tetracyclines on Weight Gains of Pigs Fed
in Two Environments**[a]

Environment and spiramycin level	Total gain		Feed efficiency[b]	
	Average (kg)	Improvement (%)	Average	Improvement (%)
First environment[c,d]				
No antibiotic	8.13		1.90	
12.5 gm/ton	9.62	18.3	1.84	3.2
25 gm/ton	10.44	28.4	1.64	13.7
50 gm/ton	10.81	33.0	1.70	10.5
Tetracycline[e]	10.71	31.7	1.78	6.3
Second environment[f,g]				
No antibiotic	4.81		2.89	
12.5 gm/ton	6.13	27.4	2.40	17.0
25 gm/ton	7.99	66.1	1.95	32.5
50 gm/ton	8.40	74.6	1.83	36.7
Tetracycline[e]	7.35	52.8	2.03	29.8

[a] Hays and Speer (1960).
[b] Unit of feed per unit of gain.
[c] Building thoroughly cleaned and disinfected before test, occupied only by pigs in test.
[d] 64 pigs fed at each level, averaging 26.3 days of age and 5.63 kg body weight, initially.
[e] 50 gm/ton of chlortetracycline or oxytetracycline in first and second environments, respectively.
[f] Building not thoroughly cleaned before test and contained older pigs before and during test.
[g] 59 pigs fed at each level, averaging 31.8 days of age and 5.69 kg body weight, initially.

fore starting the test, and only those pigs involved in the test occupied the building during the test. The building used in the other test contained older pigs preceding and during the test, and neither the building nor the individual pens were thoroughly cleaned or disinfected before the test. In the cleaned environment, spiramycin (50 gm/ton of diet) resulted in a 33% improvement in gains and a 10.5% improvement in feed efficiency; whereas in the uncleaned building, the addition of the antibiotic to the diet resulted in a 75% increase in growth rate and a 37% improvement in feed conversion. Similar responses were noted to chlortetracycline (50 gm/ton) in one of the tests and to oxytetracycline (50 gm/ton) in the other test. Though other variables, such as climatic conditions and breeding of animals, may have influenced the performance, the relative contamination of the buildings obviously had an important bearing on the response to the antibiotics. The buildup of a nonspecific infection, in buildings continuously used to house animals, can depress performance of animals without resulting in obvious symptoms of a disease problem. Such is the type of problem that the routine feeding of antibiotics aids in combating, and therapeutic usage of antibiotics is of little or no benefit, as a need for treatment is not indicated.

TABLE VII
Effect of a "Nonspecific Infection" on Chick Growth[a]

Hatch number	Average gain 0–7 days (gm)	Relative gain (%)
1	44.2	100.0
2	42.7	96.6
3	41.5	93.9
4	40.1	90.7
5	42.8	96.8
6	41.8	94.6
7	40.9	92.5
8	40.2	91.0
9	39.5	89.4
10	35.2	79.7
Depopulation and fumigation		
11	37.7	85.3
12	26.2	59.3
Depopulation and fumigation		
13	38.2	86.4
14	34.5	78.1
15	28.3	64.0

[a] Adapted from Scott, 1962.

556 Virgil W. Hays

Scott (1962) presented an excellent example of the buildup of the growth depressing effect of nonspecific infections in a chick starting facility. The performance of successive hatches of chicks was poorer than their previous counterparts (Table VII). Emptying the facility, cleaning it thoroughly and fumigating it resulted in an improvement in performance and a growth rate of chicks approaching the level of performance of first hatch. These are the kinds of problems that feed additive usage of antibiotics help to control.

The challenge experiments of Miyat and Gossett (1964) further demonstrate the prophylactic effects of antibiotics in controlling specific diseases (Table VIII). Treatment with tylosin was effective in controlling hemorrhagic dysentery, but treatment followed by prophylactic administration of the antibiotic was more effective in restoring performance to normal. These data illustrate the marked improvement in performance resulting from antibiotic supplements in severely high and, in this case, specific disease conditions. Similar observations have been reported on naturally occurring outbreaks of hemorrhagic dysentery (Gossett and Miyat, 1964).

TABLE VIII
Effect of Feeding Tylosin on Experimentally Induced Hemorrhagic Dysentery in Pigs[a]

Amount of tylosin fed		Number of pigs at		Average weight (kg)		
In water	In feed (gm/ton)	Start of trial	End of trial	Initial	Final	Feed efficiency[b]
Trial 1						
0	0	24	12	16.66	37.82	20.6
250 mg/gal[c]	40[d]	23	23	16.57	57.52	2.85
250 mg/gal[c]	0	23	20	16.66	47.31	3.84
0	100[e]	24	23	16.57	62.97	2.82
Trial 2						
0	0	23	13	35.96	59.02	
250 mg/gal[c]	40[d]	21	19	35.32	64.65	4.20
250 mg/gal[c]	0	22	20	36.37	63.97	4.90
0	100[e]	23	18	35.90	67.28	5.86

[a] Miyat and Gossett (1964).
[b] Units of feed per unit of gain.
[c] Antibiotic included in water for 6–8 days before infection and 4–5 days after infection.
[d] 40 gm/ton of feed after water treatment.
[e] 100 gm/ton of feed for 2 days before and for 33 or 15 days after infection, followed by 40 gm/ton.

TABLE IX
Relationship between Growth Rate of Control Animals and Animals Fed Antibiotics[a]

Number of tests	Daily gain in weight (gm)		Response to antibiotic: improvement (%)
	Control animals	Antibiotic-fed animals	
4	94	245	270
1	136	227	67
12	182	336	85
13	227	340	50
16	272	449	65
31	318	481	51
12	363	499	38
18	409	563	38
16	454	572	26
36	499	572	15
32	545	627	15
39	590	636	8
48	636	713	12
20	681	735	8
22	726	790	9
1	772	881	14

[a] Adapted from Braude et al. (1953b).

Braude et al. (1953b) summarized a number of experiments and concluded that the relative improvement in growth rate resulting from supplementing the diets with antibiotics was inversely related to the growth rate of the control animals (Table (IX). Similar experiments, involving the antibiotic combination of penicillin and streptomycin and conducted about 10 years after those studied by Braude, are summarized and presented in Table X. Of 61 comparisons included in the summary, 56 showed a positive response to the antibiotics in rate of gain, and 49 showed a positive response in feed conversion, with average improvements of 10.7% and 5.1% for rate of gain and feed efficiency, respectively.

The observation that degree of response is associated with degree of contamination has led to the suggestion that antibiotics are a substitute for good housekeeping and sanitation procedures. Theoretically, this is true; however, there are practical and economic limits to the amount livestock producers can invest in sanitation procedures. Experiment stations, which usually employ husbandry and sanitation practices often

TABLE X
**Relationship between Growth Rate of Control Pigs and Pigs Fed a Combination of
Penicillin and Streptomycin[a]**

Daily gain in weight of controls (gm)	Number of comparisons	Improvement over controls by pigs fed antibiotics	
		Gain in weight (%)	Feed efficiency (%)
91 to 182	2	22.0	8.2
182 to 272	3	27.0	4.5
272 to 363	4	20.4	5.6
363 to 454	7	16.1	11.1
454 to 545	9	12.3	6.4
545 to 636	9	9.4	1.9
636 to 726	20	5.6	4.7
726	7	3.8	1.8
Total	61		
Average improvement (%)		10.7	5.1

[a] Data summarized from agricultural experiment station reports, 1960 to 1967 by Hays (1969).

beyond the practical limits of producers, do, nonetheless, note responses of substantial magnitude to antibiotics.

The data used to estimate the economic benefits from the use of antibiotics are for the most part based on experiments conducted at experiment stations. These stations frequently employ management and sanitation procedures that are difficult or near impossible and certainly often impractical for the producer to use. For example, many of the tests involve only healthy pigs at the beginning, whereas the farmer must rear all of his pigs. Sainsbury (1975) presents an excellent example of the difference in response to normal healthy pigs and those he classed as "bad doers" or what we might frequently term as "runt" pigs. Antibiotic supplements to the normal pigs resulted in a 10% improvement in rate of gain, whereas antibiotic supplements to the "bad doers" resulted in a 30% improvement in gains. Thus, if unselected pigs are used, one would expect a greater response to antibiotics than if only healthy pigs are selected for the tests.

Also, researchers usually clean the facility well and at times it may set idle between groups of pigs. This practice should result in a lesser response to antibiotics as illustrated in Table VI.

It is most difficult or near impossible to thoroughly clean and sanitize many swine facilities. Another practice that undoubtedly reduces the stress on animals and hence reduces the expected response to antibiotics is the practice of using only a few animals per pen. In fact, some of the antibiotic studies involve single animals per pen and most involve only four to six animals per pen. It is rather obvious that this is not a practical management procedure. It is common practice to have 75 to 100 or more pigs per pen with limited space per pig.

Melliere *et al.* (1973) summarized sixty-nine experiments conducted under research station and farm conditions and verify that the average response is greater in the farm situation than at research stations. Their data is reported in more detail by Natz (1973) and summarized in Table XI. The average response for rate of gain and feed/gain was 5.7 and 4.7%, respectively in field trials as compared with 3.6 and 3.3% for University Experiment Station tests. In experiments carried out in facilities in which extreme care was taken to maximize sanitary conditions, the response was 1.7 and 0.3% improvement in gain and feed/gain, respectively. Thus, if one calculates economic benefits from the use of antibiotics on data from experiments in the field rather than from

TABLE XI
Effect of Tylosin on Growth Rate and Feed Conversion of Finishing Pigs

		Treatment		
Experimental unit	Number of trials	Control	Tylan 10–20	Improve- ment (%)
Average daily gain (gm/day)				
Research type 1[a]	32	790	803	1.7
Research type 2[b]	22	763	790	3.6
Field tests[c]	24	713	754	5.7
Average		755	783	3.7
Feed/gain[d]				
Research type 1[a]	32	3.36	3.35	0.3
Research type 2[b]	16	3.64	3.52	3.3
Field tests[c]	24	3.84	3.66	4.7
Average		3.61	3.51	2.8

[a] Closed herds, confinement houses thoroughly cleaned prior to test.
[b] Herd status and cleaning procedures not defined.
[c] Practical production units.
[d] Feed gain data available on only 16 of the 22 experiments for which rate of gain data were available.

Experiment Station data, the benefits would exceed the 533 million dollar estimate of Gilliam and Martin (1975) for economic returns to use of antibiotics in swine production.

It has been suggested that there is no need for feed additive usage of antibiotics if one has a Specific-Pathogen-Free (SPF) or Minimal Disease (MD) herd. SPF and MD are terms used in the United States and Great Britain, respectively, to designate animals that are free of mycoplasma pneumonia, atrophic rhinitis and possibly other diseases that are spread by direct pig-to-pig contact. Any reduction in disease problems should lower the response to antibiotics. However, there are many experiments which illustrate that SPF pigs do respond to antibiotics. Much of the data available has been summarized by Hays (1973), and indicates that there is little difference in responses to antibiotics by SPF and nonSPF pigs used by Experiment Station researchers. Sainsbury (1975) also reported that MD pigs fed antibiotic-supplemented diets grew 8% faster than their respective controls as compared with a 10% improvement for conventional pigs supplemented with antibiotics. Every practical method should be utilized to reduce the morbidity and mortality from disease; however, at present there are no methods available that would contraindicate the need for feed additives. The wise use of antibiotics is not a substitute but a complement for good husbandry, sanitation, and disease control practices.

III. CONTINUED EFFECTIVENESS

The extensive use of antibiotics as feed additives has elicited concern about potential harmful effects due to the development of resistant strains of organisms in the host animal or due to resistant organisms or allergic reactions in the consumer of the meat, milk, or eggs from animals continuously fed antibiotics. Concern should exist with the application of any new drug either as a feed additive or a medicament; but, after 25 years of usage of some of these drugs, fear should have changed to rational thinking leading to adequate evaluation of the potential harmful effects as contrasted with the proven health and economic benefits.

After more than 25 years of extensive use of antibiotics in animal feeds, discussions still deal with "potential public health hazards", as did a presentation by Goldberg (1962). Significantly, it is difficult to cite one human health problem that can be attributed to the consumption of meat from animals fed antibiotics.

It has been well established that continuous exposure of enteric organisms to an antibiotic permits the development of strains of organisms with greater tolerance for or complete resistance to that antibiotic. This is more readily demonstrated in laboratory tests with pure cultures than it is with the complex microflora that exists in the environment or in the gastrointestinal tract of domestic animals. However, an increase in multiple and transferable drug resistance has been observed in naturally occurring enteric organisms from the use of antibiotics as feed additives (Smith, 1962).

The evidence that resistant organisms in animals compromise treatment of diseases in man or animals is indirect and difficult to evaluate. For those persons concerned only with disease treatment, an idealistic decision is to limit the use of any drug to treatment of a patient. For those that are concerned with the health of a population through a plentiful food supply which involves both disease control and efficient production, the decisions are more complicated. A thorough evaluation of the human health implication of any biologically active drug is essential. When there are benefits, there are likely to be some risks involved. A more thorough discussion of this aspect of feed additive usage is covered in other papers in this symposium.

It has been suggested that antibiotics are losing their effectiveness and that higher and higher levels are being required to give the typical antibiotic response. The general explanation attached to this observation is that organisms are developing or have developed resistance to the problem organisms. It is recognized today that 40–50 gm/ton of a broad spectrum antibiotic are normally required to approach a maximum response, whereas the generally recommended level in the early 1950's was approximately 10–20 gm/ton. However, the data of Catron *et al.* (1951) illustrate that, since antibiotics were first used, the recommended feeding level has not necessarily been the level that would elicit maximum response. Even though a response was obtained with 10 or 20 gm/ton (Table XII), maximum gain was approached at 40 gm/ton, and maximum feed efficiency was realized at 80 gm/ton, the highest level tested.

The levels selected for practical use are not necessarily the levels that will elicit maximum response. The growth response increases with increasing levels of antibiotics up to 250 gm/ton or more in some cases. The rate of increase in growth response decreases, however, as the level of antibiotic increases; thus, the level selected in practice is usually a compromise based on the cost-benefit ratio.

Improved methods of producing antibiotics and competition among producers have resulted in a decline in the price of the commonly used

TABLE XII
Effect of Chlortetracycline Fed at Different Levels on Performance of Growing–Finishing Swine[a]

Level of chlortetracycline (gm/ton)	Average daily gain (gm)	Feed consumed per day (gm)	Feed efficiency[b]
0	654	2343	3.69
10	722	2443	3.49
20	726	2479	3.50
40	758	2588	3.44
80	763	2561	3.36

[a] Catron et al. (1951).
[b] Feed required per unit gain.

antibiotics, which allows consideration of the use of higher levels. Figure 1 presents price data for all antibiotics combined and Table XIII presents the price histories of penicillin, streptomycin, and tetracyclines. The prices of feed-grade penicillin and streptomycin in 1975 were only 10–15% of the 1950 price and tetracyclines were only about 20% as expensive as in 1950. These reductions in antibiotic prices were accompanied by increases in most other production costs. The evidence available suggests that these price changes have been the primary reason for higher levels being recommended rather than any decline in effectiveness. The higher levels were more effective from the beginning, but with the natural biological phenomena of a decreasing response with an increasing level, the practical optimum level changes with cost changes. It should not go unstated that prices of certain antibiotics have increased within the past 5 years. These have basically attained basic commodity status and prices will respond to ingredient, labor, transportation, and

TABLE XIII
Approximate Price per Kilogram of Feed-Grade Antibiotics for the Specified Years, 1950–1975

Year	Penicillin	Streptomycin	Tetracyclines
1950	$200	$200	$120
1955	50	55	100
1960	22	30	80
1965	20	20	80
1970	24	28	30
1975	26	29	22

other costs. Removal of these from use in livestock production will increase cost of production.

Certainly, there are tests in which little or no response is observed to a recommended level of an antibiotic. This situation is not peculiar to 1976. Similar observations have been reported since the early use of antibiotics as dietary supplements. Speer *et al.* (1950) reported that 10–20 gm of chlortetracycline per ton of diet did not improve the performance of pigs in one test and suggested that the low disease level existing could be the reason for no improvement.

Teague *et al.* (1966) reviewed the antibiotic studies conducted at the Ohio Station over the preceding 11 years. They noted variations in the response from year to year; but there was no consistent decline in antibiotic response. A similar study of the swine data from the Iowa Station for the years 1950–1959 suggests that less response to antibiotics existed (Fig. 3) in the years 1953–1956. A critical evaluation of the experiments conducted during those years shows that they were few in number and mainly involved individually fed pigs in experiments designed to study the effects of antibiotics on protein or vitamin utilization. Thus, the disease stress on the animals was minimized because of low population density of animals in the buildings, as most of the animals were individually housed in metabolism cages.

Peo (1962) summarized the long-term effects of antibiotic feeding to swine at the Nebraska Station and concluded that, after more than 10

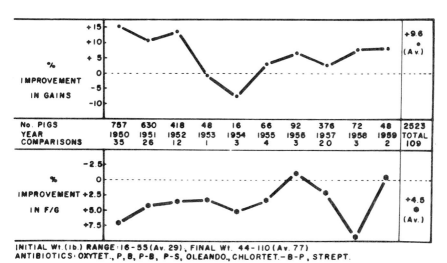

Fig. 3.   Response of growing pigs to antibiotics. (V. C. Speer, Animal Science Department, Iowa Agric. and Home Econ. Exp. Sta.).

TABLE XIV

Effect of Feeding Antibiotics on Weight Gains of Swine, in Tests on a Single Commercial Farm, 1960–1965[a,b]

Date experiment started	Average daily gain			Feed efficiency[c]		
	Controls (gm)	Plus antibiotic (gm)	Improvement (%)	Controls	Plus antibiotic	Improvement (%)
Dec. 1960	263	413	57	2.13	2.11	1.0
Mar. 1961	222	395	78	2.08	1.85	11.1
Apr. 1962	186	359	93	2.15	1.81	15.8
May 1964	191	336	76	2.99	2.18	27.1
Sep. 1964	200	322	61	2.71	2.36	12.9
Oct. 1965	250	331	32	2.77	2.28	17.7

[a] R. F. Elliott and D. D. Johnson (private communication, 1967).

[b] Antibiotic: 100 gm of chlortetracycline, 100 gm of sulfamethazine, and 50 gm of penicillin per ton of diet for pigs 3–9 weeks of age.

[c] Units of feed per unit of gain.

years of extensive use of antibiotics, a response was still being observed. His observations are particularly relevant, since, in that period of time, the Nebraska researchers had changed to a "specific pathogen-free" herd and had strived to keep disease conditions at a minimum in their herd.

Hvidsten and Homb (1961) reported the results of nine consecutive experiments on one farm in which oxytetracycline and chlortetracycline were tested at low or high levels. The antibiotic-fed pigs gained 5% faster on the average for the nine trials and the average improvement for the ninth trial was 5.3%. The lowest response to antibiotics was observed in the fourth trial and the highest in the fifth trial, suggesting that the variations in results from trial to trial was largely a result of normal variation associated with small experiments, and not a reflection of a changing response to antibiotics.

The continuous use of a single antibiotic has not been critically evaluated, as it is not general practice for a livestock producer to feed antibiotics throughout the animal's life cycle or to use the same antibiotic year after year. However, numerous experiments have been carried out that shed some light on whether the more commonly used

TABLE XV
Effect of Feeding Antibiotics at High Levels on Weight Gains of Young Pigs[a,b]

Antibiotic	Level of feeding (gm/ton)	Daily gain		Feed efficiency[c]	
		Average (gm)	Improvement (%)	Average	Improvement (%)
Control	0	318		2.30	
Pro-Strep[d]	250	454	43	1.98	13.9
ASP-250[e]	250	427	34	1.94	15.7
Pro-Strep[d]	100	395	24	2.02	12.2
Aureomycin[f]	100	396	25	2.14	7.0

[a] V. W. Hays (unpublished data, experiment 6443, Iowa Agric. Home Econ. Exp. Sta., 1965).

[b] Average initial weight of pigs, 8.67 kg; 4 pens of 10 pigs each per treatment, 34 days on test. Pigs nursed sows prior to going on experiment.

[c] Unit of feed per unit of gain.

[d] 1:3 ratio of procaine penicillin to streptomycin.

[e] 100 gm of chlortetracycline, 100 gm of sulfamethazine, and 50 gm of penicillin per ton of diet.

[f] Chlortetracycline.

antibiotics are continuing to improve the performance of animals. R. F. Elliott and D. D. Johnson reported in a private communication in 1967 that they had conducted experiments on a single commercial swine farm for a period of 6 years. A summary of their data is presented in Table XIV. This swine producer fed chlortetracycline routinely during the entire period, though other antibiotics may have been fed intermittently for short periods. The average performance and the response within any one year varied with environmental conditions, including stresses, existing at the time the experiments was conducted. But, after 6 years of testing, the combination of chlortetracycline, sulfamethazine, and penicillin resulted in a 33% improvement in rate of gain and an 18% improvement in feed efficiency.

Hays (1965) conducted an experiment on the same commercial swine farm that Elliott and Johnson had used for their tests; the results of that experiment are presented in Table XV. The response to the antibiotic combination was similar for the two studies: an improvement of 33-34% in growth rate and an improvement of 16-18% in feed conversion for the two tests conducted in 1965 (Tables XIV and XV). Table XV also shows a 7% improvement in feed conversion and a 26% improvement in rate of gain resulting from the addition of chlortetracycline, though it had been used extensively on the farm for at least 5 years. The combination of penicillin and streptomycin resulted in similar improvements in performance.

The results of similar tests using tylosin from 1959 to 1966 are summarized in Table XVI (C. E. Jordan, private communication, 1967). The rates of gain and feed conversion by the animals in the later experiments were less than in the earlier years, which Jordan attributes to change in the management program and use of a more simplified diet. The percentage of response is actually greater in 1965-1966 as compared with 1959-1962, in keeping with the previous examples of an increased response for animals under nutritional stress.

Hays and Baker (1967) conducted an experiment specifically to test the response to chlortetracycline in a confinement swine unit in which the antibiotic had been continuously used for more than 3 years. The unit housed 650-700 pigs continuously for the 3 year period, which would allow ample time for resistance problems to develop. Though the resistance patterns of the intestinal organisms were not determined, from our present knowledge of antibiotic resistance, we can state with confidence that the intestinal coliforms were solidly resistant to tetracyclines and that resistance was a multiple and transferable type. As illustrated in Table XVII, chlortetracycline (50 gm/ton) resulted in a 10.2% improvement in growth rate and a 1.0% improvement in feed efficiency.

TABLE XVI

Effect of Feeding Tylosin for a Prolonged Period on Weight Gains of Pigs[a]

Years	Number of experiments	Average daily gain			Feed efficiency[b]		
		Controls (gm)	Plus tylosin[c] (gm)	Improvement (%)	Controls	Plus tylosin[c]	Improvement (%)
1959–1960	3	445	490	10	1.98	1.92	3.0
1961–1962	1	454	499	10	2.21	2.12	4.1
1963–1964	1	254	286	13	1.90	1.80	5.3
1965–1966	3	277	327	18	2.20	2.04	7.3
1959–1960	1	409	490	20	2.33	2.15	7.7
1965–1966	1	281	304	8	2.32	2.05	11.6

[a] C. E. Jordan (private communication, 1967).

[b] Units of feed per unit of gain.

[c] 100 gm of tylosin per ton of diet, except for last 2 lines in which the level of tylosin was 40 gm/ton.

TABLE XVII
Effects of Chlortetracycline on Weight Gains of Pigs after Continued Use[a,b]

Group	Average daily gain (gm)	Improvement (%)	Feed efficiency[c]	Improvement (%)
Control (36 pigs)	577		2.97	
Fed chlortetracycline[d] (35 pigs)	636	10.2	2.94	1.0

[a] V. W. Hays and D. S. Baker (unpublished data, experiment 6708, Iowa Agric. Home Econ. Exp. Sta., 1967).
[b] Chlortetracycline had been used continuously in the building for 3 years before the test, and pigs had received chlortetracycline before the start of the experiment.
[c] Units of feed per unit of gain.
[d] 50 gm of chlortetracycline per ton of diet.

IV. APPLICATION OF ANTIBIOTICS IN FEEDING PROGRAMS

There is ample evidence that species involved, age of animal or stage of production, adequacy of diet, and environmental conditions are all important factors affecting the response to antibiotics. Each of these factors must be considered when selecting an antibiotic to use, level to feed, and duration of feeding. The previous examples in Sections II and III will also serve to illustrate effective application in feeding programs. Only a few additional illustrations of particular benefits will be presented here.

The use of a high level of antibiotics in the diet of sows at breeding time increases conception rate and litter size. Table XVIII summarizes a number of studies that involved more than 1100 sows and show an average 8% improvement in conception rate at first estrus and 0.5 more live pigs farrowed per litter. Speer (1970) summarizes additional unpublished data on both tetracycline and tylosin which in some cases show an even larger difference in conception rate than shown in Table XVIII. A rather high level of an adsorbable antibiotic seems necessary to elicit this response. This is reasonable since conception rate or litter size problems are likely associated with systemic rather than gastrointestinal problems.

Young growing pigs and calves show a markedly greater and more consistent response to antibiotics than do more mature animals. Table XIX provides a typical illustration of the greater response of very young pigs as compared with that of older pigs. Oleandomycin was fed to the two groups of pigs. In baby pigs, the antibiotic resulted in an increase in growth rate of 30–44% and an improvement in feed efficiency of 14–20%. In the older pigs, the antibiotic resulted in an improvement of 7–10% in growth rate and efficiency.

The diets used today to evaluate the effectiveness of antibiotics are, in general, more adequately balanced to meet the animals' needs than were the diets used in the early 1950's. There are two main reasons for this, one being that more information is available regarding the nutrient needs and the other being that some nutrients, particularly the vitamins, are less expensive today. The feeding of nutritionally balanced diets reduces but does not eliminate the response to antibiotics.

Though a great deal more is known about balancing diets for maximum rate and efficiency of gain, in some situations such "high performance" diets may themselves be a stress on the animal and result in a need for antibiotic supplementation. It is well recognized that antibiotics are beneficial in the adjustment by light-weight, young calves, that have been stressed by weaning, handling, and trucking to their new environments. Antibiotics are also beneficial in improving rate of gain and reducing the incidence of liver abscesses in cattle that are on high concentrate diets. Tables XX and XXI present a summary to illustrate that tylosin and tetracyclines are effective in reducing the incidence of liver abscesses.

TABLE XVIII

The Effect of Antibiotics at Breeding Time on Farrowing Rate and Litter Size

Number of sows	Farrowing rate (%)		Live pigs/litter		Reference
	Control	Treated	Control	Treated	
377	68.5	82.9[a]	9.8	10.1[a]	Messersmith et al., 1966
59	—	—	7.1	9.7[b]	Dean and Tribble, 1962
96	87.5	95.8[c]	9.0	10.3[c]	Ruiz et al., 1968
182	60.9	70.0[c]	9.8	10.0[c]	Krug, 1976
249	66.9	75.4[a]	9.9	10.2[a]	Myers and Speer, 1973
192	93.8	91.6[d]	10.9	11.3[d]	Mayrose et al., 1964
Weighted average	73.0	81.7	9.8	10.3	

[a] Chlortetracycline, 0.5–1.0 gm/sow/day.

[b] Chlortetracycline, 0.5–1.0 gm/sow/day, 0.54 gm/sow/day.

[c] Chlortetracycline, sulfamethazine, and penicillin at 0.5, 0.5 and 0.25 gm/sow/day, respectively.

[d] Tylosin phosphate, 0.6 gm/sow/day.

TABLE XIX
Effect of Feeding Oleandomycin at Different Levels on Performance of Pigs[a]

Pigs tested, and level of oleandomycin fed	Average weight (kg)		Daily gain		Feed efficiency[b]	
	Initial	Final	Average (gm)	Improvement (%)	Average	Improvement (%)
Baby pigs[c]						
No oleandomycin	4.29	8.91	163		2.02	
2.5 gm/ton	4.18	10.13	213	30.7	1.73	14.4
5 gm/ton	4.10	10.07	213	30.7	1.62	19.8
10 gm/ton	4.34	10.70	227	39.3	1.69	16.3
20 gm/ton	4.35	10.98	236	44.8	1.62	19.8
Growing pigs[d]						
No oleandomycin	13.26	34.41	527		2.82	
5 gm/ton	13.35	36.18	572	8.5	2.60	7.8
10 gm/ton	13.21	35.96	563	6.8	2.52	10.6
20 gm/ton	13.44	35.87	563	6.8	2.63	6.7

[a] Hawbaker et al. (1960).
[b] Units of feed per unit of gain.
[c] Initial age 13 days.
[d] Initial age 51 days.

TABLE XX
Effect of Tylosin on Incidence of Liver Abscesses and on
Performance of Feedlot Cattle[a]

Item	Control	Tylosin[b]
Number of trials	4	4
Animals starting trials	204	570
Completing trial (%)	91.2	92.3
Livers condemned (%)	23.1	4.2
Average daily gain (kg)	1.012	1.066
Feed/gain	7.646	7.412

[a] Adapted from Brown et al. (1973).
[b] Tylosin phosphate or tylosin urea adduct at 50–100 mg/animal/day.

Hygienic conditions in animal production have not greatly improved in recent years. Though greater knowledge about the role of hygiene in animal performance has accumulated and livestock producers are expending greater effort, some marked changes in systems of production have occurred that partially offset the advances made in sanitation practices. These changes have been necessitated by the increased value of land and a marked reduction in available labor. Livestock producers are finding it necessary to specialize in fewer livestock enterprises and to confine their animals to smaller spaces in order to release land for alternative uses and to facilitate the mechanization of feeding livestock and disposing of wastes.

TABLE XXI
Effect of Chlortetracycline (CTC) on the Incidence of Liver Abscesses in Fattening Cattle[a]

Experiment	Year	Group	Number of cattle	CTC mg/day	Abscesses Number	Percentage
1	1956	1	291	0	95	33
		2	302	75	76	25
2	1956	1	199	0	80	40
		2	200	75	8	4
3[b]	1957	1	224	0	154	69
		2	679	70	109	16

[a] Flint and Jensen, 1958.
[b] Feed per unit gain averaged 10.05 for controls and 9.33 for treated or a 6.8% improvement in efficiency.

Such intensification of livestock production accentuates some of the environmental factors effecting responses to antibiotics. The increased concentration of animals in limited space can lead to a higher incidence of clinical and subclinical disease because of the greater ease of transmittal from one animal to another. Fortunately, the extensive use of antibiotics has contributed to the success of many of these intensive units. Feed additive usage results in the greatest responses during periods of natural or imposed stresses. In pigs the greatest responses are observed at breeding or farrowing in sows, at weaning in young pigs, and during the stresses, associated with relocation, such as movement of feeder pigs. Similar situations apply to other species.

V. SUMMARY

Antibiotic feed supplements have now been used routinely and successfully in livestock production for more than 25 years. As the need for animal protein increases with the expanding world population, the use of antibiotics will become increasingly important for maintaining an efficient and competitive livestock industry. There can be no doubt that antibiotics continue to provide substantial economic benefits to the producer and consumer of meat, milk, and eggs.

The number of alternative antibiotics available that have been proven effective in improving performance is relatively small. These same antibiotics are those often found to be most effective in treatment of diseases. This observation is not inconsistent in that the bulk of the evidence supports the thesis that antibiotics result in improved performance through their control of specific or nonspecific diseases. These observations are significant in that one is not likely to find antibiotics that are particularly useful in improving performance of animals and that at the same time have no application in treatment of diseases.

The magnitude of the response to antibiotics varies with stage of life cycle or stage of production and the environmental conditions to which the animals are exposed. The response is greater in young animals than in more mature animals. The response is greater during critical stages of production such as weaning, breeding, and farrowing. Environmental stresses such as inadequate nutrition, crowding, moving and mixing of animals, and poor sanitation also contribute to increased responses to antibiotics. These are, however, ordinary stresses that are involved in intensive animal production and cannot be completely avoided. The judicious use of feed additives is essential to efficient production in today's intensive poultry and animal production units.

REFERENCES

Anderson, G. W., Cunningham, J. D., and Slinger, S. J. (1952a). Effect of protein level and penicillin on growth and intestinal flora of chickens. *J. Nutr.* **47,** 175.
Anderson, G. W., Slinger, S. J., and Pepper, W. F. (1952b). Effect of dietary microorganisms on the growth and cecal flora of chicks. *Poult. Sci.* **31,** 905.
Beacom, S. E. (1959a). Chlortetracycline and protein level in rations for market hogs. I. Effect on rate of gain and efficiency of feed utilization. *Can. J. Anim. Sci.* **39,** 71.
Beacom, S. E. (1959b). Chlortetracycline and protein level in rations for market hogs. II. Effect on carcass quality. *Can. J. Anim. Sci.* **39,** 79.
Bowland, J. P. (1956). Influence of environment on response of swine to antibiotic and/or Vigofac Supplements. *Univ. Alberta Press Bull.* **41,** 12.
Braude, R., and Johnson, B. C. (1953). Effect of aureomycin on nitrogen and water metabolism in growing pigs. *J. Nutr.* **49,** 505.
Braude, R., Kon, S. K., and Porter, J. W. G. (1953a). Antibiotics in nutrition. *Nutr. Abstr. Rev.* **23,** 473.
Braude, R., Wallace, H. D., and Cunha, T. J. (1953b). The value of antibiotics in the nutrition of swine: A review. *Antibiot. Chemother. (Washington, D.C.)* **3,** 271.
Braude, R., Coates, M. E., Davies, M. K., Harrison, G. F., and Mitchell, K. G. (1955). The effect of aureomycin on the gut of the pig. *Br. J. Nutr.* **9,** 363.
Brody, T. M., Hurwitz, M. R., and Bain, J. A. (1954). Magnesium and the effect of the tetracycline antibiotics on oxidative processes in mitochondria. *Antibiot. Chemother. (Washington, D.C.)* **4,** 864.
Brown, H., Elliston, N. G., McAskill, J. W., Muenster, O. A., and Tonkinson, L. V. (1973). Tylosin Phosphate (TP) and Tylosin Urea Adduct (TUA) for the prevention of liver abscesses, improved weight gains and feed efficiency in feedlot cattle. *J. Anim. Sci.* **37,** 1085.
Burnside, J. E., Cunha, T. J., Pearson, A. M., Glasscock, R. S., and Shealy, A. L. (1949). Effect of APF supplement on pigs fed different protein supplements. *Arch. Biochem. Biophys.* **23,** 328.
Burnside, J. E., Grummer, R. H., Phillips, P. H., and Bohstedt, G. (1954). The influence of crystalline aureomycin and vitamin B_{12} on the protein utilization of growing-fattening swine. *J. Anim. Sci.* **13,** 184.
Burroughs, W., Summers, C. E., Woods, W., and Zmolek, W. (1959). Feed additives in beef cattle rations. *Iowa State Univ., Mimeo. Rep. Am. Soc. Anim. Sci., Anim. Sci. Leafl.* **805.**
Bush, L. J., Allen, R. S., and Jacobson, N. L. (1959). Effect of chlortetracycline on nutrient utilization by dairy calves. *J. Dairy Sci.* **42,** 671.
Catron, D. V., Maddock, H. M., Speer, V. C., and Vohs, R. L. (1951). Effect of different levels of aureomycin with and without vitamin B_{12} on growing–fattening swine. *Antibiot. Chemother. (Washington, D.C.)* **1,** 31.
Catron, D. V., Jensen, A. H., Homeyer, P. G., Maddock, H. M., and Ashton, G. C. (1952). Re-evaluation of protein requirements of growing–fattening swine as influenced by feeding an antibiotic. *J. Anim. Sci.* **11,** 221.
Catron, D. V., Lane, M. D., Quinn, L. Y., Ashton, G. C., and Maddock, H. M. (1953). Mode of action of antibiotics in swine nutrition. *Antibiot. Chemother. (Washington D.C.)* **3,** 571.
Coates, M. E. (1953). The mode of action of antibiotics in animal nutrition. *Chem. Ind. (London)* **50,** 1333.
Coates, M. E., Dickensen, C. D., Harrison, G. F., Kon, S. K., Cummins, S. H., and Cuthbertson, W. F. J. (1951). Mode of action of antibiotics in stimulating growth of chicks. *Nature (London)* **168,** 332.

Coates, M. E., Davies, M. K., and Kon, S. K. (1955). The effect of antibiotics on the intestine of the chick. *Br. J. Nutr.* **9**, 110.

Dean, B. T., and Tribble, L. F. (1962). Effect of feeding therapeutic level of antibiotic at breeding on reproductive performance of swine. *J. Anim. Sci.* **21**, 207.

Flint, J. C., and Jensen, R. (1958). The effect of chlortetracycline fed continuously during fattening, on the incidence of liver abscesses in beef cattle. *Am. J. Vet. Res.* **19**, 830.

Gilliam, H. C., and Martin, J. R. (1975). Economic importance of antibiotics in feeds to producers and consumers of pork, beef and veal. *J. Anim. Sci.* **40**, 1241.

Goldberg, H. S. (1962). Evaluation of some potential public health hazards from nonmedical uses of antibiotics. *Proc. Easter Sch. Agric. Sci., Univ. Nottingham* **9.**

Gordon, H. A. (1952). "Studies on the Growth Effect of Antibiotics in Germ-free Animals," Colloq. University of Notre Dame, Lobund Inst., South Bend, Indiana.

Gordon, H. A. (1955). Morphologic characterization of germ-free life. *Bull. N.Y. Acad. Med.* [2] **31**, 239.

Gordon, H. A., Wagner, M., and Wostman, B. (1957–1958). Studies on conventional and germ-free chickens treated orally with antibiotics, *Antibiot. Annu.* p. 248.

Gossett, F. O., and Miyat, J. A. (1964). A new antibiotic in treatment of swine dysentery. *Vet. Med. & Small Anim. Clin.* **59**, 169.

Hash, J. H., Wishnick, M., and Miller, P. A. (1964). On the mode of action of the tetracycline antibiotics in *Staphylococcus aureus. J. Biol. Chem.* **239**, 2070.

Hawbaker, J. A., Diaz, F., Speer, V. C., Hays, V. W., and Catron, D. V. (1960). The effect of oleandomycin on the performance of the young growing pig. *J. Anim. Sci.* **19**, 800.

Hays, V. W. (1965). Unpublished data, experiment 6443. Iowa Agric. and Home Econ. Exp. Sta.

Hays, V. W. (1969). Biological basis for the use of antibiotics in livestock production. The Use of drugs in Animal Feeds. *Proc. Symp.* Publ. 1679, p. 11. Nat'l. Academy Sci. Wash. D.C.

Hays, V. W. (1973). SPF hogs: Do they need antibiotics? *Hog Farm Manage.* **10**, 12:30.

Hays, V. W. and D. S. Baker. (1967). Unpublished data, experiment 6708. Iowa Agric. and Home Econ. Exp. Sta.

Hays, V. W., and Speer, V. C. (1960). Effect of spiramycin on growth and feed utilization of young pigs. *J. Anim. Sci.* **19**, 938.

Hill, C. H., Keeling, A. D., and Kelley, J. W. (1957). Studies on the effect of antibiotics on the intestinal weights of chicks. *J. Nutr.* **62**, 255.

Hill, D. C., Branion, H. D., and Slinger, S. J. (1952). Influence of environment on the growth response of chicks to penicillin. *Poult. Sci.* **31**, 920.

Hogue, D. E., Warner, R. G., Loosli, J. K., and Grippin, C. H. (1957). Comparison of antibiotics for dairy calves on two levels of milk feeding. *J. Dairy Sci.* **40**, 1072.

Hvidsten, H., and Homb, T. (1961). The effect of supplementary terramycin and aureomycin at low and high levels in long-term experiments with bacon pigs. *Acta Agric. Scand.* **11**, 121.

Johansson, K. R., and Sarles, W. B. (1949). Some considerations of the biological importance of intestinal microorganisms. *Bacteriol. Rev.* **13**, 25.

Kellogg, T. F., Hays, V. W., Catron, D. V., Quinn, L. Y., and Speer, V. C. (1964). Effect of level and source of dietary protein on performance and fecal flora of baby pigs. *J. Anim. Sci.* **23**, 1089.

Kellogg, T. F., Hays, V. W., Catron, D. V., Quinn, L. Y., and Speer, V. C. (1966). Effect of dietary chemotherapeutics on the performance and fecal flora of pigs. *J. Anim. Sci.* **25**, 1102.

Krug, J. L. (1976). Effects of length of lactation and chlortetracycline on reproductive performance. Ph.D. Thesis, University of Kentucky, Lexington.

Lucas, I. A. M. (1957). Antibiotic supplements in rations for pigs. *Vet. Rec.* **69,** 233.

March, B., and Biely, J. (1952). The effect of feeding aureomycin on the bacterial content of chick feces. *Poult. Sci.* **31,** 177.

Mayrose, V. B., Speer, V. C., Hays, V. W., and McCall, J. T. (1964). Effect of an antibiotic (tylosin) and protein source on swine reproduction. *J. Anim. Sci.* **23,** 737.

Meade, R. J., and Forbes, R. M. (1956). The influence of chlortetracycline and vitamin B_{12} alone and in combination on nitrogen utilization by growing swine. *J. Nutr.* **59,** 459.

Melliere, A. L., Brown, H., and Rathmacher, R. P. (1973). Finishing swine performance and responses to tylosin. *J. Anim. Sci.* **37,** 286.

Messersmith, R. E., Johnson, D. D., Elliot, R. F., and Dean, J. J. (1966). Value of chlortetracycline in breeding rations for sows. *J. Anim. Sci.* **25,** 752.

Miyat, J. A., and Gossett, F. O. (1964). A new antibiotic in treatment of swine dysentery. *Vet. Med. & Small Anim. Clin.* **59,** 295.

Moore, P. R., Evenson, A., Luckey, T. D., McCoy, E., Elvehjem, C. A., and Hart, E. B. (1946). Use of sulfasuxidine, streptothricin and streptomycin in nutritional studies with the chick. *J. Biol. Chem.* **165,** 437.

Myers, D. J., and Speer, V. C. (1973). Effects of an antibiotic and flushing on performance of sows with short farrowing intervals. *J. Anim. Sci.* **36,** 1125.

Natz, D. (1973). Report measures economic gains from feed antibiotics. *Feedstuffs* **45,** 2:73.

Peo, E. R., Jr. (1962). Effectiveness of antibiotic supplements. *Nebr. Swine Day Rep.* **373,** 14. Anim. Husb. Dept., Univ. Nebraska, Lincoln.

Raper, K. B. (1952). A decade of antibiotics in America. *Mycologia* **44,** 1.

Ruiz, M. E., Speer, V. C., Hays, V. W., and Switzer, W. P. (1968). Effect of feed intake and antibiotic on reproduction in gilts. *J. Anim. Sci.* **27,** 1602.

Rusoff, L. L., Landogora, F. T., and Hester, H. H. (1954). Effect of aureomycin on certain blood constituents, body temperature, weights of organs and tissues and thickness of small intestines. *J. Dairy Sci.* **37,** 654.

Sainsbury, D. (1975). Making better use of antibiotics as growth promoters. *Pig Farming* **23,** 4:27.

Scott, H. M. (1962). The effect of a nonspecific infection on chick growth. *Proc. Ill. Nutr. Conf.* p. 23.

Smith, H. M. (1962). The effects of the use of antibiotics on the emergency of antibiotic-resistant disease-producing organisms in animals. *Proc. Easter Sch. Agric. Sci., Univ. Nottingham* **9.**

Speer, V. C. (1970). Maximizing the reproduction efficiency of the sow. *Feedstuffs* **42,** 46:27.

Speer, V. C., Vohs, R. L., Catron, D. V., Maddock, H. M., and Culbertson, C. C. (1950). Effect of aureomycin and animal protein factor on healthy pigs. *AMA Arch. Biochem.* **29,** 452.

Stokstad, E. L. R. (1954). Antibiotics in animal nutrition. *Physiol. Rev.* **34,** 25.

Taylor, J. H. (1957). The mode of action of antibiotics in promoting animal growth. *Vet. Rec.* **69,** 278.

Taylor, J. H., and Harrington, F. (1955). Influence of dietary antibiotic supplements on visceral weights of pigs. *Nature (London)* **175,** 643.

Teague, H. S., Griffo, A. P., Jr., and Rutledge, E. A. (1966). Response of growing-finishing swine to different levels and methods of feeding chlortetracycline. *J. Anim. Sci.* **25,** 693.

United States Tariff Commission. (1949–1973). "Synthetic Organic Chemicals." U. S. Production and Sales, Washington, D.C.

Wachholz, D. E., and Heidenreich, C. J. (1970). Effect of tylosin on swine growth in two environments. *J. Anim. Sci.* **31,** 1014.

Wallace, H. D., Milicevic, M., Pearson, A. M., Cunha, T. J., and Kroger, M. (1954). The influence of aureomycin on the protein requirement and carcass characteristics of swine. *J. Anim. Sci.* **13,** 177.

Weinberg, E. D. (1957). The mutual effects of antimicrobial compounds and metallic cations. *Bacteriol. Rev.* **21,** 46.

21

Physiological Effects of Estrogens in Animal Feeds with Emphasis on Growth of Ruminants

ALLEN TRENKLE and WISE BURROUGHS

I. INTRODUCTION

An estrogen by definition is any substance that will induce changes like those of natural estrus in the reproductive tract of female animals. Many naturally occurring compounds have estrogenic activity and are widely distributed in both plants and animals. Marshall and Jolly (1906) reported that estrus could be induced in ovariectomized dogs by injection of extracts of ovaries taken from another dog during estrus, which established that the changes associated with estrus were chemically induced. During the late 1920's, estrone, the first estrogen to be chemically identified, was isolated from human urine (Laqueur and De Jough, 1928) and later crystallized (Doisy *et al.*, 1929). Loewe and Spohr (1926) reported the presence of estrogenic activity in plants in 1926. Estrone and estriol, two of several natural estrogens found in animals, have also been isolated from plants (Butenandt and Jacobi, 1933; Skarzynski, 1933). Another source of naturally occurring estrogens was established when an estrogenic condition in swine was associated with consumption of corn infected with a fungus (McNutt *et al.*, 1928). The active compound from the mold has been isolated and identified as a resorcylic acid lactone (Stob *et al.*, 1962; Urry *et al.*, 1966). Investigations of the relationships between molecular structure and estrogenic activity resulted in the chemical synthesis of a number of compounds with estrogenic activity, including sources of estrogens with biological activity equal to or greater than that of the naturally occurring estrogens.

A feature of both natural and synthetic estrogens is the wide variety of structures that show estrogenic activity. The natural estrogens of animal origins are steroids with the cyclopentanoperhydrophenanthrene nucleus. The synthetic estrogens and those occurring in plants are not steroids, but possess similar biological characteristics of the naturally occurring animal estrogens.

The widespread distribution of compounds with estrogenic activity in both the plant and animal kingdoms makes it inevitable that estrogens are present in the food chain. One important consideration in livestock production is whether estrogens in feeds have any effects upon the productivity of animals. It became known during the 1940's that estrogens in forages might have undesirable effects upon animals when it was demonstrated that estrogenic activity in certain species of clover was great enough to adversely affect the reproductive performance of grazing sheep (Bennetts *et al.*, 1946). The lipemia and incidence of fatty livers associated with increased ovarian activity in chickens led to the use of DES in fattening poultry for market (Lorenz, 1954). Eventually experiments were conducted to study the effects of implanted DES in cattle and sheep (Andrews *et al.*, 1949; Dinusson *et al.*, 1950), but increased growth was observed rather than increased fat deposition as seen in poultry. The studies that showed that the plant estrogens were biologically active when consumed orally and the growth response of ruminants implanted with DES, an estrogen known to be active when fed, provided the rationale for feeding low levels of DES to cattle and sheep (Burroughs *et al.*, 1955; Hale *et al.*, 1955). Since then, estrogens of one form or another have been widely used in beef cattle and sheep in the United States as well as in some other countries to increase growth rate and to improve the efficiency of meat production.

It is not our intent to include all the effects of estrogens on animals in this review, but to limit it to some of the physiological responses of cattle and sheep to estrogens present in feed or implanted subcutaneously. Cattle and sheep that obtain much of their diet by grazing are the only species of domestic livestock that would be seriously affected by estrogens in pasture forages and are the only species in which estrogens are extensively used in production practices. The literature on the use of estrogens to stimulate growth of cattle and sheep is voluminous and can only be summarized. Comprehensive reviews of the effects of estrogens on performance of livestock have been published (Preston and Willis, 1974; Preston, 1975). Consideration will be given to the significance of plant estrogens, to estrogens of mycological origin, and to those estrogens deliberately added to feeds or implanted in relation to animal production.

II. PLANT ESTROGENS

The presence of estrogenic substances in plants was first reported by Loewe and Spohr (1926), and since then, more than 50 species of plants have been found to contain differing degrees of estrogenic activity (Bradbury and White, 1954). These substances from plants when consumed by animals produced effects on the reproductive system of immature female animals comparable to those manifested during estrus and can, therefore, be classified as naturally occurring estrogens similar to those of animal origin.

Because the potency of estrogens in plants is relatively low, little significance was attributed to their rather widespread occurrence in the plant kingdom. Considerable interest developed in Australia when infertility of grazing sheep was related to the estrogenic activity in certain species of subterranean clover (Bennetts *et al.*, 1946). These investigations have been extended by workers in several countries to include studies of the estrogens present in other legumes and pasture plants (Bickoff, 1968; Bickoff *et al.*, 1969).

The estrogenic activity in plants is extremely variable. Most of the early studies of the legumes dealt with environmental factors, such as level of fertilization, location, season, light and temperature, stage of growth, and genetic differences (Bickoff *et al.*, 1969). Many varieties have been studied in an attempt to find those with low estrogenic activity. It is now recognized that increased incidence of various plant diseases caused by insects, bacteria, fungi, or viruses cause higher levels of estrogenic activity (Bickoff, 1968; Rossiter, 1970; Saba *et al.*, 1972). In many of the studies in which increased estrogenic activity was related to environmental or genetic factors, the plants were also more susceptible to disease, so many of the observed differences probably have been confounded with effects caused by increased disease levels. It has been suggested that the greater estrogenic content of diseased plants may be associated with the accumulation of phenolic compounds as a mechanism of resistance of the plant to disease (Bickoff *et al.*, 1969).

A. Known Forage Estrogens

The compounds with estrogenic activity that have been isolated from forages and identified include the isoflavones, genistein, biochanin A, daidzein, formononetin, and pratensein, and the coumestans, coumestrol and 4′-methoxycoumestrol (Bickoff, 1968). The structural formulas of these compounds, along with the animal estrogen estradiol and the synthetic estrogens diethylstilbestrol and hexestrol, are shown in Fig. 1.

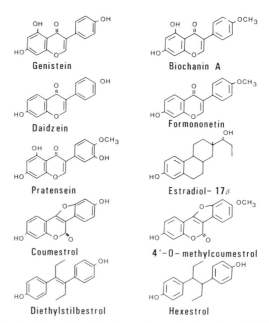

Fig. 1. Structural formulas of various plant, animal, and synthetic estrogens.

TABLE I
Concentrations of Estrogens in Certain Forages[a]

Estrogen	Forage (μg/gm dry forage)			
	Alfalfa	Ladino clover	Red clover	Subterranean clover
Biochanin A	1–5	0	1000	500
Daidzein	< 1	3	29	18
Formononetin	14	38	1700	900
Genistein	< 1	1	40	850
Coumestrol	57	49	18	26

[a] Adapted from Guggolz et al. (1961).

Genistein, formononetin, and daidzein have been found in subterranean clover, Ladino clover, red clover, and alfalfa. Biochanin A was found in subterranean and red clovers and alfalfa. Pratensein was found in red and subterranean clovers. An isoflavone glucoside, genistein, has been isolated from soybean meal. Coumestrol has been found in alfalfa, Ladino clover, and barrel medic, and 4'-methoxycoumestrol in alfalfa. In plants, the estrogens often occur as glycosides with the acidic malonate esters accounting for the predominant proportion of the glycosides (Beck and Knox, 1971). The quantities of some of the isoflavones and coumestrol in several legume forages are given in Table I. These values do not represent the extremely high levels sometimes found in pastures where daily dietary intake of the plant estrogens may be several grams. Estrogenic activity is widely distributed in different parts of plants, being found in leaves, stems, petioles, and flowers, but greatest levels of activity seem to be concentrated in the leaves (Francis and Millington, 1965).

Many other feedstuffs have been studied, but the active substances have not been isolated (Cheng et al., 1953a,b; Pieterse and Andrews, 1956a; Kitts et al., 1959). Grasses have been found to contain estrogenic activity, but usually the grasses have low levels compared with legumes. Many of the vegetable oils have measurable levels of estrogenic activity as measured by their uterotropic effect in immature mice (Booth et al., 1960). The presence of estrogenic activity in vegetable oils complicates many of the assays for plant estrogens because, often, the plant extracts or isolated estrogens have been dissolved in oil before being administered to assay animals.

Increase in uterine weight of immature or ovariectomized female mice or rats often has been used to measure the biological activity of estrogens in feeds and forages. More recently, bioassay methods using sheep have been developed to estimate the level of biological activity in some of the legumes (Braden *et al.*, 1964; Kelly, 1972). Estrogens in plant materials are first extracted with organic solvents, usually alcohol or acetone, followed by some additional purification by extraction of the estrogenic substances into ether. The extracts are incorporated into test diets and fed to assay animals, or dried, dissolved in oil, and injected into assay animals. Because many of the compounds have been isolated and identified, chromatographic procedures are available for quantitative estimation of specific plant estrogens in forages and animal tissues (Lindner, 1967). Antiserum to some of the plant estrogens, coupled to either proteins or synthetic polypeptides, have been produced in rabbits and sheep and are being used to develop radioimmunoassays for these estrogens (Bauminger *et al.*, 1969; Cox *et al.*, 1972). These sensitive assays will allow more detailed studies of the distribution and concentrations of plant estrogens in animal tissue.

The biological activities of several plant estrogens relative to DES and some of the estrogens from animals are given in Table II. Coumestrol is about 30 times more active than biochanin A, daidzein, or genistein, but only $1/3000$ as active as DES when fed to immature mice. Formononetin is quite insoluble, so a direct comparison with the other isoflavones is difficult and probably not justified in many of the reported assays. The method of administration of coumestrol or genistein to the assay animals (rodents) does not have an effect upon the estrogenic activity of these two compounds. The estrogens of animal origin are several hundred times more active than the plant estrogens, but the relative potency of the animal hormones varies considerably, depending upon the assay method and species of animal used for the assay. Estrone and estradiol are much more active when injected than when fed. Estradiol, the predominant estrogen secreted by the ovary, has biological activity similar to DES when injected, but much less activity when fed.

When given parenterally to ovariectomized ewes, the relative potencies of the plant estrogens as determined by measuring increases in uterine weights generally are similar to those measured in rodents. Genistein, biochanin A, and coumestrol are all active, and formononetin is relatively inactive. When given intraruminally, genistein, biochanin A, and coumestrol are considerably less active than when injected intramuscularly. Formononetin, however, is more active when given as an intraruminal infusion than when injected. In sheep, coumestrol is about 15 times more active than the isoflavones when given intraruminally and about 100 times more active when given by intramuscular injection. From these studies, it is evident that there are some differences in estrogenic activity of plant estrogens as determined in different species of assay

TABLE II
Estrogenic Activity of Some Estrogens[a]

Estrogen	Reference[b]									
	1	2	3	4	5	6	7	8	9	10
Biochanin A	0.000013	0.000005								
Daidzein	0.000017	0.000008								
Formononetin	0.000004	0.000003								
Genistein	0.000012	0.000010		0.000020						
Coumestrol		0.000346	0.000333							
Estrone		0.069			0.039	0.824	0.012	0.567	0.062	0.062
Estradiol					0.047	4.67	0.016	0.944	0.125	0.250
Estriol					0.100	0.047	0.032	0.063	0.333	0.025

[a] Values in μg of diethylstilbestrol activity/μg.

[b] Key to reference numbers: (1) Mouse uterine weight (Cheng et al., 1954) oral; (2) Mouse uterine weight (Bickoff et al., 1962) oral; (3) Mouse uterine weight (Bickoff et al., 1969) injected; (4) Mouse uterine weight (Cheng et al., 1953b) injected; (5) Mouse uterine cell changes (Sondern and Sealey, 1940) oral; (6) Mouse uterine cell changes (Sondern and Sealey, 1940) injected; (7) Rat uterine cell changes (Sondern and Sealey, 1940) oral; (8) Rat uterine cell changes (Sondern and Sealey, 1940) injected; (9) Rat uterine weight (Sealey and Sondern, 1941) oral; 10 Rat uterine weight (Sealey and Sondern, 1941) injected.

animals and by different routes of administration. The assays with rodents have been beneficial in directing the research effort to certain plants such as the subterranean clovers and other legumes, but are not a reliable prediction of potential problems with estrogenic activity of forages for grazing ruminants.

B. Metabolism

The isoflavones are extensively metabolized in sheep, with less than 1% being excreted as such in the feces and urine (Shutt *et al.*, 1970). In grazing animals, most of the metabolism occurs in the rumen before absorption. Both the plant estrogens and their metabolites are readily absorbed, largely from the rumen, and circulate in the plasma predominantly conjugated with glucuronic acid. When fed, measurable concentrations of free and conjugated isoflavones, coumestrol, and various metabolites are found in the plasma. Some further metabolism probably occurs in the liver and other tissues. Excretion from the body is largely in the urine, which contrasts to major excretion of the estrogens of animal and synthetic origin in the feces.

Genistein and biochanin A, which were isolated from varieties of subterranean clover implicated in causing infertility of grazing sheep, were first considered to be the active substances in as much as they were shown to be estrogenic when fed to rodents and were present in great enough concentrations in some clovers to cause problems. Later work, however, indicated that infertility of grazing sheep was more closely correlated with levels of formononetin rather than with genistein or biochanin A. This was somewhat surprising in view of the low estrogenic activity of formononetin. The differences in estrogenic activity of the isoflavones when administered to sheep by different routes, however, indicated that the metabolism of the plant estrogens was not the same when given parenterally and intraruminally (Braden *et al.*, 1967). Several studies have shown that the plant estrogens are extensively metabolized in the rumen.

The proposed metabolic pathways of the more frequently occurring plant estrogens are shown in Fig. 2. The initial step in the metabolism of biochanin A and formononetin in sheep is demethylation to genistein and daidzein, respectively. Genistein is largely degraded to p-ethylphenol, which is not estrogenic (Lindsay and Kelly, 1970). This metabolite is considered to originate in the rumen, which explains why estrogenic activity of biochanin A and genistein is much lower when given intraruminally as compared with parenterally. It has been estimated that 60–80% of the ingested biochanin A and genistein are ex-

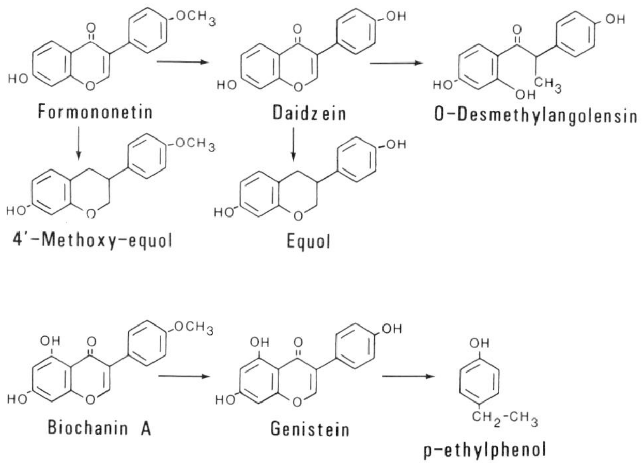

Formononetin   Daidzein   O-Desmethylangolensin

4'-Methoxy-equol   Equol

Biochanin A   Genistein   p-ethylphenol

Fig. 2. Structural formulas of formononetin, biochanin A, and their metabolites.

creted in the urine as p-ethylphenol. Daidzein, which is present in forages or arises from demethylation of formononetin, is metabolized to equol (Shutt et al., 1970), O-desmethyl-angolensin (Batterham et al., 1971), and 4'-methoxy-equol (Cox and Braden, 1974b). Equol is the predominating metabolite and accounts for about 70% of the formononetin consumed (Shutt and Braden, 1968). Because tissues of sheep do not convert daidzein to equol, its production must occur in the digestive tract. It has been shown to be produced from formononetin in ruminal fluid in vitro (Nilsson et al., 1967) and has been found in samples of rumen fluid taken from sheep grazing forages containing formononetin. Equol is readily absorbed from the rumen and mostly excreted in the urine, with a small portion in the feces. It is a weak estrogen, with about 25% of the activity of genistein in mouse assays. The concentration of equol in plasma of sheep grazing problem pastures is sufficiently high to be estrogenic and is considered to be the major compound responsible for the estrogenic response of sheep grazing forages containing high levels of formononetin (Cox and Braden, 1974a). Intraruminal infusion or intramuscular injection of coumestrol results in increased concentrations of free coumestrol as well as of coumestrol conjugated with glucuronic acid in plasma (Shutt et al., 1969). Because 4'-methylcoumestrol, which occurs in plants, is not found in plasma, it is thought to be converted to coumestrol in the rumen.

There seem to be some adaptations of the microbial population in the rumen for degradation of the plant estrogens because estrogenic effects of genistein and biochanin A can be detected within hours after sheep first consume them, but the activity decreases markedly within 2 to 4 days (Lindsay and Kelly, 1970). Estrogenic activity of coumestrol fed to ewes also decreases with increased period of intake, but at a slower rate than observed with the isoflavones. The proportion of formononetin converted to equol does not change with time after sheep consume the compound, so the estrogenic activity of plants containing formononetin remains high when consumed by grazing animals.

Qualitatively, metabolism of the plant estrogens in cattle is similar to that in sheep, but the concentrations of free estrogens and their metabolites are lower relative to the concentrations of the conjugated forms in cattle than in sheep (Braden *et al.*, 1971). These differences may account for the lower susceptibility of cattle grazing forages with relatively high levels of plant estrogens (Cox and Braden, 1974a). The factors that regulate the degradation and conjugation of plant estrogens are not known. Upon the basis of available evidence, it seems that the estrogenic response of animals grazing pastures with high concentrations of isoflavones is not due so much to the isoflavones themselves, but rather to their metabolites. The response to coumestrol seems to be more direct.

C. Physiological Effects

The biological effects of the plant estrogens are the same as the effects of the naturally occurring estrogens in mammalian species. For example, coumestrol has been found to increase the incorporation of labeled precursors into ribonucleic acid, proteins, and phospholipids of uterine cells similar to that of estradiol, differing only in degree of stimulation (Noteboom and Gorski, 1963).

A marked decrease in fertility of the female is the main symptom observed in sheep grazing estrogenic pastures. Fertility of males is not seriously affected. There are reports from Australia that indicate cattle are less susceptible than sheep to the effects of dietary intakes of high levels of plant estrogens (Cox and Braden, 1974a); the irregular cycles and decreased fertility of cattle consuming alfalfa, however, are thought by others (Adler and Trainin, 1962; Moule *et al.*, 1963) to be caused by high consumption of plant estrogens.

Ewes grazing estrogenic pastures usually have nearly normal estrous cycles and ovulation rates, but are less fertile in that they require more services per conception and have a lower lambing percentage (Underwood and Shier, 1951, 1952). There also, however, are reports of reduced estrus and ovulation rates in ewes grazing estrogenic forages (Lightfoot and Wroth, 1974). The pathological condition, cystic glandular hyperplasia, is almost always found in the cervix and uterus of sheep grazing estrogenic pastures for long periods. Similar pathological changes and infertility have been induced by prolonged administration of DES to ewes (Underwood et al., 1953; 1959). The main cause of infertility seems due to a failure of the ovulated eggs to be fertilized. It has been proposed that the increased amount and fluidity of the cervical mucus reduces the number of sperm entering the cervix. There are fewer sperm on the zona pellucida of eggs recovered from the oviducts of ewes after artificial insemination (Lightfoot and Wroth, 1974). Transport of eggs also might be affected. The histology of the pituitary, ovaries, and adrenals seems normal (Hearnshaw et al., 1972), but there is evidence that plant estrogens may affect luteal function (Lightfoot and Wroth, 1974). There is one report of decreased responsiveness of the pituitary to release of luteinizing hormone after injection of estradiol (Findlay et al., 1973). An impairment of the hypothalamus was suggested because the pituitary responded to gonadotropic-releasing hormone. In wethers, there is metaplasia of the glandular and duct epithelium of the bulbo-urethral and prostate glands and increased teat growth (Bennetts, 1947).

D. Effects on Growth

In feeding practice, beneficial effects frequently have been observed when good quality legume hay is fed to cattle and sheep. The superiority of these feeds cannot always be attributed to their nutrient composition. A series of experiments with lambs (Story et al., 1957) suggested that the estrogenic activity found in legume forages, as well as isolated genistein, caused increased rate of growth of fattening lambs. In other experiments, coumestrol increased the growth rate of wethers, but not ewe lambs (Oldfield et al., 1966). In most of these experiments, the addition of diethylstilbestrol to the diets stimulated weight gains to a greater extent than an equivalent amount of estrogenic activity from the plant estrogens as determined by assays in rodents. No beneficial responses were observed that could be related to coumestrol when sources of alfalfa containing different levels of coumestrol were fed to cattle (Stob, et al., 1963). Diethylstilbestrol and coumestrol have been compared in an experiment with steers, and daily gains were increased 12% by feeding 10 mg of DES per animal daily and only 4% by feeding 840 mg of coumestrol per animal daily (Stob et al., 1964).

Unfortunately, the studies of the effects of plant estrogens on growth of cattle and sheep were conducted before it was known that the isoflavones were extensively metabolized in the rumen. As most of the experiments have shown, it seems plausible that equivalent amounts of estrogenic activity from genistein and coumestrol should not give the same growth response as DES when fed because of the degradation of the plant estrogens. Formononetin or daidzein, which are converted to the estrogenic metabolite equol in the rumen, however, should give a growth response similar to that produced by an equivalent amount of DES, but this has not been demonstrated.

III. ESTROGENS OF MYCOLOGICAL ORIGIN

Since 1928, there have been several publications reporting the occurrence of estrogenic stimulation of animals fed moldy corn or spoiled grain (McNutt et al., 1928). A compound, which was isolated from corn infected with *Gibberella zeae*, elicited a uterotropic response in mice and was identified as a resorcylic acid lactone (Stob et al., 1962; Urry et al., 1966; Mirocha et al., 1967). It is referred to by the trivial name zearalenone (Fig. 3). Reduction of the double bond and the ketone group in the lactone ring converts the compound to zeranol. Both compounds have estrogenic activity in mice or rats. When zeranol is administered orally to immature mice or rats, it has $1/300$ to $1/400$ the estrogenic activity of diethylstilbestrol as measured by increase in uterine weight. When administered parenterally, zeranol has $1/1250$ to $1/2500$ the activity of diethylstilbestrol. Studies with sheep, however, indicate that the compound may be relatively more estrogenic in ruminants than in rodents as measured by increase in teat size, seminal vesicle weight, and pituitary weight (Table III). Compounds similar in structure have been reported to be produced by the fungi *Curvularia sp.*, *Penicillium stubii* Zalesbi and *P. Expansun* Link (Shibata et al., 1964), *Nectria radicicola* (Mirrington et al., 1964) and *Monosporium sp.* (McCapra et al., 1964). The increase in

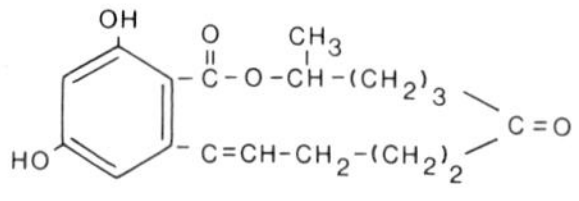

Zearalenone

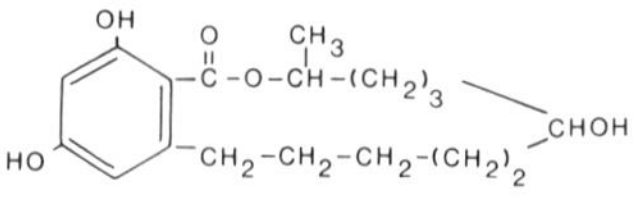

Zeranol

Fig. 3. Structural formulas of resorcylic acid lactones.

TABLE III
Effect of Estradiol-17β and Zeranol on Size of Seminal Vesicles, Pituitaries, and Teats of Wether Lambs[a]

Treatment (μg/day)	Number of animals	Seminal vesicles (gm)	Pituitary (mg)	Increase in teat size (cc)[b]	Body weight (kg)
Control (0)	20	0.91	657	0.444	51.3
Estradiol (50)	19	3.52	896	2.673	54.9
Zeranol (143)[c]	17	2.78	801	2.674	52.2

[a] Unpublished data from J. F. Wagner (personal communication, 1976).
[b] Diameter at base × length × 0.6.
[c] This level was calculated assuming total release of zeranol from the implant.

estrogenic activity of alfalfa during ensiling (Pieterse and Andrews, 1956b) suggests that estrogenic substances originate during the ensiling fermentation. These substances have not been identified, so it is not known if they are more active metabolites of some original plant estrogen present in alfalfa at the time of ensilling or if the activity is associated with compounds produced by molds or yeasts during the fermentation.

Zeranol implanted in cattle or sheep increases weight gain and improves feed efficiency. It now is commercially produced and is available as 12-mg pellets. The recommended dosage as a subcutaneous implant at the base of the ear is 12 mg for sheep and calves and 36 mg for feedlot cattle.

A. Metabolism

The known metabolism of zeranol is oxidation of the alcohol radical on the sixth carbon to a carbonyl radical, resulting in a nonestrogenic metabolite. Dehydrogenase enzymes in the liver and possibly from microorganisms in the gastrointestinal tract are thought to be involved. The metabolism and excretion of tritiated zeranol implanted subcutaneously have been studied in cattle (Sharp and Dyer, 1972). Plasma concentrations of the compound were either not detectable or present in low concentrations, but in other studies with higher doses, tritiated zeranol could be found in the plasma. Urinary excretion peaked at 10–12 days and then declined to undetectable levels at 90 days after implanting. Excretion in the feces peaked at 6–8 days and was undetectable after 85 days. Some radioactivity was still present in the bile at 125 days after implanting. Of the original activity in the implant, 10% was excreted in the urine, 45% in the feces, and 10% remained at the site of implantation. The remaining 35% was not accounted for. No residues were detected in any of the edible tissues of the body 65–126 days after implanting when an assay sensitive to about 10 ppb was used. Zeranol seems to be absorbed from the implant into the blood, cleared by the liver, and a major portion excreted into the intestine with the bile.

B. Physiological Effects

Enlarged, tense, and elevated vulvae, enlarged mammary glands, and in some instances, prolapse of the vagina and rectum have been observed in pigs fed grain infected with fungus (McNutt *et al.*, 1928). These are typical responses to estrogens and presumably are caused by the estrogenic activity present in the infected grain.

Subcutaneous implantation of zeranol, a derivative of the isolated estrogenic compound, into sheep or cattle also results in numerous endocrine and metabolic changes similar to those observed in cattle and sheep treated with DES (see Section IV, C). Increased weight of adrenal, pituitary, and seminal vesicles and increased size of teats have been reported (Borger *et al.*, 1971). Some of these data are shown in Table III. Plasma glucose and insulin concentrations tend to be greater in cattle implanted with zeranol, especially within 4 weeks of implantation (Sharp and Dyer, 1970). In another study in which measurements were made 84 days after implantation, there were no differences in plasma insulin between control and treated cattle, but serum concentrations of growth hormone were significantly greater in the implanted animals (Borger *et al.*, 1973).

C. Effects on Growth

Implanting zeranol at the level of 36 mg in cattle or 12 mg in sheep increases rate of gain and improves utilization of feed for weight gain. Feed consumption is only slightly increased (Sharp and Dyer, 1971; Wilson *et al.*, 1972; Borger *et al.*, 1973).

Differences in body composition are not always statistically significant, but usually, the treated animals have more protein and water and less fat. Use of the technique of comparative slaughter, with representative animals being slaughtered and chemical composition determined at the beginning of the experiment and animals slaughtered for determining chemical composition at the end of the experiment, indicated that both cattle and sheep implanted with zeranol retained more of the dietary nitrogen but less of the dietary energy than control animals (Sharp and Dyer, 1971). These studies suggest there is a change in nutrient metabolism that results in more efficient utilization of dietary protein for growth but less efficient use of energy. Even though the experimental data suggest that protein synthesis is accelerated, there does not seem to be a change in the relative amounts of myofibrillar, sarcoplasmic, or stromal proteins and nonprotein nitrogen fractions in skeletal muscle from treated cattle.

IV. SYNTHETIC ESTROGENS

Soon after the effectiveness of estrogens for increasing fat deposition in chickens was demonstrated, experiments were conducted with mammalian species. The results with ruminants were quite different from those obtained with poultry in that growth was increased without additional accumulation of fat. The levels of hormone implanted in the first experiments with cattle and sheep tended to decrease carcass quality and had a marked effect upon the accessory sex organs. Subsequent research indicated that adding small amounts of DES to the feed increased growth rate without undesirable effects on carcass quality. It is now known that use of lesser amounts of hormone in implants also will increase growth rate with minimal effects on carcass quality. These findings have found considerable application in growing and finishing cattle and sheep for meat production. The initial investigations were done with DES because it was relatively inexpensive and highly potent. Subsequently, the related stilbene derivatives, hexestrol and dienestrol, the dimethyl ethers of these compounds, and the natural estrogens have been evaluated for their effectiveness in stimulating growth and also have been developed for use in cattle and sheep.

Information on the development and the use of hormones in livestock production has been reviewed by Umberger (1975). The effects of estrogens on growth and performance of cattle have been extensively reviewed by Preston and Willis (1974) and Preston (1975) and provide references to many of the original experiments.

A. Effect on Body Weight Gain

A summary of the first experiments showing the beneficial effects of implanting DES on growth of cattle and sheep is given in Table IV. The results of the first experiments with the addition of small amounts of DES to the feed of beef cattle and sheep are given in Tables V and VI. As the results of these experiments show, DES significantly increased daily gain when added to the feed or when pellets containing the hormone

TABLE IV
Effect of Diethylstilbestrol Implants on Growth of Cattle and Sheep[a]

Experimental group	Number of animals	Initial weight (kg)	Daily gain (kg)	Feed per day (kg)	Feed/ gain
Heifers					
Control	5	230	0.94	7.27	7.74
Ovariectomized	5	224	0.87	7.73	8.92
DES[b]	5	232	1.05	7.83	7.44
Heifers					
Control	9	229	0.78	8.67	11.10
Ovariectomized	9	226	0.70	8.30	11.88
DES[c]	9	230	0.91	9.01	9.92
Sheep					
Control	20	32	0.159	2.11	13.26
DES[d]	20	32	0.222	2.14	9.61
DES[e]	20	33	0.227	2.13	9.38

[a] Adapted from Dinusson et al. (1950) and Andrews et al. (1949).
[b] Diethylstilbestrol, 42 mg.
[c] 48 mg.
[d] 12 mg.
[e] 24 mg.

were implanted subcutaneously. Daily feed consumption was only slightly increased while the efficiency of feed utilization for growth was significantly improved. The ovariectomized heifers in comparison with the control cattle gained less and had less efficient feed utilization (Table IV). A significant observation, although probably not fully appreciated at the time, was that growth rate seemed to be proportional to the amount of estrogen present whether of endogenous or exogenous origin. These were the first experiments to demonstrate that estrogens were anabolic in ruminants, which is contrary to much of the literature of experiments with rodents, in which estrogens often are considered to be catabolic with respect to somatic growth. There have been a few reports of increased growth in other species, but these findings have not been able to be repeated by other investigators. Some of the effects of estrogens on growth of different species has been reviewed by Trenkle (1969). In total, almost all published studies have indicated that estrogens markedly decrease the growth of rats, which has precluded their use to study the mode of action of estrogens on growth. Pigs given

TABLE V
Effect of Feeding Diethylstilbestrol on the Growth of Cattle[a]

Experimental group	DES (mg/day)	Number of animals	Initial weight (kg)	Daily gain (kg)	Feed per day (kg)	Feed/ gain
Cattle	0	8	314	1.01	9.52	9.40
	5.5	8	316	1.20	10.48	8.74
	11.0	8	316	1.39	10.50	7.56
Cattle	0	8	374	1.07	9.11	8.50
	5	8	374	1.17	9.17	7.83
	10	8	375	1.13	9.09	8.07
Cattle	0	8	396	0.92	9.20	9.98
	6	8	407	1.01	8.99	8.88
	12	8	413	1.06	9.37	8.82
Cattle	0	8	301	0.79	9.20	11.58
	10	8	282	0.92	9.53	10.34

[a] Adapted from Burroughs et al. (1955).

estrogens as implants or with the feed do not gain weight at a faster rate, but the hormone seems to be anabolic in pigs in that there is less fat and more lean in the treated animals (Plimpton and Teague, 1972). The rather high levels of DES required to produce the lipemic response in chickens result in some residues remaining in tissues, so most estrogens are not approved for use in poultry production. Only one product, estradiol-17b-monopalmitate, currently is available.

The initial observations with ruminants that estrogens increase growth rate and improve feed utilization have been confirmed in hundreds of experiments with animals of different breeds, sex, and age, as well as with animals fed many kinds of feeds and raised under different management practices (Preston and Willis, 1974). The recommended dosages of DES have been 10 mg per head daily when fed to cattle, 2 mg per head daily when fed to sheep, 24 or 36 mg when implanted in cattle, and 3 mg when implanted in sheep. Compressed pellets containing hexestrol (usually 15 mg for sheep and 60 mg for cattle) have been widely used in some countries. Combination of estrogens with other hormones have been studied extensively (Gassner et al., 1958), and several products have been developed. One pellet developed as an implant for cattle contains 24 mg of DES and 120 mg of testosterone. A combination of 20 mg of

594   Allen Trenkle and Wise Burroughs

TABLE VI
Effect of Feeding Diethylstilbestrol on Growth of Sheep[a]

Experimental group	DES (mg/kg feed)	Daily gain (kg)	Feed per day (kg)	Feed/ gain
Sheep[b]	0	0.173	1.86	10.76
	0.66	0.185	1.63	8.82
	1.32	0.196	1.74	8.87
	1.98	0.179	1.67	9.32
Sheep[b]	0	0.157	1.72	10.95
	0.66	0.196	1.82	9.28
	1.32	0.210	1.62	7.71
	1.98	0.231	1.90	8.21
Sheep[c]	0	0.157	1.42	9.02
	1.32	0.181	1.40	7.76
	2.64	0.158	1.40	8.85
Sheep[c]	0	0.134	1.33	9.90
	1.32	0.178	1.36	7.63
	2.64	0.167	1.29	7.74

[a] Adapted from Hale et al. (1955).
[b] Sheep were individually fed, 4 animals per treatment.
[c] Sheep were fed in pens, 2 pens per treatment, 40 animals per treatment.

estradiol benzoate with either 200 mg of testosterone propionate or 200 mg of progesterone in pellet form is available for implanting heifers and steers, respectively.

The greatest response to estrogen is noted in castrated males, with somewhat less response in females and often no growth response in sexually mature entire males unless much higher levels of estrogen are used. Administration of estrogens to immature bull calves does increase growth rate (Vander Wal et al., 1975a). With respect to age, there is considerable experimental variation; the more mature animals near growth stasis, however, seem to respond more than very young rapidly growing individuals. Growth rate of 3- to 4-month-old calves usually is increased by implanting estrogens, but not to the same extent observed in older animals.

The response to estrogens is an increase in normal somatic growth, with the extra weight being distributed in all parts of the body, including the carcass, bones, individual organs, and hide. The composition of the body determined by physical separation into lean, bone, and separable fat is significantly altered. Cattle or sheep given estrogen have more lean tissue and bone and less fat. Larger muscles often are found in the estrogen-treated animals. The higher concentrations of elastin, hydroxyproline, and mucoprotein hexose amine in muscle tissue are indicative of more connective tissue (McIntosh *et al.,* 1961). Meat from estrogen-treated animals, when evaluated in organoleptic tests, usually is slightly less tender, which is consistent with the chemical analysis. Evaluations of juiciness and flavor have been variable (Simone *et al.,* 1958; Forrest and Sather, 1965), but the differences have been small. Chemically, the bodies of cattle or sheep given estrogen contain more protein, water, and minerals, but less fat (Table VII). In these long-term growth studies, the increased body water must be associated with the increased amount of muscle mass because, on a fat-free basis, there is no change in the proportion of water in the body.

In all the experiments designed to study the effects of estrogens on nutrient requirements, with the exception of energy, there is no evidence of altered nutrient requirements. Cattle or sheep fed diets con-

TABLE VII
Effect of Diethylstilbestrol on Composition of Body Gain and on Utilization of Dietary Energy and Protein for Body Weight Gain of Cattle[a]

	Ration					
	Corn grain		Higher moisture corn silage		Lower moisture corn silage	
Level of DES, mg/day	0	20	0	20	0	20
Number of animals	9	9	10	10	10	10
Empty body weight gain (kg)	158	181	144	177	142	172
Composition of gain						
Moisture (%)	24.7	30.9	20.9	31.6	22.5	29.7
Protein (%)	9.5	11.7	8.2	12.1	8.6	11.1
Fat (%)	63.4	54.4	68.7	53.3	66.7	56.3
Efficiency of gain						
Energy gained/						
energy consumed × 100	33.5	29.6	34.7	30.0	32.2	30.2
Protein gained/						
protein consumed × 100	11.3	15.0	7.7	13.3	7.9	11.5

[a] Adapted from Fowler *et al.* (1970).

taining higher levels of grain usually respond relatively more than those fed diets containing high levels of roughage. In experiments in which cattle have not been fed sufficient feed to maintain body weight, administration of estrogens increased the rate of weight loss (Everitt, 1962a,b; Oltjen et al., 1973). When measured, the efficiency of converting dietary energy to body energy also is reduced (Table VII). The metabolizable energy content of these diets was not altered by feeding DES (Adeyanju et al., 1969), which indicates that digestion of the energy component of the feed is not affected. The less efficient use of energy in cattle treated with estrogen is caused by an increase in basal metabolism, which has been observed to occur as evidenced by increased respiratory and heart rates as well as by measurements by direct calorimetry (Tyrrell et al., 1975). There is an improvement of other dietary nutrients by ruminants treated with estrogens. As can be seen from the data in Table VII, the nitrogen fraction of the diet was used more efficiently for body growth by the animals fed DES. Similar results have been observed with hexestrol in cattle (Burgess and Lamming, 1960) and sheep (Gee and Preston, 1957), the combination of estradiol and progesterone in cattle (Lofgreen, 1973), and zeranol in cattle and sheep (Sharp and Dyer, 1971. Improved utilization of dietary nitrogen also has been demonstrated in nitrogen-balance studies with both cattle and sheep (Clegg and Cole, 1954; Whitehair et al., 1953; Bell et al., 1957; Trenkle, 1969; Vander Wal et al., 1975b). Representative data from an experiment with sheep are presented in Table VIII. These data, as well as those from the other experiments, indicate that digestibility of the nitrogen fraction of the diet is not changed, but rather, that there is improvement in the utilization of the absorbed nitrogen, with less being excreted in the urine. Injection of growth hormone increased nitrogen retention of sheep to an extent similar to feeding DES (Table VIII).

The effects of estrogens on mineral balance have been measured in several experiments with sheep, and there is increased retention of calcium and phosphorus (Whitehair et al., 1953; Bell et al., 1957; Braithwaite et al., 1972). Increased growth and uptake of calcium by bone also has been reported (Shroder and Hansard, 1958a; Davey et al., 1959; Braithwaite et al., 1972). Braithwaite (1975) reported that injection of growth hormone caused changes in calcium metabolism similar to estrogens.

Attention has been directed to possible effects of estrogens in altering rumen function to account for the unique effect of estrogens on increasing growth of cattle and sheep. There have been reports of increased cellulose digestion in the rumen (Brooks et al., 1954), as well as increased numbers of protozoa in the rumen of animals fed estrogens (Christiansen et al., 1964; Ibrahim et al., 1970), but there have been no

TABLE VIII

Effect of Diethylstilbestrol and Growth Hormone on Nitrogen Retention and Digestibility in Sheep [a]

Protein (%)	DES (mg/day)	No growth hormone (Period 1, 12 days)	Growth hormone (Period 2, 12 days)	No growth hormone (Period 3, 12 days)
Nitrogen retained (gm/sheep/day)				
8.5	0	2.7	4.4	2.2
8.5	2	4.5	5.0	3.9
13.0	0	3.9	5.8	2.0
13.0	2	6.0	6.8	4.6
Digestibility of protein (%)				
8.5	0	60	59	61
8.5	2	57	60	62
13.0	0	69	73	72
13.0	2	67	69	71
Digestibility of dry matter (%)				
8.5	0	72	71	71
8.5	2	72	74	75
13.0	0	71	74	72
13.0	2	72	74	75

[a] Adapted from Struempler and Burroughs (1959).

consistent effects of estrogens on digestibility of any dietary constituent that could account for the increased growth or nitrogen and mineral retention (Whitehair et al., 1953; Bell et al., 1957).

B. Metabolism

The metabolism of DES in ruminants is reviewed in more detail in another chapter (see Aschbacher, Chapter 22). The metabolism of the natural estrogens normally produced in cattle and sheep has been reviewed by Velle (1963). Suffice it to indicate here that both the natural and synthetic estrogens are readily absorbed from the gastrointestinal tract and rapidly cleared by the liver. Seemingly, the liver is somewhat less efficient in clearing DES so that sufficient quantities get into circulation to exert an estrogenic effect. The liver, as well as tissues from the small intestine and rumen mucosa, rapidly conjugate DES to form the glucuronide (Huber et al., 1972). In ruminants, the important route of elimination is in the feces (Aschbacher and Thacker, 1974). The DES excreted in the feces is found as free hormone; there are, however, indications that there may be other phenolic metabolites (Aschbacher et al., 1975). The possibility that the free hormone and metabolites may originate from microbial activity in the large intestine has not been excluded. Excretion in the feces is also the predominant route for excretion of ^{14}C-diethylstilbestrol implanted in cattle, but the proportion of the total excreted in the feces is somewhat less (Aschbacher et al., 1975). That portion excreted in the urine occurs chiefly as the glucuronide. Metabolism od DES to CO_2 probably is not a significant metabolic pathway, because no labeled CO_2 is expired after administration of labeled hormone (Ashbacher, 1972). Eventually, all the DES or hexestrol given to cattle or sheep is excreted in the feces and urine. The high concentration of the hormones in bile and gallbladder suggests that the bile is a major excretory pathway in ruminants.

Because most of the synthetic estrogens administered to ruminants are rapidly excreted in the feces and urine as free or as conjugated hormones, consideration has been given to the fate of the hormones in excreta distributed on the soil. Both DES and hexestrol are unstable in soil and disappear within a few weeks (Broom et al., 1961; Glascock and Jones, 1961; Gregers-Hansen, 1964a). Volatilization and leaching from the soil are not major losses. Bacteria and enzymes present in soil are considered to degrade the estrogens in inactive metabolites. The uptake of estrogenic activity by growing plants does not present any danger to animals or humans (Glascock and Hewitt, 1963); Gregers-Hansen, 1964b; Hacker et al., 1967).

C. Physiological Effects

Numerous experiments to study the physiological changes associated with the use of estrogens have been conducted with cattle and sheep to gain some understanding of the mode of action of estrogens on growth of ruminants and the effects of the hormone on reproductive performance. It is not surprising that continuous administration of estrogens does have some effects on the primary and secondary sex glands. Reproduction of heifers fed 10 or 20 mg of DES per day, however, does not seem to be affected, and there is no change in subsequent milk production (Reuber, 1958; Reuber et al., 1961). Reproduction of ewes, which are sensitive to low levels of estrogen, was impaired by injection of 0.09 mg or more of DES per week (Underwood et al., 1959). Higher levels caused infertility and cystic changes in the endometrium similar to the changes observed in ewes grazing estrogenic pastures. Uterine weight is increased, ovarian weight decreased, and testicular weight decreased with estrogen treatment (Preston et al., 1960). There is stimulation of the mammary gland in both males and females. Teat size is increased (Table III), and, if the levels of estrogens are high enough, some milk can be expressed from the glands. The size of the seminal vesicles and bulbo-urethrals of the castrated male are also increased (Preston and Burroughs, 1960).

Pituitary glands from estrogen-treated animals are larger relative to body weight (Clegg and Cole, 1954; Shroder and Hansard, 1958b; Struempler and Burroughs, 1959; Burgess and Lamming, 1960; Preston and Burroughs, 1960; Trenkle, 1970). The increase in size of the gland is caused by an increase in cell numbers and possibly in cell size (Martin and Lamming, 1958). The heavier glands have been found to contain more growth hormone (Clegg and Cole, 1954; Shroder and Hansard, 1958b; Struempler and Burroughs, 1959), less gonadotropins (Shroder and Hansard, 1958b; Burgess and Lamming, 1960), and similar quantities of adrenocorticotropin and thyrotropin (Clegg and Cole, 1954; Shroder and Hansard, 1958b; Burgess and Lamming, 1960). The amount of growth hormone in the pituitary relative to body weight is significantly increased. Plasma concentrations of growth hormone are greater in animals given estrogen over relatively long periods (Trenkle, 1970). Concentrations of growth hormone in plasma after shorter periods are more variable (Beck et al., 1976; Davis and Borger, 1974). The concentration of growth hormone in plasma was higher in cattle after administration of zeranol (Borger et al., 1973).

The effect of estrogens on weight of the thyroid glands of ruminants is quite variable, but in many experiments, weight of the gland tends to be decreased (Davey et al., 1959; Burgess and Lamming, 1960; Preston and Burroughs, 1960). Increased follicular epitehlial cell height has been reported (Davey et al., 1959; Burgess and Lamming, 1960), but concentration of thyroid hormones in plasma as measured by protein-bound iodine was not changed by feeding DES (Trenkle, 1969, 1970). Metabolic clearance of thyroxine was not statistically different, but tended to be greater in the treated sheep.

Cattle implanted with DES often have heavier adrenal glands, and histological examination has indicated that the increase is in the cortex (Clegg and Cole, 1954). Shroder and Hansard (1958b), Burgess and Lamming (1960), and Preston and Burroughs (1960) did not observe differences in weight of adrenal glands of cattle or sheep given estrogens. The enzyme glucose-6-phosphate dehydrogenase in adrenal tissue from cattle is inhibited by DES (McKerns, 1963). If the concentration of estrogen is high enough in adrenal tissue of treated cattle to inhibit this enzyme, there would be, in turn, decreased synthesis of glucocorticoids, which would increase adrenocorticotropin secretion. Reduction in blood eosinophils in cattle implanted with DES (Clegg and Cole, 1954) is evidence of increased adrenocorticotropin secretion. Altered secretion of adrenocorticotropin from the pituitary or secretion of steroids from the adrenal cortex has not been measured directly.

In a number of experiments, cattle and sheep treated with estrogens have had higher concentrations of insulin in the plasma (Trenkle, 1969, 1970; Davis *et al.*, 1970b; J. F. Wagner, personal communication, 1976). Concentrations of blood glucose generally are higher in the treated animals (Preston and Burroughs, 1960; Harter and Vetter, 1967; Davis *et al.*, 1970b; Riis *et al.*, 1974). The effects of estrogens on glucose metabolism of ruminants has not been extensively studied, except in one study with a limited number of calves where it seemed that estrogens increased glucose turnover rate (Riis *et al.*, 1974). It is not known if the effects of estrogens on glucose metabolism are direct or indirect through some other hormone such as growth hormone. The increased insulin secretion may be a response to the higher plasma glucose, which follows elevated growth hormone concentrations rather than being caused by a direct effect of estrogens on the pancreas or glucose metabolism. Wallace and Bassett (1966) have observed increases in plasma concentrations of glucose and insulin in sheep during infusion of growth hormone.

Concentrations of urea (Preston, 1968; Davis *et al.*, 1970b), total amino acids and essential amino acids (Oltjen and Lehmann, 1968; Oltjen *et al.*, 1973) in plasma each tend to be decreased after administration of estrogens to ruminants. Maximum response occurs within 2 to 3 weeks (Grebing *et al.*, 1970). These changes are in accordance with increased utilization of nitrogen absorbed from the digestive tract. All the nitrogen-balance studies have indicated that there is less nitrogen excreted in the urine. A more detailed study by Huber (1970) showed that there was less urea excreted in the urine of sheep treated with DES, but that there were no changes in rates of tubular reabsorption or glomerular filtration that might account for the decreased excretion of urea. In total, all the experimental evidence suggests that there is increased protein synthesis, which decreases plasma amino acids and results in less urea being produced. Many of the experiments conducted to study the effects of estrogens on blood metabolites have been of rather short duration, and sudden changes in body water could alter concentrations of metabolites in blood or body fluids. Preston (1969) measured body water in sheep given DES and found no differences that could account for the changes in blood metabolites or hormones.

D. Mode of Action of Growth-Promoting Effects of Estrogens

Proposals advanced for explaining the growth-promoting action of estrogens in ruminants include (1) increased production of androgens from the adrenal cortex (Clegg and Cole, 1954), (2) increased thyroid activity (Burgess and Lamming, 1960), (3) increased growth hormone secretion (Struempler and Burroughs, 1959), and (4) a direct effect of estrogens at the tissue level (McLaren *et al.*, 1960). There is some experimental evidence to support each of these proposals, but the evidence is indirect and quite variable for each except for proposal (3).

Higher concentrations of androgens in plasma of cattle or sheep treated with estrogens have not been demonstrated. Increased growth of the androgen-sensitive secondary sexual glands of castrated males is the strongest evidence of greater production of androgens. Administration of exogenous androgens alone usually has not resulted in increased growth of feedlot cattle or sheep (Dinusson *et al.*, 1950), so it seems unlikely that the principal mode of action of estrogens is an increase in secretion of androgens.

Changes in the epithelial cells of the follicles in the thyroid and increased metabolic rates are suggestive of the thyroid being involved, but the changes in blood metabolites, such as glucose, amino acids, urea, and insulin, are not in complete agreement with higher rates of thyroid secretion. Furthermore, the studies of the relationship between growth and thyroid secretion in sheep by Falconer and Draper (1968) would indicate that greater hormone secretion probably would decrease growth rates. Injection of thyroxine has decreased the weight gain of cattle (Brumby, 1959).

Most of the experimental data support the proposal that increased secretion of growth hormone in response to estrogens results in faster growth of ruminants. The most direct evidence is larger pituitary glands containing more growth hormone, along with higher concentrations of growth hormone in plasma. The higher concentrations of growth hormone in plasma must be interpreted with some caution because they might be caused by decreased metabolic clearance rather than increased secretion. The effects of estrogens on clearance of growth hormone from the circulatory system of ruminants have not been studied. The most supportive evidence for the involvement of growth hormone is that all the effects of estrogens on metabolism and growth of ruminants can be duplicated by administration of growth hormone. The results are summarized in Table IX. Because of the limited amounts of growth hormone available for research and the short half-life of growth hormone in the circulatory system, it has not been economical or feasible to conduct studies for long periods, so most of the experiments have been of short duration and could be criticized on that point. Injection of purified growth hormone in cattle (Brumby, 1959) and sheep (J. F. Wagner, personal communication, 1976) has increased growth rate and carcass leanness. Attempts to find compounds other than estrogens that could be

602

Allen Trenkle and Wise Burroughs

TABLE IX

Physiological Responses of Cattle and Sheep to Estrogens Which Are Duplicated by Administrat
of Growth Hormone

Effect of estrogen	Duplicated by growth hormone	Reference
Increase protein synthesis	Yes	J. F. Wagner (personal communication, 1976)
Increase nitrogen retention	Yes	Davis et al. (1970a); Struempler and Burroughs (1959)
Increase Ca and P retention	Yes	Braithwaite (1975)
Decrease blood urea	Yes	Davis et al. (1970a)
Decrease plasma amino acids	Yes	Davis et al. (1970a)
Increase blood glucose	Yes	Davis et al. (1970a); Wallace and Bassett (1966)
Increase plasma insulin	Yes	Davis et al. (1970a); Wallace and Bassett (1966)
Increase metabolic rate	Yes	Yousef and Johnson (1966)

used to increase release of growth hormone over long periods have not been successful. The concentration of growth hormone in plasma also increases in response to estrogens in other species in which estrogens are not anabolic, such as rat (Lloyd et al., 1971) and man (Frantz and Rabkin, 1965). It is not known why the higher concentrations of growth hormone following administration of estrogens are more anabolic in ruminants than other species.

It is not certain what role the higher concentrations of insulin, which probably are secondary to the increase in growth hormone, might play in the anabolic response to estrogens. Insulin is considered necessary for and to increase protein synthesis in rats, but its role in protein synthesis in ruminants is not clearly established. It may be that the total anabolic response observed with estrogens in ruminants is the result of the combined actions of insulin and growth hormone.

The possibility that estrogens have a direct effect on tissues that results in increased utilization of nutrients and growth is intriguing and cannot be ruled out as a possible explanation of the effects of estrogens on growth. There have been few attempts to demonstrate such a direct effect, but one limited study with chick myoblasts cultured in vitro (unpublished results of R. Allen, Iowa State University) indicated that DES did not significantly increase growth of these cells. Similar studies with cells from ruminants need to be conducted.

It is well known that female cattle or sheep do not grow as fast or are not as lean as the entire or castrated male. An obvious question is why do females not grow faster than males if estrogens are anabolic. In the cycling female, estrogenic secretion is increased for only a few days during the cycle, and the changes usually result in increased activity and altered feed consumption not conducive to greater growth. The metabolic effects of estrogens are evident within a few hours, but maximum reduction in plasma urea, for example, does not occur for 2–3 weeks. It seems that cyclic increases in estrogen secretion during the estrus cycle would not be as effective in causing most of the changes observed with continuous administration. Hormones secreted by the ovary, however, seem to express some anabolic effect because ovariectomy reduces growth rate of heifers. There is preliminary evidence that metabolic clearance of growth hormone is greater in female than in male cattle (Trenkle, 1971), which would keep plasma concentrations of growth hormone similar to or lower than those in males even if there was increased secretion from the pituitary. This difference in growth hormone metabolism may be related to the slower growth of females.

The decreased efficiency of utilization of dietary energy for deposition in body gain might be considered not in agreement with an anabolic response. As discussed, it has been demonstrated a number of times that one effect of estrogens in ruminants is increased growth of muscle and other lean tissues at the expense of fat. Some of the greater energy loss in estrogen-treated cattle is most likely caused by the difference in efficiency of the use of energy for synthesis of increased quantities of protein and less fat. It may be relevant that increased heat loss has been induced in mature cows after injection of growth hormone (Yousef and Johnson, 1966).

V. OVERVIEW

All the available evidence indicates that administration of low levels of estrogens on a continuous basis to increase concentrations of estrogen in the body to levels still considerably below those during peak production rates during pregnancy or estrus produces an anabolic response in cattle and sheep that is not observed in other species. The variation of response by different species to the same hormone, which has been documented many times in endocrinology, is the physiological basis for the use of estrogens in commercial production of beef cattle and sheep. The variation of response to estrogens by different species is great enought that it is not possible to extrapolate experimental findings from one species to another.

The increase in growth rate, alteration in body composition, and changes in concentrations of metabolites and hormones in plasma are qualitatively similar with all the different estrogens if molecules with estrogenic activity get into circulation. It might be possible to modify estrogen molecules so that they are more effective, or to change the methods of administering the hormones to animals so that lower levels could be used. Because estrogens can elicit many responses, some of which are undesirable, there has been interest in separating estrogenic activity from anabolic activity, but the available evidence to date is not particularly encouraging. The use of forages containing naturally occurring estrogens as a source of anabolic agents does not seem very promising because of the variability of the estrogenic activity in forages and the extensive metabolism of the plant estrogens in the rumen to compounds with differing biological activities.

REFERENCES

Adeyanju, S. A., Fowler, M. A., and Burroughs, W. (1969). Metabolizable energy of finishing beef cattle rations with and without stilbestrol. *J. Anim. Sci.* **29**, 967.

Adler, J. H., and Trainin, D. (1962). The apparent effect of alfalfa on the reproductive performance of dairy cattle. *Proc. Int. Congr. Anim. Prod., 4th, 1961* p. 451.

Andrews, F. N., Beeson, W. M., and Harper, C. (1949). The effect of stilbestrol and testosterone on the growth and fattening of lambs. *J. Anim. Sci.* **8**, 578.

Aschbacher, P. W. (1972). Metabolism of ^{14}C-diethylstilbestrol in sheep. *J. Anim. Sci.* **35**, 1031.

Aschbacher, P. W., and Thacker, E. J. (1974). Metabolic fate of oral diethylstilbestrol in steers. *J. Anim. Sci.* **39**, 1185.

Aschbacher, P. W., Thacker, E. J., and Rumsey, T. S. (1975). Metabolic fate of diethylstilbestrol implanted in the ear of steers. *J. Anim. Sci.* **40**, 530.

Batterham, T. J., Shutt, D. A., Hart, N. K., Braden, A. W. H., and Tweeddale, H. J. (1971). Metabolism of intraruminally administered [4-^{14}C]formononetin and [4-^{14}C]biochanin A in sheep. *Aust. J. Agric. Res.* **22**, 131.

Bauminger, S., Sindner, H. R., Perel, E., and Arnon, R. (1969). Antibodies to a phyto-oestrogen: Antigenicity of genistein coupled to a synthetic polypeptide. *J. Endocrinol.* **44**, 567.

Beck, A. B., and Knox, J. R. (1971). The acylated isoflavone glycosides from subterranean clover and red clover. *Aust. J. Chem.* **24**, 1509.

Beck, T. W., Smith, V. G., Seguin, B. E., and Convey, E. M. (1976). Bovine serum LH, GH and prolactin following chronic implantation of ovarian steroids and subsequent ovariectomy. *J. Anim. Sci.* **42**, 461.

Bell, M. C., Taylor, J. R., and Murphee, R. L. (1957). Effect of feeding stilbestrol and urea on ration digestibility and on retention of calcium, phosphorus and nitrogen in lambs. *J. Anim. Sci.* **16**, 821.

Bennetts, H. W. (1947). A further note on metaplasia in the sex organs of castrated male sheep on subterranean clover pastures. *Aust. Vet. J.* **23**, 10.

Bennetts, H. W., Underwood, E. J., and Shier, F. L. (1946). A specific breeding problem of sheep on subterranean clover pastures in Western Australia. *Aust. Vet. J.* **22**, 2.

Bickoff, E. M. (1968). Oestrogenic constitutents of forage plants. *Commonw. Bur. Pastures and Field Crops (G.B.), Rev. Ser.* **1**.

Bickoff, E. M., Livingston, A. L., Hendrickson, A. P., and Booth, A. N. (1962). Relative potencies of several estrogen-like compounds found in forages. *J. Agric. Food Chem.* **10**, 410.

Bickoff, E. M., Spencer, R. R., Witt, S. C., and Knuckles, B. E. (1969). Studies on the chemical and biological properties of coumestrol and related compounds. *U.S., Dep. Agric., Tech. Bull.* **1408**.

Booth, A. N., Bickoff, E. M., and Kohler, G. O. (1960). Estrogen-like activity in vegetable oils and mill by-products. *Science* **131**, 1807.

Borger, M. L., Wilson, L. L., Sink, J. D., Ziegler, J. H., and Davis, S. L. (1971). Zeranol and protein effects on finishing steers. *J. Anim. Sci.* **33**, 275 (abstr.).

Borger, M. L., Wilson, L. L., Sink, J. D., Ziegler, J. H., and Davis, S. L. (1973). Zeranol and dietary protein level effects on line performance, carcass merit, certain endocrine factors and blood metabolite levels of steers. *J. Anim. Sci.* **36**, 706.

Bradbury, R. B., and White, D. E. (1954). Estrogens and related substances in plants. *Vitam. Horm. (N.Y.)* **12**, 207.

Braden, A. W. H., Southcott, W. H., and Moule, G. R. (1964). Assessment of oestrogenic activity of pastures by means of increase of teat length in sheep. *Aust. J. Agric. Res.* **15**, 142.

Braden, A. W. H., Hart, N. K., and Lamberton, J. A. (1967). The oestrogenic activity and metabolism of certain isoflavones in sheep. *Aust. J. Agric. Res.* **18**, 335.

Braden, A. W. H., Thain, R. I., and Shutt, D. A. (1971). Comparison of plasma phyto-oestrogen levels in sheep and cattle after feeding on fresh clover. *Aust. J. Agric. Res.* **22**, 663.

Braithwaite, G. D. (1975). The effect of growth hormone on calcium metabolism in the sheep. *Br. J. Nutr.* **33**, 309.

Braithwaite, G. D., Glascock, R. F., and Riazuddin, Sh. (1972). The effect of hexoestrol on calcium metabolism in the sheep. *Br. J. Nutr.* **28**, 269.

Brooks, C. C., Garner, G. B., Muhrer, M. E., and Pfander, W. H. (1954). Effect of some steroid compounds on ovine rumen function. *Science* **120**, 455.

Broom, W. A., Gurd, M. R., Harmer, G. L. M., and Randall, S. S. (1961). The stability of hexoestrol in soil and its uptake by plants. *J. Endocrinol.* **21**, 381.

Brumby, P. J. (1959). The influence of growth hormone on growth in young cattle. *N. Z. J. Agric. Res.* **2**, 683.

Burgess, T. D., and Lamming, G. E. (1960). The effect of diethylstilbestrol, hexoestrol and testosterone on the growth rate and carcass quality of fattening beef steers. *Anim. Prod.* **2**, 93.

Burroughs, W., Culbertson, C. C., Cheng, E., Hale, W. H., and Homeyer, P. (1955). The influence of oral administration of diethylstilbestrol to beef cattle. *J. Anim. Sci.* **14**, 1015.

Butenandt, A., and Jacobi, H. (1933). Über die darstellung eines kerystallisierten pflanzlichen tokokinins (thelykinins) und seine identifizierung mit dem α-follikelhormon. *Hoppe-Seyler's Z. Physiol. Chem.* **218**, 104.

Cheng, E., Story, C. D., Payre, L. C., Yoder, L., and Burroughs, W. (1953a). Detection of estrogenic substances in alfalfa and clover hays fed to fattening lambs. *J. Anim. Sci.* **12**, 507.

Cheng, E., Story, C. D., Yoder, L., Hale, W. H., and Burroughs, W. (1953b). Estrogenic activity of isoflavone derivatives extracted and prepared from soybean oil meal. *Science* **118**, 164.

Cheng, E., Yoder, L., Story, C. D., and Burroughs, W. (1954). Estrogenic activity of some isoflavone derivatives. *Science* **120**, 575.

Christiansen, W. C., Woods, W., and Burroughs, W. (1964). Ration characteristics influencing rumen protozoal populations. *J. Anim. Sci.* **23**, 984.

Clegg, M. T., and Cole, H. H. (1954). The action of stilbestrol on the growth response in ruminants. *J. Anim. Sci.* **13**, 108.

Cox, R. I., and Braden, A. W. (1974a). The metabolism and physiological effects of phyto-oestrogens in livestock. *Proc. Aust. Soc. Anim. Prod.* **10**, 122.

Cox, R. I., and Braden, A. W. H. (1974b). A new phyto-oestrogen metabolite in sheep. *J. Reprod. Fertil.* **36**, 492.

Cox, R. I., Wong, M. S. F., Braden, A. W., Trikojus, V. M., and Lindner, H. R. (1972). The formation and specificity of antibodies to phyto-oestrogens in the sheep. *J. Reprod. Fertil* **28**, 157.

Davey, R. J., Armstrong, D. T., and Hansel, W. (1959). Studies on the use of hormones in lamb feeding. II. Tissue assays and physiological effects. *J. Anim. Sci.* **18**, 75.

Davis, S. L., and Borger, M. L. (1974). Dynamic changes in plasma prolactin, luteinizing hormone and growth hormone in ovariectomized ewes. *J. Anim. Sci.* **38**, 795.

Davis, S. L., Garrigus, U. S., and Hinds, F. C. (1970a). Metabolic effects of growth hormone and diethylstilbestrol in lambs. II. Effects of daily ovine growth hormone injections on plasma metabolites and nitrogen-retention in fed lambs. *J. Anim. Sci.* **30**, 236.

Davis, S. L., Garrigus, U. S., and Hinds, F. C. (1970b). Metabolic effects of growth hormone and diethylstilbestrol in lambs. III. Metabolic effects of DES. *J. Anim. Sci.* **30**, 241.

Dinusson, W. E., Andrews, F. N., and Beeson, W. M. (1950). The effect of stilbestrol, testosterone, thyroid alteration and spaying on the growth and fattening of beef heifers. *J. Anim. Sci.* **9**, 321.

Dodds, E. C., Goldberg, L., Lawson, W., and Robinson, R. (1938). Synthesis of DES. *Nature (London)* **141**, 247.

Doisy, E. A., Veler, C. O., and Thayer, S. (1929). Folliculin from urine of pregnant women. *Am. J. Physiol.* **90**, 329.

Everitt, G. C. (1962a). Implantation of oestrogenic hormones in beef cattle. I. Effects of winter nutritional depression following autumn implantation of hexoestrol, and of re-implantation in spring. *N. Z. J. Agric. Res.* **5**, 62.

Everitt, G. C. (1962b). Implantation of oestrogenic hormones in beef cattle. II. Effects of restricted summer grazing after implantation of hexoestrol in spring. *N. Z. J. Agric. Res.* **5**, 437.

Falconer, I. R., and Draper, S. A. (1968). Thyroid activity and growth. *In* "Growth and Development of Mammals" (G. A. Lodge and G. E. Lamming, eds.), p. 109. Plenum, New York.

Findlay, J. K., Cumming, I. A., Chamley, W. A., Buckmaster, J. M., Goding, J. R., and Hearnshaw, H. (1973). The release of luteinizing hormone by oestrodial-17B and a synthetic gonadotrophin-releasing factor in ewes affected with clover disease. *J. Reprod. Fertil.* **32**, 341 (abstr.).

Forrest, R. J., and Sather, L. A. (1965). The effect of hormones on the rate of gain and feed consumption of Holstein-Friesian steers slaughtered at 340, 522, and 703 kilograms body weight. *Can. J. Anim. Sci.* **45**, 173.

Fowler, M. A., Adeyanju, S. A., Burroughs, W., and Kline, E. A. (1970). Net energy evaluations of beef cattle rations with and without stilbestrol. *J. Anim. Sci.* **30**, 291.

Francis, C. M., and Millington, A. J. (1965). Wether bioassay of annual pasture legumes. 3. The oestrogenic potency of dry subterranean clover pastures, and of leaf blade and petiole in the green state. *Aust. J. Agric. REs.* **16**, 23.

Frantz, A. G., and Rabkin, M. T. (1965). Effects of estrogen and sex difference on secretion of human growth hormone. *J. Clin. Endocrinol. Metab.* **25**, 1470.

Gassner, F. X., Reifenstein, E. C., Jr., Algeo, J. W., and Mattox, W. E. (1958). Effects of hormones on growth, fattening, and meat production potential of livestock. *Recent Prog. Horm. Res.* **14**, 183.

Gee, I., and Preston, T. R. (1957). The effect of hexoestrol implantation on carcass composition and efficiency of food utilization in fattening lambs. *Br. J. Nutr.* **11**, 329.

Glascock, R. F., and Hewitt, E. J. (1963). The uptake of hexoestrol by the roots of plants and its retention when applied to the foliage as a spray. *Ann. Appl. Biol.* **52**, 163.

Glascock, R. F., and Jones, H. E. H. (1961). The uptake of hexoestrol by plants and its persistence in soil. *J. Endocrinol.* **21**, 373.

Grebing, S. E., Hutcheson, D. P., and Preston, R. L. (1970). Early reduction in urinary-N by diethylstilbestrol in lambs. *J. Anim. Sci.* **31**, 763.

Gregers-Hansen, B. (1964a). Decomposition of diethylstilbestrol in soil. *Plant Soil* **20**, 50.

Gregers-Hansen, B. (1964b). The uptake by plants of diethylstilbestrol and of its glucuronide. *Plant Soil* **20**, 215.

Guggolz, J., Livingston, A. L., and Bickoff, E. M. (1961). Detection of daidzein, formononetin, genistein, and biochanin A in forages. *J. Agric. Food. Chem.* **9**, 330.

Hacker, R. G., Cruea, D. D., Shimoda, W., and Hopwood, M. L. (1967). Uptake of diethylstilbestrol by edible plants. *J. Anim. Sci.* **26**, 1358.

Hale, W. H., Homeyer, P. G., Culbertson, C. C., and Burroughs, W. (1955). Response of lambs fed varied levels of diethylstilbestrol. *J. Anim. Sci.* **14**, 909.

Harter, G. D., and Vetter, R. L. (1967). Feeder lamb response to cortisone acetate and diethylstilbestrol. *J. Anim. Sci.* **26**, 1397.

Hearnshaw, H., Brown, J. M., Cumming, I. A., Goding, J. R., and Nairn, M. (1972). Endocrinological and histopathological aspects of the infertility in the ewe caused by oestrogenic clover. *J. Reprod. Fertil.* **28**, 160.

Huber, T. L. (1970). The effect of diethylstilbestrol on nitrogen excretion in sheep. *Can. J. Physiol. Pharmacol.* **48**, 573.

Huber, T. L., Horn, G. W., and Beadle, R. E. (1972). Liver and gastrointestinal metabolism of diethylstilbestrol in sheep. *J. Anim. Sci.* **34**, 786.

Ibrahim, E. A., Ingalls, J. R., and Stranger, N. E. (1970). Effect of dietary diethylstilbestrol on populations and concentrations of ciliate protozoa in dairy cattle. *Can. J. Anim. Sci.* **50**, 101.

Kelly, R. W. (1972). The oestrogenic activity of coumestans in ovariectomized ewes. *J. Reprod. Fertil.* **28**, 159.

Kitts, W. D., Swierstra, E., Brink, V. C., and Wood, A. J. (1959). The estrogen-like substances in certain legumes and grasses. II. The effect of stage or maturity and frequency of cutting on the estrogen activity of some forages. *Can. J. Anim. Sci.* **39**, 158.

Laqueur, E., and De Jough, S. E. (1928). A female (sexual) hormone menformon and standardized ovarian preparations. *J. Am. Med. Assoc.* **91**, 1169.

Lightfoot, R. J., and Wroth, R. H. (1974). The mechanism of temporary interfility in ewes grazing estrogenic subterranean clover prior to and during joining. *Proc. Aust. Soc. Anim. Prod.* **10**, 130.

Lindner, H. R. (1967). Study of the fate of phyto-oestrogens in the sheep by determination of isoflavones and coumestrol in the plasma and adipose tissue. *Aust. J. Agric. Res.* **18**, 305.

Lindsay, D. R., and Kelly, R. W. (1970). The metabolism of phyto-oestrogens in sheep. *Aust. Vet. J.* **46,** 219.

Lloyd, H. M., Meares, J. D., Jacobi, J., and Thomas, F. J. (1971). Effects of stilbestrol on growth hormone secretion and pituitary cell proliferation in the male rat. *J. Endocrinol.* **51,** 473.

Loewe, S., and Spohr, E. (1926). Nachweis und gehaltsbestimmung des weiblichen brunsthormons in weiblichen organes des pflanzenseiches. *Anz. Akad. Wiss. Wien Math-naturw. Kl.* **63,** 167.

Lofgreen, G. P. (1973). Effect of synovex and ralgro on performance and body composition. Cattle Day Report. *Calif., Agric. Exp. Stn. Rep.* p. 4.

Lorenz, F. W. (1954). Effects of estrogens on domestic fowl and applications in the poultry industry. *Vitam. Horm. (N.Y.)* **12,** 235.

McCapra, F., Scott, A. I., Delmotte, P., Delmotte-Plaquee, J., and Bhacca, N. W. (1964). The constitution of monorden, an antibiotic with tranquilizing action. *Tetrahedron Lett.* No. 15, p. 869.

McIntosh, E. N., Acker, D. C., and Kline, E. A. (1961). Influence of orally administered stilbestrol on connective tissue of skeletal muscle of lambs fed varying levels of protein. *J. Agric. Food Chem.* **9,** 418.

McKerns, K. W. (1963). The regulation of adrenal function by estrogens and other hormones. *Biochim. Biophys. Acta* **71,** 710.

McLaren, G. A., Anderson, G. C., Welch, J. A., Campbell, C. D., and Smith, G. S. (1960). Diethylstilbestrol and length of preliminary period in the utilization of crude biuret and urea by lambs. II. Various aspects of nitrogen metabolism. *J. Anim. Sci.* **19,** 44.

McNutt, S. H., Purwin, P., and Murray, C. (1928). Vulvovaginitis in swine. *J. Am. Vet. Med. Assoc.* **73,** 484.

Marshall, F. H. A., and Jolly, W. A. (1906). V. Contributions to the physiology of mammalian reproduction. Part I. The oestrus cycle in the dog. Part II. The ovary as an organ of internal secretion. *Philos. Trans. R. Soc. London, Ser. B* **198,** 99.

Martin, E. M., and Lamming, G. E. (1958). The effect of hexoestrol on the nucleic-acid content of the anterior pituitary gland of yearling male sheep. *Proc. Nutr. Soc.* **17,** 48.

Mirocha, C. J., Christensen, C. M., and Nelson, G. H. (1967). Estrogenic metabolite produced by Fusarium Graminearum in stored corn. *Appl. Microbiol.* **15,** 497.

Mirrington, B. N., Ritchie, E., Shoppee, C. W., Taylor, W. C., and Sternhell, S. (1964). The constitution of radicicol. *Tetrahedron Lett.* No. 7, p. 365.

Moule, G. R., Braden, A. W. H., and Lamond, D. R. (1963). The significance of oestrogens in pasture plants in relation to animal production. *Anim. Breed. Abstr.* **31,** 139.

Nilsson, A., Hill, J. L., and Davies. H. L. (1967). An "in vitro" study of formononetin and biochanin-A metabolism in rumen fluid from sheep. *Biochim. Biophys. Acta* **148,** 92.

Noteboom, W. D., and Gorski, J. (1963). Estrogenic effect of genistein and coumestrol diacetate. *Endocrinology* **73,** 736.

Oldfield, J. E., Fox, C. W., and Bahn, A. V. (1966). Coumestrol in alfalfa as a factor in growth and carcass quality in lambs. *J. Anim. Sci.* **25,** 167.

Oltjen, R. R., and Lehmann, R. P. (1968). Effect of diethylstilbestrol on the blood plasma amino acid patterns of beef steers fed finishing diets. *J. Nutr.* **95,** 399.

Oltjen, R. R., Swan, H., Rumsey, T. S., Bolt, D. J., and Weinland, B. T. (1973). Feedlot performance and blood plasma amino acid patterns in beef steers fed diethylstilbestrol under ad libitum, restricted, and compensatory conditions. *J. Nutr.* **103,** 1131.

Pieterse, P. J. S., and Andrews, F. N. (1956a). The estrogenic activity of alfalfa and other feedstuffs. *J. Anim. Sci.* **15,** 25.

Pieterse, P. J. S., and Andrews, F. N. (1956b). The estrogenic activity of legume, grass, and corn silage. *J. Dairy Sci.* **39**, 81.

Plimpton, R. F., Jr., and Teague, H. S. (1972). Influence of sex and hormone treatment on performance and carcass composition of swine. *J. Anim. Sci.* **35**, 1166.

Preston, R. L. (1968). Reduction of plasma urea-N by diethylstilbestrol in ruminants. *Proc. Soc. Exp. Biol. Med.* **129**, 250.

Preston, R. L. (1969). Influence of diethylstilbestrol on body water space in ruminants. *Proc. Soc. Exp. Biol. Med.* **132**, 401.

Preston, R. L. (1975). Biological responses to estrogen additives in meat producing cattle and lambs. *J. Anim. Sci.* **41**, 1414.

Preston, R. L., and Burroughs, W. (1960). Physiological actions of diethylstilbestrol in lambs fed varying levels of protein and energy. *J. Appl. Physiol.* **15**, 97.

Preston, T. R., and Willis, M. B. (1974). "Intensive Beef Production," 2nd ed. Pergamon, Oxford.

Preston, T. R., Greenhalgh, I., and MacLeod, N. A. (1960). The effect of hexoestrol on growth, carcass quality, endocrines and reproductive organs of ram, wether and female lambs. *Anim. Prod.* **2**, 11.

Reuber, H. W. (1958). Effects of diethylstilbestrol feeding on the bovine reproductive tract. *Am. J. Vet. Res.* **19**, 585.

Reuber, H. W., Pearson, C. C., and Pope, L. S. (1961). Genital effects of implanted and oral diethylstilbestrol on heifers. *J. Am. Vet. Med. Assoc.* **138**, 72.

Riis, P. M., Suresh, T. P., Rattan, P. S., and Bouffault, J. C. (1974). Metabolic effects of estradiol and trienbelone. *J. Anim. Sci.* **39**, 164.

Rossiter, R. C. (1970). Factors affecting the oestrogen content of subterranean clover pastures. *Aust. Vet. J.* **46**, 141.

Saba, N., Drane, H. M., Hebert, C. N., Newton, J. E., and Betts, J. E. (1972). Effect of disease on the oestrogenic activity and coumestrol content of white clover and lucerne. *J. Agric. Sci.* **78**, 471.

Sealey, J. L., and Sondern, C. W. (1941)). Comparative estrogenic potency of diethylstilbestrol, estrone, estradiol, and estriol. *Endocrinology* **29**, 356.

Sharp, G. D., and Dyer, I. A. (1970). Metabolic responses to zearalanol implants. *Proc., West. Sect., Am. Soc. Anim. Sci.* **21**, 1.

Sharp, G. D., and Dyer, I. A. (1971). Effect of zearalanol on the performance and carcass composition of growing–finishing ruminants. *J. Anim. Sci.* **33**, 865.

Sharp, G. D., and Dyer, I. A. (1972). Zearalanol metabolism in steers. *J. Anim. Sci.* **34**, 176.

Shibata, S., Natori, S., and Udagana, S. (1964). "List of Fungal Products." Univ. of Tokyo Press, Tokyo.

Shroder, J. D., and Hansard, S. L. (1958a). Effects of orally administered stilbestrol upon growth and upon calcium and phosphorus metabolism in lambs. *J. Anim. Sci.* **17**, 343.

Shroder, J. D., and Hansard, S. L. (1958b). Effects of dietary stilbestrol upon certain endocrine organs in lambs, *J. Anim. Sci.* **17**, 569.

Shutt, D. A., and Braden, A. W. H. (1968). The significance of equol in relation to the oestrogenic responses in sheep ingesting clover with a high formononetin content. *Aust. J. Agric. Res.* **19**, 545.

Shutt, D. A., Braden, A. W. H., and Lindner, H. R. (1969). Plasma coumestrol levels in sheep following administration of synthetic coumestrol or ingestion of medic hay (*Medicago Littoralis*). *Aust. J. Agric. Res.* **20**, 65.

Shutt, D. A., Weston, R. H., and Hogan, J. P. (1970). Quantitative aspects of phytooestrogen metabolism in sheep fed on subterranean clover (*Trifolium Subterranean* Cultivar Clare) or red clover (*Trifolium Pratense*). *Aust. J. Agric. Res.* **21**, 713.

Simone, M., Clegg, M. T., and Carroll, F. (1958). Effect of methods of stilbestrol administration on quality factors of beef. *J. Anim. Sci.* **17**, 834.
Skarzynski, B. (1933). An oestrogenic substance from plant material. *Nature (London)* **131**,
766.
Sondern, C. W., and Sealy, J. L. (1940). The comparative estrogenic potency of diethylstilbestrol, estrone, estradiol, and estriol. *Endocrinology* **27**, 670.
Stob, M., Baldwin, R. S., Tuite, J., Andrews, F. N., and Gillette, K. G. (1962). Isolation of
an anabolic, uterotrophic compound from corn infected with *Gibberella zea*. *Nature
(London)* **196**, 1318.
Stob, M., Beeson, W. M., and Perry, T. W. (1963). Effect of low and high coumestrol
dehydrated alfalfa meal and double stilbestrol treatment (implant and oral) on the
gain and feed efficiency of steer calves. Cattle Day Report. *Purdue Univ., Agric. Exp.
Stn., Rep.* p. 29.
Stob, M., Beeson, W. M., Perry, T. W., and Mohler, M. T. (1964). Effect of coumestrol, oral
and implanted progesterone, and ethylene diamine dihydroiodide on gain and feed
efficiency of steer calves. Cattle Day Report. *Indiana, Agr. Exp. Stn. Rep.* p. 1.
Story, C. D., Hale, W. H., Cheng, E. W., and Burroughs, W. (1957). The effect of low levels
of diethylstilbestrol and plant estrogens upon performance of fattening lambs. *Proc.
Iowa Acad. Sci.* **64**, 259.
Struempler, A. W., and Burroughs, W. (1959). Stilbestrol feeding and growth hormone
stimulation in immature ruminants. *J. Anim. Sci.* **18**, 427.
Trenkle, A. H. (1969). The mechanisms of action of estrogens in feeds on mammalian and
avian growth. *N. A. S.—N. R. C. Publ.* **1679**.
Trenkle, A. (1970). Plasma levels of growth hormone, insulin, and plasma protein-bound
iodine in finishing cattle. *J. Anim. Sci.* **31**, 389.
Trenkle, A. (1971). Growth hormone secretion rates in cattle. *J. Anim. Sci.* **32**, 115.
Tyrrell, H. F., Rumsey, T. S., Moe, P. W., and Oltjen, R. R. (1975). Effect of DES on fasting
metabolism of beef steers. *J. Anim. Sci.* **41**, 423 (abstr.).
Umberger, E. J. (1975). Products marketed to promote growth in food-producing animals:
Steroid and hormone products. *Toxicology* **3**, 3.
Underwood, E. J., and Shier, F. L. (1951). The permanence of the oestrogenic effects of
subterranean clover grazing on the ewe. *Aust. Vet. J.* **27**, 63.
Underwood, E. J., and Shier, F. L. (1952). The incidence of oestrus in ewes grazing on
subterranean-clover pastures. *Aust. Vet. J.* **28**, 157.
Underwood, E. J., Shier, F. L., and Peterson, J. E. (1953). The effects of prolonged
injections of stilbestrol on the ewe. *Aust. Vet. J.* **29**, 206.
Underwood, E. J., Shier, F. L., Davenport, N., and Bennetts, H. W. (1959). Further studies
of the effects of prolonged injections of stilbestrol on the ewe. *Aust. Vet. J.* **35**, 84.
Urry, W. H., Wehrmeister, H. L., Hodge, E. G., and Hidy, P. H. (1966). The structure of
zearalenone. *Tetrahedron Lett.* No. 27, p. 3109.
Vander Wal, P., Berende, P. L. M., and Spietsma, J. E. (1975a). Effect of anabolic agents on
performance of calves. *J. Anim. Sci.* **41**, 978.
Vander Wal, P., Van Weerden, E. J., Spietsma, J. E., and Huisman, J. (1975b). Effect of
anabolic agents on nitrogen retention of calves. *J. Anim. Sci.* **41**, 986.
Velle, W. (1963). Metabolism of estrogenic hormones in domestic animals. *Gen. Comp.
Endocrinol.* **3**, 621.
Wallace, A. L. C., and Bassett, J. M. (1966). Effect of sheep growth hormone on plasma
insulin concentration in sheep. *Metab. Clin. Exp.* **15**, 95.

Whitehair, C. K., Gallup, W. D., and Bell, M. C. (1953). Effect of stilbestrol on ration digestibility and on calcium, phosphorus and nitrogen retention in lambs. *J. Anim. Sci.* **12,** 331.

Wilson, L. L., Varela-Alvarez, H., Rugh, M. C., and Broger, M. L. (1972). Growth and carcass characteristics of rams, cryptorchids, wethers and ewes subcutaneously implanted with zeranol. *J. Anim. Sci.* **34,** 336.

Yousef, M. K., and Johnson, H. D. (1966). Colorigenesis of cattle as influenced by growth hormone and environmental temperature. *J. Anim. Sci.* **25,** 1076.

22

Distribution and Fate of Growth-Promoting Drugs Used in Animal Production*

P. W. ASCHBACHER

*Mention of a trade name, proprietary product, or specific equipment does not constitute a guarantee or warranty by the United States Department of Agriculture and does not imply its approval to the exclusion of other products that may be suitable.

613

I. INTRODUCTION

In the past 30 years, animal scientists have observed that exposure of growing animals to relatively small amounts of certain compounds will produce economically significant improvement in the rates of body weight gain or in the efficiencies of feed conversion, or in both. These compounds are not nutrients in the classic sense (e.g., minerals or vitamins), and, in general, their mode of action is not well understood. The compounds all have some other demonstrable biological activity, but often the knowledge is not available how or if this biological activity is related to the growth-promoting properties of the compound. Before these growth promotants could be used in animal production, residues that might remain in edible tissues of the animals exposed under the ordinary practical conditions of animal production had to be determined. Initially, biological assays were commonly used for quantitation of residues and studies of rates and routes of excretion. Although these bioassays were relatively sensitive for the parent compound, they were often laborious and lacked specificity. Also, they could not reveal the ultimate metabolic fate of the compound.

In recent years, the use of growth-promoting drugs in animal production has become more complicated for several reasons. Public concern with the implications of use of chemicals in food production has definitely increased. In addition, technological advances make possible the detection of lower levels of residues than those previously detected, and assessing the possible hazard posed by these low levels of residues is difficult. Questions are being asked about the ultimate metabolic fate of the compounds and the significance of the metabolites. New methods of disposal or utilization of animal wastes necessitate knowledge about the presence and fate of parent compounds and metabolites in the excreta (Bhattacharya and Taylor, 1975; Elmund et al., 1971; Morrison et al., 1969; Webb and Fontenot, 1975).

The objective of this paper is to review the published information concerning the metabolic fate of growth-promoting compounds used in animal production. Computer-aided searches of several data bases were used to find pertinent references; however, citation tapes were available for only the past 7–8 years. Earlier literature was not searched systematically. Efforts were made to select those data most applicable to the way animals are exposed to the compounds in actual practice. In general, those compounds in widest usage and with the most recent information are discussed; however, the selection will be somewhat arbitrary. (For a previous review with similar objectives, see Sykes et al., 1960).

In this paper, growth-promoting compounds are classified into three groups: hormonally active, antibiotics, or arsenic-containing. This classification is not entirely satisfactory because within a group the chemical nature may vary widely. Therefore, each compound is treated individually.

II. COMPOUNDS POSSESSING HORMONAL ACTIVITY

Compounds in this group (Table I) all have some degree of sex hormone activity, and their efficacy as growth promotants is restricted primarily to ruminants. The synthetic estrogens, diethylstilbestrol (DES), dienestrol, and hexestrol, may be described as derivatives of diphenylethanes. With the exception of zeranol, all other compounds in the group have steroid-type structures. Zeranol, a resorcylic acid lactone, is quite different structurally from the other compounds in this group. It is a slight modification of zearalenone, a compound produced by the mold, *Gibberella zeae*, and it is a weak estrogen.

A. Diethylstilbestrol

DES has been the most widely used growth promotant in ruminants. It is effective both orally and as an implant. In early studies of the metabolic fate of DES, assays for estrogenic activity were used as the analytical method to detect DES. These assays quantitated 1-2 ppb of DES, but they lacked specificity and would not detect nonestrogenic metabolites. More recently, radiotracer, chromatographic, and spectral techniques have been used to study the metabolic fate of DES, and results of these studies will be reviewed here. (For a somewhat more extensive review, see Aschbacher, 1976).

Mitchell *et al.* (1959) were the first to use radiolabeled DES to study metabolic fate of DES in ruminants (later extended by Hinds *et al.*, 1965). These investigators used tritium-labeled DES ([^{3}H]DES), and data from subsequent research generally agree with their results. The major limitation of the interpretation of the studies with [^{3}H]DES is the low recovery of administered radioactivity (approximately 50%). Recoveries of ^{3}H may have been incomplete because quantitation in tissues and feces was dependent upon solvent extractions. Recoveries of radioactivity have been more complete in several studies in which DES labeled with ^{14}C in the number one carbon atom of an ethyl side chain ([^{14}C]DES) was fed to ruminants. In these studies, [^{14}C] DES was given via a gelatin cap-

TABLE I
Hormonally Active Compounds with Growth-Promoting Actions in Some Meat Animals

Common Name	Structure
trans-Diethylstilbestrol[a]	
Dienestrol	
Hexestrol	
Estradiol-17β benzoate[b]	
Zeranol[b]	
Progesterone[b]	
Melengestrol acetate[b]	

(continued)

TABLE I, *continued*

Common Name	Structure
Trenbolone acetate[c]	$O-\overset{\overset{O}{\|}}{C}-CH_3$ H_3C (steroid structure with ketone)
Testosterone propionate[b]	$O-\overset{\overset{O}{\|}}{C}-CH_2CH_3$ H_3C H_3C (steroid structure with ketone)

[a] Future status in the United States is under discussion (Anonymous, 1976).
[b] Presently approved for use in the United States (Umberger, 1975).
[c] Registered trade name.

sule to animals that had been fed DES for a period of time immediately before the radioactive dose. The [^{14}C]DES was given as a single dose to wether sheep (Aschbacher, 1972) and steers (Aschbacher and Thacker, 1974) and as three consecutive daily doses to steers and heifers (Rumsey *et al.*, 1975a). The animals were slaughtered at various time intervals after the [^{14}C]DES dose, and urine and feces were collected during the period from dosing to slaughter. The results of these three studies were generally similar, and data presented from one study can be taken as representative unless otherwise indicated.

The distribution of ^{14}C at various time intervals after a single oral dose was given to steers is shown in Table II. Total recoveries of ^{14}C averaged 97% (range for individual steers was 90.8 to 103.7%). Urine and feces were the only significant routes of elimination of ^{14}C. In the studies with sheep (Aschbacher, 1972) and in the preliminary work with steers (Rumsey *et al.*, 1975a), no ^{14}CO$_2$ was detected in the expired air. The system used to monitor ^{14}CO$_2$ expiration by sheep would have quantitated 0.2% of the total dose of ^{14}C if expired in an 8-hour period.

Cattle given [^{14}C]DES orally excreted two to three times more ^{14}C in feces than in urine (Aschbacher and Thacker, 1974; Rumsey *et al.*, 1975a). Wether sheep excreted approximately fourteen times more ^{14}C in feces than in urine, and increasing the intake of DES from 3 to 100 mg

618

P.W. Aschbacher

TABLE II
Distribution of ^{14}C in Steers after Single Oral Dose of [^{14}C]DES[a]

	Hours from dosing until sacrifice (% of dose)					
Location	24	48	72	120	168	240
Rumenoreticulum	38.00	19.40	2.74	0.69	0.90	ND[b]
Omasum	13.30	5.09	1.83	0.20	0.04	ND
Abomasum	0.59	0.77	0.18	0.02	0.03	ND
Small intestine	3.10	2.13	0.65	0.10	0.05	0.01
Large intestine	8.38	6.86	1.30	0.29	0.39	ND
Feces	21.7	52.8	72.75	73.55	63.75	70.7
Urine	7.98	14.65	22.30	21.00	31.90	20.2
Organs and carcass	0.96	0.29	0.26	0.01	<0.01	<0.01
Total recovery	94.0	102.0	102.0	95.9	97.1	90.9

[a] From Aschbacher and Thacker (1974). Each value is an average of two steers. Values for gastrointestinal tract include contents and tissue. Total mass of [^{14}C]DES dose was 10 mg. Steers were ingesting 20 mg of DES per day before radioactive dose.
[b] ND, not detected.

per day or continued feeding of unlabeled DES during the collection period did not have a dramatic effect on the route or rate of excretion; however, the number of animals per treatment (two) was small (Aschbacher, 1972).

More than 85% of the ^{14}C in feces of steers given [^{14}C]DES orally had solubility and thin-layer chromatographic (TLC) properties similar to those of DES (Aschbacher and Thacker, 1974). However, in a later study (Aschbacher and Feil, 1975), the ^{14}C excreted in feces was characterized more completely (expedited by a larger dose) by gas-liquid chromatographic (GLC) and mass-spectral analyses; only 64% of the ^{14}C was DES. Approximately 23% was characterized as 3-(p-hydroxyphenyl)-2-hexen-4-one (mass spectral and nuclear magnetic resonance analysis). Also, a small amount (< 1%) of the ^{14}C was identified as p-hydroxypropiophenone (comparative GLC and mass spectral data). Both of these compounds had the solubility properties of DES, and the R_f of the hexenone was similar to that of trans-DES with the TLC systems used in the previous study; therefore, the hexenone would not have been differentiated when characterization was based on only solubility and TLC data.

When [^{14}C]DES was added to fresh ruminant feces, degradation was extensive upon standing at ambient temperature for 7 days (P. W. Aschbacher and V. J. Feil, unpublished data). Less than 5% of the ^{14}C remained as DES; other radioactive compounds isolated included dienestrol (nonestrogenic isomer), 3,4-bis-(*p*-hydroxyphenyl)-2-hexene, 3-(*p*-hydroxyphenyl)-2-hexen-4-one, *p*-hydroxypropiophenone, acetic acid, and propionic acid. More than 50% of the ^{14}C was not characterized. Degradation was similar in the feces from ruminants receiving DES when the feces remained at ambient temperature (Aschbacher and Feil, 1975). We have not determined whether DES is degraded in the gastrointestinal tract.

Only one radioactive fraction was isolated from the urine of steers given [^{14}C]DES orally, and this radioactivity chromatographed (TLC) as DES-monoglucuronide (DES-G) (Aschbacher and Thacker, 1974). Approximately 85% of the radioactivity in the urine was recovered in this fraction, and other discrete fractions were not observed. The presence of DES-G in the urine of a cow fed 200 mg of DES per day was confirmed by mass spectral analysis (P. W. Aschbacher, unpublished data). DES-G in urine hydrolyzed extensively at room temperature (Aschbacher and Thacker, 1974), presumably a result of microbial activity.

Biliary secretion of DES has not been quantitated in intact ruminants; however, the relatively high concentrations of radioactivity in bile after an oral dose of [^{14}C]DES suggests that bile is a secretory route. Sheep liver perfusion studies by Huber *et al.* (1972) indicated that the liver conjugates DES efficiently. Biliary secretion and enterohepatic circulation of DES-G has been shown in humans and rats (Fischer *et al.*, 1976) and in the Rhesus monkey (Mroszczak, 1974).

The ^{14}C in the bile of steers given [^{14}C]DES orally did not exhibit the properties of DES; however, a hydrolysis product (β-glucuronidase-arylsulfatase) was identified as [^{14}C]DES by isotopic dilution (80 and 43% of the ^{14}C in the bile from gallbladders of steers slaughtered 24 and 168 hours, respectively, after a [^{14}C]DES dose) (Aschbacher and Thacker, 1974). The contents of the small intestine of steers slaughtered 48 hours after dosing with [^{14}C]DES contained ^{14}C with solubility and chromatographic properties of DES-G (38% of ^{14}C present); however, radioactivity with properties of DES-G was not found in any other part of the gastrointestinal tract. At least 80% of the ^{14}C compounds in the large intestinal contents partitioned and chromatographed (TLC) as DES. Hydrolysis of DES conjugates in the lower intestines of rats has been reported by Fischer *et al.* (1976).

When compared with the amount of radioactivity in the total dose, the amount in organs and tissues after oral [^{14}C]DES was always very small, and the major part of the unexcreted ^{14}C was in the gastrointestinal contents. Concentrations of ^{14}C in liver, kidney, and bile of steers are shown in Table III. Values in the table are expressed as DES equivalents (to facilitate comparisons among animals), but they should be regarded

TABLE III
Concentrations of ^{14}C in Steer Tissues (Expressed as DES
Equivalents) after Single Oral Dose of [^{14}C]DES[a]

Hours from dosing until sacrifice	Tissue (ppb)		
	Liver	Kidney	Gallbladder and contents
24	3.4	5.5	112
	4.3	1.9	125
48	3.1	4.5	65
	2.0	2.0	64
72	1.1	2.5	21
	0.34	0.36	8.5
120	0.57	0.90	11
	0.11	0.07	2.5
168	0.13	0.75	0.44
	0.37	0.21	12.0
240	0.08	0.09	0.08
	0.08	0.09	ND[b]

[a] From Aschbacher and Thacker (1974). DES equivalents were
calculated by dividing dpm/gm of fresh tissue by the specific activity
of the dose for that steer. Values are for individual steers.
[b] ND, not detected.

as quantitation of ^{14}C and not DES. Samples from internal organs, other
than liver, kidney, and bile, occasionally contained radioactivity slightly
above background, but preferential accumulation in these tissues was
not indicated. Sheep were an exception because the highest tissue concentration of ^{14}C was often in the adrenal gland (Aschbacher, 1972).

Liver and kidney are the only tissues in which DES (or a DES conjugate) has been identified after oral DES. Data in Table IV show concentrations in livers of steers as determined by isotopic dilution methods
(Rumsey et al., 1975a). These results (and similar data from Aschbacher
and Thacker, 1974) suggest that the proportion of radioactivity in the
liver as [^{14}C]DES (or DES conjugates) decreases with time after ingestion
of [^{14}C]DES. Extraction with acetone:water (80:20) recovered 62% of the
^{14}C in the liver of a steer slaughtered 168 hours after a single dose, but
less than half of the extracted radioactivity was recovered as DES after
hydrolysis, partitioning, and recrystallization (Aschbacher and Thacker,
1974). The concentrations of ^{14}C in the liver were so low that further
characterization would have been extremely difficult.

Data on metabolic fate of DES implanted subcutaneously in steers are
from collaborative studies by Aschbacher et al. (1975) and Rumsey et al.

TABLE IV

Characterization of ^{14}C in Liver of Steers after Withdrawal of [^{14}C]DES[a]

Hour of withdrawal	Percentage of ^{14}C in liver as		DES equivalents in wet tissue[b] (ppb)
	Free DES (%)	Conjugated DES (%)	
18	14.7	63.3	13.65
36	16.4	38.2	2.15
120	12.2	21.0	0.27
168	1.5	3.1	0.04

[a] From Rumsey et al. (1975a). Values are from isotope dilution and recrystallization procedures.
[b] Free DES and DES conjugates.

(1975b). Steers were implanted with two 14 mg [^{14}C]DES pellets that had been formulated similarly to commercial DES implants. Excretion of ^{14}C was monitored, and individuals were slaughtered at 30, 60, 90, and 120 days after implantation. The ^{14}C observed in blood plasma and excretions indicated that absorption of DES from the pellets was continuous throughout the study. Levels of ^{14}C in plasma and excretions plateaued by the second week after implantation and then gradually declined; at the end of the trial, levels were approximately 50% of the initial plateau. Data obtained when nonradioactive implants were used generally agree with the data obtained when radiolabeled implants were used (Hale et al., 1959).

The distribution of ^{14}C at various times after implantation is shown in Table V. Tissues other than the ear contained no more than 0.05% of the ^{14}C originally in the implant. Concentrations of ^{14}C were thirty to sixty times greater in the bile than in blood plasma; and concentrations were two to ten times greater in salivary glands, lungs, livers, and kidneys (in order of decreasing concentration) than in blood plasma. The concentration of ^{14}C in muscle (from the round), fat, spleen, and heart was lower than in blood plasma. The relatively high concentration of ^{14}C in the salivary glands apparently does not indicate salivary secretion because no ^{14}C was found in the rumen. Ferrando et al. (1974) also reported no DES in saliva of sheep implanted with DES.

Radiochemical purity of the [^{14}C]DES in the pellets recovered from the ears when the steers were slaughtered ranged from 92.6 to 95.1% on the basis of isotopic dilution procedures (Aschbacher et al., 1975). Radiopurity at the time of implantation (one pellet selected randomly

TABLE V
Distribution of ^{14}C after [^{14}C]DES Was Implanted in Ears of Steers[a]

Days after implantation	Location (% of ^{14}C implanted)				
	Feces	Urine	Ear[b]	GI tract	Total recovery (% of ^{14}C implanted)
30	17.2[c]	7.5	65.9	0.21	90.9
	21.3[d]	22.8	33.6	0.2	77.9
	9.5[d]	10.5	65.2	0.1	85.3
60	39.8[c]	17.0	27.3	0.18	84.3
	25.8[d]	11.3	47.9	0.1	85.1
	17.6[d]	14.3	52.4	0.1	84.4
90	40.1[c]	12.4	30.0	0.16	82.7
	15.8[d]	21.0	48.3	0.1	85.2
	28.0[d]	17.4	33.5	0.1	79.0
120	60.5[c]	24.4	4.2	0.1	89.3
	35.6[d]	22.9	19.2	0.1	77.8
	28.9[d]	26.4	16.5	0.1	71.8

[a] Each steer was implanted with two pellets that contained a total of approximately 28 mg of [^{14}C]DES. Values are for individual steers. Radioactivity in other tissues was insignificant when compared with total ^{14}C in the implant.
[b] Includes residual implant and ear tissue.
[c] From Aschbacher *et al.* (1975).
[d] From Rumsey *et al.* (1975b).

from the lot) was 96%. Less than 50% of the ^{14}C in feces was recovered as [^{14}C]DES (isotopic dilution); and GLC analysis of the silyl derivatives of the radioactive compounds isolated from feces revealed a radioactive component with a retention time similar to that of a compound isolated from feces after oral dosing with [^{14}C]DES (identified as 3-(*p*-hydroxyphenyl)-2-hexen-4-one). After enzymatic hydrolysis (β-glucuronidase-arylsulfatase) of ^{14}C compounds from urine, 60–75% of the ^{14}C was recovered as [^{14}C]DES. The other ^{14}C was not characterized, and additional metabolites in urine cannot be ruled out.

The percentages of ^{14}C in liver that were isolated as DES or a DES conjugate and the concentrations of DES equivalents in fresh tissue are given in Table VI (isotopic dilution data). The variations are so great that conclusions about the relationship between concentrations of DES or DES conjugates and time after implanting are not possible. Also, a major part (average of 48%) of the ^{14}C was not characterized. In the study by Aschbacher *et al.* (1975), approximately 75% of the ^{14}C in livers

TABLE VI

Characterization of ^{14}C in Livers of Steers Implanted in the Ear with [^{14}C]DES[a]

| Days after implantation | ^{14}C recovered as DES + DES conjugates expressed as: | |
	Percentage of ^{14}C in liver	DES equivalent in fresh tissue (ppb)
30	32.7[b]	0.13
	24.3[c]	0.15
	37.8[c]	0.19
60	17.3[b]	0.07
	27.8[c]	0.14
	36.3[c]	0.21
90	15.9[b]	0.07
	52.5[c]	0.36
	21.4[c]	0.11
120	16.4[b]	0.11
	11.5[c]	0.03
	23.1[c]	0.07

[a] Each value is for an individual liver and is based on isotopic dilution procedures.
[b] From Aschbacher *et al.* (1975).
[c] From Rumsey *et al.* (1975b). In this study, more than 99% of the DES equivalents were as conjugates of DES.

was extracted with acetone, and nearly all of this ^{14}C was recovered by ether extraction after hydrolysis. However, a large proportion of this ^{14}C would not partition into sodium hydroxide from chloroform, thus it had neither water solubility nor phenolic character.

Hydroxylated and methoxylated metabolites of DES have been reported in the urine of rats and hamsters after intraperitoneal injection (Metzler, 1975, 1976). Similar metabolites were isolated after DES was incubated with liver homogenates of several mammalian species including cattle (Engel *et al.*, 1976; Masarcchia, 1969). Possibly, such metabolites of DES are present in excreta and tissues of ruminants; however, the hydroxylated and methoxylated metabolites reported would retain their phenolic character and should have been detected (with the possible exception of methoxylation in both phenyl rings).

The use of DES as a growth promotant has been questioned on the basis of public health. Various regulatory and legal steps have been undertaken, and the future status of DES is under discussion as of this writing (Anonymous, 1976). While these questions are being resolved, DES is being used as a growth promotant in commercial production of sheep and cattle. Reliable estimates of the proportion of animals receiving DES are not available. Cattle may be fed 10–20 mg of DES per day (depending on body weight), and current regulations require a 14-day withdrawal period before slaughter (Anonymous, 1975a). Cattle may be implanted subcutaneously with 15–30 mg of DES, and the directions on the label state that the animals should not be slaughtered for 120 days after implantation. Extrapolating from the data reviewed in this paper, one would expect the liver to contain the highest concentration of DES (or its metabolites) to be found in edible tissues of feedlot cattle that had been given DES in the prescribed manner. The expected concentration of DES plus DES metabolites in liver after prescribed oral use would be less than 0.1 ppb of DES equivalents. Livers of cattle implanted with DES would be expected to contain of the order of 0.1 ppb of DES equivalents as DES plus conjugates of DES (primarily conjugates). Similar concentrations of other metabolites of DES may also be present in liver of implanted cattle. The only metabolic products of DES identified in edible tissues of cattle are DES and conjugates of DES (from liver). In the studies reviewed, animals were under dosage and temporal relationships that were similar to DES usage in actual practice; however, some other conditions were obviously different. Also, the number of animals observed was too small to adequately measure individual variation.

A large proportion of the DES administered to cattle is excreted either in the feces as DES or in the urine as DES-G. Under some conditions, degradation of DES was extensive in feces after excretion; however, the eventual environmental fate of DES excreted by cattle in a feedlot is not certain. Rumsey et al. (1975c) analyzed feedlot wastes and found that 52% of the DES fed to the cattle was still present in the waste after storing for 3 months in a concrete pit (0.35–0.83 ppm, wet basis); this was approximately 75% of the amount of DES in the fresh waste. Results from the study of Rumsey et al. (1975c) and others (Gregers-Hansen, 1964a,b; Hacker et al., 1967) indicate that spreading waste from DES-fed cattle on land as fertilizer does not create a problem with respect to movement of DES into plants or runoff water. However, when considering disposal methods for wastes from cattle fed DES, one should be aware that the concentration of DES may be of the same order of magnitude as that found in the feed.

B. Estradiol

The benzoate ester of estradiol-17β is combined with either progesterone (for steers) or testosterone propionate (for heifers) and administered as an implant for growth promotion. Metabolism of endogenous estradiol in ruminants has been reviewed by Velle (1963) and Mellin and Erb (1965). Estradiol-17β is the ovarian estrogen and the major metabolites are estradiol-17α and estrone.

The kinetics of estradiol and estrone metabolism in the circulating blood of sheep has been studied by Challis *et al.* (1973) and Kazama and Longcope (1972). They reported metabolic clearance rates for estradiol-17β and estrone and interconversion rates of estradiol-17β and estrone in nonpregnant, pregnant, and lactating ewes. It is not clear to me how these data can be applied to assessing the metabolic fate of implanted estradiol.

Fecal excretion of radioactivity by a cow was approximately 1.75 times the amount eliminated in urine after a series of subcutaneous injections of [^{3}H]estradiol-17β (25 μg/kg body weight twice daily for 7 days) (Willett *et al.*, 1976). Total excretion of ^{3}H in 28 days was 88.7% of the dose. Mellin and Erb (1966) reported that excretion of radioactivity in urine after intravenous administration (150 μg) of ^{14}C-labeled estradiol-17β (in 500 ml of 10% ethanolic solution over a 2-hour period) reached a maximum rate in 6–9 hours (average of eight injections in the same female bovine). Approximately 30% of the ^{14}C was excreted in the first 24 hours (range 23–35%); thereafter, the rate of excretion decreased rapidly. In the period 48–72 hours after dosing, approximately 2% of the dose was excreted for an average 72-hour total of 35%. Excretion in feces was not measured. Approximately 5% of the ^{14}C in the urine (0–24 hours after injection) was ether-extractable. After hydrolysis (enzymatic and acid), the combined organic-soluble ^{14}C compounds were characterized by countercurrent distribution, paper chromatography, TLC, and recrystallization with known standards. Radioactive estradiol-17α, estradiol-17β, and estrone were identified. Estradiol-17α was the major metabolite.

Sheep rapidly excreted radioactivity after intravenous administration of ^{3}H-labeled estradiol-17β (Terqui, 1972). Radioactivity in the feces accounted for 52–67% of the dose; urinary excretion accounted for 32–36% of the dose. (No time frame was given.) Pregnancy did not appear to affect the route of excretion (injections were at 70, 90, and 131 days of gestation and during anestrus). After enzymatic hydrolysis of the urine, the radioactive compounds shown in Table VII were characterized by partitioning, chromatography, and recrystallization. Fecal metabolites were not characterized. Excretions of radioactivity and radiolabeled compounds in urine after injections of [^{14}C]estrone were similar to those observed from injections of [^{3}H]estradiol-17β.

Biliary metabolites after intravenous injection of [4-^{14}C]estradiol-17β in a bull were reported by Pearson and Martin (1966). Concentration of

TABLE VII
Relative Amounts of Radioactivity in Various
Metabolites Found in Urine of Pregnant Ewe
Dosed Intravenously with [^{3}H]Estradiol-17β[a]

Metabolite	Amount (%)
Estradiol-17α	56
Estrone	21
17-Epiestriol	12
16-Epiestriol	3
16-α-Hydroxyestrone	3
2-Methoxyestrone	2
Estriol	1
Unidentified	2

[a] After enzymatic hydrolysis of urine (from Terqui, 1972).

radioactivity in the bile (collected from the gallbladder) was maximum 12 minutes after injection. Within 3 hours, 53% of the dose was excreted in the bile and 4% in the urine. Radioactivity in bile was not ether-extractable until after hydrolysis (β-glucuronidase). Radioactive estrone and estradiol-17α were identified (recrystallization with a carrier to a constant specific activity) and constituted 94% of the ^{14}C in the bile collected during the first 30 minutes after injection. In a similar experiment, Leung and Martin (1972) used column and paper chromatography to separate radioactivity in the bile into three components which they identified as 17α-estradiol-3β-D-glucuronide, estradiol-3, 17α-β-D-diglucuronide, and estrone-3β-D-glucuronide. Basis for the identification was characterization of the aglycone and glycone portions of the conjugate after enzymatic hydrolysis. Leung *et al.* (1975) have shown both enterohepatic circulation of [^{14}C]estrone in the bull and conversion of estrone to estradiol-17α.

Data on tissue levels of estradiol (or its metabolites) after exogenous estradiol are limited. Vogt *et al.* (1972) implanted two male calves (4.5 and 7 weeks old) with 20 mg estradiol benzoate plus 200 mg of progesterone either intramuscularly in the shoulder or subcutaneously at the base of the ear and slaughtered them 4 weeks later. Quantitation of estrogens (estradiols and estrone) was by fluorometric techniques after extraction, hydrolysis, and purification. Recovery of estrogens (expressed as a percentage of estradiol in the pellet implanted) in the unabsorbed pellet, in urine, and in feces was as follows: from the intramuscular implant, 63.7, 8.5, 13.6, respectively; from the subcutaneous implant, 72, 1.6, and 5.1, respectively. Estrogens were not detected in the tissues (liver, kidney, and buttocks) of either calf except within 15 cm of the intramuscular implants (limit of detection 0.2–0.9 ppb). Characterization of the excreted estrogen by TLC and chemical reactions indicated that estradiol-17α was the principal excretory product.

The results of similar experiments by Ferrando *et al.* (1973) generally agree with those of Vogt *et al.* (1972). A visible piece of the implanted pellet could be found in four of thirty-nine calves slaughtered 50–70 days after being implanted in the neck region. Estradiol was detected only in the tissues near the site of the implant. Excretion was not monitored. In the United States, animal producers are directed to implant estradiol in the ear (a nonedible tissue) and not in the neck or shoulder.

The level of endogenous estradiol in blood plasma of female bovine in various reproductive stages has been determined by radioimmunoassay (Echternkamp and Hansel, 1973; Henricks *et al.*, 1972; Monk *et al.*, 1975; V. G. Smith *et al.*, 1973; Wettemann *et al.*, 1972). Efforts to use radioimmunoassays to quantitate tissue levels of estrogens encountered difficulties (Henricks, 1976), and little published data are available. However, progress is being made, and some data should soon be available. With an assay measuring estradiol-17β plus estrone, D. M. Henricks (personal communication) has observed concentrations of 0.03 to 0.07 ppb in liver and kidney of steers. Muscle contained 20–25% of the level in kidney and liver. From experiments in which similar assays were used, Hoffmann and Karg (1973) reported that levels of estradiol-17β in tissues of calves treated with estradiol benzoate were approximately ten times the levels in tissues of control calves. The specific tissues assayed and details of estradiol treatment were not given.

Kaltenbach *et al.* (1976) studied the fate of ^{14}C-labeled estradiol-17β and its benzoate ester injected subcutaneously at the base of the ear of steers and heifers. The animals received either nonradioactive estrogen for 11 days (1 mg per day) followed by three daily injections of [4-^{14}C]estradiol-17β (1 mg per day) or [4-^{14}C]estradiol-17β-3-benzoate (2.16 mg per day). All injections were made in a propylene glycol:peanut oil (30:70) carrier. Animals were slaughtered 3 hours after the last dose. Preliminary work had shown that blood plasma levels would be maximum approximately 3 hours after an injection of either hormone and that a larger amount of estradiol benzoate had to be injected to produce plasma levels equal to those resulting from estradiol. Table VIII gives the concentrations of ^{14}C in various tissues expressed as estradiol equivalents. Note that the values in the table are only mea-

TABLE VIII

Tissue Radioactivity Expressed as Estradiol Equivalents after Subcutaneous Injections of [4-^{14}C]Estradiol-17β or [4-^{14}C]Estradiol-17β-3-Benzoate[a]

	Concentrations (ppb)	
Tissue	Estradiol-17β	Estradiol-17β-3-benzoate
Rump muscle	0.37 ± 0.07[b]	0.23 ± 0.03[c]
Neck muscle	0.40 ± 0.07	0.34 ± 0.06
Rump fat	1.19 ± 0.16	0.78 ± 0.08
Neck fat	1.21 ± 0.16	0.79 ± 0.10
Mesenteric fat	1.96 ± 0.17	0.89 ± 0.10
Kidney fat	2.01 ± 0.3	0.98 ± 0.10
Kidney	4.02 ± 0.54	4.70 ± 1.34
Liver	5.42 ± 0.48	5.49 ± 1.39

[a] From Kaltenbach et al. (1976). Values were calculated by dividing the dpm per gm of tissue by the dpm per gm of the [^{14}C]estradiol-17β. (Specific activity of the estradiol-17β and estradiol-17β-3-benzoate injected were both 54.5 mCi per mM.) See text for additional details.
[b] $\bar{\chi}$ ± standard error; N = 5 (3 steers and 2 heifers).
[c] $\bar{\chi}$ ± standard error; N = 6 (3 steers and 3 heifers).

surements of radioactivity even though an effort has been made to put them in some kind of perspective by expressing them as estradiol equivalents. Steers had higher concentrations in neck muscles whereas heifers had higher concentrations in livers. Rump and kidney fat from steers treated with estradiol had higher concentrations than those tissues from steers treated with estradiol benzoate or from heifers treated with either estrogen (all differences significant at $p < 0.05$).

The tissues were extracted with ethanol, and the extracted radioactivity was characterized by partitioning and chromatography (column, TLC, and paper). More than 90% of the radioactivity extracted from muscle and fat were ether-soluble, and most of the ^{14}C in this fraction chromatographed as estradiol-17β (50–67%) or estrone (17–35%). Small amounts of radioactivity chromatographed as estradiol-17α and estriol. Approximately 70% of the activity in the livers and kidneys extracted with ethanol and approximately 75% of the extracted ^{14}C was not ether-soluble. Most of the ^{14}C in the polar fraction from liver and kidney had chromatographic properties similar to those of glucuronides. The patterns of metabolites in tissues from animals treated with estradiol-17β and estradiol-17β-3-benzoate were similar. No estradiol benzoate was found in tissues of animals treated with that estrogen. The published report of this work is stated as preliminary.

Definite conclusions about the metabolic fate of estradiol implanted in ruminants cannot be made from the published information. Feces are probably the principal excretory route, but almost nothing is known about the nature of fecal metabolites. Significant quantities are excreted via the urine, and there is considerable evidence that the principal urinary metabolites are conjugates of estradiol-17α and estrone. Some preliminary information about levels of tissue metabolites is available but relating these data to what would result from use of estradiol in animal production is difficult. Preliminary work suggests that estradiol benzoate injected subcutaneously has a different distribution and/or excretion rate than that of estradiol. Also, exogenous extradiol may be metabolized differently by heifers and steers.

C. Progesterone

In the United States, an implant of progesterone (200 mg) and estradiol benzoate (20 mg) is used for growth promotion in steers. The levels of endogenous circulating progesterone in blood of female sheep and cattle in various states of reproduction has been reported (Henricks *et al.*, 1972; Short and Moore, 1959; Stabenfeldt *et al.*, 1969; Thorburn *et al.*, 1969). Metabolic clearance rates were similar in cows and ewes (Bedford *et al.*, 1972; Heap *et al.*, 1975). The major known metabolite of progesterone in plasma and livers is 20α-hydroxypregn-4-en-3-one, and liver concentrations of this metabolite and progesterone are similar (Bedford *et al.*, 1972; Short and Moore, 1959).

After intravenous injection of [^{14}C]-labeled progesterone to a cow, excretion of ^{14}C in feces was approximately fifteen times that in urine (Williams, 1962). A similar urinary fecal ratio was observed in excreta of a cow after seven daily subcutaneous injections of tritium-labeled progesterone (0.125 mg/kg body weight/day in two injections) (Willett *et al.*, 1976). By the end of the seventh day (when injections ceased), approximately 41% of the total dose had been excreted. An additional 35% of the ^{3}H was excreted in the next 7 days and then excretion began to plateau. Radioactivity in feces was indistinguishable from background by 14 days after the last injection and in urine by 21 days. Total recovery was 94% of the dose. Stupnicki *et al.* (1969) observed the excretion of ^{14}C in bile and urine after intravenous injections of [^{14}C]progesterone to ewes. In the first 24 hours after injections, an average of 60% of the radioactivity was found in the bile and 22% in the urine.

A preliminary report (Smith *et al.*, 1975) indicated that 2–3 hours after the last of a series of subcutaneous injections of [^{14}C]progesterone in sesame oil at the base of the ear, the concentration of radioactivity in fat of cows and steers was approximately seven times that in muscle. McCracken (1964) has also reported that during the luteal phase of the estrous cycle, endogenous progesterone concentrations in the fat of a cow are approximately six times the blood plasma level.

Stupnicki and Williams (1968) characterized the ^{14}C-labeled urinary metabolites from a ewe after a large intravenous dose (1 gm) of [4-^{14}C]progesterone. Radioactive metabolites characterized included seven pregnanediols and three pregnanolones. The major metabolites were 5β-pregnane-3α,20α-diol and 5β-pregnane-3β,20α-diol.

Miller *et al.* (1956) identified (melting point and infrared spectral comparisons) 1,4-androstadiene-3,17-dione in the feces of a pregnant cow that had been injected subcutaneously with 1 gm of progesterone each day for 5 days. 5α-Androstane-3,17-dione, 5β-androstane-3,17-dione, and 4-androstene-3,17-dione were tentatively identified. These latter steroids were present in much smaller quantities.

In summary, progesterone administered subcutaneously is excreted primarily in the feces (probably via the bile). Progesterone (and possibly metabolites) has an affinity for body fat. Data on urinary and fecal metabolites may or may not be applicable under the conditions in which progesterone is used as a growth promotant.

D. Testosterone

Testosterone propionate (200 mg) combined with estradiol benzoate (20 mg) is used as an implant in beef heifers in the United States. Very little information is available about metabolism of testosterone in female bovine. According to the English summary of a Russian paper (Epshtein and Uchurova, 1975), dehydroepiandrosterone sulfate, etiocholanolone, and etiocholandione were found in the urine of female bovine after introduction of testosterone propionate. Dehydroepiandrosterone sulfate was present in greatest amount. These steriods were not found in the urine of untreated animals.

Gassner *et al.* (1962) injected two steers subcutaneously at the base of the ear with either [4-^{14}C]testosterone (120 mg) or [4-^{14}C]testosterone enanthate (262 mg). (The vehicle was not stated; however, in other work, a "polyglycolic" paste was used.) Radioactivity was measured in feces, urine, and blood plasma and in biopsies of muscle and liver. Quantitation of radioactivity depended upon extraction of acid hydrolyzed samples. For both steers, approximately ten times as much radioactivity was excreted in feces as in the urine. Total recovery in excreta was 98.4% for testosterone and 84.5% for testosterone enanthate. The rate of excretion declined rapidly during the first 7–10 days; thereafter the decline was gradual. At slaughter, no radioactivity was detected at the site of injection of testosterone (119 days after injection), but 1.6% of the original dose remained at the site of the testosterone enanthate injection (94 days). Concentrations of radioactivity in blood plasma were highest 4 hours after injection (expressed in testosterone equivalents: approximately 120 ppb after testosterone injection and 43 ppb after testosterone enanthate). The highest concentration in muscle was 0.8 ppb 11 days after the testosterone injection. No radioactivity was detected in muscle and plasma of either steer at the time of slaughter. At the time of slaughter, the liver from the enanthate-injected steer contained traces of radioactivity and the bile (240 ml) collected contained 5.7 μg equivalents of testosterone. Also, kidney fat contained 5 ppb equivalents; whereas no radioactivity was detected in subcutaneous fat.

Martin (1966) made an effort to characterize the metabolites in the feces collected from a steer during the first 24 hours after subcutaneous injection of [¹⁴C]testosterone (samples were from the experiment of Gassner *et al.*, 1962). At least six radioactive fractions were isolated. 17α-Hydroxyandrost-4-en-3-one (epitestosterone) and 17α-hydroxy-5β-androstan-3-one were identified by chromatographic and recrystallization techniques. These metabolites represented 37 and 17%, respectively, of the radioactivity in the feces. There was some evidence for 5β-androstane-3,17-dione.

From available data, the primary route of excretion of subcutaneous testosterone by bovine is via feces. Two fecal metabolites identified from a steer accounted for approximately 50% of the fecal metabolites. No information on fecal metabolites from females is available. Testosterone esters may have a different distribution in the body than the nonesterified compound.

E. Zeranol

This compound is used as an implant for sheep (12 mg) and beef cattle (36 mg) in the United States. Very little information concerning the metabolism of zeranol (also known as zearalanol) is available. Sharp and Dyer (1972) implanted five steers at the base of the ear with 72 mg of tritium-labeled zeranol and then monitored excretion until slaughter 65–125 days later. The distribution of radioactivity at the time of slaughter is summarized in Table IX. All excreta were collected for only 22 days; thereafter, excretion of radioactivity was calculated from concentrations in weekly "grab" samples and estimates of mass (based on data from the total collection period). Radioactivity could be detected in the excreta for approximately 90 days after implantation. Radioactivity was

TABLE IX
Distribution of Radioactivity after Implantation of Tritium-Labeled
Zeranol in Steers[a]

	Days after implantation (%)[b]				
Location	65	80	95	110	125
Residual pellet	14.7	14.7	14.4	11.5	12.6
Urine	7.2	10.1	8.0	7.9	10.9
Feces	38.2	47.8	46.1	33.7	37.4
Total recovery	60.1	72.7	68.5	53.0	61.0

[a] From Sharp and Dyer (1972). Each value represents one animal.
Implants were at the base of the ear.
[b] Values are a percentage of the radioactivity in the implanted pellet.

detected in only 6 of 55 blood samples analyzed, and 5 of these samples were drawn 8–10 days after implantation. Radioactivity was not detected in tissues at time of sacrifice except in bile and in one pancreas sample.

Sharp and Dyer (1972) did not indicate the limits of detection in their assays, but on the basis of the description of the procedures and a 50% efficiency of tritium counting, the calculated concentrations of zeranol equivalents that would have produced a count rate of 10 cpm over background in the liquid-scintillation vials were as follows: fresh tissue, 140 ppb; blood and urine, 35 ppb; and feces, 15 ppb. Routine counting time was 10 minutes. In this experiment, the specific activity of the zeranol and the assay methods limited the ability to quantitate the distribution of zeranol and its metabolites.

There are essentially no data available on metabolites of zeranol in ruminants. David et al. (1973) indicated no increase in estrogenic activity (immature mouse uterine response) in tissues from neck, shoulder, and liver of calves slaughtered 89 days after implantation with 36 mg of zeranol. This result is not surprising because zeranol is a rather weak estrogen, but the data may also suggest that metabolites with high estrogenic activity were not present.

F. Trenbolone Acetate

Grandadam et al. (1975) have reported that implants of trenbolone acetate in combination with estradiol-17β increase rate and efficiency of gain in various meat animals. The use of this compound is not permitted in the United States at present.

Only one paper was found in which the metabolic fate of trenbolone acetate was described. Pottier et al. (1975) reported that absorption from a 300-mg pellet of tritium-labeled trenbolone acetate implanted at the base of the ear was gradual and continuous for as long as 150 days. The blood plasma concentrations of radioactivity averaged 2.2 ppb of trenbolone equivalents at the time of slaughter of two cows (nonpregnant-nonlactating) 90 days after implantation and 1.8 ppb in two cows (lactating) 150 days after implantation. Approximately 20% of the radioactivity remained at the implant site after 150 days. The concentrations of radioactivity in liver and kidney were approximately twice the concentration in plasma. In all other tissues, the concentrations were approximately half of the concentration in the plasma. Approximately 25% of the radioactivity in tissues could be extracted with ethyl acetate except for kidneys and liver from which only 10% could be extracted. From 33 to 50% of the activity extracted from tissue was trenbolone (unesterified). Perineal fat was different from other tissues in that over 80% of the radioactivity was extractable and over half of this was the parent trenbolone acetate.

When radiolabeled trenbolone acetate was injected intravenously, only 2% of the radioactivity in blood plasma drawn 6 minutes after injection was trenbolene acetate; 70% was trenbolene which indicated rapid hydrolysis. After 2 hours, most of the radioactivity in blood plasma could no longer be extracted.

The urine and feces (indicated by level of radioactivity in bile) appear to be the routes of excretion. Radioactivity in milk could be detected (concentrations lower than plasma) but the milk was not a significant route of excretion. The authors indicated that trenbolene with the hydroxy group at carbon-17 oxidized (estra-4,9,11-trien-3,17-one) was also a metabolite, but they did not present data concerning identification or occurrence.

In summary, trenbolone implanted in the ear absorbs slowly over several months. Total residues in muscle 150 days after implantation are of the order 0.5 ppb of trenbolone equivalents (based on measurements of radioactivity). Very little is known about the nature of the residues except that a small part (approximately 10%) has chromatographic properties similar to those of trenbolone. In the study described, the experimental animals were all mature female bovines whereas reports of growth promotion from trenbolone usually involved male bovine in some stage of growth.

III. ANTIBIOTICS

The use of compounds with antimicrobial activity in animal production has at least three logical bases. They may be used therapeutically to treat a specific infection, prophylactically against a specific organism or

TABLE X
Antibiotics Used as Growth Promotants[a]

Compound	Specie	Level[b]
Bacitracin	Chickens and turkeys	4–50 gm/ton
	Swine	10–50 gm/ton
	Beef cattle	35 mg/head/day
Bacitracin Methylene-disalicylate	Chickens and turkeys	4–50 gm/ton
	Swine	10–50 gm bacitracin activity/ton
Bacitracin, zinc	Chickens and turkeys	4–50 gm/ton
	Swine	10–50 gm/ton
	Cattle	35–70 mg/head/day
Bambermycins	Chickens	1–2 gm/ton
Carbadox	Swine	10–25 gm/ton (0.0011–0.00275%)
Chlortetracycline	Chickens and turkeys	10–50 gm/ton
	Swine	10–50 gm/ton
	Calves (< 250 lb)	0.1 mg/lb body wt/day
	Beef cattle	70 mg/head/day
	Sheep	20–50 gm/ton
Erythromycin	Chickens	4.6–18.5 gm/ton
	Turkeys (< 12 weeks)	9.25–18.5 gm/ton
	Starter pigs	10–70 gm/ton
	Growing-finishing pigs	10 gm/ton
	Cattle	37 mg/head/day
Lincomycin	Chickens and turkeys	1–2 gm/ton of complete poultry ration
	Swine	5–11.25 gm/ton of complete feed
Oxytetracycline	Chickens and turkeys	5–7.5 gm/ton
	Swine (10–30 lb)	25–50 gm/ton
	Swine (30–200 lb)	7.5–10 gm/ton
	Calves (< 12 weeks)	0.005–0.1 mg/lb body wt/day
	Calves	25–75 mg/head/day
	Beef cattle	75 mg/head/day
	Sheep	10–20 gm/ton
Penicillin	Chickens and turkeys	2.4–50 gm/ton
	Swine	10–50 gm/ton
Tylosin	Chickens	4–50 gm/ton
	Swine (finishing feeds)	10–20 gm/ton
	Swine (grower feeds)	20–40 gm/ton
	Swine (starter and pre-starter feeds)	20–100 gm/ton
Virginiamycin	Swine	10 gm/ton

[a] From Anonymous (1975c).
[b] Levels are those recognized as effective for growth promotion. Chronic intake of higher levels often permitted for prophylactic purposes.

group of organisms, or as a growth promotant where the mode of action is often not certain. This paper will deal with the growth promotant use of antimicrobials; however, the same compound may be used in all three ways. Use of antibiotics as growth promotants involves chronic oral exposure, and the predominant use is in nonruminants. In Table X some of the antibiotics commonly used for growth promotion are listed.

Microbiological growth inhibiting procedures are usually used to detect possible residues of the antibiotics and their distribution in the body. In this paper no attempt will be made to review reports of inhibitory substances found in commercial meat products. Reports of inhibitory substances in the animal tissues after controlled exposure to an antibiotic will be selected to the extent that they demonstrate distribution and rate of excretion. For many antibiotics only limited data are available concerning the ultimate fate of the molecule, particularly in farm animals. The emphasis in this paper will be on the tetracycline group because of their widespread use and available information.

A. Tetracyclines

The tetracycline group of antibiotics shown in Fig. 1 are widely used as growth promotants. These complex molecules are good chelating agents and degrade under relatively mild conditions. In aqueous solutions at pH 2–6, tetracyclines epimerize at carbon-4 (Fig. 2); in strong acids they dehydrate to give anhydrotetracyclines. In alkaline solutions, the tetracyclines, particularly chlortetracycline (CTC), isomerize to give isotetracyclines (Clive, 1968; Hughes and Wilson, 1973; Katz and Fassbender, 1967; Katz et al., 1969; McCormick et al., 1957; Schlecht and Frank, 1975). Antimicrobial potency of these degradation products is very low.

Data from food-producing animals on the rates and routes of excretion of tetracycline (TC) and its metabolites are not available. Considerable data are available on the concentrations of CTC in tissues of chick-

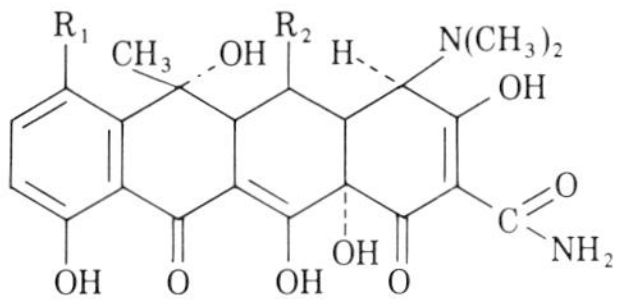

	R₁	R₂
Tetracycline (TC)	H	H
Chlortetracycline (CTC)	Cl	H
Oxytetracycline (OTC)	H	OH

Fig. 1. Tetracycline antibiotics used as growth promotants.

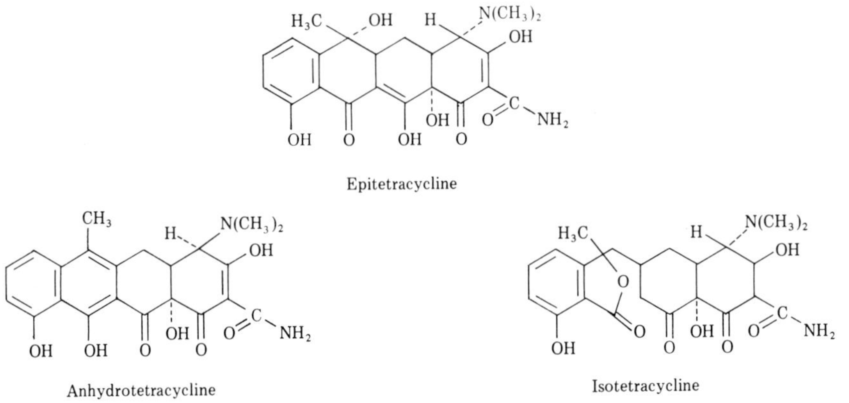

Epitetracycline

Anhydrotetracycline   Isotetracycline

Fig. 2.   Degradation products of tetracyclines.

ens, swine, and cattle after ingestion of various amounts; somewhat less data are available for oxytetracycline (OTC).

CTC was detected in tissues and eggs from chickens after ingesting levels of 50 gm per ton of feed (Katz *et al.*, 1972a,b). Concentrations were near the lower level of sensitivity of the assay (25 ppb in tissue and 20 ppb in eggs) and were not detectable 1 day after withdrawal of CTC from the feed. These workers and others (Broquist and Kohler, 1953–1954; Durbin *et al.*, 1953–1954; Filson *et al.*, 1965; Meredith *et al.*, 1965; Raica *et al.*, 1956; Shor *et al.*, 1967; Yoshida *et al.*, 1971) have reported detectable CTC in tissues and eggs from chickens ingesting higher levels. Inhibition of a CTC-sensitive bacteria was the basis for assays in all studies. The concentrations were eight to ten times higher in the kidney than in liver; concentrations were always lower in muscle and blood than in liver. CTC could be detected in kidney of chickens 3 days after withdrawal of feed containing 100 gm per ton; no activity could be detected in blood, muscle, or liver of chickens 1 day after withdrawal of feed containing 200 mg per ton. When young chicks were fed a constant level of CTC, concentrations gradually increased in tissue for approximately 3 weeks, then declined (Durbin *et al.*, 1953–1954; Katz *et al.*, 1972b; Yoshida *et al.*, 1971). There is no tested hypothesis to explain this observation. Filson *et al.* (1965) reported higher blood serum levels of CTC in laying hens than in nonlaying birds. The marked difference in calcium metabolism between egg laying birds and nonlayers was thought to be related to differences in serum CTC levels; however, the authors did not exclude the possibility that higher estrogen levels in laying birds could affect serum CTC levels directly.

The proportion of ingested CTC that is excreted unchanged by chickens is unknown; however, an average of 12.5 ppm CTC was found in litter of broilers receiving CTC continuously (Webb and Fontenot, 1975). The level in feed was not stated. CTC may epimerize in the gastrointestinal tract. Katz *et al.* (1972a) reported approximately equal amounts of CTC and epi-CTC in the contents of the small intestine of birds receiving CTC in their feed. Epi-CTC would be found in the feed but at a lower level (Katz and Fassbender, 1967). There is no information on epi-CTC absorption or tissue distribution.

CTC metabolism data from cattle and swine are limited. Elmund *et al.* (1971) estimated that 75% of the CTC (70 mg per day) ingested by yearling steers was excreted as CTC. CTC levels were 14 ppm in fresh manure and 0.34 ppm in what was described as aged manure. The half-life in the manure was estimated as greater than 20 days at 4° or 28°C. Gale *et al.* (1967) reported steers (250–350 kg body weight) fed 70 mg CTC per day for 28 days had CTC levels in kidney and liver that were near lower limits of sensitivity of the assay (25–40 ppb). Steers ingesting 5 mg of CTC per lb of body weight had concentrations of 2.5 ppm CTC in the kidney, 1.0 ppb in the liver, and 0.22 ppb in the muscle. CTC could be detected (0.05 ppm) in the kidney 10 days after withdrawal of the CTC. Brüggemann *et al.* (1972) reported that after ingestion of CTC, calves weighing 75–120 kg exhibited higher serum CTC levels than calves weighing under 75 kg or over 125 kg. CTC could also be detected for a longer time (80 hours after the last of 12 twice-a-day feedings of milk replacer containing 400 mg/kg CTC) in this weight class. Brüggemann *et al.* (1972) suggested that there was retention of CTC in the rumen of these animals. Other workers have observed a very rapid decline in CTC levels in ruminal fluids of calves after ingestion of 40 mg of CTC via a gelatin capsule (Bush *et al.*, 1957; Lodge *et al.*, 1956). They noted higher CTC levels in young animals (age range 79–148 days), but these could have been caused by a dilution factor because the total dose was the same for all animals. A rapid decrease in CTC activity was observed when CTC was incubated with mixed suspensions of rumen bacteria *in vitro* (Jurtshuk *et al.*, 1954).

CTC levels in swine tissue after ingestion of feed containing 100 mg of CTC per ton have been reported by Gale *et al.* (1967) and Messersmith *et al.* (1967). CTC was not detected in fat, and relative levels in muscle, liver, and kidney were similar to those in cattle.

The available data concerning oxytetracycline (OTC) in chickens are similar to those concerning CTC (Katz *et al.*, 1973; Meredith *et al.*, 1965; Webb and Fontenot, 1975). In a preliminary report, Alderson *et al.*

(1975) reported that 21% of the OTC administered orally to swine was recovered in feces.

Quantitative data on the metabolic fate of TC and CTC in rats and dogs are available from studies with radiolabeled compounds (Buyske *et al.*, 1960; Eisner and Wulf, 1963; Kelly and Buyske, 1960; Kelly and Kanegis, 1967). After an oral dose of [^{14}C]CTC to rats, the recovery of radioactivity was 92.3% of the dose in feces and 4.7% in urine. With TC, the recovery of radioactivity in feces was 75.8% of the dose and 4.2% in urine. When the radiolabeled compounds were given intravenously, the respective fecal and urinary excretions of radioactivity were 41.2 and 35.4% for CTC and 19.5 and 69.2% for TC. Observation of excretion in rats with ligated bile ducts or ureters indicated that CTC is eliminated readily via the bile. Apparently, the predominant fecal excretion of CTC is not caused entirely by lack of absorption.

CTC and TC are adsorbed by bone. Kelly and Buyske (1960) estimated that 1 week after an intraperitoneal dose of [^{14}C]CTC (60 mg/kg of body weight) to rats, 3–6% of the dose was adsorbed by the skeleton. After a similar oral dose, they estimated that only 0.1% of the dose was adsorbed. The concentration in bone appeared to be directly related to concentration in blood. After a 250-mg/kg intraperitoneal dose of CTC was given, the CTC levels in bone decreased rapidly for approximately 3 to 4 days and then decreased gradually over the next 28 weeks of observation. The CTC levels in femora 28 weeks after dosing were approximately 20 ppm for female rats and 65 ppm for male rats. The sex difference may have been more apparent than real because the male rats were in a more rapid phase of their growth curve and preferential adsorption occurs on new bone growth. TC is also adsorbed by bone but to a lesser extent than CTC is adsorbed. This finding is consistent with the stronger chelating properties of CTC.

The radioactivity in rat urine collected in the first 24 hours after dosing with [^{14}C]CTC was characterized by paper chromatography. Most of the radioactivity migrated similarly to CTC (44–65%) and epi-CTC (23–35%). A small amount (0–11%) migrated as TC; however, TC was a known radiolabeled contaminant of the dosing material. From 2 to 11% was unidentified. Results were similar with dogs. Chromatography of fecal radioactivity was more difficult. CTC and epi-CTC were characterized; and occasionally there was suggestive evidence for iso-CTC. The iso-CTC could have been an artifact of the extraction and clean-up procedures. TC was the only radioactive compound characterized in feces and urine of rats dosed with radioactive TC.

In summary, the tetracyclines ingested by farm animals are absorbed to some extent, but quantitative data are not available. Some of the ingested material is excreted unchanged. One would expect to find epi-CTC in excreta on the basis of reports with chickens, rats, and dogs. There is evidence that animals continue to excrete very low levels of tetracyclines for some time after withdrawal from the feed. Retention by bone is a possible reservoir supporting this continued excretion, but other factors such as enterhepatic circulation cannot be ruled out. Residues in soft tissues decrease quickly upon withdrawal of tetracyclines from the feed; however, under some conditions residues can be detected in the kidney for several days.

B. Penicillin

Oral administration of penicillin did not result in detectable residues in tissues of swine (Messersmith *et al.*, 1967) nor in tissue or eggs of chickens (Katz *et al.*, 1974). Assays were based on inhibition of penicillin-sensitive organisms, and sensitivity was 0.04 unit per gm or lower. Penicillin is rapidly inactivated in the digestive tract of chickens (Bare *et al.*, 1965; Katz *et al.*, 1974). Several metabolites were identified (cochromatography on TLC) in the digestive tract of chickens (18 hours without feed) given 250 mg of benzylpenicillin procaine (sodium salt) via a gelatin capsule placed in the crop passage. These included penicilloic acid, penicillamine, and penillic acid (Katz *et al.*, 1974). Penicillin was not found beyond the duodenum. These workers observed a shift in the resistance patterns of lactose fermenting organisms in the feces of chickens receiving penicillin and made the interesting observation that a similar shift in resistance patterns was observed when only penicilloic acid (50 gm per ton) was fed to chickens. No possible mechanisms were suggested by which a substance without inhibitory properties could influence resistance patterns of microorganisms.

C. Monensin

Monensin (Fig. 3) is a compound that has been recently approved for use as a growth promotant for ruminants (Anonymous, 1975b). It has also been used for some time as a coccidiostat in broilers. Monensin is effective as a growth promotant in ruminants only, and its mode of action is believed to involve alterations in microbial metabolism in the rumen. A preliminary report of the metabolic fate of monensin has been presented (Donoho *et al.*, 1976). Excretion of radioactivity by steers and rats after a single oral dose of [^{14}C]monensin was rapid and essentially quantitative. Less than 0.5% of the dose was excreted via the urine. Monensin was metabolized extensively, and some twenty radioactive

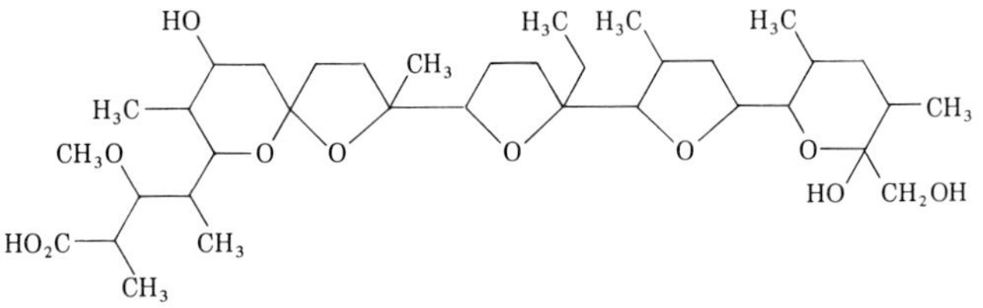

Fig. 3. Structure of monensin (from Agtarap and Chamberlin, 1967).

fractions were isolated from feces. Six metabolites have been characterized, one involved demethylation and decarboxylation and the other five resulted from O-demethylation and hydroxylation. Liver was the only tissue in which radioactivity could be detected (0.59 ppm of monensin equivalents) 12 hours after the last dose of [^{14}C]monensin, and only 3% of the ^{14}C in the liver was identified as monensin.

Rates and routes of excretion of radioactivity by chickens fed tritiated monensin have also been reported (Herberg and Van Duyn, 1969). More than 99% of the activity was excreted in the feces, and the proportion of ^{3}H in feces exhibiting the properties of monensin decreased rapidly with time after dosing. Some radioactivity was absorbed as indicated by tissue assays; however, much of this activity was associated with tissue water. Liver and kidney contained the highest concentration of ^{3}H not associated with water.

IV. ARSENIC-CONTAINING COMPOUNDS

The two compounds listed in Table XI are commonly referred to as arsanilic acid and 3-nitro-4-hydroxyphenylarsonic acid. Arsanilic acid is also recognized as a coccidiostat. The fact that some forms of arsenic are toxic makes the fates of these additives important.

A. 4-Aminobenzenearsonic Acid (Arsanilic Acid)

Total arsenic levels in tissues of chickens are increased by feeding of arsanilic acid (Frost, 1953; Frost *et al.*, 1955). Tissue arsenic levels did not continue to increase with length of time in birds fed arsanilic acid. For the first 48 hours after withdrawal, levels decreased sharply; thereafter, the decrease was gradual. Liver had the highest concentration of the tissues examined (two to three times muscle levels).

Moody and Williams (1964a) reported that all of the arsenic excreted by hens fed a dose of arsanilic acid was as arsanilic acid. No other proba-

TABLE XI

Arsenic Compounds Recognized as Growth Promotants in the United States[a]

Name	Specie	Level in feed (%)
4-Aminobenzenearsonic acid	Chickens, turkeys, and swine	0.005 – 0.01
4-Hydroxy-3-nitrobenzenearsonic acid	Chickens and turkeys	0.025 – 0.005
	Swine	0.0025 – 0.0075

[a] From Anonymous (1975c).

ble metabolites could be detected by extraction and TLC. Approximately 75% of the dose (50–100 mg/kg) was excreted within 3 days after dosing. Experiments in which chickens were dosed with arsanilic acid double-labeled with ^{74}As and ^{14}C indicate the C-As bond is not broken extensively (Overby and Fredrickson, 1963; Overby and Straube, 1965). The ratios of ^{14}C to ^{74}As in several tissues and excreta were similar to the ratio in the dose of the double-labeled arsanilic acid. The authors concluded less than 1% of the C-As bonds were cleaved.

Patterns of tissue levels of total arsenic after oral arsanilic acid in swine were similar to those observed in chickens (Hanson et al., 1955). However, Overby and Frost (1960) reported that unchanged arsanilic acid (found only in feces) represented only approximately 5% of the arsanilic acid consumed by swine. After 10 days of arsanilic acid feeding at 30 or 60 gm per ton of feed, excretion and intake were approximately equal. Excretion in the feces averaged three times that in the urine (range 1.2–5.5 times), and there was a tendency for the proportion excreted in the urine to increase with high levels of intake (60–90 gm per ton).

B. 4-Hydroxy-3-nitrobenzenearsonic Acid (4H3NBA)

Tissue concentrations of arsenic in chickens after oral 4H3NBA are similar to those after feeding arsanilic acid (Frost et al., 1955; Kerr et al., 1963, 1969). The levels rose quickly after initiation of feeding and plateaued after approximately 1 week. After withdrawal, the arsenic levels decreased rapidly for 3 to 4 days and thereafter more gradually. Liver contained the highest concentration, followed by kidney, skin, and muscle. Carpenter (1951) measured levels of arsenic in liver and kidney of swine fed 0.005% 4H3NBA in their diet for 40 days. After withdrawal, levels decreased rapidly; and by 7 days, they were too low for accurate determination (< 0.5 ppb).

The arsenic in a single dose of 4H3NBA (75 mg/kg) given to hens was quantitatively recovered in the excreta in 11 days (Moody and Williams, 1964b). The crop was the major location of unexcreted arsenic during the first 48 hours after dosing (37.5 mg/kg); 72 hours after dosing, the amount in the large intestine (6.8% of the dose) was similar to amounts in the crop (5.0%). A major metabolite in the excreta was the reduction product 4-hydroxy-3-aminobenzenearsonic acid (3-amino). This compound represented from 19 to 29% of the arsenic recovered in excreta during the first 3 days after a single oral dose (75–78.9 mg/kg). The parent compound plus the "3-amino" metabolite accounted for more than 90% of the arsenic excreted in this experiment. A major site of formation of the "3-amino" metabolite was the crop.

Interest in the use of poultry litter as a feed for ruminants has raised the question as to the fate of arsenic residues that may be present in the litter. Calvert (1975) has reviewed this subject. Because arsanilic acid is excreted by poultry without extensive metabolism, the fate of this compound in ruminants is of interest. L. W. Smith et al. (1973) fed arsanilic acid to sheep (0–273 ppm in the diet) and observed tissue levels of arsenic after 28 days of feeding and until 6 days after withdrawal. Residues could be detected in liver, kidney, muscle, and blood in patterns similar to those observed in chickens receiving arsanilic acid. Excretion of arsenic by sheep after ingestion of poultry litter from chickens receiving 4H3NBA was also studied. During the last 5 days of a 15-day feeding experiment, the excreta contained an average of 87% of the arsenic in the ingested poultry litter. The ratio of fecal to urinary arsenic was approximately 3:1. Tissue levels were not measured.

Morrison (1969) has reported that application of poultry litter containing arsenic residues to soil as a fertilizer does not measurably affect the arsenic content of the soil or plants grown on the soil.

In summary, considerable data are available on the metabolic fate of arsanilic acid and 4H3NBA in chickens. Arsanilic acid is excreted essentially quantitatively unmetabolized. 4-Hydroxy-3-aminobenzenearsonic acid is a major metabolite of 4H3NBA and over 90% of the excreted arsenic can be accounted for by the parent compound plus this metabolite. In contrast, little data are available on the fate of arsenicals in swine (other than tissue levels of arsenic after feeding arsanilic acid). More than 90% of the arsanilic acid was metabolized to unknown compounds. No data were available concerning fate of 4H3NBA in swine.

V. CONCLUSIONS

Making generalizations about the metabolic fate of growth-promoting chemicals is difficult; however, a few statements may have some common validity. When animals are exposed to the chemicals in the prescribed manner, some level (usually ppb range) of the parent compounds can be detected in tissues of the animals. In the case of arsenic-containing compounds, increases in total arsenic content of some tissues in the ppm range are observed. Animals are able to excrete the compounds by conventional mechanisms. The initial decline in tissue residues after withdrawal of an orally administered chemical is rapid, but this is followed by a period in which the decline is much slower. Although no quantitative evidence is available, we can reasonably assume that with some chemicals enterohepatic circulation may be involved in the period of slow decline.

Absorption from subcutaneous implants used in animal production is slow and continuous for at least 100 days. After an initial sharp decline, the rate of absorption (as indicated by excretion and blood levels) decreases very gradually. Considerable individual variations exist in the rate of absorption from a subcutaneous implant.

REFERENCES

Agtarap, A., and Chamberlin, J. W. (1967). Monensin, a new biologically active compound. IV. Chemistry. *Antimicrob. Agents Chemother.* pp. 359–362.

Alderson, N. E., Knight, W. M., Robinson, R., Colaianne, J., and Bradley, B. (1975). Ovine absorption and excretion of oxytetracycline. *J. Anim. Sci.* **41**, 388–389.

Anonymous. (1975a). *Fed. Regist.* **40**, 6323.

Anonymous. (1975b). *Fed. Regist.* **40**, 58289–58290.

Anonymous. (1975c). "Feed Additive Compendium." Miller Publishing Co., Minneapolis, Minnesota.

Anonymous. (1976). *Fed. Regist.* **41**, 1804–1807.

Aschbacher, P. W. (1972). Metabolism of ^{14}C-diethylstilbestrol in sheep. *J. Anim. Sci.* **35**, 1031–1035.

Aschbacher, P. W. (1976). Diethylstilbestrol metabolism in food-producing animals. *J. Toxicol. Environ. Health, Suppl.* **1**, 45–59.

Aschbacher, P. W., and Feil, V. J. (1975). Degradation of diethylstilbestrol in feces. *J. Anim. Sci.* **41**, 263 (abstr.).

Aschbacher, P. W., and Thacker, E. J. (1974). Metabolic fate of oral diethylstilbestrol in steers. *J. Anim. Sci.* **39**, 1185–1192.

Aschbacher, P. W., Thacker, E. J., and Rumsey, T. S. (1975). Metabolic fate of diethylstilbestrol implanted in the ear of steers. *J. Anim. Sci.* **40**, 530–538.

Bare, L. N., Wiseman, R. F., and Abbott, O. J. (1965). Levels of antibiotics in the intestinal tract of chicks fed bacitracin and penicillin. *Poult. Sci.* **44**, 489–491.

Bedford, C. A., Harrison, F. A., and Heap, R. B. (1972). The metabolic clearance rate and production rate of progesterone and the conversion of progesterone to 20α-hydroxypregn-4-en-3-one in the sheep. *J. Endocrinol.* **55**, 105–118.

Bhattacharya, A. N., and Taylor, J. C. (1975). Recycling animal wastes as a feedstuff: A review. *J. Anim. Sci.* **41**, 1438–1457.

Broquist, H. P., and Kohler, A. R. (1953–1954). Studies of the antibiotic potency in the meat of animals fed chlortetracycline. *Antibiot. Annu.* pp. 409–415.

Brüggemann, V. J., Lösch, U., and Knall, G. (1972). Über die Chlortetracyclin-Konzentration und-Verweildauer im Serum von Kälbern nach peroraler

Chlortetracyclin-Verabreichung. *Z. Tierphysiol., Tierernaehr. Futtermittelkd.* **29**, 230–238.

Bush, L. J., Jacobson, N. L., and Hartman, P. A. (1957). Levels of chlortetracycline in the rumen fluid of dairy calves following oral administration of the antibiotic. *Antibiot. Chemother. (Washington, D.C.)* **7**, 9–12.

Buyske, D. A., Eisner, H. J., and Kelly, R. G. (1960). Concentration and persistence of tetracycline and chlortetracycline in bone. *J. Pharmacol. Exp. Ther.* **130**, 150–156.

Calvert, C. C. (1975). Arsenicals in animal feeds and wastes. *Am. Chem. Soc., Symp. Ser.* **7**, 70–80.

Carpenter, L. E. (1951). The effect of 3-nitro-4-hydroxy phenyl arsonic acid on the growth of swine. *Arch. Biochem. Biophys.* **32**, 181–186.

Challis, J. R. G., Harrison, F. A., and Heap, R. B. (1973). The kinetics of oestradiol-17β metabolism in the sheep. *J. Endocrinol.* **57**, 97–110.

Clive, D. L. J. (1968). Chemistry of tetracyclines. *Q. Rev., Chem. Soc.* **22**, 435–456.

David, C., Grandadam, A., Pipin, F., Szumowski, P., Théret, M., Vaissaire, J., Vuillaume, R., and Wyers, M. (1973). Recherche des résidus oestrogènes dans les viandes de veaux traités au zéranol. *Rec. Med. Vet.* **149**, 503–506.

Donoho, A. L., Herberg, R. J., Manthey, J. A., and Occolowitz, J. L. (1976). Excretion and metabolism of monensin in cattle and rats. *172nd Meet., Am. Chem. Soc. Agric. Food Chem. Div., San Francisco.* Pap. 164.

Durbin, C. G., DiLorenzo, J. J., Randall, W. A., and Wilner, J. (1953–1954). Antibiotic concentration and duration in animal tissues and fluids. II. Chicken blood, tissue, and eggs. *Antibiot. Annu.*, pp. 428–432.

Echternkamp, S. E., and Hansel, W. (1973). Concurrent changes in bovine plasma hormone levels prior to and during the first postpartum estrous cycle. *J. Anim. Sci.* **37**, 1362–1370.

Eisner, H. J., and Wulf, R. J. (1963). The metabolic fate of chlortetracycline and some comparisons with other tetracyclines. *J. Pharmacol. Exp. Ther.* **142**, 122–131.

Elmund, G. K., Morrison, S. M., Grant, D. W., and Nevins, M. P. (1971). Role of excreted chlortetracycline in modifying the decomposition process in feedlot waste. *Bull. Environ. Contam. Toxicol.* **6**, 129–132.

Engel, L. J., Weidenfel, J., and Merriam, G. R. (1976). The metabolism of diethylstilbestrol by rat liver. A preliminary report. *J. Toxicol. Environ. Health,Suppl.* 37–44.

Epshtein, N. A., and Uchurova, A. S. (1975). On metabolites of testosterone in cattle urine. *Izv. Timiryazevsk. Skh. Akad.* **2**, 176–183.

Ferrando, R., Cumont, G., Richou-Bac, L., and Valette, J.-P. (1973). Recherche de réidus d'oestradiol dans les viandes de veaux implantes à l'oestradiol-progestérone. *Rec. Med. Vet.* **149**, 1319–1325.

Ferrando, R., Valette, J.-P., LeBars, H., and Brugère, H. (1974). Economie rurale—recherche du diethylstilboestrol (DES) et de la progésterone dans la salive de la chèvre et du mouton soumis à des implants renfermant ces composés. *C. R. Hebd. Seances Acad. Sci.* **278**, 1091–1093.

Filson, D. R., Weiser, H. H., Meredith, W. E., and Winter, A. R. (1965). Absorption of chlortetracycline from the alimentary tract in White Leghorn hens. *Poult. Sci.* **44**, 761–767.

Fischer, L. J., Weissinger, J. L., Rickert, D. E., and Hintze, K. L. (1976). Studies on the biological disposition of diethylstilbestrol in rats and humans. *J. Toxicol. Environ. Health* **1**, 587–605.

Frost, D. V. (1953). Considerations on the safety of arsanilic acid for use in poultry feeds. *Poult. Sci.* **32**, 217–227.

Frost, D. V., Overby, L. R., and Spruth, H. C. (1955). Studies with arsanilic acid and related compounds. *J. Agric. Food Chem.* **3**, 235–243.

Gale, G. O., Abbey, A., and Shor, A. L. (1967). Disappearance of chlortetracycline residues from edible tissues of animals fed rations containing the drug. I. Cattle and swine. *Antimicrob. Agents Chemother.* **7**, 749–756.

Gassner, F. X., Martin, R. P., Shimoda, W., and Algeo, J. W. (1962). Metabolism of radioactive steroid esters in the bovine male and female. *Fertil. Steril.* **45**, 49–73.

Grandadam, J. A., Scheid, J. P., Jobard, A., Dreux, H., and Boisson, J. M. (1975). Results obtained with trenbolone acetate [R] in conjunction with estradiol-17β in veal calves, feedlot bulls, lambs, and pigs. *J. Anim. Sci.* **41**, 969–977.

Gregers-Hansen, B. (1964a). Decomposition of diethylstilboestrol in soil. *Plant Soil* **20**, 50–58.

Gregers-Hansen, B. (1964b). The uptake by plants of diethylstilboestrol and of its glucuronide. *Plant Soil* **20**, 215–220.

Hacker, R. G., Cruea, D. D., Shimoda, W., and Hopwood, M. L. (1967). Uptake of diethylstilbestrol by edible plants. *J. Anim. Sci.* **26**, 1358–1362.

Hale, W. H., Sherman, W. C., White, E. A., Kuhn, G., Schnell, R. B., Reynolds, W. M., and Luther, H. G. (1959). Adsorption of diethylstilbestrol pellets in steers. *J. Anim. Sci.* **18**, 1201–1207.

Hanson, L. E., Carpenter, L. E., Aunan, W. J., and Ferrin, E. F. (1955). The use of arsanilic acid in the production of market pigs. *J. Anim. Sci.* **14**, 513–524.

Heap, R. B., Henville, A., and Linzell, J. L. (1975). Metabolic clearance rate, production rate, and mammary uptake and metabolism of progesterone in cows. *J. Endocrinol.* **66**, 239–247.

Henricks, D. M. (1976). Estrogen concentrations in bovine and porcine tissues. *J. Toxicol. Environ. Health* **1**, 617–639.

Henricks, D. M., Dickey, J. F., Hill, J. R., and Johnston, W. E. (1972). Plasma estrogen and progesterone levels after mating and during late pregnancy and postpartum in cows. *Endocrinology* **90**, 1336–1342.

Herberg, R. J., and Van Duyn, R. L. (1969). Excretion and tissue distribution studies in chickens fed 3^H-monensin (Na salt). *J. Agric. Food Chem.* **17**, 853–856.

Hinds, F. C., Draper, H. H., Mitchell, G. E., and Neumann, A. L. (1965). Metabolism of labeled diethylstilbestrol in ruminants. *J. Agric. Food. Chem.* **13**, 256–259.

Hoffmann, B., and Karg, H. (1973). Determination of tissue levels of steroid-oestrogens in the bovine using a radioimmunological technique. *Acta Endocrinol. (Copenhagen), Suppl.* **177**, 44 (abstr.).

Huber, T. L., Horn, G. W., and Beadle, R. E. (1972). Liver and gastrointestinal metabolism of diethylstilbestrol in sheep. *J. Anim. Sci.* **34**, 786–790.

Hughes, D. W., and Wilson, W. L. (1973). Chemical and physical analysis of antibiotics. Part I. *Can. J. Pharm. Sci.* **8**, 67–74.

Jurtshuk, P., Doetsch, R. N., McNeill, J. J., and Shaw, J. C. (1954). *In vitro* studies of the effect of aueromycin and terramycin on mixed suspensions of bovine rumen bacteria. *J. Dairy Sci.* **37**, 1466–1472.

Kaltenbach, C. C., Dunn, T. G., Koritnik, D. R., Tucker, W. F., Batson, D. B., Staigmiller, R. B., and Niswender, G. D. (1976). Isolation and identification of metabolites of ^{14}C-labeled estradiol in cattle. *J. Toxicol. Environ. Health* **1**, 607.–616.

Katz, S. E., and Fassbender, C. A. (1967). Studies on the stability of chlortetracycline in mixed feeds: Epimerization of chlortetracycline. *J. Assoc. Off. Anal. Chem.* **50**, 821–827.

Katz, S. E., Fassbender, C. A., and Hain, L. J. (1969). Stability of chlortetracycline in pelleted feeds. *J. Assoc. Off. Anal. Chem.* **52**, 920.-929.

Katz, S. E., Fassbender, C. A., and Dowling, J. J. (1972a). Chlortetracycline residues in eggs from hens on chlortetracyclien supplemented diet. *J. Assoc. Off. Anal. Chem.* **55**, 128-133.

Katz, S. E., Fassbender, C. A., Dorfman, D., and Dowling, J. J. (1972b). Chlortetracycline residues in broiler tissue and organs. *J. Assoc. Off. Anal. Chem.* **55**, 134-138.

Katz, S. E., Fassbender, C. A., and Dowling, J. J. (1973). Oxytetracycline residues in tissue, organs, and eggs of poultry fed supplemented rations. *J. Assoc. Off. Anal. Chem.* **56**, 77-81.

Katz, S. E., Fassbender, C. A., Dinnerstein, P. S., and Dowling, J. J. (1974). Effects of feeding penicillin to chickens. *J. Assoc. Off. Anal. Chem.* **57**, 522-526.

Kazama, N., and Longcope, C. (1972). Metabolism of estrone and estradiol-17β in sheep. *Endocrinology* **91**, 1450-1454.

Kelly, R. G., and Buyske, D. A. (1960). Metabolism of tetracycline in the rat and the dog. *J. Pharmacol. Exp. Ther.* **130**, 144-149.

Kelly, R. G., and Kanegis, L. A. (1967). Tissue distribution of tetracycline and chlortetracycline in the dog. *Toxicol. Appl. Pharmacol.* **11**, 114-120.

Kerr, K. B., Cavett, J. W., and Thompson, O. L. (1963). The toxicity of an organic arsenical, 3-nitro-4-hydroxyphenylarsonic acid. 1. Acute and subacute toxicity. *Toxicol. Appl. Pharmacol.* **5**, 507-525.

Kerr, K. B., Narveson, J. R., and Lux, F. A. (1969). Toxicity of an organic arsenical, 3-nitro-4-hydroxyphenylarsonic acid residues in chicken tissues. *J. Agric. Food Chem.* **17**, 1400.-1402.

Leung, B. S., and Martin, R. P. (1972). Biliary metabolites of 17β-estradiol in the bovine. *Fed. Proc., Fed. Am. Soc. Exp. Biol.* **31**, 880 (abstr.).

Leung, B. S., Pearson, J. R., and Martin, R. P. (1975). Enterohepatic cycling of ³H-estrone in the bull. Identification of estrone-3-glucuronide. *J. Steroid Biochem.* **6**, 1477-1481.

Lodge, J. R., Miles, J. T., Jacobson, N. L., and Quinn, L. Y. (1956). Influence of chlortetracycline on *in vitro* cellulose digestion by bovine rumen microorganisms. *J. Dairy Sci.* **39**, 303-311.

McCormick, J. R. D., Fox, S. M., Smith, L. L., Bitler, B. A., Reichenthal, J., Origoni, V. E., Muller, W. H., Winterbottom, R., and Doerschuk, A. P. (1957). Studies of the reversible epimerization occurring in the tetracycline family. The preparation, properties, and proof of structure of some 4-epi-tetracyclines. *J. Am. Chem. Soc.* **79**, 2849-2858.

McCracken, J. A. (1964). Progesterone in the body fat of the dairy cow. *J. Endocrinol.* **28**, 339-340.

Martin, R. P. (1966). Fecal metabolites of testosterone-4-¹⁴C in the bovine male castrate. *Endocrinology* **78**, 907-913.

Masarcchia, R. (1969). Interactions of diethylstilbestrol with mammalian systems *in vitro*. Ph.D. Thesis, University of Massachusetts, Amherst [*Diss. Abstr. Int.* **30**, 3021-B (1970)].

Mellin, T. N., and Erb, R. E. (1965). Estrogens in the bovine—a review. *J. Dairy Sci.* **48**, 687-700.

Mellin, T. N., and Erb, R. E. (1966). Estrogen metabolism and excretion during the bovine estrous cycle. *Steroids* **7**, 589-606.

Meredith, W. E., Weiser, H. H., and Winter, A. R. (1965). Chlortetracycline and oxytetracycline residues in poultry tissues and eggs. *Appl. Microbiol.* **13**, 86-88.

Messersmith, R. E., Sass, B., Berger, H., and Gale, G. O. (1967). Safety and tissue residue evaluations in swine fed rations containing chlortetracycline, sulfamethazine, and penicillin. *J. Am. Vet. Med. Assoc.* **151**, 719-724.

Metzler, M. (1975). Metabolic activation of diethylstilbestrol: Indirect evidence for the formation of a stilbene oxide intermediate in hamster and rat. *Biochem. Pharmacol.* **24,** 1449–1453.

Metzler, M. (1976). Metabolic activation of carcinogenic diethylstilbestrol in rodents and man. *J. Toxicol. Environ. Health Suppl.* **1,** 21–35.

Miller, W. R., Turner, C. W., Fukushima, D. K., and Salamon, I. I. (1956). The identification of C_{19} steroids in bovine feces. *J. Biol. Chem.* **220,** 221–225.

Mitchell, G. E., Neumann, A. L., and Draper, H. H. (1959). Metabolism of tritium-labeled diethylstilbestrol by steers. *J. Agric. Food Chem.* **7,** 509–512.

Monk, E. L., Erb, R. E., and Mollett, T. A. (1975). Relationship between immunoreactive estrone and estradiol in milk, blood, and urine of dairy cows. *J. Dairy Sci.* **58,** 34–40.

Moody, J. P., and Williams, R. T. (1964a). The fate of arsanilic acid and acetylarsanilic acid in hens. *Food Cosmet. Toxicol.* **2,** 687–693.

Moody, J. P., and Williams, R. T. (1964b). The metabolism of 4-hydroxy-3-nitrophenyl-arsonic acid in hens. *Food Cosmet. Toxicol.* **2,** 707–715.

Morrison, J. L. (1969). Distribution of arsenic from poultry liver in broiler chickens, soil and crops. *J. Agric. Food. Chem.* **17,** 1288–1290.

Morrison, S. M., Grant, D. W., Nevins, M. P., and Elmund, K. (1969). Role of excreted antibiotic in modifying microbial decomposition of feedlot waste. *Proc. Cornell Univ. Conf. Agric. Waste Manag., 1969* pp. 336–339.

Mroszczak, E. (1974). The biliary excretion and enterohepatic circulation of diethylstilbestrol and diethylstilbestrol monoglucuronide in the Rhesus monkey. Ph.D. Thesis, University of California, San Francisco. [*Diss. Abstr. Int.* 36 114-B (1975)].

Overby, L. R., and Frederickson, R. L. (1963). Metabolic stability of radioactive arsanilic acid in chickens. *J. Agric. Food Chem.* **11,** 378–381.

Overby, L. R., and Frost, D. V. (1960). Excretion studies in swine fed arsanilic acid. *J. Anim. Sci.* **19,** 140–145.

Overby, L. R., and Straube, L. (1965). Metabolism of arsanilic acid. I. Metabolic stability of doubly labeled arsanilic acid in chickens. *Toxicol. Appl. Pharmacol.* **7,** 850–854.

Pearson, J. R., and Martin, R. P. (1966). Biliary metabolites of 17β-estradiol-4-^{14}C in the bull. *Endocrinology* **78,** 914–918.

Pottier, J., Busigny, M., and Grandadam, J. A. (1975). Plasma kinetics excretion in milk and tissue levels in the cow following implantation of trenbolone acetate$^{(R)}$. *J. Anim. Sci.* **41,** 962–968.

Raica, N., Heywang, B. W., and Kemmerer, A. R. (1954). Antibiotic concentration in eggs from hens on chlortetracycline supplemented diets. *Poult. Sci.* **35,** 884–888.

Rumsey, T. S., Oltjen, R. R., Daniels, F. L., and Kozak, A. S. (1975a). Depletion patterns of radioactivity and tissue residues in beef cattle after the withdrawal of oral ^{14}C-diethylstilbestrol. *J. Anim. Sci.* **40,** 539–549.

Rumsey, T. S., Oltjen, R. R., Kozak, A. S., Daniels, F. L., and Aschbacher P.W. (1975b). Fate of radiocarbon in beef steers implanted with ^{14}C-diethylstilbestrol. *J. Anim. Sci.* **40,** 550–560.

Rumsey, T. S., Dinius, D. A., and Oltjen, R. R. (1975c). DES, antibiotic and ronnel in beef feedlot waste. *J. Anim. Sci.* **41,** 275 (abstr.).

Schlecht, K. D., and Frank, C. W. (1975). Dehydration of tetracycline. *J. Pharm. Sci.* **64,** 352–354.

Sharp, G. D., and Dyer, I. A. (1972). Zearalanol metabolism in steers. *J. Anim. Sci.* **34,** 176–179.

Shor, A. L., Abbey, A., and Gale, G. O. (1967). Disappearance of chlortetracycline residues from edible tissues. II. Chickens and turkeys. *Antimicrob. Agents Chemother.* **7,** 757–762.

Short, R. V., and Moore, N. W. (1959). Progesterone in blood. V. Progesterone and 20α-hydroxypregn-4-en-3-one in the placenta and blood of ewes. *J. Endocrinol.* **19**, 288–293.

Smith, D. L., Estergreen, V. L., Martin, E. L., Lin, M. T., Moss, G. E., Frandle, K. A., Klicker, R. K., Luedemen, R. L., Branen, A. L., Luedecke, L. O., and Shimoda, W. (1975). Distribution of ^{14}C-progesterone in cattle tissue fluids and excreta. *J. Anim. Sci.* **41** 380 (abstr.).

Smith, L. W., Calvert, C. C., and Menear, J. R. (1973). Dehydrated poultry manure as a crude protein supplement for sheep. *Proc. Md. Nutr. Conf., 1973* p. 35.

Smith, V. G., Edgerton, L. A., Hafs, H. D., and Convey, E. M. (1973). Bovine serum estrogens, progestins, and glucocorticoids during late pregnancy, parturition, and early lactation. *J. Anim. Sci.* **36**, 391–396.

Stabenfeldt, G. H., Holt, J. A., and Ewing, L. L. (1969). Peripheral plasma progesterone levels during the ovine estrous cycle. *Endocrinology* **85**, 11–15.

Stupnicki, R., and Williams, K. I. H. (1968). Urinary metabolites of 4-^{14}C-progesterone in the ewe. *Steroids* **12**, 581–587.

Stupnicki, R., McCracken, J. A., and Williams, K. I. H. (1969). Progesterone metabolism in the ewe. *J. Endocrinol.* **45**, 67–74.

Sykes, J. F., Thomas, J. W., Bitman, J., and Winchester, C. F. (1960). Antibiotics, hormones, and tranquilizers in animals. *U. S., Dep. Agric., Agric. Res. Serv. [Publ.]* **20**-9.

Terqui, M. (1972). Métabolisme des oestrogènes chez labrebis gravide. *Ann. Biol. Anim., Biochim., Biophys.* **12**, 47–56.

Thorburn, G. D., Bassett, J. M., and Smith, I. D. (1969). Progesterone concentration in the peripheral plasma of sheep during the oestrous cycle. *J. Endocrinol.* **45**, 459–469.

Umberger, E. J. (1975). Products marketed to promote growth in food-producing animals: Steroid and hormone products. *Toxicology* **3**, 3–21.

Velle, W. (1963). Metabolism of estrogenic hormones in domestic animals. *Gen. Comp. Endocrinol.* **3**, 621–635.

Vogt, K., Waldschmidt, M., and Karg, H. (1972). Detection of excretion and residues of estradiol in calves after intramuscular and subcutaneous implantation of pellets containing adequate doses of estrogen. *Arch. Lebensmittelhyg.* **23**, 70–76.

Webb, K. E., and Fontenot, J. P. (1975). Medicinal drug residues in broiler litter and tissues from cattle fed litter. *J. Anim. Sci.* **41**, 1212–1217.

Wettemann, R. P., Hafs, H. D., Edgerton, L. A., and Swanson, L. V. (1972). Estradiol and progesterone in blood serum during the bovine estrous cycle. *J. Anim. Sci.* **34**, 1020–1024.

Willett, L. B., Smith, K. L., Schanbacher, F. L., Erb, R. E., and Malven, P. V. (1976). Hormone induced lactation in the bovine. III. Dynamics of injected and endogenous hormones. *J. Dairy Sci.* **59**, 504–514.

Williams, W. F. (1962). Excretion of progesterone and its metabolites in milk, urine, and feces. *J. Dairy Sci.* **45**, 1541–1542.

Yoshida, M., Yonezawa, S., Nakamura, H., Azecki, H., Terakado, N., and Horiuchi, T. (1971). Residue of dietary chlortetracycline and spiramycin in blood, muscles, and liver of growing chicks. *Jpn. Poult. Sci.* **8**, 94–102.

Note Added in Proof

The proceedings of a "Symposium on Natural Hormones in Edible Products" held at the 68th annual meeting of the American Society of Animal Science appear in *J. Anim. Sci.* **45**, 609–674, 1977. These papers are very relevant to this review.

23

Antibiotics in Animal Feeds: An Assessment of the Animal and Public Health Aspects

RICHARD P. SILVER and H. DWIGHT MERCER

I. INTRODUCTION

Antibiotics have been used commercially in animal feed for improving weight gain and feed efficiency for almost 30 years. However, it became clear, as early as 1957, that this practice gave rise to large populations of resistant bacteria. Smith and Crabb (1957) showed that feeding diets containing tetracycline to pigs and to poultry led to high levels of tetracycline-resistant *Escherichia coli* which complicated the satisfactory control of *E. coli* infections. Yet, not until several years after the discovery in 1959 (Watanabe, 1963) by Japanese investigators that resistance to antibiotics was transferable, did scientists begin to question the practice of supplementing animal feeds with antibiotics for growth stimulation. Scientists feared that resistant bacteria could be transmitted to humans making treatment of certain infections difficult, constituting a possible hazard to human health.

Because of the public health concerns restrictions were placed on the use of antibiotics in feeds in Britain in 1969 (Swann, 1969). The Swann Committee of Great Britain grouped antibiotics into "feed" and "therapeutic" categories and recommended that antibiotics which are used as feed additives not include drugs used for treatment of disease in man or animals. In 1970, the Food and Drug Administration organized a task force to study the human and animal health hazards associated with antibiotics in animal feeds. The main recommendations of the task force were basically the same as outlined by the Swann Committee (VanHouweling, 1972). Antibiotics used in human clinical medicine that failed to meet the guidelines established by the task force in regard to safety were to be prohibited from growth promotion and subtherapeutic use in animals by July 1973.

Subsequent to the task force report, however, regulations were published which allowed drug sponsors to submit evidence, by April 1975, to conclusively show that the use of antibiotics in animal feeds presents no human or animal health hazard (Gardner, 1973). These data have been submitted and are now being evaluated by a subcommittee of the National Food and Drug Advisory Committee and its consultants.

The guidelines considered by the task force to establish the presence of a hazard to human health are listed below.

1. A hazard to human health is present if a drug given to animals results in a significant increase in the animal reservoir of gram-negative bacilli capable of causing human disease and capable of being transmitted through the feed chain to man. Gram-negative bacilli with R factors that are resistant to drugs used systemically in human medicine are particularly undesirable.

2. The use of antibacterial agents that promote a significant increase of gram-negative bacilli in animals that are resistant to antibacterial agents used systemically in clinical human medicine present a potential hazard to human health.

3. Antibacterial agents that may enhance pathogenicity of gram-negative bacilli in animals by increasing the development and linkage of genetic elements that produce for example, toxins, with R factors are undesirable for use in animals if transmitted through food to man.

4. Any increase in the human florae of pathogenic bacteria resistant to antibacterial agents used to treat human disease and caused by the ingestion of biologically active antibacterial agents in foodstuffs is undesirable.

Documentation of the factors which were considered in establishing these guidelines and subsequent recommendations of the task force are published in an appendix to its report (VanHouweling, 1972). The purpose of this report is to summarize some recent data which we think relative to these important issues.

II. RELEVANT NEW INFORMATION

Guideline 1 (listed above) refers in essence to the ecology of *Salmonella* in food-producing animals. The task force clearly felt that when resistance involves *Salmonella* a potential threat to human health exists. Although most *Salmonella* infections will not require antibiotic therapy, the systemic ones will, and it is here that the problem of antibiotic resistance arises. Their recommendations were based in part on the following points: (1) *Salmonella* strains of animal origin cause illness and death in humans; (2) *Salmonella* contiminates food products; (3) antibiotics in feed selects for resistant *Salmonella* in animals; (4) a high number of human isolates of *S. typhimurium* carry R factors; (5) antibiotics may enhance colonization and increase the carriage and quantity of *Salmonella* shed in man and animals. Thus, an important objective recommended by the task force was to determine the effect of feed antibiotics on the *Salmonella* reservoir in animals.

The data from a number of studies indicate that the feeding of antibiotics to animals infected with *Salmonella* may result in either no change, an increase, or a decrease in the *Salmonella* reservoir. A decrease in the *Salmonella* reservoir was observed in those instances in which animals were infected with an antibiotic-sensitive organism; i.e., the antibiotic had a protective effect (Evangelisti *et al.*, 1975; Gutzmann *et al.*, 1976; Jarolmen *et al.*, 1976; Williams *et al.*, 1977). In contrast, an increase in both the quantity and duration of *Salmonella* shed was generally seen in animals infected with *Salmonella* resistant to the drug being used (Dey *et al.*, 1977a; Williams *et al.*, 1977). The severity of the disease also increased in those experimental infections which produced clinical signs (Dey *et al.*, 1977b).

To determine the impact of antibiotics on the *Salmonella* reservoir it is also necessary to consider the antibiotic susceptibility of *Salmonella* as isolated from man and animals. A number of surveys throughout the world have noted an increase in the resistance of enteric organisms (Dulaney and Laskin, 1971; Falkow, 1975) with particular interest focused on *Salmonella* (Bissett *et al.*, 1974; Pocurull *et al.*, 1971; Voogd *et al.*, 1973). The results of a recent study by Neu *et al.* (1975) "clearly demonstrate that resistance to antibiotics is increasing in *Salmonellae* isolated from both humans and animals."

Guideline 2 states that antibiotics fed to animals shall not significantly increase gram-negative bacilli in animals resistant to agents used in human clinical medicine. No one now really questions the fact that antibiotics in animal feeds lead to a high level of resistant coliforms. This has been well documented (Mercer *et al.*, 1971; Siegel *et al.*, 1974; Smith, 1967; Loken *et al.*, 1971; Smith and Crabb, 1957). The major question and bone of contention since the task force has been whether the large reservoir of resistant *E. coli* in domestic animals is a source of resistant strains commonly isolated from humans. This is perhaps one of the most controversial and yet most difficult aspects of R factor ecology to assess.

At one level we can examine the direct extension of resistant organisms from animals to man. A number of studies have shown that humans in contact with animals receiving medicated feed have a higher incidence of drug-resistant organisms in their flora than do control populations (Linton *et al.*, 1972; Fein *et al.*, 1974; Siegel *et al.*, 1975; Levy *et al.*, 1976b). Indeed, a recent study by Levy *et al.* (1976a) showed the direct spread of resistant organisms from chickens to chickens and from chickens to man. A temperature-sensitive chloramphenicol-resistant gene was used as a marker to identify a particular plasmid.

One can appreciate, however, the difficulties involved in this type of experiment. *E. coli,* unlike *Salmonella,* is a normal inhabitant of the human and animal intestinal tract. Moreover, the methods of identifying *E. coli* are not as developed as those for *Salmonella* species. Yet it has been claimed that human and animal *E. coli* strains are distinct (Bettleheim *et al.*, 1974). In order to determine whether *E. coli* strains from human and animal sources can indeed be distinguished, Hartley *et al.*, 1975; Howe *et al.*, 1976; Howe and Linton, 1976 have serotyped a large number of resistant and sensitive isolates. The important point of these studies is that many "O" serotypes which carry R plasmids are common to both animals and man. Moreover, the same preferential resistant serotypes of *E. coli* from human and animal fecal sources were also prevalent among R$^+$ strains from clinical material (Petrocheilou and Richmond, 1976). While these studies do not prove that resistant *E. coli* which cause disease in man originate in animals, they do not exclude the possibility.

At yet another level we can examine the R factors themselves to see if one can distinguish "animal" and "human" R plasmid types. Fein *et al.* (1974) showed a strong association between the resistance patterns of *E. coli* isolated from people and those isolated from their livestock. Human exposure to animal *E. coli* via home-raised meat was suggested as the most plausible explanation for interspecies crossover of transferable drug resistance on these farms (Dorn *et al.*, 1975). It is not enough, however, to simply follow the phenotypic properties which plasmids confer on their bacterial hosts since the same resistance pattern may be determined by unrelated plasmids.

The most common way of genetically classifying plasmids is on the basis of their ability to coexist with each other in the same bacterium. Unrelated plasmids can peacefully coexist in the same host; they are compatible. On the other hand, related plasmids cannot coexist; they are incompatible (Datta, 1975; Falkow, 1975). In practice, if a cell is infected with two related plasmids, either one of the two is lost or they may recombine to form a single replicon, sort of a biochemical squatters rights between related plasmids. R plasmids are now divided into more than twenty compatibility groups (Coatzee *et al.*, 1972; Datta and Hedges, 1971; Datta, 1975; Chabbert *et al.*, 1972; Grindley *et al.*, 1972). F, I, and N represent the most common classes found in *E. coli*, *Salmonella* and *Shigella* isolates. In this context we have examined the compatibility properties of more than 100 R plasmids from *E. coli* and *Salmonella* isolated from animals (N. Datta, See Food and Drug Administration, 1977). The R plasmid incompatibility groups seen in animal isolates show the same distribution as those found in human isolates. The data *do not suggest* separate animal and human R factor populations.

A more direct approach, however, to study the relationship between plasmids is to measure the proportion of DNA sequences, that is, the number of genes which are common between any two plasmids. Theoretically, one would expect that plasmids of the same group, which share common mechanisms of replication and maintenance within the bacterial cell, would have similar genetic fine structure. DNA–DNA hybridization experiments show that this is indeed the case. As shown in Table I, R plasmids from the same group have extensive DNA sequences in common with each other but are only minimally related to other R plasmids. Thus DNA from different members of the same group hybridize extensively whereas DNA from unrelated groups will not (Guerry and Falkow, 1971; Grindley *et al.*, 1973; So *et al.*, 1974a,b).

R factors also know no geographic boundaries (Table II). W plasmids independently isolated from Japan, Greece, and England, came from different bacterial genera and have different resistance patterns. Yet each of these plasmids hybridizes with each other to at least 75% of its DNA content (Table I). Clearly, plasmids from the same group are drawn from a common pool. This is true whether the R factor containing bacteria is isolated from animals or man. F, I, or N group R factors isolated from humans are the same as F or I or N group R factors isolated from animal sources (Anderson *et al.*, 1975).

This raises the question as to the origin of the resistance gene themselves. Unrelated plasmids can carry similar resistances. Is there a single

TABLE I
Nucleotide Sequence Relationships among R Plasmids[a]

R plasmid	Compatibility group	Mol. wt. ($\times 10^6$)	Percentage sequences in common with			
			R1	R144	N3	Sa
R1	FII	62	100	—	—	—
222	FII	68	74	6	6	5
F	FI	62	37	—	—	—
R144	I	65	16	100	1	1
R64	I	66	8	86	—	—
ColI	I	62	8	78	—	—
N3	N	33	8	2	100	8
R15	N	38	—	—	75	—
RM430	N	33	—	—	60	—
Sa	W	25	4	5	8	100
R388	W	21	—	—	—	79
R7K	W	21	—	—	—	75

[a] Data from So et al. (1974b).

pool or reservoir of drug resistance genes that transfer factors drawn upon or is there a number of distinct pools? It now seems clear that the drug resistance genes found in human and animal isolates are essentially the same.

Recent studies have shown that the genes specifying resistance to ampicillin, tetracycline, kanamycin, chloramphenicol, trimethoprim, and streptomycin reside on DNA sequences that can translocate from plas-

TABLE II
W Plasmids[a]

R factor	Resistance patterns[b]	Origin
S-a	SmCmKmSu	Shigella flexneri (Japan)
R7K	ApSm	Proteus rettgeri (Greece)
R388	SuTp	Escherichia coli (England)

[a] Data from Datta (1975).
[b] Abbreviations: Sm, streptomycin; Cm, chloramphenicol; Km, kanamycin; Su, sulfonamide; Ap, ampicillin; Tp, trimethoprim.

mid to plasmid as a discrete unit independent of host function (Berg *et al.*, 1975; Barth *et al.*, 1976; Foster *et al.*, 1975; Gottesman and Rosner, 1975; Hedges and Jacob, 1974; Heffron *et al.*, 1975; Kleckner *et al.*, 1975; Kopecko and Cohen, 1975). Simply stated, resistance genes can "hop" from one plasmid to another plasmid, or from a plasmid to the bacterial chromosome. This is perhaps the most significant addition to our understanding of R factor biology in recent years. We now have to be concerned not only with the direct transfer of resistant bacteria or R plasmids from animals to man but must be aware that the genes themselves can migrate from plasmid to plasmid by translocation. Moreover, an R factor does not have to be stably maintained within a cell to donate its resistance genes to a recipient chromosome or an indiginous plasmid; it need only be a transiet encounter.

In this context it is important to realize that most species of bacteria possess indigenous plasmid gene pools. In fact, plasmids have been found in all species of bacteria which have been examined. The function of these plasmids are often "cryptic" but they could serve as effective recipients for the insertion of translocatable genes. The most striking example of this has been the emergence of ampicillin-resistant strains of *Haemophilus influenzae* causing meningitis, acute epiglotitis, otitis, and other infections primarily in young children (Khan *et al.*, 1974; Tomeh *et al.*, 1974). The ampicillin resistance genes in *Haemophilus* are plasmid-mediated and are identical to those previously found only in *E. coli* and other enteric organisms (Elwell *et al.*, 1975; De Graaff *et al.*, 1976). Resistance to tetracycline, kanamycin, and chloramphenicol has also been reported in *Haemophilus* (Dang Van *et al.*, 1975a,b; van Klingeren *et al.*, 1977).

More recently β-lactamase producing penicillin-resistant strains of *Neisseria gonorrhoeae* have been described (Ashford *et al.*, 1976; Phillips, 1976). The resistance is plasmid-mediated and once again the genes are the same translocatable DNA sequence found in other gram-negative organisms (Elwell *et al.*, 1977). This is yet another example of the extension, either direct or indirect, of the R factor gene pool.

Human health guideline 3 states that antibiotics should not enhance the pathogenicity of gram-negative bacilli. It is now clear that plasmids contribute significantly to an organism's capacity to produce disease and to survive within the host organism (Falkow, 1975). For example, the production of an enterotoxin is an essential factor in the pathogenicity of *E. coli* strains of porcine origin. Smith and Halls (1968) showed that this property was governed by a plasmid, termed ENT. Similarly, the genetic determinants for enterotoxin production in *E. coli* isolated from calves and lambs have also been shown to be controlled by transmissible plasmids (Smith and Linggood, 1972). Recent studies support the idea that enterotoxin-producing strains of *E. coli* are also responsible for a significant proportion of previously undiagnosed human diarrheal disease (Gorbach, 1970; Gorbach and Khurana, 1972; DuPont *et al.*, 1971). In parallel with the studies in domestic animals, the ability of *E. coli* strains of human origin to elaborate enterotoxin has now been shown to be mediated by a transmissible plasmid (Skerman *et al.*, 1972; Smith and Linggood, 1971b).

Guideline 3 called for a study of the association of such plasmid-mediated toxin production with R plasmids both *in vitro* and *in vivo*. This subject has been investigated by Dr. Stanley Falkow of the University of Washington who demonstrated in an *in vitro* mating that ENT and R plasmids do cotransfer (Food and Drug Administration, 1977). Drug selection for the R plasmid and subsequent clonal screening for ENT was an adequate laboratory tool for detection of cotransfer. Furthermore, cotransfer of ENT and R plasmids was detected in the intestinal tract of calves receiving medicated feeds. Transfer did not take place in control animals. Falkow has also been able to show the translocation of antibiotic resistance genes to ENT plasmids *in vitro*, demonstrating that ENT plasmids can acquire resistance genes from R plasmids if they inhabit the same cell. Translocation is the primary mechanism for the dissemination of resistance genes *in vivo*. Su, Sm, Ap plasmids constructed *in vitro* by translocation are indistinguishable from Su, Sm, Ap plasmids from clinical isolates of *E. coli* and *Salmonella* (Heffron *et al.*, 1977).

Many toxigenic strains of *E. coli* are also miltiply resistant. During a recent hospital outbreak of infantile diarrhea in Texas, plasmid-mediated toxin production and multiple antibiotic resistance was demonstrated (Wachsmuth *et al.*, 1976). Transfer of 67×10^6 and 30×10^6 dalton plasmids was associated with the transfer of resistances and enterotoxin production respectively. When antibiotics were used to select *E. coli* K 12 recipients from a one step bacterial cross, all the resistances were concurrently transferred. In addition, 36% of the resistant recipient organisms produced enterotoxin (Wachsmuth *et al.*, 1976).

In addition to toxins, other plasmid-mediated virulence factors have been described. One of the characteristics of the diarrheal disease caused by enterotoxigenic *E. coli* in man or animals is colonization of the small bowel by large numbers of the bacteria. There is evidence for a surface associated antigen on *E. coli* toxigenic for pigs, termed K88 which functions to overcome gut motility and other clearing mechanisms (Ørskov *et al.*, 1961, 1964; Smith and Linggood, 1971a; Jones and Rutter, 1972; Hohmann and Wilson, 1975). Ørskov and Ørskov (1966) showed that K88 production was governed by a transmissible plasmid. A similar antigen, K99, has been described for calves (Smith and Linggood, 1972; Ørskov *et al.*, 1975; Burrows *et al.*, 1976). These K antigens seem to play a role in the host specificity of these pathogens; the K88 antigen from porcine isolates is unable to produce adhesion to the calf intestine, and the K99 calf antigen is unable to adhere to the pig intestine (Smith and Linggood, 1972). A similar plasmid-controlled surface antigen has recently been described in a strain of *E. coli* causing severe human diarrheal disease (Evans *et al.*, 1975).

Another way plasmids can contribute to virulence is exemplified by the Col V plasmid (Smith, 1974). Colicin V is the most common colicin produced by *E. coli*. Pathogenic *E. coli* that contain the Col V plasmid have a greater ability to resist the defense mechanisms of the host (Smith, 1974). They tend to be more refractory to the bactericidal effects of undefined components in serum. In addition, experiments in chickens and in humans revealed that Col V confers on organisms an increased ability to survive in the alimentary tract as well as in the tissue (Smith and Huggins, 1976). Other plasmid-mediated factors which enhance pathogenicity may well be found in the future.

Although pathogenicity is generally determined by more than one factor, one can see that the addition of a single specific character can endow an organism with virulence. The potential dangers of this character being mediated by a transmissible element are apparent. R factors and virulence plasmids can reside in the same bacterial cell. We must be aware of the possibility, as was pointed out by the task force, that plasmids which contribute to the pathogenicity may become more widely disseminated among bacterial species because of the selection of the large reservoir of R factors within enteric organisms.

III. CONCLUSIONS

Although *Salmonella* infections are a hazard to human health the danger of a widespread epidemic occurring in this country appears remote. Poor sanitation and the lack of health care facilities contribute to the occurrence of epidemics. The greater hazard to human health of antibiotics in feed appears to be the large reservoir of plasmid-mediated resistance genes in the normal flora of animals; resistance which can be transferred from a non-pathogen to a pathogenic organism. We have seen in recent years the emergence of resistance in dangerous pathogens. Antibiotic resistance in *Haemophilus* and *Neisseria* has already been discussed. A strain of *Salmonella typhi* carrying an R factor mediating resistance to chloramphenicol caused an epidemic of typhoid fever in Mexico (Olarte and Galindo, 1973). Transferable chloramphenicol resistance has also become common in S. typhi isolated in India, Vietnam, and Thailand (Anderson, 1975; Anderson and Smith, 1972). The recent epidemic of drug-resistant Shigella dysenteriae infection in Central America is another example of an epidemic disease which was no longer susceptible to antibiotics that had previously been used for its treatment (Mata et al., 1970).

Plasmid-mediated resistance has also been reported in strains of Bordatella bronchiseptica (Terakado et al., 1973; Terakado and Mitsuhashi, 1974) and we have recently demonstrated plasmid-determined resistance to ampicillin, tetracycline, streptomycin, and sulfonamide in strains of Pasturella multocida and Pasturella haemolytica (Silver et al., 1977; R. P. Silver, unpublished observation). Are these plasmids the same as found in enteric organisms? We do not know yet although it does seem apparent that antibiotics select from a pool of genetic elements common and available to all species. Ampicillin resistance in the strain of Shigella dysenteriae which caused the epidemic in Central America was due to a small (5.5×10^6 dalton) nontransmissible plasmid (Crosa et al., 1977). The identical plasmid was isolated in the S. typhimurium type 29 outbreak in England which was influential in the Swann Committee recommendations (Anderson, 1968; S. Falkow, personnel communication). The same plasmid was found in S. panama isolated from calves in Holland and from S. panama isolated in France. The identical plasmid was isolated in S. typhimurium in humans and calves in the United States (Crosa et al., 1977; S. Falkow, personnel communication).

The situation has become even more complex. Transmissible resistance has now been described in strains of streptococci isolated from man and from animals (Clewell and Franke, 1974; Clewell et al., 1974; Jacob and Hobbs, 1974; Courvalin et al., 1972; Silver et al., 1976; Horodniceanu et al., 1976). Antibiotic resistance is not a problem unique to gram-negative organisms. The emergence of widespread resistance to penicillin in Group A streptococci or in the pneumococcus would probably dwarf the concerns of resistance in Salmonella and in E. coli.

Of course, the safety aspects which are under consideration must be dealt with in light of the benefits. The relatively narrow avenue between real safety concerns and desirable or essential benefits does not lend itself well to emotional, political, or economic considerations. The true test in the decision making process regarding the ultimate program of agricultural antimicrobial usage will depend upon the ability of knowledgable scientists to interpret results of fractional data and to project its impact to the next decade. If this is done well, then the benefits as well as hazards may be more contained within acceptable margins.

REFERENCES

Anderson, E. S. (1968). The ecology of transferable drug resistance in the enterobacteria. *Annu. Rev. Microbiol.* **22**, 131–180.

Anderson, E. S. (1975). The problem and implications of chloramphenicol resistance in the typhoid bacillus. *J. Hyg.* **74**, 289–299.

Anderson, E. S., and Smith, H. R. (1972). Chloramphenicol resistance in the typhoid bacillus. *Br. Med. J.* **3**, 329–331.

Anderson, E. S., Humphreys, G. O., and Willshaw, G. A. (1975). The molecular related-ness of R factors in enterobacteria of human and animal origin. *J. Gen. Microbiol.* **91**, 376–382.

Ashford, W. A., Golash, R. G., and Hemming, V. G. (1976). Penicillinase-producing *Neisseria gonorrhoeae. Lancet* **2**, 657–658.

Barth, P. T., Datta, N., Hedges, R. W., and Grinter, N. J. (1976). Transposition of a deoxyribonucleic acid sequence encoding trimethoprim and streptomycin resistances from R483 to other replicons. *J. Bacteriol.* **125**, 800–810.

Berg, D. E., Davies, J., Allet, B., and Rochaix, J. D. (1975). Transposition of R Factor genes to bacteriophage λ. *Proc. Natl. Acad. Sci. U.S.A.* **72**, 3628–3632.

Bettleheim, K. A., Bushrod, A. M., Chandler, E., Cooke, E. M., O'Farrell, S., and Shooter, R. A. (1974). *Escherichia coli* serotype distribution in man and animals. *J. Hyg.* **73**, 467–471.

Bissett, M. L., Abbott, S. L., and Wood, R. M. (1974). Antimicrobial resistance and R factors in *Salmonella* isolated in California (1971–1972). *Anitmicrob. Agents & Chemother.* **5**, 161–168.

Burrows, M. R., Sellwood, R., and Gibbons, R. A. (1976). Haemagglutinating and adhesive properties associated with the K99 antigen of bovine strains of *Escherichia coli. J. Gen. Microbiol.* **96**, 269–275.

Chabbert, Y. A., Scavizzi, M. R., Gerbaud, J. L., and Bouanchaud, D. H. (1972). Incom-patibility groups and the classification of fi⁻resistance factors. *J. Bacteriol* **112**, 666–675.

Clewell, D. B., and Franke, A. E. (1974). Characteristization of a plasmid determining resistance to erythromycin, lincomycin, and vernamycin B in a strain of *Streptococcus pyogenes. Antimicrob. Agents & Chemother.* **5**, 534–537.

Clewell, D. B., Yagi, Y., Dunny, G. M., and Schultz, S. K. (1974). Characterization of three plasmid deoxyribonucleic acid molecules in a strain of *Streptococcus faecalis:* Identifica-tion of a plasmid determining erythromycin resistance. *J. Bacteriol.* **117**, 283–289.

Coatzee, J. N., Datta, N., and Hedges, R. W. (1972). R factors from *Proteus rettgeri J. Gen. Microbiol.* **72**, 543–552.

Courvalin, P. M., Carlier, C., and Chabbert, Y. A. (1972). Plasmid-linked tetracycline and erythromycin resistance in group D «streptococcus». *Ann. Inst. Pasteur, Paris* **123**, 755–759.

Crosa, J. H., Olarte, J., Mata, L. J., Luttrop, L. K., and Pénaranda, D. (1977). Characteriza-tion of an R plasmid associated with ampicillin resistance in *Shigella dysenteriae* Type I. *Antimicrob. Agents & Chemother.* **11**, 553–558.

Dang Van, A., Goldstein, F., Acar, J. F., and Bouanchaud, D. H. (1975a). A transferable kanamycin resistance plasmid isolated from *Haemophilus influenzae*. *Ann. Microbiol. (Paris)* **126**, 397–399.

Dang Van, A., Bieth, G., and Bouanchaud, D. H. (1975b). Resistance plasmidique à la tetracycline chez *H. influenza*. *C. R. Held. Seances Acad. Sci., Ser. D* **280**, 1321–1323.

Datta, N. (1975). Epidemiology and classification of plasmids. *In* "Microbiology-1974" (D. Schlessinger, ed.), pp. 9–15. Am. Soc. Microbiol., Washington, D.C.

Datta, N., and Hedges, R. W. (1971). Compatibility groups among fi⁻ R factors. *Nature (London)* **234**, 222–223.

de Graaff, J., Elwell, L. P., and Falkow, S. (1976). Molecular nature of two beta-lactamase-specifying plasmids isolated from *Haemophilus influenzae* type B. *J. Bacteriol* **126**, 439–446.

Dey, B. P., Blenden, D. C., Burton, G. C., Mercer, H. D., and Tsutakawa, R. K. (1977a). Influence of continuous chlortetracycline feeding on experimentally induced salmonellosis in calves. I. Rate and duration of shedding of *Salmonellae*. *J. Infect. Dis.* (submitted for publication).

Dey, B. P., Blenden, D. C., Burton, G. C., Mercer, H. D., and Tsutakawa, R. K. (1977b). Influence of continuous chlortetracycline feeding on experimentally induced salmonellosis in calves II. Clinical response to challenge. *J. Infect. Dis.* (submitted for publication).

Dorn, C. R., Tsutakawa, R., Fein, D., Burton, G. C., and Blenden, D. C. (1975). Antibiotic resistance patterns of *Escherichia coli* isolated from farm families consuming home-raised meat. *Am. J. Epidemiol.* **102**, 319–326.

Dulaney, E. L., and Laskin, A. I., eds. (1971). The problem of drug resistant pathogenic bacteria. *Ann. N.Y. Acad. Sic.* **182**, 1–415.

DuPont, H. L., Formal, S. B., Hornick, R. B., Snyder, M. J., Libonati, J. P., Sheahan, D. G., LeBrec, E. H., and Kalas, J. P. (1971). Pathogenesis of *Escherichia coli* diarrhea. *N. Engl. J. Med.* **285**, 1–9.

Elwell, L. P., de Graaff, J., Seibert, D., and Falkow, S. (1975). Plasmid-linked ampicillin resistance in *Haemophilus influenzae* type B. *Infect. Immun.* **12**, 404–410.

Elwell, L. P., Roberts, M., Mayer, L. W., and Falkow, S. (1977). Plasmid mediated B-lactamase production in *Neisseria gonorrheae*. *Antimicrob. Agents & Chemother.* **11**, 528–533.

Evangelisti, D. G., English, A. R., Girard, A. E., Lynch, J. E., and Solomons, I. A. (1975). Influence of subtherapeutic levels of oxytetracycline on *Salmonella typhimurium* in swine, calves and chickens. *Antimicrob. Agents & Chemother.* **8**, 664–672.

Evans, D. G., Silver, R. P., Evans, D. J., Jr., Chase, D. G., and Gorbach, S. L. (1975). Plasmid-controlled colonization factor associated with virulence in *Escherichia coli* enterotoxigenic for humans. *Infect. Immun.* **12**, 656–667.

Falkow, S. (1975). "Infectious Multiple Drug Resistance." Pion Ltd., London.

Fein, D., Burton, G., Tsutakawa, R., and Blenden, D. (1974). Matching of antibiotic resistance patterns of *Escherichia coli* of farm families and their animals. *J. Infect. Dis.* **130**, 274–279.

Food and Drug Administration. (1977). "Study to Define the Interrelationship Between Transmissible Elements and Pathogenicity of Enteric Microorganisms" (Dr. S. Falkow, Principal Investigator). Contract 223-73-7210. University of Washington, School of Medicine, Seattle.

Foster, T. J., Howe, T. G. B., and Richmond, M. H. (1975). Translocation of the tetracycline resistance determinant from R100-1 to the *Escherichia coli* K-12 chromosome. *J. Bacteriol.* **124**, 1153–1158.

Gardner, S. (1973). Statements of policy and interpretation regarding animal drugs and medicated feeds. *Fed. Regist.* **38,** 9811-9814.

Gorbach, S. L. (1970). Acute diarrhea—"toxin" disease? *N. Engl. J. Med.* **283,** 44-45.

Gorbach, S. L., and Khurana, C. M. (1972). Toxigenic *Escherichia coli:* A cause of infantile diarrhea in Chicago. *N. Engl. J. Med* **287,** 791-795.

Gottesman, M. M., and Rosner, J. L. (1975). Acquisition of a determinant for chloramphenicol resistance by coliphage lambda. *Proc. Natl. Acad. Sci. U.S.A.* **72,** 5041-5045.

Grindley, N. D. F., Grindley, J. N., and Anderson, E. S. (1972). R factor compatibility groups. *Mol. Gen. Genet.* **119,** 287-297.

Grindley, N. D. F., Humphreys, G. O., and Anderson, E. S. (1973). Molecular studies of R factor compatibility groups. *J. Bacteriol.* **115,** 387-398.

Guerry, P., and Falkow, S. (1971). Polynucleotide sequence relationships among some bacterial plasmids. *J. Bacteriol.* **107,** 372-374.

Gutzmann, F., Layton, H., Simkins, K., and Jarolman, H. (1976). Influence of antibiotic-supplemented feed on occurrence and persistance of *Salmonella typhimurium* in experimentally infected swine. *Am. J. Vet. Res.* **37,** 649-655.

Hartley, C. L., Howe, K., Linton, A. H., Linton, K. B., and Richmond, M. H. (1975). Distribution of R plasmids among the O-antigen types of *Escherichia coli* isolated from human and animal sources. *Antimicrob. Agents & Chemother.* **8,** 122-131.

Hedges, R. W., and Jacob, A. E. (1974). Transposition of ampicillin resistance from RP4 to other replicons. *Mol. Gen. Genet.* **132,** 31-40.

Heffron, F., Sublett, R., Hedges, R. W., Jacob, A., and Falkow, S. (1975). Origin of the TEM Beta-lactamase gene found on plasmids. *J. Bacteriol.* **122,** 250-256.

Heffron, F., Rubens, C., and Falkow, S. (1977). Transposition of a plasmid deoxyribonucleic acid sequence that mediates ampicillin resistance; identity of laboratory constructed plasmids and clinical isolates. *J. Bacteriol.* **129,** 530-533.

Hohmann, A., and Wilson, M. R. (1975). Adherence of enteropathogenic *Escherichia coli* to intestinal epithelium *in vivo. Infect. Immun.* **12,** 866-880.

Horodniceanu, T., Bouanchaud, D. H., Bieth, G., and Chabbert, Y. A. (1976). R plasmids in *Streptococcus agalactiae* (Group B). *Antimicrob. Agents & Chemother.* **10,** 795-801.

Howe, K., and Linton, A. H. (1976). The distribution of O-antigen types of *Escherichia coli* in normal calves, compared with man, and their R plasmid carriage. *J. Appl. Bacteriol.* **40,** 317-330.

Howe, K., Linton, A. H., and Osborne, A. D. (1976). A longitudinal study of *Escherichia coli* in cows and calves with special reference to the distribution of O-antigen and antibiotic resistance. *J. Appl. Bacteriol.* **40,** 331-340.

Jacob, A. E., and Hobbs, S. J. (1974). Conjugal transfer of plasmid-borne multiple antibiotic resistance in *Streptococcus faecalis* var. *zymogenes. J. Bacteriol.* **117,** 360-372.

Jarolmen, H., Shirk, R. J., and Langworth, B. F. (1976). Effect of chlortetracycline feeding on the *salmonella* reservoir in chickens. *J. Appl. Bacteriol.* **40,** 153-161.

Jones, G. W., and Rutter, J. M. (1972). Role of the K88 antigen in the pathogenesis of neonatal diarrhea caused by *Escherichia coli* in piglets. *Infect. Immun.* **6,** 918-927.

Khan, W., Ross, S., Rodriguez, W., Controni, G., and Saz, A. K. (1974). *Haemophilus influenzae* type B resistant to amicillin. *J. Am. Med. Assoc.* **229,** 298-301.

Kleckner, N., Chan, R. K., Tye, B. K., and Botstein, D. (1975). Mutagenesis by insertion of a drug resistance element carrying an inverted repetition. *J. Mol. Biol.* **97,** 561-575.

Kopecko, D. J., and Cohen, S. N. (1975). Site-specific RecA independent recombination between bacterial plasmids: Involvement of palinodromes at the recombination loci. *Proc. Natl. Acad. Sci. U.S.A.* **72,** 1373-1377.

Levy, S. B., Fitzgerald, G. B., and Macone, A. B. (1976a). Spread of antibiotic resistant plasmids from chicken to chicken and from chicken to man. *Nature (London)* **260**, 40–42.

Levy, S. B., Fitzgerald, G. B., and Macone, A. B. (1976b). Changes in intestinal flora of farm personnel after introduction of a tetracycline-supplemented feed or a farm. *N. Engl. J. Med.* **295**, 583–588.

Linton, K. B., Lee, P. A., Richmond, M. H., Gillespie, W. A., Rowland, A. J., and Baker, V. N. (1972). Antibiotic resistance and transmissible R factors in the intestinal coliform flora of healthy adults and children in an urban and rural community. *J. Hyg.* **70**, 99–104.

Loken, K. I., Wagner, L. W., and Henke, C. L. (1971). Transmissible drug resistance in Enterobacteriaceae isolated from calves given antibiotics. *Am. J. Vet. Res.* **32**, 1207–1212.

Mata, L. J., Gangarosa, J., Caceres, A., Perara, D. R., and Mejicanos, M. L. (1970). Epidemic *Shiga* bacillus dysentery in Central America. I. Etiological investigations in Guatamala, 1969. *J. Infect. Dis.* **122**, 170–180.

Mercer, H. D., Pocurull, D., Gaines, S., Wilson, S., and Bennett, J. V. (1971). Characteristics of antimicrobial resistance of *Escherichia coli* from animals: Relationship to veterinary and management uses of antimicrobial agents. *Appl. Microbiol.* **22**, 700–705.

Neu, H. C., Cherubin, C. E., Longo, E. D., Flouton, B., and Winter, J. (1975). Antimicrobial resistance and R factor transfer among isolates of *salmonella* in the northeastern United States: A comparison of human and animal isolates. *J. Infect. Dis.* **132**, 617–622.

Olarte, J., and Galindo, E. (1973). *Salmonella typhi* resistant to chloramphenicol, ampicillin, and other antimicrobial agents: Strains isolated during an extensive typhoid fever epidemic in Mexico. *Antimicrob. Agents & Chemother.* **4**, 597–601.

Ørskov, I., and Ørskov, F. (1966). Episome-carried surface antigen K88 of *Escherichia coli*. I. Transmission of the determinant of the K88 antigen and influence on the transfer of chromosomal markers. *J. Bacteriol.* **91**, 69–75.

Ørskov, I., Ørskov, F., Sojka, W. J., and Leach, J. M. (1961). Simultaneous occurrence of *Escherichia coli* B and L antigens in strains from diseased swine. *Acta Pathol. Microbiol. Scand.* **53**, 404–422.

Ørskov, I., Ørskov, F., Sojka, W. J., and Wittig, W. (1964). K antigens K88ab(L) and K88ac(L) in *E. coli*. A new O antigen: 0141 and a new K antigen (K89(B). *Acta Pathol. Microbiol. Scand.* **62**, 439–447.

Ørskov, I., Ørskov, F., Smith, H. W., and Sojka, W. J. (1975). The establishment of K99, a thermolabile, transmissible *Escherichia coli* K antigen, previously called "Kco", possessed by calf and lamb enteropathogenic strains. *Acta Pathol. Microbiol. Scand.* **83**, 31–36.

Petrocheilou, V., and Richmond, M. H. (1976). Distribution of R plasmids among the O-antigen types of *Escherichia coli* isolated from various clinical sources. *Antimicrob. Agents & Chemother.* **9**, 1–5.

Phillips, I. (1976). B-lactamase-producing penicillin resistant gonococcus. *Lancet* **2**, 656–657.

Pocurull, D. W., Gaines, S. A., and Mercer, H. D. (1971). Survey of infectious multiple drug resistance among *Salmonella* isolated from animals in the United States. *Appl. Microbiol.* **21**, 358–362.

Siegel, D., Huber, W. G., and Enloe, F. (1974). Continuous nontherapeutic use of antibacterial drugs in feed and drug resistance of the gram-negative enteric flora of food-producing animals. *Antimicrob. Agents & Chemother.* **6**, 697–701.

Siegel, D., Huber, W. G., and Drysdale, S. (1975). Human therapeutic and agricultural uses of antibacterial drugs and resistance of the enteric flora of humans. *Antimicrob. Agents & Chemother.* **8,** 538–543.

Silver, R. P., Leming, B., Cohen, E., and Rollins, L. D. (1976). Effect of antibiotics in animal feed on plasmid determined drug resistance in group D streptococci *Abstr., 76th Annu. Meet. Am. Soc. Microbiol.* p. 258.

Silver, R. P., Leming, B., and Hjerpe, C. A. (1977). R plasmids in *Pasteurella multocida.* *Abstr., 77th Annu. Meet. Am. Soc. Microbiol.* p. 141.

Skerman, F. J., Formal, S. B., and Falkow, S. (1972). Plasmid-associated enterotoxin production in a strain of *Escherichia coli* isolated from humans. *Infect Immun.* **5,** 622–624.

Smith, H. W. (1967). The effect of the use of antibacterial drugs, particularly as food additives, on the emergence of drug resistant strains of bacteria in animals. *N. Z. Vet. J.* **15,** 153–166.

Smith, H. W. (1974). A search for transmissible pathogenic characters in invasive strains of *Escherichia coli:* The discovery of a plasmid-controlled toxin and a plasmid-controlled lethal character closely associated, or identical, with colicine V. *J. Gen. Microbiol.* **83,** 95–111.

Smith, H. W., and Crabb, W. E. (1957). The effect of the continuous administration of diets containing low levels of tetracyclines on the incidence of drug-resistant *Bacterium coli* in the faeces of pigs and chickens: The sensitivity of *Bact. coli* to other chemotherapeutic agents. *Vet. Rec.* **69,** 24–30.

Smith, H. W., and Halls, S. (1968). The transmissible nature of the genetic factor in *Escherichia coli* that controls enterotoxin production. *J. Gen. Microbiol.* **52,** 319–334.

Smith, H. W., and Huggins, M. B. (1976). Further observations on the association of the colicine V plasmid of *Escherichia coli* with pathogenicity and with survival in the alimentary tract. *J. Gen. Microbiol.* **92,** 335–350.

Smith, H. W., and Linggood, M. A. (1971a). Observations on the pathogenic properties of the K88 Hly and ENT plasmids of *Escherichia coli* with particular reference to porcine diarrhea. *J. Med. Microbiol.* **4,** 467–485.

Smith, H. W., and Linggood, M. A. (1971b). The transmissible nature of enterotoxin production in a human enteropatogenic strain of *Escherichia coli.* *J. Med. Microbiol.* **4,** 301.-305.

Smith, H. W., and Linggood, M. A. (1972). Further observations on *Escherichia coli* enterotoxins with particular regard to those produced by atypical piglet strains and by calf and lamb strains: The transmissible nature of these enterotoxins and of a K antigen possessed by calf and lamb strains. *J. Med. Microbiol.* **5,** 243–250.

So, M., Crosa, J. H., and Falkow, S. (1974a). Polynucleotide sequence relationship among *E. coli* ENT plasmids and the relationship between ENT and other plasmids. *J. Bacteriol.* **121,** 234–238.

So, M., Crosa, J. H., Gyles, C., and Falkow, S. (1974b). Polynucleotide sequence relationships among *E. coli* ENT plasmids. *Proc. Joint Cholera Res. Conf., 9th, 1974* Dept. State Publ. 8762, pp. 324–335.

Swann, M. M. (1969). "Report of the Joint Committee on the Use of Antibiotics in Animal Husbandry and Veterinary Medicine." HM Stationery Office, London.

Terakado, N., and Mitsuhashi, S. (1974). Properties of R factors from *Bordetella bronchiseptica.* *Antimcrob. Agents & Chemother.* **6,** 836–840.

Terakado, N., Azechi, H., Ninomiya, K., and Shimizu, T. (1973). Demonstration of R factors in *Bordetella bronchiseptica* isolated from pigs. *Antimcrob. Agents & Chemother.* **3,** 555–558.

Tomeh, M. O., Starr, S. E., McGowan, J. E., Terry, P. M., and Nahmias, A. J. (1974). Ampicillin-resistant *Haemophilus influenzae* type B infection. *J. Am. Med. Assoc.* **229,** 295–297.

VanHouweling, C. D. (1972). "Report to the Commissioner of the Food and Drug Administration by the FDA Task on the Use of Antibiotics in Animal Feeds." Food and Drug Admin., Rockville, Maryland.

Van Klingeren, B., van Embden, J. D. A., and Dessens-Kroon, M. (1977). Plasmid-mediated chloramphenicol resistance in *Haemophilus influenzae, Antimicrob. Agents & Chemother.* **11,** 383–387.

Voogd, C. E., Guinée, P. A. M., Manten, A., and Valkenburg, J. J. (1973). Incidence of resistance to tetracycline, chloramphenicol and ampicillin among *Salmonella* species isolated in the Netherlands in 1969, 1970, and 1971. *J. Microbiol. Serol.* **39,** 321–329.

Wachsmuth, I. K., Falkow, S., and Ryder, R. W. (1976). Plasmid-mediated properties of an enterotoxigenic *Escherichia coli* associated with infantile diarrhea. *Infect. Innum.* **14,** 403–407.

Watanabe, T. (1963). Infective heredity of multiple drug resistance in bacteria. *Bacteriol. Rev.,* **27,** 87–115.

Williams, R. D., Rollins, L. D., Selwyn, M., Pocurull, D. W., and Mercer, H. D. (1977). The effect of feeding chlortetracycline on the fecal shedding of *Salmonella typhimurium* by experimentally infected swine. (In preparation.)

Section IV

USE OF NUTRIENTS AND
FOODS AS DRUGS

24

Some Aspects of Pharmacologic Use
and Abuse of Water-Soluble Vitamins

WILLIAM B. BEAN

I. REVIEW OF VITAMINS

Vitamins are essential but can cause trouble in many ways. Whenever a diet contains none, or only a scant supply of one or more vitamins, a nutritional deficiency syndrome or disease results. In rare circumstances a normal or slightly increased amount of one vitamin will speed certain metabolic activities and precipitate or disclose another vitamin deficiency. Such a special but fortunately rare case was the harmful effect of adding folic acid to vitamin tablets before vitamin B_{12} was available. Although folic acid improved the hematological status of patients with pernicious anemia, it did not prevent development of the disasterous central and peripheral nervous system manifestations which can occur in vitamin B_{12} deficiency. This sequence was especially likely if the pernicious anemia had not been accurately diagnosed. This phenomenon resembles the disorders produced after an infarct in the pituitary decreases the functions of the thyroid, adrenals, and gonads, but only

667

the low thyroid function is observed and treated. Thyroid treatment may then overwhelm the adrenals and produce a crisis of adrenal cortical insufficiency.

In our mania for mega it is not surprising that an additional danger of damage by vitamins comes from the simple faith many have in using colossal amounts of these nutrients for a variety of minor and meager problems, or for serious disorders for which we know no remedy. The misuse of routine vitamin tablets as putative tonic or placebo for the walking worried I have called "vitaminia" (Bean, 1955).

Unwise addition of vitamins to emergency military rations may cause serious problems. Some nutritional advisors for the American Army in World War II must have been in considerable dread of beriberi, pellagra, and scurvy. The designers of emergency rations felt obliged to introduce into every meal one day's vitamin allowances even if this required the use of brewer's yeast, soybean flour, and liver extract. The result of this practice was a ration which had such a high satiety value that it became unpalatable after a few days of consumption. When asked to write a critique of Army emergency rations, I suggested that what was needed were familiar, simple foods which would be accepted and eaten, and to use considerable dietary variety. If the food was to be used only for a short time, vitamin, minerals, and protein could be ignored. The main requirements in those circumstances would be for caloric content and palatability.

During a ration test in the Pacific in the last year of World War II, I had an opportunity to make casual observations on the use of vitamin C. Vitamin C for soldiers, using prepared garrison rations, was provided largely in the form of powder to make lemonade. The American soldiers soon discovered that this powder made a very effective tooth cleanser, and, indeed, was splendid for polishing brass buttons or even rifles. In most circumstances where the supply of this powder was adequate, its use did not follow official instructions but was a function of the availability of ice to cool the drink. Even when most soldiers had some degree of water deficit, their consumption of fluids or beverages was related directly to the availability of ice to cool drinks. Thus the amounts of vitamin C provided to the troops may have been large enough to allow intakes beyond the physiological range; actual consumption of this vitamin may well have been suppressed.

The administration of vitamin C in amounts greatly in excess of physiological requirements usually produces no significant effect. Very large doses may produce diarrhea. When the urine is acidified by massive doses of vitamin C, cystine and oxalate may be precipitated and produce renal calculi. Vitamin C can alter the excretion of drugs which are given concurrently. Scurvy has been reported in infants of mothers who consumed very large doses during pregnancy.

Thiamin was the first B-complex vitamin to be identified, isolated, and synthesized. In ordinary doses it is devoid of any pharmacological action. When it is injected rapidly, intravenously, there may be a sense of warmth, some dermal vasodilation, and a fall in blood pressure. Some people complain of a sulfur-like taste after injection. Presumably there may be instances of hypersensitivity to the vitamin or the vehicle in which it is dispensed. It has been used to treat many incurable or troublesome neurological symptoms and diseases. They are still incurable and troublesome. Whatever improvement occurred was a placebo effect.

Riboflavin is not known to have any pharmacological action whether taken by mouth or injected: presumably huge overdoses may be toxic and sensitivity reactions may occur.

The name nicotinic acid was enough like that of nicotine to frighten some physicians and nutrition experts. It was changed to niacin, but this name has never been uniformly accepted. The clinical effects of nicotinic acid in large doses include vasodilatation, flushing, headache, pruritus, gastrointestinal distress, increased secretion of hydrochloric acid and, if taken in very large doses over long periods of time, hepatotoxicity and activation of peptic ulcer.

Pyridoxine has no significant pharmacological activity when given to humans or experimental animals. It comes close to being completely nontoxic.

Biotin is without pharmacological action in large oral or intravenous doses.

Choline has the same type of action as acetylcholine, but to a lesser extent. It is nontoxic compared to some of its esters. Single oral doses of as much as 10 gm have produced no obvious pharmacological effects.

Inositol has no known pharmacological action.

Since most water-soluble vitamins serve directly or indirectly in enzyme and metabolic functions we must study whether the notion of a supercharging effect, a health bonus from megavitamin doses, can do what is claimed. Very large amounts of water-soluble vitamins taken in one large oral dose or by one large bolus injected intravenously are very promptly eliminated by the body's detoxifying mechanisms, or are excreted in the urine. The body deals with a vast vitamin overload as it does with overloads of most naturally occurring materials: the excess is treated as a poison and detoxicated or excreted. This is not the case with the fat-soluble vitamins which may accumulate and cause serious damage, as Dr. Arnrich tells us in Chapter 27.

Another fallacy is the naive belief that because some is good, an enormous amount is proportionately better. Here I think the analogy of an automobile and its internal combustion mechanism might be used. Because a small amount of tetraethyl lead keeps the engine from knocking, there is no reason to put in twenty, a hundred, or a thousand times as much of it. Indeed, doing so will cause much harm to the engine.

II. NICOTINIC ACID

During the 1930's, what originally had been thought to be a single water-soluble vitamin B turned out to be a series of separate chemicals. Each new factor was discovered because it was found to be essential for the growth of bacteria, yeast, molds, or certain experimental animals. It was a time of much excitement and considerable clinical confusion because very few physicians with experience in clinical research knew anything significant about vitamin deficiency diseases. Even nutrition experts were sorely puzzled. There was a great rush to try to discover which of the new factors did what. The first fraction of the B-complex to be understood was thiamin when its relation to beriberi was worked out in detail. Early advances in understanding vitamin B_1 deficiency in fowls helped to remove beriberi from the realm of disorders caused by toxins, poisons, or infections, and to identify it as a vitamin deficiency state.

The crucial advance in pellagra came when Elvehjem and his colleagues (1937) reported that nicotinic acid and some related pyridine compounds given to dogs with blacktongue disease promptly relieved the clinical manifestations of the experimental model of pellagra. Nicotinic acid also prevented the occurrence of blacktongue if added to the deficient diet. Thus a chemical which had been available for many decades was suddenly lifted from the obscurity of the laboratory shelf to a place of honor at the new vitamin feast.

When Elvehjem and his colleagues reported their findings there was little information about the pharmacological action of pyridine compounds in humans. These compounds had to be tested before they could be used to treat patients with pellagra. Many investigators volunteered to try these new drugs. Fairly small doses, 10 mg or so, were taken with water on an empty stomach. Soon after the dose, the test subjects experienced intense flushing on the face; some developed headaches and mild sniffles. One had a particularly distressing feeling of perianal warmth. Added to the pharmacological effects was the anxiety that this compound, a close chemical relative of nicotine, might be the end of them all.

To the great relief of all, the symptoms abated after a number of minutes and no one was worse for the experience.

In the course of a series of subsequent studies which I conducted, it turned out that nicotinamide did not produce the flushing but was as efficacious as nicotinic acid in preventing or curing the manifestations of pellagra (Bean and Spies, 1940). I designed and conducted experiments on vasodilatation in forty-seven men, seven women and four children, using a large variety of pyridine and pyrazine compounds. Each of these substances was tested on myself and sometimes on other colleagues. We decided that an oral dose of 200 mg or 20 mg given intravenously would be used for the test. All patients were studied in a postabsorptive state after they had spent at least an hour, and usually two, lightly clothed in an unpleasantly cool (20° C) constant temperature room. This environment stabilized vasoconstriction; the skin temperature remained substantially constant after treatment with the pyridine compound being investigated. It turned out that the face and neck were the most vasolabile regions, so I selected the fifteen areas illustrated in Fig. 1 to measure the skin temperature changes with a simple electrode. The substances studied were nicotinic acid and its sodium, ammonium, and monoethanolamine salts; ethylnicotinic, quinolinic, dinicotinic, 2,6-dimethyldinicotinic, 6-methylnicotinic, and isonicotinic acids; nicotinic acid amide; nicotinamide hydrochloride; nicotinic acid N-diethylamide

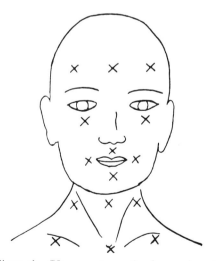

Fig. 1. Crosses indicate the fifteen spots on the face and neck where temperature readings were made. From Bean and Spies (1940).

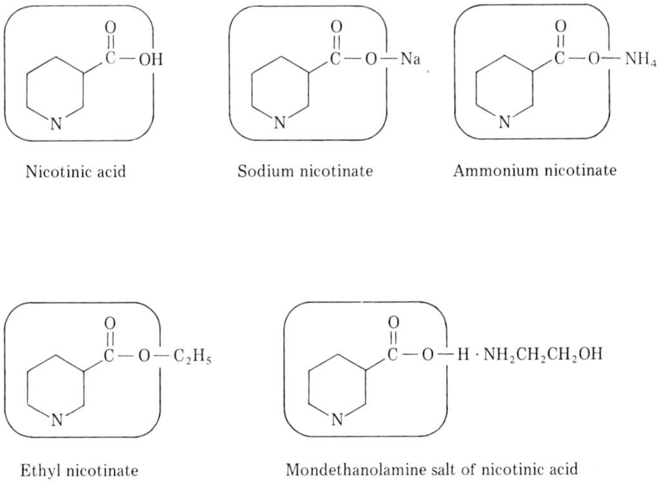

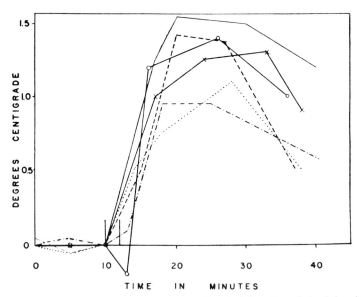

Fig. 2.   Formulas for pyridine compounds which produced vasodilatation. Specific radical involved is enclosed in the box.   From Bean and Spies (1940).

Fig. 3.   Variations in facial temperature after the administration of nicotinic acid. Continuous line, sodium nicotinate. Line with x's connected, ammonium nicotinate. Dotted line, ethyl nicotinate. Lower dashed line, monoethanolamine salt of nicotinic acid. Upper dashed line, irradiated nicotinic acid. Connected circles, sodium nicotinate. From Bean and Spies (1940).

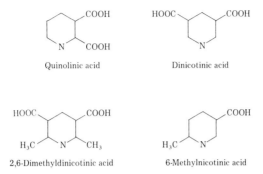

Quinolinic acid   Dinicotinic acid

2,6-Dimethyldinicotinic acid   6-Methylnicotinic acid

Fig. 4. Pyridine compounds with additional radicals not producing vasodilatation. From Bean and Spies (1940).

(coramine); pyridine; 3-aminopyridine; sodium sulfapyridine; vitamin B_6 (2-methyl-3-hydroxy-4,5-dihydroxymethylpyridine); and pyrazine mono- and 2,3-dicarboxylic acids. It each case the material was dissolved in 20 ml of physiological saline or sterile water. The injection was completed within 1 to 3 minutes. No untoward reaction occurred with any of these compounds.

The results were as follows. Every salt of nicotinic acid containing the radical blocked off in Figs. 2 and 3 produced vasodilatation. The addition of other radicals to the pyridine ring in the 2-, 5-, or 6-positions, in any two or all three, caused the loss of the vasodilatating property (Figs. 4 and 5). If additional radicals were added, as in quinolinic, dinicotinic,

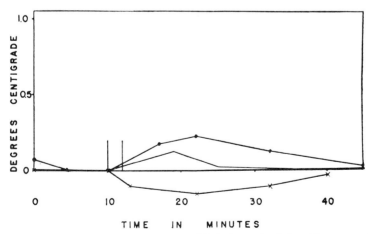

Fig. 5. X's, dinicotinic acid; connected solid circles, quinolinic acid; connected dots, 6-dimethyldinicotinic acid. The variations are not significant. From Bean and Spies (1940).

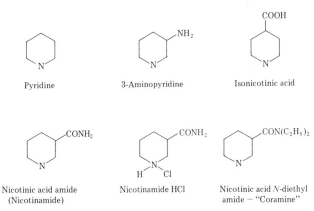

Fig. 6.   Pyridine compounds without vasodilatile potency. From Bean and Spies (1940).

2,6-dimethylnicotinic, and 6-methylnicotinic acids, no vasodilatation was produced.

No pyridine compound without the free carboxyl group in the 3-position, as in nicotinic acid, caused vasodilatation (Figs. 6 and 7). Pyrazine compounds produced no flushing (Fig. 8), although they were somewhat effective as antipellagra agents.

Because it took longer for nicotinic acid compounds taken orally to produce the flushing and because a larger amount was needed, we ordinarily compared 20 mg given intravenously with 200 mg given orally. It was found that when epinephrine was given first, the vasoconstriction almost completely prevented the vasodilatation usually produced by

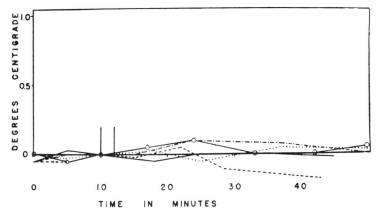

Fig. 7.   Temperature changes after inert compounds shown in Fig. 6 were given. From Bean and Spies (1940).

Pyrazine-2,3-dicarboxylic
acid

Pyrazinemonocarboxylic
acid

Fig. 8. Pyrazine compounds without vasodilator effect.   From Bean and Spies (1940).

nicotinic acid (Fig. 9). It was also found that a meal slowed the onset of vasodilatation and considerably lessened the height of the increase in skin temperature in comparison with tests in the fasting state (Fig. 10). Sixty grams of glycine had a particularly strong effect in neutralizing or reducing the vasodilatation response (Fig. 11).

In general we did not encounter much trouble with nausea, epigastric distress, vomiting, or throbbing headache. The urticarial rashes described by several observers were nothing but the intense vasodilatation that in some instances was associated with definite but transient edema of the skin. Ruffin and Smith (1939) observed lassitude, depression, palpitation, cyanosis, substernal oppression, headache, nausea, vomiting, and dyspnea in addition to the flushing in several normal subjects who took oral doses of 250 mg of nicotinic acid four times a day. These effects were not observed in comparable magnitudes by other workers. Since the effect of an injection of nicotinic acid was similar to but less intense than the effect of ordinary injection of histamine, we speculated

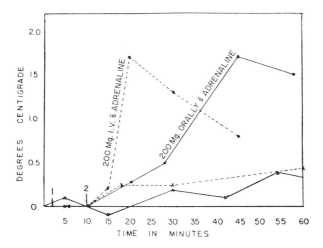

Fig. 9. Temperature response after oral and intravenous administration of nicotinic acid with and without injection of epinephrine. Upper lines indicate temperature rise without epinephrine.   From Bean and Spies (1940).

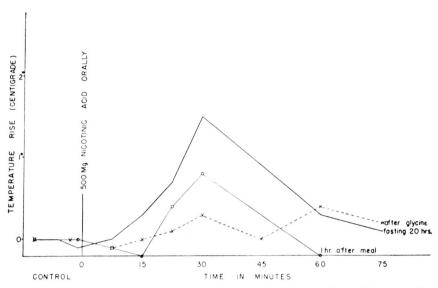

Fig. 10. Comparison of temperature response to 500 mg of nicotinic acid given orally to a fasting subject, just after a meal, after 30 gm of glycine during the preceding half hour. From Bean and Spies (1940).

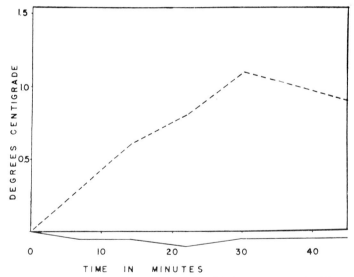

Fig. 11. Two hundred milligrams of nicotinic acid given ten normal subjects. Dashed line, without 60 gm of glycine half an hour before nicotinic acid; solid line, with glycine given during the half hour before nicotinic acid. From Bean and Spies (1940).

that nicotinic acid might produce vasodilatation by liberating histamine. We also found that injection of nicotinic acid gave rise to a definite increase in the secretion of gastric hydrochloric acid but not to the extent produced by histamine. We tried using the weak antihistamine preparations available at that time and were not able to show that they had any effect in reducing the effect of either histamine or nicotinic acid on the secretion of hydrochloric acid.

Physicians treating peripheral vascular disease had high hopes that nicotinic acid would produce vasodilatation and increase blood flow to the extremities of those suffering from the effects of atherosclerosis and other forms of vascular disease. Unfortunately, most of the vasodilatation is in the skin and not in the muscles. Nicotinic acid is thus not of any value in the treatment of vascular disease.

Flushing doses of nicotinic acid increase spinal fluid pressure, but there is apparently no net increase in cerebral blood flow. It has proved of no value in treating cerebral atherosclerosis in its chronic form or in acute episodes of hemiparesis and hemiplegia.

The notion that nicotinic acid might be of some specific help in treating mental disorders, particularly schizophrenia, evolved as follows. When nicotinic acid is used in high doses it theoretically should produce an excess of nicotinamide adenine dinucleotide, an active metabolite of nicotinic acid, a methyl acceptor. The hypothesis has been studied in detail by Mosher (1970). The presence of an extra supply of methyl acceptors was postulated to completely inhibit aberrant transmethylation processes. The hypotheses is a good example of self-contradiction and, of course, there is no uniformity of supporting results.

Very high doses of nicotinic acid used in rats have been reported to produce fatty liver; other workers have reported no changes. Large doses in dogs may produce weight loss, enteric bleeding, convulsions, and death. A number of congeners of nicotinic acid such as 6-aminonicotinamide and N-ethylnicotinamide are teratogens. Their effect can be reduced or prevented by the use of nicotinic acid or nicotinamide.

In a few patients given very high doses, 3 gm a day or more of niacin for at least a year, biochemical tests disclosed deterioration in liver function. Hyperglycemia has been reported in half to a third of nondiabetics taking large doses of nicotinic acid. There are no reports of birth defects produced by nicotinic acid or its analogues, though in humans most studies of high doses have been in older persons. Minor hepatic dysfunctions and a tendency to peptic ulceration are the most likely draw-backs to a long-term megavitamin treatment of schizophrenia, but it is likely that many metabolic systems are under strain. The significance of their altered mechanisms is not understood. Serum cholesterol falls, and blood sugar and blood uric acid rise. There are some indications that very large doses of nicotinamide, although it does not produce flushing, may be more toxic than equivalent doses of nicotinic acid. A serious discrepancy in the clinical reports has been the almost uniform failure of psychiatrists to record the side-effects stressed in reports by nutritionists and medical investigators. In short, nicotinic acid is still of unproved value in megavitamin doses for schizophrenia. At present the toxic side-effects and metabolic derangements make it wise to use great caution in employing nicotinic acid therapeutically.

The relationship of nicotinic acid to isoniazid used in treatment of tuberculosis led to testing a series of related compounds for possible value. McKenzie et al. (1948) related the antituberculosis effect of nicotinamide and other compounds of pyridine carboxylic acid derivatives to their therapeutic value in pellagra. They did not pursue the subject very much further when they found nicotinamide was the most effective.

A recent study reports that mongrel dogs subjected to 40% body area burns lost significantly less plasma if treated with 10 mg of nicotinic acid per kilogram of body weight before or, less effectively, within 10 minutes after the burn (Hilton and Wells, 1976).

III. VITAMIN C

A notable foible of the human mind is the belief that if one has symptoms, one must take medicine. The corollary is that if the symptoms cease, taking medicine should cease. This accounts for many therapeutic failures in chronic diseases which require maintenance therapy.

The advent of vitamins and the availability of many in abundance made them relatively cheap. Two misuses followed: One was the widespread use of vitamins as superchargers. In our age of prevailing— though often mild—depression, lack of "the old zip" was attacked with a pill. Usually nothing happened. The worry increased. This do-it-yourself treatment had an adverse effect, mainly on the pocketbook.

Another more formidable misuse was the prescribing of the injection of vitamins by physicians who hoped they might cure incurable disorders or eliminate all manner of complaints. As an example, far more vitamin B_{12} is dispensed today than would be needed to control all existing cases of pernicious animia. Large amounts of thiamin, nicotinic acid, folic acid and other water-soluble vitamins, as well as the more dangerous fat-soluble vitamins, have been added to what we eat or drink, or are needled into us.

One of the surprising by-products of vitamin research is the synthesis of compounds closely related to vitamins which compete for an active site in an enzyme complex. The effective part of the vitamin antagonist is inert and does not serve the vitamin's usual function. Thus an enzyme is rendered inactive. The division and development of rapidly growing cells, as in cancers, leukemias, and lymphomas, may be greatly slowed or completed stopped by these inhibitors. Of course, bone marrow and other vital tissues may be damaged too. Just before going on active duty in World War II, I had been doing some experiments to determine whether pyridine-3-sulfonic acid, an antagonist of nicotinic acid, would induce pellagra (Bean *et al.*, 1944). The experiments had not progressed very far when they were interrupted by my military duty. When I resumed civilian life, the folic acid antagonists already had introduced a new chapter in chancer chemotherapy. To solve some of the remaining problems such as what the vitamins pyridoxine and pantothenic acid do, we employed the corresponding vitamin antagonists.

A. Vitamin C and the Common Cold

In 1970 Linus Pauling, twice a Nobel Prize winner, started a conflagration with his book "Vitamin C and the Common Cold". He thus became, almost overnight, the most spectacular of the megavitamin postulants. Now the blaze of controversy has diminished, but its embers keep smoldering.

One may summarize the situation confidently as follows: Vitamin C has no obvious effect on any of the perhaps one-hundred viruses which produce the common cold. Thus any effect vitamin C might have toward preventing or ameliorating the common cold must be an effect on the host. It is logical to suppose that this would be primarily a prophylactic enhancement of resistance. Among the questions that have been asked are the following: If there is an effect, is it a specific physiological or biological effect, or is it a placebo effect? Is it pharmacological or is it related to the known vitamin C functions? How did a gigantic requirement arise which bypassed the natural environment of man? Are megadoses necessary or is minor supplementation satisfactory? If large doses are required, are the dangerous side-effects worth the risk when the target itself is relatively harmless? In the light of frequent failure of patients to take prescribed medication, will more than a small number of those for whom the vitamin is prescribed follow their program rigorously? The complexity of such problems related to ascorbic acid seems to increase rather than decrease. The New York Academy of Sciences held in 1974 their second conference on vitamin C. The results of their deliberations and ruminations were published in a book of 552 pages which contains the first reference, among others, in this chapter.

Among the functions of ascorbic acid is its role in the detoxification of histamine as reported by Chatterjee *et al.* (1975) in their study of the synthesis and major functions of vitamin C in animals. Large doses of ascorbic acid circulating in the blood favor the development of hyperglycemia in animals deficient in vitamin C (Chatterjee *et al.*, 1975). In animals deficient in vitamin C the metabolism of many drugs is decreased. Guinea pigs with scurvy have a reduced capacity to biodegrade pesticides, as reported by Street and Chadwick (1975). DDT and lipid-soluble pesticides are powerful inducers of hepatic microsomal enzymes, including the biosynthetic ascorbic acid pathways. Such pesticides given to rats may enhance the formation and excretion of L-ascorbic acid (Fox and Spivey, 1975). Japanese quail growers know that cadmium is very toxic to these birds. Small amounts of ascorbic acid protect them (Fox and Spivey, 1975). Ascorbic acid may reduce convulsions produced by metrazole in guinea pigs. When chickens are exposed to high environmental temperatures, egg production falls off, the egg becomes smaller and the shells thinner. Ascorbic acid reduces body temperature in such chickens and corrects these malfunctions (Scott, 1975). Pelletier's report on vitamin C and cigarette smokers (1975) indicates that ascorbic acid is effective in reducing the formation of nitrosamines from sodium nitrate both *in vivo* and *in vitro*. The major action appears to take place in the stomach (Kamm *et al.*, 1975). High oral doses of vitamin C diminish the resistance to high altitudes of normal subjects as is manifest by the inability to perform mental arithmetic as well under controlled circumstances (Schrauzer *et al.*, 1975). Large doses of vitamin C in pregnant women may give rise to symptoms of scurvy in the newborn, as reported by Norkus and Rosso (1975). Ascorbic acid deficiency significantly inhibits the transformation of cholesterol into bile salts in guinea pigs, thus increasing the plasma cholesterol concentration. Patients with such inborn errors as cystinuria, oxalosias, and gout may need special warnings. Conflicting testimony has appeared about the effect of ascorbic acid on vitamin B_{12}. It has been suggested that vitamin B_{12} is destroyed by massive doses of vitamin C, thus creating a dietary deficiency, but this has been contradicted by other work. False negative tests for occult blood in the stools has been reported (Jaffe *et al.*, 1975).

B. Large-Scale Studies on Vitamin C

Terence Anderson condensed and summarized three large-scale studies on vitamin C he and his colleagues performed in Toronto, Canada in 1971–1972, 1972–1973, and 1973–1974 (Anderson, 1975). They found no evidence to support Linus Pauling's claim that one gram of vitamin C per day would reduce the frequency of common colds by 45% and the days of illness by 60%. One of the very praiseworthy conditions of their regimen was that the placebo and vitamin C supplement were indistinguishable even by the shrewdest and most suspicious subjects. They had subject dropout rates of around 20–33% which sounds appalling but are fairly common in large-scale studies of this kind. A labeling error caused serious confusion in two groups. There was some concern about whether to include the results of both protracted illnesses and very short ones. The difference between the treatments were disappointingly small and, although some differences such as days of chest symptoms, days of feeling feverish, days of shivering, and days spent indoors, achieved "statistical significance" this disappeared when symptoms lasting 2–14 days only were analyzed.

Such things as the introduction of a sustained release form of ascorbic acid brought another variable into the last test, causing difficulty in comparing it with the others. Shortcomings of the study, though hard to avoid in large field studies, include the absence of records of other medications or of independent spontaneous supplementation with vitamin C or other vitamins, and absence of a check to determine whether the placebo or vitamin C were taken according to plan.

Another study by Lewis, Karlowski and their colleagues, a controlled clinical trial of ascorbic acid for the common cold, shows signs of haste in planning and reporting (Lewis et al., 1975). There was a breakdown in the separation of placebo and vitamin subjects; many subjects were able to detect which group they were in by tasting the powder in the capsules supplied. A large percentage correctly identified the substance they were taking. The statement in their opening paragraph that "the study was conducted so that nurses, physicians and volunteers did not know who received placebo and who received ascorbic acid" reflects how the study was planned, not actually how it was carried out. The tone of the paper suggests that the authors were anticipating the results of the experiment. Even if one agrees with their conclusions, the information on which they are based is more testimonial than evidential. The final conclusion was that "with a large population of well-motivated volunteers taking two or three capsules three times a day was too much bother for the possible small benefit received". This should not be regarded as a triumph of investigation.

In a double-blind study among Navajo school children, Coulehan and his colleagues (1975) reported that prophylaxis with vitamin C in 1 and 2 gm doses daily for 14 weeks reduced days of morbidity by one-third, compared with a group taking placebo. They found about a quarter fewer "symptom days" of cough and nasal discharge as observed in the classroom. Children were observed during 5 days only. On holidays and the weekends they were given packets of pills to take at home.

After this preliminary evaluation of their 1973 double-blind study among Navajo school children had indicated a significant reduction in days of morbidity and cough and nasal complaints, the final evaluation of a second trial done in 1974 by Coulehan *et al.* (1975) revealed "no difference in number becoming ill, number of episodes of mean illness duration between the groups" receiving 1 or 2 gm of vitamin C per day and those receiving placebo. There was no difference in the overall complicated illness rate. "Children with high plasma ascorbic acid concentration had longer mean illness than those with low levels." The final conclusion was that "vitamin C does not seem to be an effective prophylactic or therapeutic agent for upper respiratory illness."

Coulehan's conclusion from studies done in two places in two different years with significantly and mysteriously different results was that "the conflicting results indicate that this method is not sensitive enough to detect the pharmacological action of ascorbic acid in a dose of one gram daily, if indeed such an action does exist. We anticipate that analysis of biochemical data and the clinical episode data, reflecting actual 'illness' rather than more evanescent 'symptoms', may clarify the matter. A specific symptomatic benefit, for example, could explain the conflicting findings in various studies in that methodology, population, and the syndromes prevalent at the time of the study could all influence whether and to what extent benefit was observed in a given investigation. Nevertheless, this suggests that *vitamin C is unlikely to have widespread usefulness as a cold remedy.*"

IV. CONCLUSIONS

The arguments, contradictions, and the questions left unsettled indicate a degree of indeterminism and confusion which would be amusing to the innocent bystander if clear answers were not so important in preventive medicine and therapy. Experience in field tests or large nutritional studies reminds us that compliance with instructions, taking or not taking a tablet, capsule or pill, if not carefully supervised is erratic and uncertain. Biochemical tests for placebos with chemical markers as well as the test substance to demonstrate that what was supposed to have been taken was taken as directed are never mentioned.

Rapid decreases in compliance with advice and instruction among office or clinic patients given maintenance medication introduces possibly large errors of unknown dimensions. If comparisons are made based on groups in which significant numbers of subjects took nothing, results are triply-blind. Suppose a study could be done in which vitamin C could be added to the food of half of the people in a military camp, an isolated school, or custodial institution while the other half received nothing. Such manipulative intervention may not be ethical, but it would be better than having clinically illiterate zealots corrupt the public. At any rate, such a test has never been done.

In addition to their better studied effects in nutrition and malnutrition, vitamins have a number of effects as drugs. These have been studied less than the natural function of vitamins. It is unfortunate that nutritional studies have to be done in the field under circumstances where supervision would interpose impossible logistic problems and greatly complicate interpretation. Thus they lack the precision of studies in physics or chemistry. This has always been true of biological problems. So we have confusion, false hopes, outlandish propaganda, folklore, and quackery. These continue to vex workers in the field of clinical nutrition and clinical medicine who strive to make the condition of the "common man" not only tolerable but better.

REFERENCES

Anderson, T. W. (1975). Large-scale trials of vitamin C. Second Conference on Vitamin C. *Ann. N. Y. Acad. Sci.* **258,** 498–504.
Banic, S. (1972). Prevention of rabies by vitamin C. *Nature (London)* **258,** 153–154.
Bean, W. B. (1974–1975). Drugs for nutritional disorders. *In* "Drugs of Choice," pp. 106–132. Mosby, St. Louis, Missouri.
Bean, W. B. (1955). Vitamania, polypharmacy, and witchcraft. *Arch. Intern. Med.* **96,** 137–141.
Bean, W. B., and Spies, T. D. (1940). A study of the effects of nicotinic acid and related pyridine and pyrazine compounds on the temperature of the skin of human beings. *Am. Heart J.* **20,** 62–75.
Bean, W. B., Spies, T. D., and Blankenhorn, M. A. (1944). Secondary pellagra. *Medicine (Baltimore)* **23,** 1–77.
Chatterjee, A. K., Majumder, A. K., Nandi, B. K., and Subramanian, N. (1975). Synthesis and some major functions of vitamin C in animals. Second Conference on Vitamin C. *Ann. N. Y. Acad. Sci.* **258,** 24–47.

684   William B. Bean

Cochrane, W. A. (1965). Over nutrition in prenatal and neonatal life: problem? *Can. Med. Assoc. J.* **93**, 893–899.

Conney, A. H., Bray, G. A., Evans, C., and Burns, J. J. (1961). Metabolic interactions between L-ascorbic acid and drugs. *Ann. N. Y. Acad. Sci.* **92**, 115–127.

Coulehan, J. L., Kapner, L., and Eberhard, S. (1975). Vitamin C and upper respiratory illness in Navajo children: Preliminary observations. Second Conference on Vitamin C. *Ann. N. Y. Acad. Sci.* **258**, 513–522.

Coulehan, J. L., Eberhard, S., Kapner, L., Taylor, F., Rogers, K., and Garry, P. (1976). Vitamin C in acute illness in Navajo school children. *N. Engl. J. Med.* **295**, 973–977.

Crandon, J. H., Lund, C. C., and Dill, D. B. (1940). Experimental human scurvy. *N. Eng. J. Med.* **223**, 353–369.

Elvehjem, C. A., Madden, R. J., Strong, F. M., and Woolley, D. W. (1937). The relationship of nicotinic acid and nicotinic acid amide to canine black tongue. *J. Am. Chem. Soc.* **59**, 1767.

Fox, H. H. (1953). Chemical attack on tuberculosis. *Trans. N. Y. Acad. Sci.* [2] **15**, 234–242.

Fox, H. H., and Spivey, M. R. (1975). Protective effects of ascorbic acid against toxicity of heavy metals. Second Conference on Vitamin C. *Ann. N. Y. Acad. Sci.* **258**, 144–150.

Hilton, J. G., and Wells, C. H. (1976). Nicotinic acid reduction of plasma volume loss after thermal trauma. *Science* **191**, 861–862.

Jaffe, R. M., Kasten, B., Young, D. S., and MacLowry, J. D. (1975). False-negative stool occult blood tests caused by ingestion of ascorbic acid (vitamin C). *Ann. Intern. Med.* **83**, 824–826.

Kamm, J. J., Dashman, T., Conney, A. H., and Burns, J. J. (1975). Effect of ascorbic acid on amine-nitrite toxicity. Second Conference on Vitamin C. *Ann. N. Y. Acad. Sci.* **258**, 169–174.

Klevay, L. (1976). Hypercholesterolemia due to ascorbic acid. (39263). *Proc. Soc. Exp. Biol. Med.* **151**, 579–582.

Lewis, T. L., Karlowski, T. R., Kapikian, A. Z., Lynch, J. M., Shaffer, G. W., and George, D. A. (1975). A controlled clinical trial of ascorbic acid for the common cold. Second Conference on Vitamin C *Ann. N. Y. Acad. Sci.* **258**, 505–512.

McKenzie, D., Malone, L., Kushner, S., Oleson, J. J., and SubbaRow, Y. (1948). The effect of nicotinic acid amide on experimental tuberculosis of white mice. *J. Lab. Clin. Med.* **33**, 1249.

Mosher, L. T. (1970). Nicotinic acid side effects and toxicity: A review. *Am. J. Psychiatry* **126**, 1290–1296.

Norkus, E. P., and Rosso, P. (1975). Changes in ascorbic acid metabolism of the offspring following high maternal intake of this vitamin in the pregnant guinea pig. Second Conference on Vitamin C. *Ann. N. Y. Acad. Sci.* **258**, 401–409.

Pelletier, O. (1975). Vitamin C and cigarette smokers. Second Conference on Vitamin C. *Ann. N. Y. Acad. Sci.* **258**, 156–168.

Ruffin, J. M., and Smith, D. T. (1939). Treatment of pellagra with special reference to nicotinic acid. *South. Med. J.* **32**, 40.

Schrauzer, G. N., Ishmael, D., and Kiefer, G. W. (1975). Some aspects of current vitamin C usage: Diminished high-altitude resistance following overdosage. Second Conference on Vitamin C. *Ann. N. Y. Acad. Sci.* **258**, 377–381.

Scott, M. L. (1975). Environmental influences on ascorbic acid requirements in animals. Second Conference on Vitamin C. *Ann. N. Y. Acad. Sci.* **258**, 151–155.

Spies, T. D. (1932). Pellagra: Improvement while taking so-called "pellagra-inducing diet." *Am. J. Med. Sci.* **184**, 837–845.

Spies, T. D., Bean, W. B., and Stone, R. E. (1938). Treatment of subclinical and classic pellagra. *J. Am. Med. Assoc.* **111,** 584.

Stein, B., Hasan, A., and Fox, I. H. (1976). Ascorbic acid-induced uriscoria. A consequence of megavitamin therapy. *Ann. Intern. Med.* **84,** 4.

Street, J. C., and Chadwick, R. W. (1975). Ascorbic acid requirements and metabolism in relation to organochlorine pesticides. Second Conference on Vitamin C *Ann. N. Y. Acad. Sci.* **258,** 132–143.

Unna, K. (1939). Studdies on the toxicity and pharmacology of nicotinic acid. *J. Pharmacol. Exp. Ther.* **65,** 95.

25

Uses and Function of Vitamin K

WALTER H. SEEGERS

I. HISTORICAL SKETCH

In a short while it will be a half century since vitamin K was discovered by Dam (1929, 1935). It was one of the last vitamins to be found during an era when vitamin studies were fashionable, and biochemistry was emerging from the field of nutrition. Subsequently, vitamins became regarded as a special class of drugs. Thus, in concert with pharmacology, industry, and clinical applications, attention became broad in scope. Vitamin K deficiency proved to be associated with prothrombin deficiency (Dam *et al.*, 1936), but the original data were not especially convincing. Vitamin K was isolated (Dam *et al.*, 1939; Doisy *et al.*, 1939) and was conveniently available for research purposes.

In the clinics the vitamin became especially important (Owen, 1974) for its usefulness in obstructive jaundice, hemorrhagic disease of the newborn, poor absorption syndromes, and liver diseases. A little later it was demonstrated in clinical work that the hypoprothrombinemia induced with dicumarol could be reversed with vitamin K (Overman *et al.*, 1942; Davidson and MacDonald, 1943).

The background for the discovery of dicumarol relates to nutrition problems in agriculture. Spoiled sweet clover silage consumed by cows induced a bleeding tendency that was fatal in many herds (Schofield, 1922, 1924). The problem was not related to infection, and serum or defibrinated blood temporarily stopped the hemorrhage. This work was confirmed (Roderick, 1929) and extended (Roderick, 1931) to record that the prothrombin level was depressed in cattle with spoiled sweet clover disease.

The toxic agent was isolated and induced to crystallize (Campbell and Link, 1941). It was synthesized (Stahmann *et al.*, 1941) and related compounds were also synthesized, tested, and introduced for clinical trials. These dramatic events are vividly described in the Harvey Lecture by Link (1944). Basic to the whole clinical enterprise was the demonstration that withdrawal of Dicumarol was followed by a restoration of prothrombin concentration and there was no damage at the manufacturing site which was known to be the liver.

To learn about the effect of vitamin K on blood coagulation, it was essential to know more about these mechanisms. For that purpose, vitamin K and Dicumarol, considered as a family of compounds, served as convenient prime modifiers for experiments in blood coagulation. Like the rapid proliferation of vitamins at one time, the discovery of new coagulation factors was equally exciting and occurred during the mid-century period. It was essential to isolate each of the previously recognized ones, as well as the ones that very likely existed.

The main problem with purification was the low concentration of coagulation factors in blood, their lability, the estimation of concentration, and the state of technology in protein chemistry. The progressive conquest of these obstacles followed the introduction of ion exchange resins, polyacrylamide gel electrophoresis, gel filtration, amino acid analysis, new molecular weight determination methods, and advances in general protein chemistry. Spectacular developments related to our knowledge of blood coagulation occurred during the past 15 years. Very early in the purification of prothrombin, it was possible to show that vitamin K is not a prosthetic group associated with the prothrombin molecule (Seegers, 1962).

Today we know that there are five proteins in plasma that require vitamin K for their synthesis by the liver. These are quite similar in structure; in fact, they are so similar that my evidence for their origin in prothrombin was not easily set aside. I shall outline a useful and hopefully accurate way to study the nature of these mechanisms. The function of the vitamin K-dependent proteins can then be seen up to the time of our present knowledge.

In the synthesis of prothrombin, one of the functions of vitamin K is at the postribosomal level (Suttie et al., 1974). Ten glutamic acid residues are converted to γ-carboxyglutamic acid and serve as calcium ion binding sites (Stenflo et al., 1974; Magnusson et al., 1974; Nelsestuen et al., 1974). The other four vitamin K-dependent proteins also contain a certain number of γ-carboxyglutamic acid residues.

II. BLOOD COAGULATION MECHANISMS

A. Introduction

The need to understand the function of vitamin K in terms of blood coagulation was expressed by Suttie (1969) when he stated, "... it has been possible for workers interested in the mechanism of action of vitamin K to proceed even though details of the coagulation process are unresolved." I presume by now he has taken much satisfaction from the recent developments.

The literature on the subject of blood coagulation is so vast that very few can keep up with it and still have time to write themselves. In order to keep the references at a sensible level and to avoid selective credit to contributors, I shall only indicate a few valuable sources, such as Biggs (1972), Bradshaw and Wessler (1975), Fearnley (1965), Johnson (1971), Koch-Weser and Sellers (1971a,b), Olson (1975), Quick (1942), Reich et al. (1975), Seegers (1962, 1967), Seegers et al. (1975), and Wintrobe (1974).

B. Blood Coagulation Nomenclature

Each specialty in science has its own language and in the field of blood coagulation, plasma components are referred to as factors and have been given Roman numerals to serve as an equivalent to diverse common names. Platelet factors are given Arabic numbers. The list below has been stable for several years. Note that the vitamin K-dependent factors are II, VII, IX, X and XIV.

Factor I	Fibrinogen
Factor II	Prothrombin
Factor III	Thromboplastin, tissue factor
Factor IV	Calcium ions
Factor V	Ac–globulin, labile factor, proaccelerin
Factor VI	Not verified
Factor VII	Cothromboplastin, stable factor, proconvertin, serum prothrombin conversion accelerator (SPCA)
Factor VIII	Antihemophilic factor A or globulin, platelet cofactor I, hemophilia A factor, thromboplastinogen
Factor IX	Antihemophilia B factor, autoprothrombin II, Christmas factor, platelet cofactor II
Factor X	Autoprothrombin III, Auto–III, Stuart–Prower factor, prothrombokinase
Factor XI	Plasma thromboplastin antecedent (PTA), antihemophilic factor C
Factor XII	Hageman factor, glass factor, contact factor
Factor XIII	Fibrinoligase, plasma transglutaminase, fibrin stabilizing factor

The above system has been expanded to designate active enzymes as follows: Factor IIa (thrombin); Factor IXa; Factor Xa (autoprothrombin C, thrombokinase) and variants of the latter have been described. Other active forms are Factor XIa, Factor XIIIa, and Factor XIVa. It is not correct to write Factor Va because no enzyme activation occurs when thrombin potentiates the activity of Factor V, and the same seems to be true for Factor VIIIa as modified by thrombin.

C. Three Basic Reactions of Blood Coagulation

In this cybernetic system, the controlling components consist of positive and negative feedback, controlled chain reactions, multiple enzyme involvement, apparent stoichiometric reactions, and there is integration with organ function. It is convenient to consider inhibitors last, and to begin by dividing the blood coagulation system into three basic events as follows:

(1) the formation of autoprothrombin C (Factor Xa);
(2) the formation of thrombin;
(3) the formation of fibrin.

These reactions involve formation of the clot and the activity of two enzymes. The events most likely occur in sequence and each successive reaction depends upon the preceding one (Fig. 1).

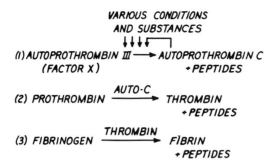

Fig. 1. Three basic chemical reactions of blood coagulation. The first occurs under various conditions. The second is due to the specific formation of thrombin and fragments. In the third, the visible clot is formed.

D. Formation of Fibrin

Purified fibrinogen or the fibrinogen of plasma with a molecular weight near 340,000 has three polypeptide chains. Two are susceptible to limited proteolysis by thrombin. The process removes fibrinopeptide A and fibrinopeptide B from each fibrinogen molecule. This amounts to about 3% of the large molecule. The fibrinopeptides are split from the $A\alpha$ and $B\beta$ chains, but nothing is removed from the γ chain. Each one of the three chains of fibrinogen is duplicated in the fibrinogen molecule. The function of thrombin being considered can thus be represented as follows:

$$(A\alpha \cdot B\beta \cdot \gamma)_2 \xrightarrow{\text{Thrombin}} (\alpha \cdot \beta \cdot \gamma)_2 + 2A + 2B$$
$$\downarrow$$
$$[(\alpha \cdot \beta \cdot \gamma)_2]_n$$

The fibrinogen, without fibrinopeptides, is referred to as a fibrin monomer and by a process of self-assembly, the monomer forms polymers. The molecules align end-to-end and side-to-side, and the fibrin has interconnecting branches. The resulting gel is of variable strength and consistency depending primarily upon the concentration of the protein and pH of the reaction. The rate of fibrin formation is dependent on pH, ionic strength of the medium, fibrinogen concentration, thrombin concentration, calcium ion concentration, temperature, and many other variables.

E. Cross-Linking of Fibrin

Artificial fibrin obtained by clotting purified fibrinogen with purified thrombin has several characteristics that distinguish it from the true or genuine fibrin obtained from whole blood clots. The main property generally featured is solubility in urea as a characteristic of fibrin from purified systems (fibrin-s) and insolubility for the fibrin (fibrin-i) from the natural clot. The conversion of fibrin-s to fibrin-i is brought about by the activated cross-linking enzyme of plasma. It functions after it has been converted by thrombin and/or autothrombin C to its active form (Factor XIIIa). The enzyme forms peptide bonds between preferred glutamic acid and lysine residues. The formation of cross-linked fibrin can be indicated as follows:

$$[(\alpha \cdot \beta \cdot \gamma)_2]_n \xrightarrow[\text{Factor XIIIa}]{\substack{\text{Factor XIII} \\ \downarrow \text{Thrombin}}} [(\alpha \cdot \beta \cdot \gamma)]_n^x + NH_3$$

Plasma Factor XIII, with a molecular weight of 340,000, is composed of two pairs of nonidentical polypeptide chains A and B. The respective molecular weights are 75,000 and 88,000. The formula for the tetramer can be written as A_2B_2. The A chains contain the catalytic function and are the only chains found in the crystalline protein obtained from platelets. Activation occurs in two steps as follows:

$$A_2B_2 \xrightarrow{\text{Thrombin}} \begin{array}{c} A_2'B_2 \\ + \\ 2 \text{ Peptides} \end{array} \xrightarrow{Ca^{2+}} \begin{array}{c} A_2' \\ + \\ B_2 \end{array}$$

The $A_2'B_2$ structure is not active, but dissociation occurs in the presence of calcium ions. An active center A'—SH is unmasked to generate the active protein while the B chains then no longer serve as carriers.

F. Formation of Thrombin

Prothrombin was the first one found to be vitamin K-dependent for its synthesis. About half of the molecule is needed for the thrombin structure (Fig. 2). For many years, data completely supported the view that the formation of thrombin is a process in which prothrombin is degraded. It was only recently, however, that functions for the nonthrombin portion of prothrombin were found. It is the region where phospholipids, calcium ions, and Ac–globulin bind to form complexes, and

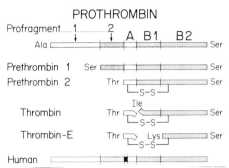

Fig. 2.   The prothrombin molecule, with a molecular weight near 73,000, is drawn to scale as a single polypeptide chain. In experiments, prothrombin fragment 1 is removed by thrombin, yielding prethrombin 1. Prothrombin fragment 2 is removed by autoprothrombin C, yielding prethrombin 2. Alternatively, prothrombin fragment 1·2 can be removed by autoprothrombin C and later divided into prothrombin fragment 1 and prothrombin fragment 2 by thrombin. Autoprothrombin C breaks an Arg–Ile bond in prethrombin 2 to develop thrombin activity. By a slow autolysis process, the B1 chain of thrombin is lost and practically only thrombin esterase activity remains. The degradation of human prothrombin is the same, except that thrombin splits an A1 peptide (13 amino acids) from the A chain of thrombin. This split involves an Arg–Thr bond. In the bovine material, the corresponding bond is Lys–Thr and is not attacked by thrombin.

thus make the activation process efficient. The binding sites in the prothrombin molecule are primarily provided by the recently discovered γ-carboxyglutamic acid residues at the NH_2-terminal region. Without vitamin K, an incomplete prothrombin is produced in which the corresponding residues are glutamic acid. Among the degradation fragments of prothrombin produced during activation are accelerators and inhibitors.

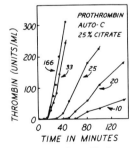

Fig. 3.   This illustrates the conversion of purified prothrombin (1,000 U/ml), in 25% sodium citrate solution, with only autoprothrombin C in various amounts (U/ml on each curve). There is a lag phase, followed by the generation of thrombin.

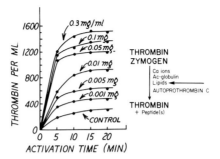

Fig. 4. This illustrates the generation of thrombin from a system of purified prothrombin, purified Ac-globulin, purified autoprothrombin C, calcium ions, and crude
cephalin. With all else kept constant, a decrease in phospholipid concentration is associated
with a decrease in yield of thrombin. Similarly, with all else constant, any one of the
reactants can be decreased to decrease the yield of thrombin. Compare with Fig. 3 to
appreciate that the presence of lipids, Ac-globulin, and calcium ions introduces more
rapid activation and mechanisms for control of rate at which thrombin generates.

For the conversion of prothrombin to classical thrombin, only autoprothrombin C (Factor Xa) is essential. Very favorable conditions are
provided by a 25% sodium citrate solution (Fig. 3). The powerful enzyme is, nevertheless, not sufficiently active nor present in high enough
concentration under physiological conditions to function adequately. To
compensate for this and to introduce a means to control the enzyme,
support is supplied from accessories; namely, plasma Ac-globulin (Factor V), calcium ions, and platelet factor 3 (Fig. 4). A condensed equation
for thrombin formation, recorded in two nomenclatures, follows:

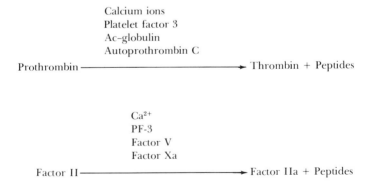

The five-component system outlined above yields all of the thrombin
possible from the selected amount of prothrombin. By reducing the

concentration of platelet factor 3 stepwise, the yield of thrombin can be reduced. Reducing the prothrombin, autoprothrombin C, Ac–globulin, or calcium ion concentration stepwise is associated with a correspondingly reduced yield of thrombin. Thrombin initially makes Ac–globulin more active but that is not a prerequisite for the function of Ac–globulin. On the basis of this complex way to obtain thrombin, five different deficiencies in thrombin formation are clearly possible: namely, a deficiency for prothrombin, for autoprothrombin III, for Ac–globulin, for platelet factor 3, and for calcium ions. In addition, the apparent stoichiometric nature of the reaction is the basis for buffering the generation of thrombin activity.

Important facts for thrombin generation can be summarized (Fig. 5): Prothrombin is a substrate which is degraded by autoprothrombin C as enzyme. The enzyme can function by itself, but to control its function and to make it more effective than by itself, Ac–globulin and phospholipids from platelets are involved. Lipids serve as a surface on which the molecular interactions take place. Calcium ions presumably enable the formation of complexes involving calcium binding sites on prothrombin (Henriksen and Jackson, 1975). Lipids bind directly to prothrombin in cooperation with calcium ions and γ-carboxyglutamic acid binding sites. Ac–globulin binds at the profragment 2 area in prothrombin and prethrombin 1.

Calcium binding sites of prothrombin are at the NH_2-terminal end of prothrombin. These are incomplete when the function of vitamin K is depressed. These are also not there when prethrombin 1 is used as a

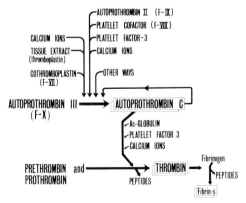

Fig. 5. Three basic reactions of blood coagulation, illustrating formation of thrombin by autoprothrombin C and accessories and the formation of autoprothrombin C by multiple ways.

source of thrombin. Ignored has been the fact that prethrombin 1 activates perfectly well if sufficient procoagulant material is used (Baker and Seegers, 1967). Until now the abnormal prothrombin molecule isolated under vitamin K-deficient conditions has not been studied adequately from the standpoint of its activation with biological materials.

G. Formation of Autoprothrombin C (Factor Xa)

The formation of autoprothrombin C occurs under a variety of conditions and with the support of several different substances. Based on their origin, at least four main classifications of substances can be made; namely, as follows:

    1. Extrinsic group
        a. Calcium ions
        b. Tissue thromboplastin
        c. Factor VII (cothromboplastin)
    2. Intrinsic group
        a. Calcium ions
        b. Platelet cofactor (Factor VIII)
        c. Platelet factor 3
        d. Autoprothrombin II (Factor IXa)
    3. Autocatalysis
    4. Enzymes and enzymes from snake venom
        a. Trypsin, papain, cathepsin C
        b. Russell's viper, *Echis carinatus*, etc.

The *autocatalytic* formation of autoprothrombin C from purified autoprothrombin III occurs most rapidly in strong salt solutions such as 25% sodium citrate solution. It also occurs in physiological saline solutions.

The yield of autoprothrombin C by the *extrinsic* and *intrinsic* groups of procoagulants is usually less than with snake venoms such as Russell's viper venom. As a consequence, the sera of most species contain appreciable amounts of residual or unactivated autoprothrombin III. Thromboplastin of the extrinsic system is structurally and functionally different from PF-3 of the intrinsic system. When the two systems are in operation at the same time, the result is a synergistic function.

The mechanics of autoprothrombin C formation by the intrinsic system are similar to thrombin formation. In both cases, an enzyme creates an active enzyme in the presence of accessory substances. In the case of autoprothrombin C formation, Factor IXa, platelet factor 3, Factor VIII, and calcium ions are involved. A reduction in concentration of a reactant from its optimum concentration limits the yield of active enzyme. As done previously for thrombin formation, the requirements for intrinsic autoprothrombin C formation (Fig. 5) are stated in two nomenclatures as follows:

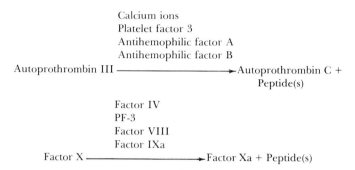

One view, which has become dogma, accounts for the formation of Factor IXa. Hageman factor becomes activated upon contact with certain surfaces, then produces Factor XIa from its precursor. Factor XIa can then produce Factor IXa. Factor XI seems to have a molecular weight near 160,000. Factor IXa is also produced by thrombin when the latter is in the optimum concentration, and this may be an important way to account for coagulation in Factor XII deficiency.

Under conditions of extrinsic autoprothrombin C formation, only four components are involved; namely, the substrate (autoprothrombin III), tissue thromboplastin, Factor VII and calcium ions. Presumably, Factor VII is the enzyme. Tissue thromboplastin consists of phospholipid bound to protein. Equations are given in two nomenclatures:

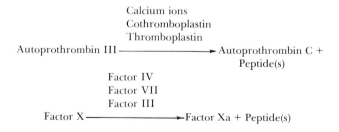

III. ROLE OF VITAMIN K-DEPENDENT PROTEINS

The discussion of the nature of the blood coagulation mechanisms up to this point has considered procoagulant effects. Anticoagulant effects are equally important but need not be taken up extensively to comprehend the role of vitamin K-dependent proteins and the effects of

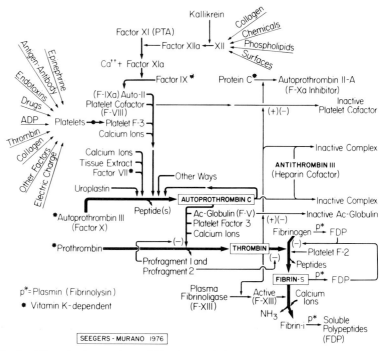

Fig. 6. Three basic reactions of blood coagulation. Same as Fig. 5, with additions to illustrate inhibition of procoagulants, the role of platelets, the formation of Factor IXa, the lysis of fibrinogen and fibrin by plasmin. Antithrombin III inactivates thrombin, autoprothrombin C, Factor IXa, and Factor VII. The place of the five vitamin K-dependent proteins is marked. (Seegers and Murano, 1976.)

drugs. A diagram of the procoagulant system has been projected (Fig. 5) and repeated to include the anticoagulant effects extensively discussed in the literature, but not elaborated on in this paper (Fig. 6).

The central protein in these mechanisms is prothrombin, without which a clot cannot form unless bacteria, snake venoms, or other extraneous materials come to bear on the situation. Prothrombin activation is dependent upon autoprothrombin C which itself is derived from the vitamin K-dependent proenzyme called Factor X. For the conversion of Factor X to Factor Xa, one mechanism involves Factor VII and another, Factor IX. Both of these are vitamin K-dependent proteins. Thus, four proteins at the very center of the blood coagulation mechanisms are required. Removal of any one of them from the blood is associated with a bleeding tendency. One enigma which remains is quite evident. Why are Factor VII and Factor IX essential for proper hemostasis when each one, in purified systems, participates in the separate system that is quite adequate for the formation of active Factor X?. The *intrinsic* and *extrinsic* systems are represented as redundant systems on the basis of excellent laboratory data, but in clinical cases they are not.

IV. INACTIVATION OF VITAMIN K-DEPENDENT PROTEINS BY ANTITHROMBIN III

Antithrombin III is more closely related to the inhibition of active vitamin K-dependent proteins than any other inhibitor. Antithrombin III is a plasma protein already known at the beginning of this century and there are extensive literature resources, as for example, Dombrose *et al.* (1971) and Bradshaw and Wessler (1975). This plasma protein has been obtained in purified form recently in several laboratories. Antithrombin III neutralizes the active forms of all four vitamin K-dependent enzymes considered in the discussion thus far.

A mutual depletion system is involved, in which there is a one-to-one molecular neutralization. In the case of thrombin, the active serine center is required, as well as arginine residues of the inhibitor. The mutual inactivation process is accelerated by heparin, and for that function, lysyl residues of the inhibitor probably serve as binding sites for heparin. In both cases of inhibition, the activity of antithrombin III is also diminished because complexes form which represent enzyme plus inhibitor. Antithrombin III also reduces the activity of plasmin, but only limited information about the mechanism is available. The fact that a deficiency of antithrombin III is accompanied by a thrombosing tendency is evidence that it is one of the most important inhibitors of the active vitamin K-dependent enzymes.

V. A FIFTH VITAMIN K-DEPENDENT PROTEIN

Attention to a fifth protein was primarily due to work in this laboratory. The names given to it are Protein C and autoprothrombin II-A. Neither name is entirely satisfactory. Autoprothrombin II-A is an inhibitor produced by thrombin. In fact, it was discovered when purified prothrombin complex was activated by small amounts of purified thrombin. Instead of the expected generation of thrombin, an inhibitor was produced (Mammen *et al.*, 1960). Ten years later, Marciniak (1970) concluded that it is not derived from prothrombin. It is a competitive inhibitor of autoprothrombin C, and is composed of two polypeptide chains with tentatively arrived at apparent molecular mass of 40,000 and 22,000 daltons (Murano *et al.*, 1974).

During the 15 years that work on autoprothrombin II-A was progressing in this laboratory, we were unable to prove that it was distinct from other members of the prothrombin complex (vitamin

700   Walter H. Seegers

K-dependent proteins). Our attempts were nearing success when Stenflo
(1976) isolated Protein C and differentiated it from all the others. By
using an antibody to Protein C, which Stenflo supplied and by applying
other criteria, it was possible to prove that autoprothrombin II-A is an
active form of Protein C (Seegers *et al.*, 1976).

Stenflo (1976) surveyed the recent literature and presented the evidence that all five vitamin K-dependent proteins are homologous (Fig. 7)
and presumably this conclusion will gain further experimental support.
This implies that there was a common ancestral gene and that all five
proteins are the result of genetic divergence. Only prothrombin has a
high molecular weight (73,000), as compared with the others (circa
55,000). This is because prothrombin has internal molecular homology
(Hewett-Emmett *et al.*, 1974) as a result of partial gene duplication. This
genetic event must have occurred after there were five vitamin
K-dependent proteins. To get an idea as to how long ago that occurred,
consider the following: Chicken prothrombin, like bovine prothrombin,
has a molecular weight near 73,000 (Walz *et al.*, 1974b), and let us *assume*
that internal homology will be found, due to partial gene duplication.
Then, we can go on to say that five proteins existed longer than 300 million
years, because mammals (cow) diverged from birds (chicken) 300 million
years ago. It is not a wild use of the imagination to suppose that vitamin
K was required in those times.

Another interesting fact is that autoprothrombin II-A serves to induce
fibrinolysis in addition to its anticoagulant function. It is thus a unique
protein, with a dual function. The molecular basis for its function in
fibrinolysis is only to a minor degree due to activation of profibrinolysis
(plasminogen). The major portion of the induced fibrinolysis is due to
the suppression of inhibitors of fibrinolysis (Zolton and Seegers, 1973.)

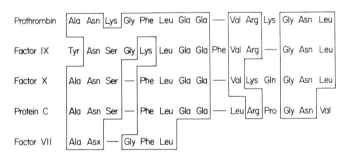

Stenflo J.B.C. 251 355 (1976)

Fig. 7. Indication for homology of five vitamin K-dependent proteins. Modified from
arrangement of Stenflo (1976). Gla = γ-carboxyglutamic acid.

It remains for future work to determine whether drastic reduction of Protein C concentration with oral anticoagulants seriously impairs much desired fibrinolysis. The position of Protein C in blood coagulation is included on Fig. 6, and the following functions are known: (1) Inhibitor of blood coagulation; (2) competitive inhibitor of autoprothrombin C; (3) promotes fibrinolysis by depressing inhibitors; (4) cofactor for epinephrine in platelet aggregation; and (5) inhibits activation of prethrombin 1 by trypsin.   .

VI. DEPRESSION OF VITAMIN K ACTIVITY

There are numerous valuable papers, books, and reviews about vitamin K deficiency and its depression with Dicumarol and related drugs. To illustrate the main points, I am presenting a previously unpublished illustration from the series of Müller-Berghaus and Seegers (1966). A 1.5 kg of rabbit was given 4 mg Coumadin intravenously on 4 successive days (Fig. 8). The prothrombin concentration, as measured by two-stage assay, dropped over a period of 4 days. The same assay was called the prethrombin assay when supplemented with purified autoprothrombin C and gave a higher yield of thrombin. This higher yield became proportionately greater as the prothrombin concentration decreased. Something built up in the plasma that was resistant to the generation of thrombin, but formed thrombin in the presence of much autoprothrombin C.

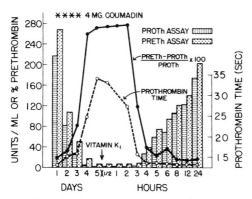

Fig. 8.   A 1.6 kg rabbit was treated with 4 mg coumadin on 4 successive days. Then a single dose of 15 mg vitamin K_1 was given on the fifth day. Histograms represent prethrombin 1 and prothrombin assays. The percentage of prethrombin 1 (prethrombin 1–prothrombin/prothrombin × 100), and the prothrombin time are represented by curves.

A large dose of vitamin K_1 was given intravenously and within 2 hours a response was noted as follows: (a) the material responsive to the prethrombin assay decreased relative to the material responsive to the two-stage assay; (b) the prothrombin time decreased dramatically; and (c) the prothrombin concentration increased over a period of 24 hours. The experiment gives a crude indication of the half-life of prothrombin. The rapid rate of response to vitamin K, and there is evidence that something was in plasma that was difficult to convert to thrombin but did so in the presence of large amounts of autoprothrombin C. This substance, as will now be discussed below, must have been, or at least included, an abnormal prothrombin molecule.

VII. VITAMIN K FUNCTION AND THE STRUCTURE OF PROTHROMBIN

A series of contributions appeared in several laboratories and some of these are referenced (Carlisle *et al.*, 1975; Davidson and MacDonald, 1943; Esmon *et al.*, 1975a,b; Emson and Suttie, 1975; Fernlund and Stenflo, 1975; Ganrot and Niléhn, 1968; Ganrot and Stenflo, 1970; Gitel *et al.*, 1973; Heldebrant *et al.*, 1973; Hemker *et al.*, 1963; Johnston and Olson, 1972; Josso *et al.*, 1968; Malhotra and Carter, 1971; Nelsestuen and Suttie, 1972a,b, 1973; Olsen *et al.*, 1974; Shah and Suttie, 1971, 1972, 1974; Skotland *et al.*, 1974; Stenflo, 1970, 1972, 1973, 1974, 1976; Stenflo and Ganrot, 1972, 1973; Stenflo *et al.*, 1974; Suttie, 1969, 1970, 1973, Walz *et al.*, 1975).

From this work, one can conclude that vitamin K deprivation is associated with the production of an abnormal prothrombin molecule. A previously unrecognized amino acid was discovered in prothrombin (Stenflo *et al.*, 1974; Magnusson *et al.*, 1974; Nelsestuen *et al.*, 1974). This is γ-carboxyglutamic acid. The abnormal prothrombin produced under conditions of partial vitamin K deprivation contains glutamic acid in place of the γ-carboxyglutamic acid. In amino acid analysis of prothrombin, the latter is converted to glutamic acid upon hydrolysis and thus is not detected. The vitamin functions in the mechanics of introducing the carboxyl group after the incomplete prothrombin is synthesized.

Beginning in 1967, Magnusson and his associates worked on determining the amino acid sequence of bovine prothrombin and the complete sequence has been presented (Magnusson *et al.*, 1975a,b). Included was the positioning of the disulfide bonds, as well as locations of carbohydrate (Figs. 9 and 10). In this laboratory we contributed data on the nonthrombin portion of thrombin, as well as for the A chain of thrombin

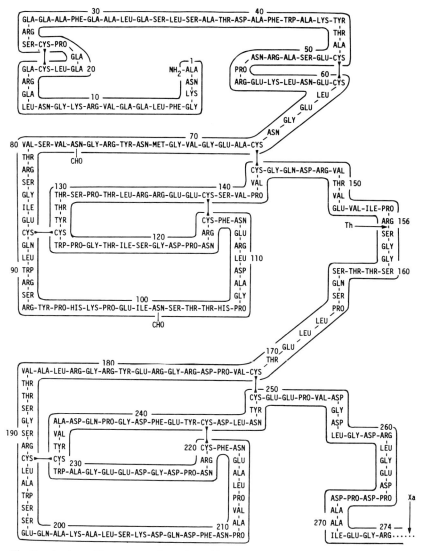

Fig. 9. Amino acid sequence of nonthrombin portion of bovine prothrombin. The first 156 amino acid residues are called the prothrombin fragment 1 portion. The next 118 compose the prothrombin fragment 2. Th = thrombin and Xa = Factor Xa or autoprothrombin C. Note ten γ-carboxyglutamic acid at positions 7, 8, 15, 17, 20, 21, 26, 27, 30, and 33. Data of Reuterby *et al.* (1974), Hewett-Emmett *et al.* (1974, 1975), and Magnusson *et al.* (1974, 1975a,b).

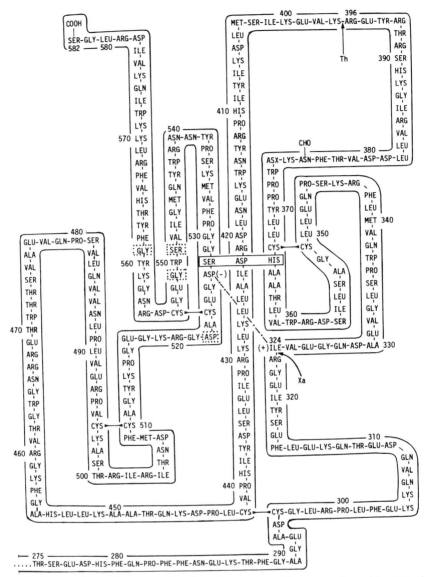

Fig. 10. Amino acid sequence for thrombin portion of bovine prothrombin. Note A chain of 49 residues below, the B1 chain up to residue 397, the Ser, Asp, His active center, and the Ile to Asp salt bridge. Loss of B1 includes active His and the resulting thrombin-E has only esterase activity. B chain structure represents almost exclusively the data of Magnusson *et al.* (1975a,b), and all positions of disulfide bonds in bovine prothrombin originated in that work. Table I gives structure of human prothrombin fragment 1.

(Walz and Seegers, 1974; Walz *et al.*, 1974a; Reuterby *et al.*, 1974; Hewett-Emmett *et al.*, 1974, 1975). Heldebrant and associates (1973) also contributed partial sequences. We are in the process of completing the sequencing of the nonthrombin portion of human prothrombin, and have presented the amino acid sequence of the A chain of human thrombin (Walz and Seegers, 1974).

There are ten γ-carboxyglutamic acid residues in bovine prothrombin located at positions 7, 8, 15, 17, 20, 21, 26, 27, 30, and 33. These are also found in human prothrombin (Table I). These positions have glutamic acid in the abnormal bovine prothrombin isolated from plasma when vitamin K activity is depressed. The γ-carboxyglutamic acid residues are calcium binding sites and function in phospholipid-binding. A complex consisting of prothrombin, Ac–globulin, phospholipid, autoprothrombin C, and calcium ions then constitutes the mixture out of which thrombin activity is generated.

If the bovine prothrombin molecule is degraded to prethrombin 1 by thrombin, the prothrombin fragment 1, with the γ-carboxyglutamic acid residues, is out of the reactions. Nevertheless, like prothrombin, the prethrombin 1 is converted to thrombin in a complex mixture consisting of prethrombin 1, Ac–globulin, phospholipid, autoprothrombin C, and calcium ions. The main difference between the generation of thrombin from prethrombin 1 and prothrombin is the requirements in the larger amounts of procoagulants for prethrombin (Baker and Seegers, 1967; Barthels and Seegers, 1969; Seegers *et al.*, 1972). Prethrombin 1 requires much more autoprothrombin C and Ac–globulin than prothrombin. If the purified prothrombin fragment 1 is added to the prethrombin activation mixture, it functions as an accelerator (Seegers *et al.*, 1976). It serves its function without being covalently bound as it is in prothrombin. It is not correct to say (Magnusson *et al.*, 1975a) that prethrombin 1 is not further activated to thrombin. Unfortunately, there is really very little information on the activation of the abnormal Dicumarol-induced prothrombin. Malholtra (1975) has published an abstract and wrote to me as follows: "I have had difficulty in convincing others that thrombin can be generated from Dicumarol-induced atypical prothrombin by biological accelerators. As a matter of fact, some of the reviewers thought that bioactivities of atypical proteins could be due to the presence or normal prothrombin molecules in our purified preparations. In view of this predicament, your recent letter is a great source of encouragement and confidence. I am, therefore, very grateful to you." Presumably, the other vitamin K-dependent proteins also have their function impaired but not completely lost during vitamin K deficiency.

TABLE I
Comparison of Amino Acid Sequences of Human and Bovine Prothrombin Fragment 1[a]

	1	2	3	4	5	6	7	8	9	10	11	12	13	14	15
NH₂-	Ala	-Asn-			Thr-	Phe	-Leu-	Gla	-Gla-	Val	-Arg-	Lys	-Gly-	Asn	-Leu-Gla-
NH₂-	Ala	-Asn-	Lys	-Gly-	Phe	-Leu-	Gla	-Gla-	Val	-Arg-	Lys	-Gly-	Asn	-Leu-Gla-	

	16	17	18	19	20	21	22	23	24	25	26	27	28	29	30
H:	Arg	-Gla-	Cys	-Val-	Gla	-Gla-	Thr	-Cys-	Ser	-Tyr-	Gla	-Gla-	Ala	-Phe-Gla-	
B:	Arg	-Gla-	Cys	-Leu-	Gla	-Gla-	Pro	-Cys-	Ser	-Arg-	Gla	-Gla-	Ala	-Phe-Gla-	

	31	32	33	34	35	36	37	38	39	40	41	42	43	44	45
H:	Ala	-Leu-	Gla	-Ser-	Ser	-Gly-	Ala	-Thr-	Asp	-Val-	Phe	-Trp-	Ala	-Lys-	Tyr-
B:	Ala	-Leu-	Gla	-Ser-	Leu	-Ser-	Ala	-Thr-	Asp	-Ala-	Phe	-Trp-	Ala	-Lys-	Tyr-

	46	47	48	49	50	51	52	53	54	55	56	57	58	59	60
H:	Thr	-Ala-	Cys	-Glu-	Thr	-Ala-	Arg	-Thr-	Pro	-Arg-	Asp	-Lys-	Leu	-Ala-	Ala-
B:	Thr	-Ala-	Cys	-Glu-	Ser	-Ala-	Arg	-Asn-	Pro	-Arg-	Glu	-Lys-	Leu	-Asn-	Glu-

	61	62	63	64	65	66	67	68	69	70	71	72	73	74	75
H:	Cys	-Leu-	Glu	-Gly-	Asn	-Cys-	Ala	-Glu-	Gly	-Leu-	Gly	-Thr-	Asn	-Tyr-Arg-	
B:	Cys	-Leu-	Glu	-Gly-	Asn	-Cys-	Ala	-Glu-	Gly	-Val-	Gly	-Met-	Asn	-Tyr-Arg-	

	76	77	78	79	80	81	82	83	84	85	86	87	88	89	90
H:	Gly	-Asn-	Val	-Ser-	Ile	-Thr-	Arg	-Ser-	Gly	-Ile-	Glu	-Cys-	Gln	-Leu-Trp-	
B:	Gly	-Asn-	Val	-Ser-	Val	-Thr-	Arg	-Ser-	Gly	-Ile-	Glu	-Cys-	Gln	-Leu-Trp-	

	91	92	93	94	95	96	97	98	99	100	101	102	103	104	105
H:	Arg	-Ser-	Arg	-Tyr-	Pro	-His-	Lys	-Pro-	Glu	-Ile-	Asn	-Ser-	Thr	-Thr-His-	
B:	Arg	-Ser-	Arg	-Tyr-	Pro	-His-	Lys	-Pro-	Glu	-Ile-	Asn	-Ser-	Thr	-Thr-His-	

	106	107	108	109	110	111	112	113	114	115	116	117	118	119	120
H:	Pro	-Gly-	Ala	-Asp-	Leu	-Gln-	Glu	-Asn-	Phe	-Cys-	Arg	-Asn-	Pro	-Asp-Ser-	
B:	Pro	-Gly-	Ala	-Asp-	Leu	-Arg-	Glu	-Asn-	Phe	-Cys-	Arg	-Asn-	Pro	-Asp-Gly-	

	121	122	123	124	125	126	127	128	129	130	131	132	133	134	135
H:	Ser	-Ile-	Thr	-Gly-	Pro	-Trp-	Cys	-Tyr-	Thr	-Thr-	Asp	-Pro-	Thr	-Ala-	Arg-
B:	Ser	-Ile-	Thr	-Gly-	Pro	-Trp-	Cys	-Tyr-	Thr	-Thr-	Ser	-Pro-	Thr	-Leu-	Arg-

	136	137	138	139	140	141	142	143	144	145	146	147	148	149	150
H:	Arg	-Gln-	Glu	-Cys-	Ser	-Thr-	Pro	-Val-	Cys	-Gly-	Gln	-Asp-	Gln	-Val-	Thr-
B:	Arg	-Glu-	Glu	-Cys-	Ser	-Val-	Pro	-Val-	Cys	-Gly-	Gln	-Asp-	Arg	-Val-	Thr-

(continued)

TABLE I, *continued*

151	152	153	154	155	156

H: Val -*Met*- Val -*Thr*- Pro -Arg-COOH
B: Val -*Glu*- Val -*Ile*- Pro -Arg-COOH

a The numbering system corresponds to bovine (B) profragment 1. A single deletion occurs in human (H) profragment 1 at residue 4. Underlined residues correspond to the differences between the two species. γ-Carboxyglutamic acid residues are designated Gla. Carbohydrate is attached to aspartic acid at positions #77 and 101 of both the bovine and human fragments. Unpublished data from this laboratory by Daniel A. Walz, David Hewett-Emmett, and Walter H. Seegers.

The γ-carboxyglutamic acids in human prothrombin fragment 1 are at exactly the same place as in the bovine species (Table I). Presumably, they function exactly as has been found with bovine material. In the human protein, there are 155 amino acid residues in place of 156, because of a deletion and substitution at positions 3 and 4. In other parts of the molecule, there is remarkable similarity between human and bovine prothrombin fragment 1.

VIII. FIVE DISTINCT VITAMIN K-DEPENDENT MOLECULES

At the midcentury period, when prothrombin was known to require vitamin K for its synthesis, four other activities became recognized as being vitamin K-dependent. These activities were all present in my prothrombin preparation, which appeared to be homogeneous by the criteria available for testing at that time. I, therefore, postulated that these activities were derived from a single prothrombin molecule (Seegers, 1962). This was especially likely because treatment of the prothrombin preparation inactivated the prothrombin (it formed prethrombin 1) and other activities appeared. Today, we know that activities were derived from prothrombin fragments and also from separate molecules distinct from prothrombin, but having homology in their amino acid sequence (Enfield *et al.*, 1974, 1975; Fujikawa *et al.*, 1973; McCoy *et al.*, 1973; Titani *et al.*, 1972, 1975). The molecules do not come from prothrombin, but we can postulate a common ancestral gene which once coded for a protein. By genetic divergence, eventually five proteins were produced.

To see whether there would be five distinct proteins by the criterion of immunology, we prepared each one except Factor VII in purified form

TABLE II
Bovine Antibodies Tested against Antigens[a,b]

Antigens	Prothrombin	Prethrombin 1	Profragment 1	Profragment 2	Thrombin	Auto-III	Auto-II-A	Protein C	Factor IX	Plasma	Serum	Plasma[c]
Prothrombin	+	±	+	±	−	−			−	+	+	±
Prethrombin 1	±	+	±	±	±	−			−	+	+	+
Profragment 1	+	±	+	±	−	−			−	+	+	±
Profragment 2	±	+	±	+	−	−			−	+	+	+
Thrombin	−	±	−	−	+	−			−	+	−	−
Auto-III	−	−	−	−	−	+			−	+	+	−
Auto-II-A	−	−	−	−	−	−	+	+	−	+	+	−
Protein C	−	−	−	−	−	−	+	+	−	+	+	−
Factor IX	−	−	−	−	−	−			+	+	+	−

[a] Immunology data by Houria I. Hassouna, and proteins prepared by Eduardo Novoa and Daniel A. Walz.
[b] ±, Partial identity; +, identity; −, no identity (cross reaction).
[c] Plasma three times adsorbed with barium carbonate.

(Novoa *et al.*, 1976). These preparations were most likely of the best quality ever prepared and were used to immunize rabbits. Not a single one of the antibodies recognized another one of the vitamin K-dependent proteins (Table II). We feel that this generalization could have included Factor VII, if we had tested it, and because other reactions of the antibodies with plasma were consistent with that conclusion. There are, thus, at least five immunologically distinct vitamin K-dependent proteins.

It is not the purpose to extend this discussion (Table II), but it can be stated that prothrombin has at least four antigenic determinant sites, one of these is probably covered because the antibody to thrombin does not recognize prothrombin nor does the antibody to prothrombin recognize thrombin. On the other hand, prothrombin, prethrombin 1, prothrombin fragment 1, and prothrombin fragment 2 show cross reactions. These can, in part, be accounted for on the basis of internal homology in prothrombin (Fig. 6).

IX. SOME POSSIBILITIES AND NEEDS FOR INVESTIGATION

The prothrombin molecule has been in the vanguard of the search for information about the function of vitamin K. There are many uncertainties about the activation of the Dicumarol-induced prothrombin. It is readily activated by *Echis carinatus* venom, and that fact was properly used as an experimental convenience. Activation studies with clotting factors are needed. How will it activate in 25% sodium citrate solution? If the molecule is devoid of γ-carboxyglutamic acid residues, it probably can be converted to thrombin with autoprothrombin C alone or with the enzyme plus accessories. Perhaps autoprothrombin C without γ-carboxyglutamic acid residues can also be isolated to find out how those residues function (Nelsestuen *et al.*, 1974). The Dicumarol-induced prothrombin was usually isolated from animals given a dose that lowered the plasma concentration of prothrombin only partially. Perhaps higher doses would be associated with reduction of even the abnormal prothrombin. In the case of some preliminary experiments with dogs, prolonged administration of coumadin in large amounts removed entirely the prothrombin complex as measured and detected by immunological techniques. The nature of species variation is not entirely decided by the fact that human and bovine prothrombin have the same γ-carboxyglutamic acid residues at the same position. The isolation of the other four vitamin K-dependent proteins in abnormal form should be possible, and their function would thus serve as models for information on modified enzymes and proenzymes.

I have not discussed the role of vitamin K in the incorporation of carbohydrate. This aspect has received much attention (Pereira and Couri, 1971, 1972a,b).

A valuable old nutrition experiment from this laboratory is related to blood coagulation and has apparently been forgotten (Guest *et al.*, 1947). Chickens were placed on a diet deficient in pteroylglutamic acid and developed an increase in antiplasmin activity. This increase was prevented by feeding the crystalline vitamin. This probably correlates with the fact that methotrexate is an inhibitor of folic acid and a well known neoplastic suppressant, used with much success as a chemotherapeutic agent in the treatment of neoplastic trophoblastic diseases (Hertz *et al.*, 1958, 1961). I suggest that the therapy is also associated with an increased inhibitor titer which retards fibrinolysis. In the opposite direction, the observations of Reich (1975) deal with facts related to increased fibrinolysis. He finds that tumor cells have an increased production of plasminogen activator in neoplasia. Similarly, we find that autoprothrombin II-A promotes fibrinolysis by depressing inhibitors of fibrinolysis. This opens the possibility that Dicumarol and related compounds, by decreasing Protein C concentration, do not favor fibrinolysis.

The function of vitamin K in the carboxylation of glutamic acid is aided by the use of radioactive bicarbonate (Esmon *et al.*, 1975a). It is only logical to suppose that enzymes are involved, and that the vitamin itself might be modified during its function. The question has been raised whether vitamin K participates in the metabolism of normal bone development, on the basis that γ-carboxyglutamate was identified in proteins isolated from mineralized tissue (Hauschka *et al.*, 1975). Protein containing the amino acid has also been found in pathologically mineralized kidney stones (Lian and Prien, 1976). All this points in the direction of an increased interest in vitamin K.

ACKNOWLEDGMENT

This work was supported by research grant HL 03424-19 from the National Heart and Lung Institute, National Institutes of Health, U.S. Public Health Service. I am grateful to Dr. Houria I. Hassouna for her assistance with the references and discussion.

REFERENCES

Baker, W. J., and Seegers, W. H. (1967). The conversion of prethrombin to thrombin. *Thromb. Diath. Haemorrh.* **17,** 205-213.

Barthels, M., and Seegers, W. H. (1969). Substitution of lipids with bile salts in the formation of thrombin. *Thromb. Diath. Haemorrh.* **22,** 13-27.

Biggs, R., ed. (1972). "Human Blood Coagulation, Haemostasis and Thrombosis." Blackwell, Oxford.

Bradshaw, R. A., and Wessler, S., eds. (1975). " Heparin. Structure, Function and Clinical Implications," Adv. Exp. Med. Biol., Vol. 52. Plenum, New York.

Campbell, H. A., and Link, K. P. (1941). Studies on the hemorrhagic sweet clover disease. IV. The isolation and crystallization of the hemorrhagic agent. *J. Biol. Chem.* **138,** 21-33.

Carlisle, T. L., Shah, D. V., Schlegel, R., and Suttie, J. W. (1975). Plasma abnormal prothrombin and microsomal prothrombin precursor in various species (38492). *Proc. Soc. Exp. Biol. Med.* **148,** 140-144.

Dam, H. (1929). Cholesterinstoffwechsel in Hühnereiern und Hühnchen. *Biochem. Z.* **215,** 475-492.

Dam, H. (1935). The antihaemorrhagic vitamin of the chick. *Biochem. J.* **29,** 1273-1285.

Dam, H., Schønheyder, F., and Tage-Hansen, E. (1936). Studies on the mode of action of vitamin K. *Biochem. J.* **30,** 1075-1079.

Dam, H., Geiger, A., and Glavind, J. (1939). Isolierung des Vitamins K in hochgereinigter Form. *Helv. Chim. Acta* **22,** 310-313.

Davidson, C. S., and MacDonald, H. (1943). The effect of vitamin K_1 oxide on hypoprothrombinemia induced by dicoumarol. *N. Engl. J. Med.* **229,** 353-355.

Doisy, E. A., MacCorquadale, D. W., Thayer, S. A. *et al.* (1939). The isolation, constitution and synthesis of vitamin K_1. *Science* **90,** 407 (abstr.).

Dombrose, F. A., Seegers, W. H., and Sedensky, J. A. (1971). Inhibition of thrombin and autoprothrombin C (F-Xa) as a mutual depletion system. *Thromb, Diath. Haemorrh.* **26,** 103-123.

Enfield, D. L., Ericsson, L. H., Fujikawa, K., Titani, K., Walsh, K. A., and Neurath, H.

(1974). Bovine factor IX (Christmas factor). Further evidence of homology with factor X (Stuart factor) and prothrombin. *FEBS Lett.* **47**, 132–135.

Enfield, D. L., Ericsson, L. H., Walsh, K. A., Neurath, H., and Titani, K. (1975). Bovine factor X_1 (Stuart factor). Primary structure of the light chain. *Proc. Natl. Acad. Sci. U.S.A.* **72**, 16–19.

Esmon, C. T., and Suttie, J. W. (1975). The functional significance of vitamin K action. Difference in phospholipid binding between normal and abnormal prothrombin. *J. Biol. Chem.* **250**, 4095–4099.

Esmon, C. T., Sadowski, J. A., and Suttie, J. W. (1975a). A new carboxylation reaction. The vitamin K-dependent incorporation of $H^{14}CO_3^-$ into prothrombin. *J. Biol. Chem.* **250**, 4744–4748.

Esmon, C. T., Grant, G. A., and Suttie, J. W. (1975b). Purification of an apparent rat liver prothrombin precursor: Characterization and comparison to normal rat prothrombin. *Biochemistry* **14**, 1595–1600.

Fearnley, G. R. (1965). "Fibrinolysis." Williams & Wilkins, Baltimore, Maryland.

Fernlund, P., and Stenflo, J. (1975). Vitamin K and the biosynthesis of prothrombin. V. γ-carboxyglutamic acids, the vitamin K-dependent structures in prothrombin. *J. Biol. Chem.* **250**, 6125–6133.

Fujikawa, K., Coan, M. H., Enfield, D. L., Titani, K., Ericsson, L. H., and Davie, E. W. (1973). A comparison of bovine prothrombin, factor IX (Christmas factor), and factor X (Stuart factor). *Proc. Natl. Acad. Sci. U.S.A.* **71**, 427–430.

Ganrot, P. O., and Niléhn, J. E. (1968). Plasma prothrombin during treatment with dicumarol. II. Demonstration of an abnormal prothrombin fraction. *Scand. J. Clin. Lab. Invest.* **22**, 23–28.

Ganrot, P. O., and Stenflo, J. (1970). Prothrombin derivatives in human serum. Isolation and some properties of the non-thrombin fragments. *Scand. J. Clin. Lab. Invest.* **26**, 161–168.

Gitel, S. N., Owen, W. G., Esmon, C. T., and Jackson, C. M. (1973). A polypeptide region of bovine prothrombin specific for binding phospholipids. *Proc. Natl. Acad. Sci. U.S.A.* **70**, 1344–1348.

Guest, M. M., Ware, A. G., and Seegers, W. H. (1947). A quantitative study of antifibrinolysis in chick plasma: Increase in antifibrinolysin activity during pteroylglutamic acid deficiency. *Am. J. Physiol.* **150**, 661–669.

Hauschka, P. V., Lian, J. B., and Gallop, P. M. (1975). Direct identification of the calcium binding amino acid, γ-carboxyglutamate, in mineralized tissue. *Proc. Natl. Acad. Sci. U.S.A.* **72**, 3925–3929.

Heldebrant, C. M., Noyes, C., Kingdom, H. S., and Mann, K. G. (1973). The activation of prothrombin. III. The partial amino acid sequences at the amino terminal of prothrombin and the intermediates of activation *Biochem. Biophys. Res. Commun.* **54**, 155–160.

Hemker, H. C., Veltkamp, J. J., Hensen, A., and Loeliger, E. A. (1963). Nature of prothrombin biosynthesis preprothrombinaeia in vitamin K deficiency. *Nature (London)* **200**, 589–590.

Henriksen, R. A., and Jackson, C. M. (1975). Cooperative calcium binding by the phospholipid binding region of bovine prothrombin: A requirement for intact disulfide bridges. *Arch. Biochem. Biophys.* **170**, 149–159.

Hertz, R., Bergenstal, D. M., Lipsett, M. B., Price, E. G., and Hilbish, T. (1958). Chemotherapy of choriocarcinoma and related trophoblastic tumors in women. *J. Am. Med. Assoc.* **168**, 845–854.

Hertz, R., Lewis, J., Jr., and Lipsett, M. B. (1961). Five years experience with the chemotherapy of metastatic choriocarcinoma and related trophoblastic tumors in women. *Am. J. Obstet. Gynecol.* **82,** 631–640.

Hewett-Emmett, D., McCoy, L. E., Hassouna, H. I., Reuterby, J., Walz, D. A., and Seegers, W. H. (1974). A partial gene duplication in the evolution of prothrombin? *Thromb. Res.* **5,** 421–430.

Hewett-Emmett, D., Walz, D. A., Reuterby, J., McCoy, L. E., and Seegers, W. H. (1975). The amino acid sequence of PR fragment (NH₂-terminal fragment) of bovine prothrombin. *Thromb. Res.* **7,** 227–234.

Johnson, S. A., ed. (1971). "The Circulating Platelet." Academic Press, New York.

Johnston, M. F. M., and Olson, R. E. (1972). Studies of prothrombin biosynthesis in cell-free systems. III. Regulation by vitamin K and warfarin of prothrombin biosynthesis in rat liver microsomes. *J. Biol. Chem.* **247,** 4001–4007.

Josso, F., Lavergne, J. M., Gouault, M., Prou-Wartelle, O., and Soulier, J. P. (1968). Differents états moléculaires du facteur II (prothrombine). Leur étude à l'aide de la staphylocoagulase et d'anticorps anti-facteur II. I. Le facteur II chez les sujets traités par les antagonistes de la vitamin K. *Thromb. Diath. Haemorrh.* **20,** 88–98.

Koch-Weser, J., and Sellers, E. M. (1971a). Drug interactions with coumarin anticoagulants. (First of two parts.) *N. Engl. J. Med.* **285,** 487–498.

Koch-Weser, J., and Sellers, E. M. (1971b). Drug interactions with coumarin anticoagulants. (Second of two parts.) *N. Engl. J. Med.* **285,** 547–558.

Lian, J. B., and Prien, E. L., Jr. (1976). γ-Carboxyglutamic acid in the calcium binding matrix of certain kidney stones. *Fed. Proc., Fed. Am. Soc. Exp. Biol.* **35,** 1763 (abstr.).

Link, K. P. (1944). The anticoagulant from spoiled sweet clover hay. *Harvey Lect.* **39,** 162–216.

McCoy, L. E., Walz, D. A., Agrawal, B. B. L., and Seegers, W. H. (1973). Isolation of L-chain polypeptide of autoprothrombin III (factor X): Homology with prothrombin indicated. *Thromb. Res.* **2,** 293–296.

Magnusson, S., Sottrup-Jensen, L., Petersen, T. E., Morris, H. R., and Dell, A. (1974). Primary sturcture of the vitamin K-dependent part of prothrombin. *FEBS Lett.* **44,** 189–193.

Magnusson, S., Petersen, T. E., Sottrup-Jensen, L., and Claeys, H. (1975a). Complete primary structure of prothrombin: Isolation, structure and reactivity of ten carboxylated glutamic acid residues and regulation of prothrombin activation by thrombin. *In* "Proteases and Biological Control" (E. Reich, D. B. Rifkin, and E. Shaw, eds.), pp. 123–149. Cold Spring Harbor Lab., Cold Spring Harbor, New York.

Magnusson, S., Sottrup-Jensen, L., Petersen, T. E., and Claeys, H. (1975b). The primary structure of prothrombin, the role of vitamin K in blood coagulation and a thrombin catalyzed "negative feed-back" control mechanism for limiting the activation of prothrombin. *In* "Prothrombin and Related Coagulation Factors" (H. C. Hemker and J. J. Veltkamp, eds.), pp. 25–46. Leiden Univ. Press, Leiden, The Netherlands.

Malhotra, O. P. (1975). Radioactivity of dicoumarol-induced prothrombins. *Fed. Proc., Fed. Am. Soc. Exp. Biol.* **34,** 221 (abstr.).

Malhotra, O. P., and Carter, J. R. (1971). Isolation and purification of prothrombin from dicoumarolized steers. *J. Biol. Chem.* **246,** 2665–2671.

Mammen, E. F., Thomas, W. R., and Seegers, W. H. (1960). Activation of purified prothrombin to autoprothrombin I or autoprothrombin II (platelet cofactor II) or autoprothrombin II-A. *Thromb. Diath. Haemorrh.* **5,** 218–217.

Marciniak, E. (1970). Coagulation inhibition elicited by thrombin. *Science* **170,** 452–453.

Müller-Berghaus, G., and Seegers, W. H. (1966). Some effects of purified autoprothrombin C in blood clotting. *Thromb. Diath. Haemorrh.* **16,** 707–722.

Murano, G., Seegers, W. H., and Zolton, R. P. (1974). Autoprothrombin II-A: A competitive inhibitor of autoprothrombin C. (factor Xa). A review with additions. *Thromb. Diath. Haemorrh., Suppl.* **57**, 305–314.

Nelsestuen, G. L., and Suttie, J. W. (1972a). Mode of action of vitamin K. Calcium binding properties of bovine prothrombin. *Biochemistry* **11**, 4961–4964.

Nelsestuen, G. L., and Suttie, J. W. (1972b). The purification and properties of an abnormal prothrombin protein produced by dicoumarol-treated cows. A comparison to normal prothrombin. *J. Biol. Chem.* **247**, 8176–8182.

Nelsestuen, G. L., and Suttie, J. W. (1973). The mode of action of vitamin K. Isolation of a peptide containing the vitamin K-dependent portion of prothrombin. *Proc. Natl. Acad. Sci. U.S.A.* **70**, 3366–3370.

Nelsestuen, G. L., Zytkovicz, T. H., and Howard, J. B. (1974). γ-Carboxyglutamic acid. Identification and distribution in vitamin K-dependent proteins. *Mayo Clin. Proc.* **49**, 941–944.

Novoa, E., Seegers, W. H., and Hassouna, H. I. (1976). Improved procedures for the purification of selected vitamin K-dependent proteins. *Prep. Biochem.* **6**, 307–338.

Olson, R. E. (1975). New concepts relating to the mode of action of vitamin K. *Vitam. Horm. (N.Y.)* **32**, 483–511.

Olson, R. E., Kipfer, R. K., Morrissey, J. J., and Goodman, S. R. (1974). Function of vitamin K in prothrombin synthesis. *Thromb. Diath. Haemorrh., Suppl.* **57**, 31–44.

Overman, R. S., Stahmann, M. A., and Link, K. P. (1942). Studies on the hemorrhagic sweet clover disease. VIII. The effect of 2-methyl-1,4-naphthoquinone and L-ascorbic acid upon the action of 3,3′-methylenebis (4-hydroxycoumarin) on the prothrombin time of rabbits. *J. Biol. Chem.* **145**, 155–162.

Owen, C. A. (1974). The discoveries of vitamin K and dicumarol and their impact on our concepts of blood coagulation. *Mayo Clin. Proc.* **49**, 912–917.

Pereira, M. A., and Couri, D. (1971). Studies on the site of action of dicoumarol on prothrombin biosynthesis. *Biochim. Biophys. Acta* **237**, 348–355.

Pereira, M. A., and Couri, D. (1972a). Effect of dicoumarol on rat liver slice glycoprotein synthesis. *Experientia* **28**, 1170–1171.

Pereira, M. A., and Couri, C. (1972b). Site of inhibition by dicoumarol of prothrombin biosynthesis: Carbohydrate content of prothrombin from dicoumarol-treated rats. *Biochim. Biophys. Acta* **261**, 375–378.

Quick, A. J. (1942). "The Hemorrhagic Diseases and the Physiology of Hemostasis." Thomas, Springfield, Illinois.

Reich, E. (1975). Plasminogen activator: Secretion by neoplastic cells and macrophages. *In* "Proteases and Biological Control" (E. Reich, D. B. Rifkin, and E. Shaw, eds.), pp. 333–341. Cold Spring Harbor Lab., Cold Spring Harbor, New York.

Reich, E., Rifkin, D. B., and Shaw, E., eds. (1975). "Proteases and Biological Control." Cold Spring Harbor Lab., Cold Spring Harbor, New York.

Reuterby, J., Walz, D. A., McCoy, L. E., and Seegers, W. H. (1974). Amino acid sequence of 0 fragment of bovine prothrombin. *Thromb. Res.* **4**, 885–890.

Roderick, L. M. (1929). The pathology of sweet clover disease in cattle. *J. Am. Vet. Med. Assoc.* **74**, 314–326.

Roderick, L. M. (1931). A problem in the coagulation of the blood: "Sweet clover disease of cattle." *Am. J. Physiol.* **96**, 413–425.

Schofield, F. W. (1922). A brief account of a disease in cattle simulating hemorrhagic septicaemia due to feeding sweet clover. *Can. Vet. Rec.* **3**, 74–78.

Schofield, F. W. (1924). Damaged sweet clover: The cause of a new disease in cattle simulating hemorrhagic septicemia and black leg. *J. Am. Vet. Med. Assoc.* **64**, 553–572.

Seegers, W. H. (1962). "Prothrombin." Harvard Univ. Press, Cambridge, Massachusetts.

Seegers, W. H., ed. (1967). "Blood Clotting Enzymology." Academic Press, New York.

Seegers, W. H., Sakuragawa, N., McCoy, L. E., Sedensky, J. A., and Dombrose, F. A. (1972). Prothrombin activation: Ac-globulin, lipid, platelet membrane, and auto-prothrombin C (factor Xa) requirements. *Thromb. Res.* **1**, 293–310.

Seegers, W. H., Hassouna, H. I., Hewett-Emmett, D., Walz, D. A., and Andary, T. J. (1975). Prothrombin and thrombin: Selected aspects of thrombin formation, properties, inhibition, and immunology. *Semin. Thromb. Hemost.* **1**, 211–283.

Seegers, W. H., Novoa, E., Walz, D. A., Andary, T. J., and Hassouna, H. I. (1976). Effects of prothrombin fragments on thrombin, on thrombin formation, and separation from Ac-globulin (factor V). *Thromb. Res.* **8**, 83–97.

Shah, D. V., and Suttie, J. W. (1971). Mechanism of action of vitamin K: Evidence for the conversion of a precursor protein to prothrombin in the rat. *Proc. Natl. Acad. Sci. U.S.A.* **68**, 1653–1657.

Shah, D. V., and Suttie, J. W. (1972). The effect of vitamin K and warfarin on rat liver prothrombin concentrations. *Arch. Biochem. Biophys.* **150**, 91–95.

Shah, D. V., and Suttie, J. W. (1974). The vitamin K dependent, in vitro production of prothrombin. *Biochem. Biophys. Res. Commun.* **60**, 1397–1402.

Shah, D. V., Suttie, J. W., and Grant, G. A. (1973). A rat liver protein with potential thrombin activity: Properties and partial purification. *Arch. Biochem. Biophys.* **159**, 483–491.

Skotland, T., Holm, T., Østerud, B., Flengsrud, R., and Prydz, H. (1974). The localization of a vitamin K-induced modification in an N-terminal fragment of human prothrombin. *Biochem. J.* **143**, 29–37.

Stahmann, M. A., Hubner, C. F., and Link, K. P. (1941). Studies on the hemorrhagic sweet clover disease. V. Identification and synthesis of the hemorrhagic agent. *J. Biol. Chem.* **138**, 513–527.

Stenflo, J. (1970). Dicoumarol-induced prothrombin in bovine plasma. *Acta. Chem. Scand.* **24**, 3762–3763.

Stenflo, J. (1972). Vitamin K and the biosynthesis of prothrombin. II. Structural comparison of normal and dicoumarol induced bovine prothrombin. *J. Biol. Chem.* **247**, 8167–8175.

Stenflo, J. 1973. Vitamin K and the biosynthesis of prothrombin. III. Structural comparison of an NH$_2$-terminal fragment from normal and from dicoumarol-induced bovine prothrombin. *J. Biol. Chem.* **248**, 6325–6332.

Stenflo, J. (1974). Vitamin K and the biosynthesis of prothrombin. IV. Isolation of peptides containing prosthetic groups from normal prothrombin and the corresponding peptides from dicoumarol-induced prothrombin. *J. Biol. Chem.* **249**, 5527–5535.

Stenflo, J. (1976). A new vitamin K-dependent protein. Purification from bovine plasma and preliminary characterization. *J. Biol. chem.* **251**, 355–363.

Stenflo, J., and Ganrot, P. O. (1972). Vitamin K and the biosynthesis of prothrombin. I. Identification and purification of a dicoumarol-induced abnormal prothrombin from bovine plasma. *J. Biol. Chem.* **247**, 8160–8166.

Stenflo, J., and Ganrot, P. O. (1973). Binding of Ca^{2+} to normal and dicoumarol-induced prothrombin. *Biochem. Biophys. Res. Commun.* **50**, 98–104.

Stenflo, J., Fernlund, P., Egan, W., and Roepstorff, P. (1974). Vitamin K dependent modifications of glutamic acid residues in prothrombin. *Proc. Natl. Acad. Sci. U.S.A.* **71**, 2730–2733.

Suttie, J. W. (1969). Control of clotting factor biosynthesis by vitamin K. *Fed. Proc., Fed. Am. Soc. Exp. Biol.* **28**, 1696–1701.

Suttie, J. W. (1970). The effect of cycloheximide administration on vitamin K-stimulated prothrombin formation. *Arch. Biochem. Biophys.* **141,** 571–578.

Suttie, J. W. (1973). Vitamin K and prothrombin synthesis. *Nutr. Rev.* **31,** 105–109.

Suttie, J. W., Grant, G. A., Esmon, C. T., and Shah, D. V. (1974). Post ribosomal function of vitamin K in prothrombin synthesis. *Mayo Clin. Proc.* **49,** 933–940.

Titani, K., Hermodson, M. A., Fujikawa, K., Ericsson, L. H., Walsh, K. A., Neurath, H., and Davie, E. W. (1972). Bovine factor X_{1a} (activated Stuart factor). Evidence of homology with mammalian serine proteases. *Biochemistry* **11,** 4899–4903.

Titani, K., Fujikawa, K., Enfield, D. L., Ericsson, L. H., Walsh, K. A., and Neurath, H. (1975). Bovine factor X_1 (Stuart factor): Amino acid sequence of heavy chain. *Proc. Natl. Acad. Sci. U.S.A.* **72,** 3082–3088.

Walz, D. A., and Seegers, W. H. (1974). Amino acid sequence of human thrombin A chain. *Biochem. Biophys. Res. Commun.* **60,** 717–722.

Walz, D. A., Seegers, W. H., Hassouna, H. I., and Reuterby, J. (1974a). Human and bovine prothrombin similarities. *Thromb. Res.* **4,** 875–878.

Walz, D. A., Kipfer, R. K., Jones, J. P., and Olson, R. E. (1974b). Purification and properties of chicken prothrombin. *Arch. Biochem. Biophys.* **164,** 527–535.

Walz, D. A., Kipfer, R. K., and Olson, R. E. (1975). Effect of vitamin K deficiency, warfarin, and inhibitors of protein synthesis upon the plasma levels of vitamin K dependent clotting factors in the chick. *J. Nutr.* **105,** 972–981.

Wintrobe, M. M. (1974). "Clinical Hematology." Lea & Febiger, Philadelphia, Pennsylvania.

Zolton, R. P., and Seegers, W. H. (1973). Autoprothrombin II-A: Thrombin removal and mechanism of induction of fibrinolysis. *Thromb. Res.* **3,** 23–33.

26

Vitamin D: Metabolism, Drug Interactions and Therapeutic Applications in Humans

Abbreviations

PTH   parathyroid hormone
CT   calcitonin
CaBP   calcium-binding protein
25-(OH)D_3 25-hydroxyvitamin D_3 or 25-hydroxycholecalciferol

25-(OH)D$_2$ 25-hydroyvitamin D$_2$ or 25-hydroxyergocalciferol
1,25-(OH)$_2$D$_3$ 1,25-dihydroxyvitamin D$_3$ or 1,25-dihydroxycholecalciferol
1,25-(OH)$_2$D$_2$ 1,25-dihydroxyvitamin D$_2$ or 1,25-dihydroxyergocalciferol
1α-(OH)D$_3$ 1α-hydroxyvitamin D$_3$ or 1α-hydroxycholecaliferol
1α-OHase   25-hydroxyvitamin D-1α-hydroxylase
24,25-(OH)$_2$D$_3$ 24,25-dihydroxyvitamin D$_3$
1,24,25-(OH)$_3$D$_3$ 1,24,25-trihydroxyvitamin D$_3$.
          When no subscript is present after the D, both D$_2$ and D$_3$ are implied.
    S.m.   Solanum malacoxylon.

I. INTRODUCTION

Major advances have been achieved in the past decade in the quest to delineate the metabolism and mechanism of action of vitamin D. These discoveries have considerably enhanced our understanding of a variety of metabolic bone diseases and have illuminated a new endocrine pathway comprised of the controlled metabolism of vitamin D to a novel sterol hormone and the action of this hormone at target cells to regulate the transport of calcium and phosphate. Thus vitamin D is actually a prohormone, which under appropriate physiologic conditions is converted metabolically into its hormonal product. This product affects vitamin D-responsive tissues, such as intestine, bone and kidney, to promote extracellular calcium and phosphorus homeostasis as well as skeletal integrity.

The prevention of rickets involves the maintenance of the ion product of calcium and phosphate in the blood at a level which is consistent with normal bone mineralization. Although the endoskeleton contains 99% of the body's calcium, the other 1% which is present in the extracellular fluids serves many important functions and must be stringently regulated. Calcium plays a role in some of life's most fundamental processes such as nerve conduction, muscle contraction, blood clotting, enzyme catalysis and hormone release. Figure 1 illustrates the control of plasma calcium via the interplay of vitamin D, parathyroid hormone (PTH), and calcitonin (CT) at three organs: intestine, bone, and kidney. Plasma calcium is maintained at 10 mg% primarily via absorption from the diet, a process which is dependent upon vitamin D. The vitamin also acts in concert with PTH to mediate the resorption of calcium from bone and kidney, but these actions of vitamin D are less well understood than its classic operation on intestinal calcium absorption. Should plasma calcium fall below 10 mg%, the parathyroid glands release PTH which functions as a (rapidly acting) calcium raising hormone. Should hypercalcemia ensue, CT from the thyroid acts as the mirror-image hormone

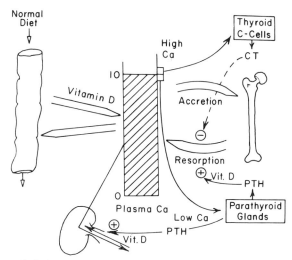

Fig. 1. Control of plasma calcium. Adapted from Copp (1968), by courtesy of Excerpta Medica Foundation.

of PTH and inhibits calcium mobilization from bone. The net result of these controlling actions is the strict maintenance of plasma calcium at the normal level. Vitamin D is essential in this homeostatic system as well as in the control of extracellular phosphate, accounting for the pivotal position of this sterol in regulating skeletal and mineral metabolism.

Man's main natural supply of vitamin D is not derived from his diet (Harrison and Harrison, 1975) and his dependency on the ultraviolet rays of the sun for endogenous conversion of 7-dehydrocholesterol in the skin is well documented. Normal exposure to the sun prevents rickets in individuals who maintain a diet adequate in calcium and phosphorus. Rickets first appeared in environmental settings of sunlight deprivation, such as during the Industrial Revolution when air pollution filtered out ultraviolet light, and crowded urban areas consisted of sunless streets and dark homes. However, the synthetic production of vitamin D has provided modern man with an independence from the sun. Supplementation of multiple food products in the United States has virtually eliminated classical vitamin D deficiency rickets. However, in world-wide perspective, deficiency rickets and nutritional osteomalacia still represent a health problem, as reflected in the current medical literature. Reports from the United Kingdom indicate that rickets is a significant problem among the migrant Asian population (Holmes *et al.*, 1973); and in Glasgow, an early urban pocket of rickets, 9% of young children demonstrate radiographic characteristics of rickets (Richards *et* *al.*, 1968). Rickets also occurs in sun-rich areas (Salimpour, 1975) and is usually related to social customs, such as the practice of purdah,* and to the consumption of diets high in phytate.

Contemporary clinical and basic research in vitamin D is now focused on the comprehension of bone diseases resembling rickets or osteomalacia which are resistant to treatment with physiologic doses of vitamin D. Notable among these disorders are renal osteodystrophy, familial (hypophosphatemic) vitamin D-resistant rickets and vitamin D-dependent rickets. Moreover, there is hope that our increased knowledge of vitamin D and its relationship to other calcium and phosphorus regulating hormones, such as parathyroid hormone and calcitonin, will aid in our understanding of a myriad of diseases of mineral metabolism including parathyroid malfunctions, osteoporosis, and renal stone formation. With the discovery of the obligatory metabolism of vitamin D to its hormonal form, an emerging chapter in vitamin D research has been the study of possible effects of drugs such as anticonvulsants and oral contraceptives on circulating concentrations of active vitamin D metabolites. The vitamin itself could be considered a drug, since it is toxic if given repeatedly in large doses and thus hypervitaminosis D must be characterized in the context of vitamin D metabolism. Finally, with assays now being developed for measuring the blood levels of active vitamin D metabolites in humans, it is possible to identify patients with defects in this metabolic pathway and to administer the appropriate synthetic sterol to correct the deficiency and ultimately bring the patient back into proper mineral balance. Such therapy has been dramatically successful in cases of renal rickets, hypoparathyroidism, vitamin D-dependent rickets (Fraser *et al.*, 1973), and anticonvulsant-induced osteomalacia.

This chapter will discuss the metabolism, drug interactions, and therapeutic applications of vitamin D in humans by first reviewing the current status of the metabolism and mode of action of vitamin D as elucidated via experiments in animal models. The resulting physiologic and biochemical principles, along with actual measurement of the hormonal form of vitamin D in humans, will be applied to the clarification of the pathophysiology of vitamin D-related diseases. In addition, the exciting new area of calcinogenic plants and the surprising occurrence of the vitamin D hormone in the plant world will be included along with a projection of which facets of vitamin D research will probably receive attention in the immediate future.

*A practice employed by Muslims and Hindus involving the seclusion of women from public observation by concealing clothing and high-walled enclosures within the home.

II. METABOLISM OF VITAMIN D

Our current understanding of the metabolism of vitamin D is illustrated in Fig. 2. The native vitamin, obtained either via diet or sunlight, is first converted to 25-hydroxyvitamin D_3 [25-(OH)D_3]. Blunt *et al.*, (1968) characterized 25-(OH)D_3 and it was subsequently shown to be formed primarily in the liver (Ponchon *et al.*, 1969). More recent work by Tucker *et al.* (1973) indicates that at least in the chick, 25-(OH)D_3 can also be biosynthesized in the intestine and kidney. At the subcellular level, the vitamin D-25-hydroxylase enzyme exists in the smooth endoplasmic reticulum (microsomes) fraction (Bhattacharyya and DeLuca, 1974). Although the possible regulation of the vitamin D-25-hydroxylase has been the subject of some debate, initial reports of a "feedback control" of this enzyme (DeLuca, 1971) are not supported by later findings (Tucker *et al.*, 1973). Moreover, measurement of circulating 25-(OH)D in rats and humans given excess vitamin D indicates that this reaction is not tightly controlled (Hughes *et al.*, 1976, 1977). Thus, 25-(OH)-D con-

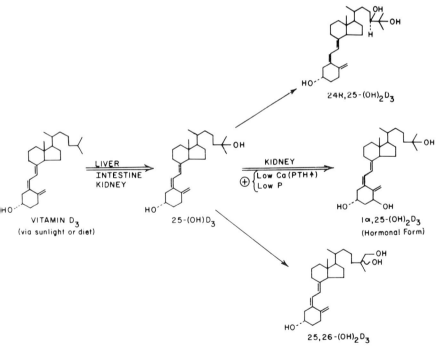

Fig. 2.   Metabolism of vitamin D.

centration is primarily a function of vitamin D intake or sunlight exposure (McLaughlin et al., 1974) and the most important function of this sterol may be to serve as an intermediate in the biosynthesis of dihydroxylated forms of vitamin D.

As is depicted in Fig. 2, 25-(OH)D$_3$ is converted into at least three dihydroxy D-vitamins. At present, little is known about the significance of the 26-hydroxylated D-vitamins; 25, 26-dihydroxyvitamin D$_3$ is not found in the main vitamin D target organs after administration of labeled vitamin D (Haussler and Rasmussen, 1972). All 24-hydroxylated forms of vitamin D are less active than their non-24-hydroxylated precursors, especially in the chick (Taylor et al., 1976). It is therefore possible that 24- and 26-hydroxylation or 25-(OH)D represent inactivation and the initial steps in excretory pathways. On the other hand, 24,25-dihydroxyvitamin D$_3$ [24,25-(OH)$_2$D$_3$] has considerable activity in rats (DeLuca, 1976), a finding which suggests that this sterol, or a metabolite thereof, may have importance in mammals. Recent work by DeLuca (1976) has shown that the natural form of 24,25-(OH)$_2$D$_3$ is the 24R-epimer and this sterol is considerably more active than the 24S-epimer.

By far the most important vitamin D metabolite discovered to date is 1,25-dihydroxyvitamin D$_3$ [1,25-(OH)$_2$D$_3$]. This metabolite was originally detected by Norman and colleagues in chick intestinal chromatin (Haussler et al., 1968) and proposed as the active form of vitamin D (Haussler, 1968). Subsequent work by Kodicek's group indicated that this sterol was formed exclusively in the kidney (Fraser and Kodicek, 1970), and the metabolite was isolated from incubations of 25-(OH)D$_3$ with renal homogenates and identified by Lawson et al. (1971). Independently, Holick et al. (1971) purified the active vitamin D metabolite from the chick gut and identified it as 1,25-(OH)$_2$D$_3$.

1,25-(OH)$_2$D$_3$ satisfies numerous criteria for its being the functional metabolite of vitamin D. Chronic administration to animals on a vitamin D-deficient diet demonstrates that it prevents rickets and maintains normal mineral metabolism (McNutt and Haussler, 1973). On a weight basis, 1,25-(OH)$_2$D$_3$ is five times as biologically active as vitamin D$_3$ or 25-(OH)D$_3$ and it functions three times faster than either of its precursors in promoting calcium absorption (Haussler et al., 1971). When assayed for bone calcium resorption activity in vitro, 1,25-(OH)$_2$D$_3$ is at least 100 times as active as 25-(OH)D$_3$ (Raisz et al., 1972). These findings, along with the original observation (Haussler et al., 1968) that 1,25-(OH)$_2$D$_3$ is the major vitamin D$_3$ form present in the intestinal mucosa subsequent to injection of labeled vitamin D$_3$ (but prior to initiation of calcium absorption), provide compelling evidence that this sterol is the active form of vitamin D$_3$. In addition to its action on calcium and phosphate translocation at gut and bone, this metabolite may also operate at the kidney (Puschett *et al.*, 1975), parathyroid glands (Brumbaugh *et al.*, 1975), and possibly other sites, such as muscle.

Unique biosynthesis of 1,25-$(OH)_2D_3$ in kidney and its action at distant target sites such as intestine suggest that this sterol can be considered a hormone. Since the production of a particular hormone is usually regulated by an endocrine feedback loop manifested by the product of the hormone's action, the discovery that the formation of 1,25-$(OH)_2D_3$ in kidney was regulated by calcium, phosphorus, and vitamin D status of animals provided major impetus for classifying 1,25-$(OH)_2D_3$ as a true sterol hormone. Thus the renal 25-(OH)D-1α-hydroxylase enzyme (1α-OHase), which is a mitochondrial P-450-mediated hydroxylase (Ghazarian *et al.*, 1974) like the 20α- or 11β-hydroxylase enzymes of adrenal cortex, plays a crucial part in the controlled biosynthesis of the 1,25-$(OH)_2D_3$ hormone. DeLuca and co-workers, based upon *in vivo* conversion of radioactive 25-$(OH)D_3$ to 1,25-$(OH)_2D_3$ have shown that hypocalcemia in the rat stimulates the production of 1,25-$(OH)_2D_3$ (Boyle *et al.*, 1971) and that this stimulation is dependent upon the parathyroid glands (Garabedian *et al.*, 1972). Also, Tanaka and DeLuca (1973) have reported that hypophosphatemia represents another stimulator of the formation of the 1,25-$(OH)_2D_3$ hormone. Hughes *et al.* (1975) conclusively showed that the actual circulating concentration of the 1,25-$(OH)_2D_3$ hormone was dramatically enhanced by hypocalcemia or hypophosphatemia. Using radioreceptor assays to quantitate the sterol in rat serum, Hughes and associates found that limited dietary availability of either calcium or phosphate elicited a fivefold increase in 1,25-$(OH)_2D_3$. The enhancement of 1,25-$(OH)_2D_3$ in calcium deficiency is dependent on the presence of the parathyroid and/or thyroid glands, which is consistent with PTH mediation of this effect. In contrast, the response to phosphate deficiency is independent of these glands and may result from a direct action of low phosphate on the renal synthesis of 1,25-$(OH)_2D_3$.

The dual control by calcium and phosphate in modulating the plasma concentration of 1,25-$(OH)_2D_3$ is reasonable in terms of homeostatic regulation of plasma ions. Calcium and phosphate are mobilized from bone and absorbed from the intestine in response to this vitamin D hormone; when plasma levels of these ions are not satisfactory, their absence triggers an increase in the hormone concentration. Figure 3 is an interpretation of the experimental results of Hughes *et al.* (1975) and of DeLuca and associates (DeLuca, 1974), in the form of a model for the dual feedback control of calcium and phosphate metabolism. Two signals, namely low plasma calcium and low plasma phosphate, are postulated as primary initiators of this hormonal system. Low circulating cal-

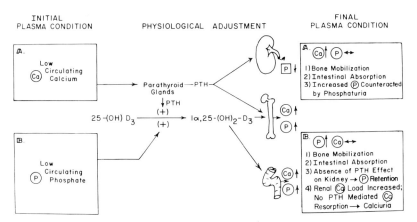

Fig. 3. Proposed model for the homeostatic control of calcium and phosphate by the integrated functioning of PTH and 1,25-(OH)₂D₃. When either calcium (A) or phosphate (B) becomes depleted, there is a stimulation of the conversion (in the kidney) of the major circulating D-vitamin, 25-(OH)D₃, to the hormone product, 1,25-(OH)₂D₃. The differential action of PTH on renal electrolyte excretion permits 1,25-(OH)₂D₃ to function in a dual capacity to regulate calcium and phosphate. From Haussler *et al.* (1976a), by courtesy of Blackwell Scientific Publications.

cium acts via an increase in PTH to enhance the 1,25-(OH)₂D₃ concentration in the plasma. The sterol then acts at the bone and intestine to increase the circulating calcium and phosphate. Parathyroid hormone also acts on bone in concert with 1,25-(OH)₂D₃ to mobilize calcium and phosphate and in kidney to stimulate phosphaturia. Since the enhanced renal excretion of phosphate counterbalances the augmented plasma phosphate, the net result produced from the original hypocalcemic stimulus is a selective increase in plasma calcium (Fig. 3).

On the other hand, low circulating phosphate apparently acts directly to stimulate the plasma level of 1,25-(OH)₂D₃. 1,25-(OH)₂D₃ in turn increases gut absorption of both calcium and phosphate and bone liberation of both ions. The consequent elevation of plasma calcium leads to a depression of PTH secretion, which together with the hypercalcemia results in an increase in urine calcium but a decrease in urine phosphate excretion. Accordingly, the net result of the initial hypophosphatemic stimulus is a selective increase in plasma phosphate (Fig. 3). The critical concept of this physiological adjustment appears to be the distinctly dissimilar physiologic mechanisms by which low phosphate and low calcium enhance the concentration of 1,25-(OH)₂D₃. Low phosphate appears to have a direct compensation mechanism, whereas low calcium operates via a separate loop involving PTH to counteract phosphatemia which would be produced by 1,25-(OH)$_2$D$_3$ alone. It is noteworthy that in the correction of calcium deficiency the extra phosphate is excreted in the urine and in the correction of phosphate deficiency the extra calcium is excreted in the urine. Thus the action of PTH at kidney emerges as the key element in the dual control of calcium and phosphate by 1,25-(OH)$_2$D$_3$.

It is probable that physiologic regulators of the renal 1α-OHase other than PTH, calcium, and phosphate exist and that these as yet uncharacterized modulators regulate 1,25-(OH)$_2$D$_3$ production during periods of calcium stress, such as growth and reproduction. One documented factor which controls the biosynthesis of 1,25-(OH)$_2$D$_3$ but is not shown in either Fig. 2 or 3 is the sterol itself. MacIntyre *et al.* (1976) have demonstrated that administration of 1,25-(OH)$_2$D$_3$ to animals causes a marked inhibition of the renal 1α-OHase activity and the concomitant induction of renal 24-hydroxylase enzyme activity; Tanaka and DeLuca (1974) have reported similar results. Since 24,25-(OH)$_2$D$_3$ is considerably less active than 1,25-(OH)$_2$D$_3$, the effect of the hormone to simultaneously shut down the 1α-OHase and stimulate the 24-hydroxylase is apparently a mechanism whereby the hormone both inhibits its own synthesis and shunts precursor 25-(OH)D$_3$ into a possible excretory pathway.

By examining Fig. 2 and considering the present understanding of the catabolism and excretion of sterols and steroids, it is evident that the pathway pictured for vitamin D metabolism is incomplete. The dihydroxylated D-vitamins and (perhaps) 25-(OH)D are most likely further metabolized and eventually excreted as water-soluble glucuronides or sulfates. To date, only one further vitamin D metabolite has been identified. DeLuca and associates (Holick *et al.*, 1973; Kleiner-Bossaller and DeLuca, 1974) have shown that 1,24,25-trihydroxyvitamin D$_3$ [1,24,25-(OH)$_3$D$_3$] can be formed either from 24,25-(OH)$_2$D$_3$ or 1,25-(OH)$_2$D$_3$. This new metabolite is less active than 1,25-(OH)$_2$D$_3$ and has not been demonstrated as yet in normal humans. However, 1,24,25-(OH)$_3$D$_3$ does have some properties in common with the hormonal sterol and its formation accounts for the biologic potency of 24,25-(OH)$_2$D$_3$ in such animals as the rat (Taylor *et al.*, 1976). Therefore, additional research is required to determine if 1,24,25-(OH)$_3$D$_3$ has physiologic relevance or simply represents an intermediate in the degradation of the 1,25-(OH)$_2$D$_3$ hormone. Recent work by Kumar *et al.* (1976) suggests that 1,25-(OH)$_2$D$_3$ may indeed be further metabolized via side chain cleavage. They have shown that radioactive CO$_2$ is lost rapidly from [26,27^{14}C]1,25-(OH)$_2$D$_3$ after injection into rats. It is not clear whether 24- or 26-hydroxylation of 1,25-(OH)$_2$D$_3$ precedes the apparent scission of the side chain or whether the further metabolism of 1,25-(OH)$_2$D$_3$ is in any fashion related to the function of the hormone. However, as is detailed in the next section, considerable evidence from *in vitro* experiments with 1,25-(OH)$_2$D$_3$ indicate that it is not further metabolized in conjunction with its molecular action at the intestine. Side chain cleavage therefore most probably represents a degradation pathway.

III. BIOCHEMICAL MODE OF ACTION OF 1,25-DIHYDROXYVITAMIN D

Since it is now considered that 1,25-(OH)$_2$D mediates normal calcium, phosphorus, and bone metabolism and apparently performs all functions heretofore ascribed to vitamin D, research is focused on elucidating the cellular mode of action of this sterol hormone. Only the mechanism of action of 1,25-(OH)$_2$D$_3$ in the intestine will be discussed in this chapter, since the most progress has been made in this target tissue. The action of 1,25-(OH)$_2$D$_3$ to stimulate intestinal calcium transport has been found to be sensitive to transcriptional inhibitors such as actinomycin D (Tsai *et al.*, 1973) and α-amanitin (Corradino, 1973a). Corradino (1973b) has developed a procedure for growing chick duodena in organ culture and these cultured intestines respond to very low concentrations of 1,25-(OH)$_2$D$_3$ to increase both calcium uptake and the formation of calcium binding protein (CaBP). This isolated system provides verification of the work of Wasserman and Taylor (1968) on the existence of a specific CaBP induced by vitamin D. The fact that 1,25-(OH)$_2$D$_3$-mediated calcium binding protein induction and increase in calcium uptake in this *in vitro* system are both sensitive to transcriptional inhibitors (Corradino, 1973a), strongly suggests that the hormone functions via mRNA synthesis. In addition, Emtage *et al.* (1973) demonstrated that vitamin D causes the appearance of polysomal mRNA specifically translated into CaBP. Formation of CaBP in this rabbit reticulocyte lysate system was monitored by specific CaBP antibody. Since CaBP is considered to be one of the functional end point proteins induced by vitamin D [1,25-(OH)$_2$D$_3$], this study provides the first definitive experimental link between 1,25-(OH)$_2$D$_3$-manifested proteins and DNA transcription. In addition, a recent experiment by Corradino *et al.* (1976), showing that addition of purified CaBP can reinitiate calcium uptake in vitamin D-deficient cultured duodena, strongly supports the role of CaBP in the overall effect of vitamin D at the gut.

Fundamental research into the mode of action of hormones, especially the steroids, is based upon the concept that high affinity receptors exist in target cells to retain and mediate the functioning of the particular hormone. Such a receptor system has been identified for 1,25-(OH)$_2$D$_3$ binding in chick intestinal mucosa (Haussler, 1974). Indirect evidence (Brumbaugh and Haussler, 1974a), such as the earliness of the hormone–receptor binding event and the correlation between the dose of hormone required to saturate the receptor and to maximally stimulate calcium absorption, suggests that hormone–receptor association is an integral part of the induction of calcium transport. Also, the properties of the chick intestinal cytoplasmic receptor for 1,25-(OH)$_2$D$_3$ are strikingly similar to those of classic steroid hormone receptors. Brumbaugh and Haussler (1974a,b, 1975) have demonstrated the following properties for this cytoplasmic receptor; (a) sediments at 3.7 S in high salt–sucrose gradients, (b) apparent molecular weight of 47,000 via gel filtration, (c) sensitive to proteases and temperatures above 25°C, (d) specific for 1,25-(OH)$_2$D and not found in nontarget tissues, (e) $K_d = 2 \times 10^{-9} M$ for 1,25-(OH)$_2$D$_3$, and (f) migrates into the nucleus and binds to chromatin in a temperature-dependent process. Thus the function of the cytoplasmic receptor appears to be to transport the hormone to its site of action in the nucleus, and the properties and the initial events in the action of this hormone receptor resemble those of steroid hormones such as estradiol-17β (Jensen and DeSombre, 1973) and progesterone (O'Malley and Schrader, 1976).

The next critical question is what is the 1,25-(OH)$_2$D–receptor complex doing in the nucleus and how might it be operating to ultimately induce the synthesis of CaBP and other possible end point proteins. Preliminary *in vivo* work intimated that the sterol is effecting transcriptional alterations in the target intestine. Tsai and Norman (1973) observed that [^{3}H]uridine incorporation into rapidly labeled intestinal RNA is enhanced by 1,25-(OH)$_2$D$_3$ administration *in vivo*. Zerwekh *et al.* (1974a) have found that the activity of DNA-dependent RNA polymerase II, the nucleoplasmic enzyme which catalyzes the synthesis of mRNA, is enhanced in activity after treatment of rachitic chicks with 1,25-(OH)$_2$D$_3$. This stimulation of RNA polymerase II occurs in concert with saturation of the intestinal chromatin with 1,25-(OH)$_2$D$_3$–receptor complex and prior to any significant increase in calcium absorption. Moreover, the increase in RNA polymerase is evident when the enzyme is assayed using exogenous template (calf thymus DNA), indicating that the intrinsic activity of the enzyme is increased.

More recent work by Zerwekh *et al.* (1976) has shown increased template efficiency of intestinal chromatin following administration of 1,25-(OH)$_2$D$_3$ to rachitic chickens. This shows that the chromatin has an increased capacity for biosynthesis of RNA. The hormone-mediated increase in template activity has been reconstructed *in vitro* by adding hormone–receptor complex to chromatin from vitamin D-deficient animals. This effect is exceedingly well correlated with the properties of the intestinal receptor protein. These correlative parameters include tissue and sterol specificity, temperature dependence, and saturability (dose response). These data are therefore consistent with the concept that the hormone–receptor complex is uncovering specific areas of the intestinal genome and permitting the synthesis of new RNA.

The above findings are incorporated into the model for 1,25-(OH)₂D action in intestine which is pictured in Fig. 4. The salient features of this mechanism are the binding of the hormone to the cytoplasmic receptor protein, migration to the nuclear chromatin, postulated exposure of a unique gene or set of genes which are transcribed into new mRNA(s) and, ultimately, translation of the new mRNA(s) into functional protein(s), such as calcium binding protein. More direct evidence for this model needs to be accumulated, especially evidence for specific new nuclear species of mRNA (e.g., CaBP mRNA), as has been accomplished in the cases of estrogen and progesterone induction of ovalbumin mRNA (O'Malley and Schrader, 1976). If this mechanism is correct, it provides the final impetus for the classification of 1,25-(OH)₂D₃ as a true sterol hormone.

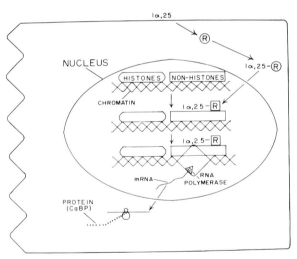

Fig. 4. Postulated mechanism of action of 1,25-(OH)₂D (1α,25) on the intestinal mucosa cell. Circled R equals cytoplasmic receptor protein; R in square equals nuclear receptor protein.

IV. DRUG AND DISEASE-RELATED ABERRATIONS IN VITAMIN D METABOLISM AND THERAPEUTIC APPLICATION OF VITAMIN D-STEROLS

A. Assay of 25-Hydroxyvitamin D and 1,25-Dihydroxyvitamin D

It was of obvious clinical importance to develop workable assay techniques for the measurement of active vitamin D sterols in human plasma. In the past 5 years, numerous diagnostically relevant assays for 25-(OH)D and 1,25-(OH)$_2$D have been created.

Several types of assays for 25-(OH)D have been devised. The most common variety is the competitive binding method which is based upon high affinity association of labeled 25-(OH)D$_3$ with various specific binding proteins. An unknown concentration of 25-(OH)D in a plasma sample is quantitated by virtue of its competition with the labeled sterol. Haddad and Chyu (1971) utilized a cytoplasmic binding protein found in all nucleated cells, while Belsey et al. (1971) employed a serum protein from rats. Hughes et al. (1976) have utilized the 1,25-(OH)$_2$D$_3$ receptor system from chick intestine to quantitate 25-(OH)D by its ability to displace labeled 1,25-(OH)$_2$D$_3$ from the protein. Physical methods are also available for the measurement of 25-(OH)D$_3$ and include gas chromatography (Sklan et al., 1973), high pressure liquid chromatography (Koshy and VanDerSlik, 1976), and a novel technique utilizing mass fragmentography (Björkhem and Holmberg, 1976). All assays have yielded normal plasma concentrations of 25-(OH)D ranging from 10 to 80 ng/ml. These values are dependent upon diet and degree of sunlight exposure and exhibit an appropriate seasonal variation. Dramatic suppression of circulating 25-(OH)D occurs in Asian immigrants to Britain (Preece et al., 1973), and even the normal level in the United Kingdom (4–20 ng/ml) is approximately one-fourth that seen in sun-rich areas of the United States, such as Tucson, Arizona and Albuquerque, New Mexico.

Brumbaugh et al. (1974a,b) and Hughes et al. (1976) have developed a radioligand receptor assay for 1,25-(OH)$_2$D which is based upon competition of unlabeled hormone from plasma with radioactive 1,25-(OH)$_2$D$_3$ for the chick intestinal receptor system. As outlined previously in this chapter, this receptor system consists of a two-step binding process involving initial association of the hormone with the high affinity cytoplasmic receptor and subsequent binding of the hormone–receptor complex to chromatin. The receptor has been shown to be equally sensitive to

1,25-$(OH)_2D_2$ and 1,25-$(OH)_2D_3$ and therefore the assay measures total 1,25-$(OH)_2D$ (Hughes *et al.*, 1976). In the procedure, 20 ml of plasma are required for triplicate assay and each plasma sample must be purified by chromatography on three successive columns. Studies in humans indicate that the normal range is 2.1 to 4.5 ng/dl, although children under 10 display an elevated level of the hormone, possibly due to increased requirements for calcium during the growing period (see Table I). This level does not exhibit a seasonal variation and is not subject to fluctuations resulting from increases in dietary vitamin D or sunlight exposure. Bioassay measurements of Hill *et al.* (1975) and a newly developed competitive protein binding assay (Eisman *et al.*, 1976) have confirmed the normal circulating concentration of 1,25-$(OH)_2D$. With these assays now available, researchers have turned to the identification of patients with defects in vitamin D metabolism. The following sections will discuss vitamin D metabolite profiles in patients with various drug-related and pathologic disorders of vitamin D and mineral metabolism, and provide possible explanations of the pathophysiology of these diseases. Table I is a summary of the levels of the 1,25-$(OH)_2D$ hormonal metabolite in these disorders as determined by the author and his collaborators.

B. Pathogenesis of Hypervitaminosis D

Although the metabolism of vitamin D to 1,25-$(OH)_2D$ is regulated, the fact that severe hypercalcemia and its deleterious consequences can occur in patients treated with pharmacologic doses of vitamin D (Chaplin *et al.*, 1951) indicates that the control of vitamin D metabolism is not absolute. The first clue to the possible etiology of vitamin D intoxication was the finding of Brumbaugh and Haussler (1973) that 25-$(OH)D_3$ could simulate the 1,25-$(OH)_2D_3$ hormone at the receptor when present in excessive amounts. When this fact was coupled with the known absence of regulation of the liver 25-hydroxylase, it suggested that 25-$(OH)D$, rather than the 1,25-$(OH)_2D$ hormone, was responsible for the symptoms of hypervitaminosis D. This hypothesis was verified both by showing that anephric patients, incapable of biosynthesizing 1,25-$(OH)_2D$, can become vitamin D intoxicated (Counts *et al.*, 1975), and that intoxicated patients with intact kidneys have normal circulating levels of 1,25-$(OH)_2D$ and strikingly enhanced levels of 25-$(OH)D$ (Hughes *et al.*, 1976).

Figure 5 depicts the metabolite profile in normal individuals and in a typical patient with hypervitaminosis D_2. The normal population (Tucson adults) had an average circulating 25-$(OH)D$ of 32 ng/ml and a 1,25-$(OH)_2D$ hormone level of 3.5 ng/dl and, notably, all metabolites

TABLE I
Summary of Circulating 1,25-(OH)$_2$D in Human Disorders of Mineral Metabolism

General group	Disease state	Number of patients	Plasma 1,25-(OH)$_2$D (ng/dl ± S.D.)
Normal	Normal (>18 years old)	58	3.4 ± 0.8
	Normal (5–10 years old)	4	6.4 ± 0.9
	Normal (adult females taking oral contraceptives)	10	4.7 ± 2.2
Renal disease	Nephrectomy	8	0.3 ± 0.2
	Chronic renal failure	50	0.4 ± 0.4
	Polycystic kidneys	5	0.8 ± 0.5
Parathyroid related disorders	Hypoparathyroidism	11	2.8 ± 0.9
	Pseudohypoparathyroidism	8	2.9 ± 1.4
	Primary hyperparathyroidism	26	5.4 ± 2.1
Osteomalacia and osteoporosis	Nutritional osteomalacia	3	1.4 ± 0.5
	Anticonvulsant-induced osteomalacia	25	4.7 ± 3.6
	Familial hypophosphatemic rickets	11	3.3 ± 1.4
	Juvenile osteoporosis (10–15 years old)	5	3.4 ± 0.4
	Postmenopausal osteoporosis	15	3.4 ± 1.2
Hypercalcemia and hypercalciuria	Sarcoidosis	4	3.6 ± 1.3
	Idiopathic hypercalciuria	40	5.0 ± 1.6
	Hypervitaminosis D	5	3.6 ± 1.5

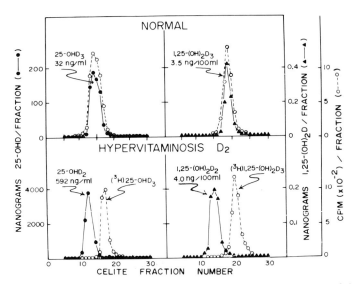

Fig. 5. Celite column chromatographic resolution and radioreceptor assay of vitamin D metabolites in normal subjects and in a patient with hypervitaminosis D_2. At the time of this study, the intoxicated patient was receiving 250,000 I. U. vitamin D_2 per day and had a serum calcium level of 14 mg%. Further experimental details are available in Hughes *et al.* (1976). Reprinted by courtesy of Rockefeller University Press.

were in the vitamin D_3 form. This finding is somewhat surprising since many of the normal individuals tested were taking approximately 400 I.U. of vitamin D_2 daily. In contrast, a typical case of hypervitaminosis D_2 exhibited approximately a fifteenfold increase in plasma 25-(OH)D concentration and a dramatic changeover to virtually all metabolites existing in the form of D_2 vitamins. Unlike 25-(OH)D however, 1,25-(OH)$_2$D was not substantially enhanced during vitamin D intoxication. These data in man verify the concept that the production of 25-(OH)D is not tightly regulated, and therefore point to 25-(OH)D as the causative agent in hypervitaminosis D.

C. Anticonvulsant-Induced Osteomalacia

Anticonvulsant drugs, particularly diphenylhydantoin and phenobarbital, are thought to affect calcium metabolism and to cause rickets or osteomalacia (Sotaniemi *et al.*, 1972; Tolman *et al.*, 1975). The mechanism of these effects is not understood but alteration in the metabolism of vitamin D, presumably secondary to induction of hepatic microsomal enzymes, has been postulated as the cause of the calcium

and bone abnormalities (Hahn and Avioli, 1975). Although gastrointestinal absorption of vitamin D is normal (Schaefer *et al.*, 1972) and conversion of vitamin D to 25-(OH)D is increased (von Herrath *et al.*, 1972),
the circulating level of 25-(OH)D is unquestionably depressed in patients
on anticonvulsants (Hahn *et al.*, 1972; Stamp *et al.*, 1972). This depressed
plasma 25-(OH)D has been linked to the reported occurrence of osteomalacia in such patients and raised the question of whether there
existed a concomitant decrease in circulating 1,25-(OH)$_2$D.

   Recent studies by Jubiz *et al.* (1977), as depicted in Fig. 6, show that
1,25-(OH)$_2$D is normal or in some cases increased in patients on anticonvulsant drugs. These data demonstrate that the suppressed levels of
25-(OH)D seen in the patients (Fig. 6) are not sufficiently low to preclude the normal synthesis of the 1,25-(OH)$_2$D hormone.

   Therefore, another mechanism must explain anticonvulsant-induced
osteomalacia. Studies in rats, as well as chick duodena in organ culture
(Corradino, 1976), indicate that the site of action of anticonvulsant drugs
may in part reside in the gastrointestinal tract, the primary effect being a
suboptimal absorption of calcium. Another tissue possibly affected by

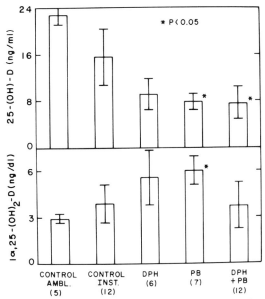

Fig. 6.   Circulating vitamin D metabolites in patients on anticonvulsant drugs. Number
of cases is shown in parentheses and bars represent standard error of mean. Patients were
age-matched, with controls being either ambulatory or institutionalized. DPH,
diphenylhydantoin; PB, phenobarbital.

anticonvulsants is bone itself, and Dilantin has been shown to inhibit PTH- and 25-(OH)D_3-induced calcium resorption in organ-cultured mouse calvaria (Jenkins et al., 1974). Thus it is conceivable that there is drug-elicited end organ hyporesponsiveness to 1,25-(OH)$_2$D in the gut and/or bone, a phenomenon which is manifested as classic osteomalacia.

However, one additional finding leaves open the question of the etiology of anticonvulsant-induced osteomalacia. Administration of vitamin D (Christiansen et al., 1973) or 25-(OH)D_3 (Stamp et al., 1972) has been reported to correct symptoms of osteomalacia in patients on anticonvulsant drugs. This may suggest that in fact these patients do have a relative deficiency of active vitamin D metabolites, or that 25-(OH)D itself has some role in bone mineral metabolism and that all effects on bone in humans are not accounted for by 1,25-(OH)$_2$D.

Another type of drug which has been shown to alter the active levels of other vitamins is the oral contraceptive. These agents appear to reduce levels of the water-soluble vitamins such as B_{12} (Wertalik et al., 1972) and ascorbic acid (McLeroy and Schendel, 1973). On the other hand, fat-soluble vitamins such as A and E are slightly elevated (Yeung and Chan, 1975). As can be seen from Table I, as in the case of anticonvulsants, oral contraceptives do not depress the level of the 1,25-(OH)$_2$D hormone and may even slightly raise it. Thus oral contraceptives apparently influence vitamin D in the same fashion in which they affect other fat-soluble vitamins.

D. Renal Disease

It had been known for many years that patients with renal failure, even those on hemodialysis, often develop serious and painful bone disease in part resembling rickets. This renal osteodystrophy is refractory to treatment with vitamin D. When Fraser and Kodicek (1970) discovered that the active 1,25-(OH)$_2$D form was biosynthesized exclusively in the kidney of experimental animals, it became clear that the pathophysiology of renal rickets involved a defect in vitamin D metabolism and a presumed deficiency of the active hormone in patients. This set into motion an explosion of experiments both in treatment of renal failure patients with 1,25-(OH)$_2$D$_3$ and its analogues, and in actual measurement of the hormone in varying states of renal disease.

1. Circulating 1,25-Dihydroxyvitamin D

In confirmation of Kodicek's animal experiments, Table I shows that nephrectomized patients have undetectable circulating concentrations of 1,25-(OH)$_2$D (Haussler, 1974). Furthermore, intact kidneys in patients

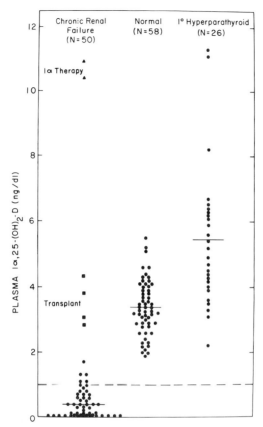

Fig. 7. Circulating 1,25-(OH)$_2$D in humans as measured by radioreceptor assay. Four renal patients receiving successful kidney transplants are shown (squares), as are two patients with chronic renal failure treated with 2 μ g/day 1α-hydroxyvitamin D$_3$ for 1 week (triangles). The dashed line indicates the lower limit of the accuracy of the assay.

with chronic renal failure are apparently incapable of biosynthesizing 1,25-(OH)$_2$D because virtually all the cases studied display 1,25-(OH)$_2$D levels below the minimum sensitivity of the assay (see Fig. 7, Table I, and Brumbaugh *et al.,* 1974b). Another renal disorder, namely polycystic kidneys, is also associated with depressed circulating 1,25-(OH)$_2$D levels. These data clearly indicate that a deficiency of the 1,25-(OH)$_2$D hormone is a likely cause of renal osteodystrophy. As can be seen from Fig. 7, successful renal transplantation returns the plasma 1,25-(OH)$_2$D level to the normal physiologic range. Thus, when possible, renal grafting is the treatment of choice, but often times compatible donors are difficult to locate. Therefore, drug therapy with exogenous 1,25-(OH)$_2$D$_3$ or an appropriate analogue has been initiated in many patients with renal failure.

2. Treatment of Renal Osteodystrophy

Brickman *et al.* (1972) first successfully treated the hypocalcemia and negative calcium balance of chronic renal failure with 1,25-$(OH)_2D_3$. Recent evidence also suggests that long-term administration of 1,25-$(OH)_2D_3$ elicits a reversal of the histologic signs of rickets and osteitis fibrosa cystica produced by excess PTH (Henderson *et al.*, 1974; Brickman *et al.*, 1974).

An effective analogue of 1,25-$(OH)_2D_3$ is 1α-hydroxyvitamin D_3[1α-$(OH)D_3$] and it has also been used by clinicians to treat renal osteodystrophy (Pierides *et al.*, 1976). Work by Zerwekh *et al.* (1974b) first showed that 1α-$(OH)D_3$ functions by conversion to 1,25-$(OH)_2D_3$. Since the 25-hydroxylase is an uncontrolled enzyme, one might expect 1α-$(OH)D_3$ therapy to produce unphysiologically high levels of 1,25$(OH)_2D_3$. Data on two patients pictured in Fig. 7 verify this notion. Therefore carefully chosen doses of the 1,25-$(OH)_2D_3$ hormone itself may be the preferred drug in treating renal osteodystrophy and should probably be included as a standard supplement for all patients on hemodialysis.

E. Parathyroid Disease

An interrelationship between PTH and vitamin D has been evident from numerous studies in animals and in man. Vitamin D is known to be necessary for many of the functions of PTH in terms of calcium metabolism (Rasmussen *et al.*, 1963). Also excessive doses of vitamin D correct some of the symptoms of hypoparathyroidism in humans. Moreover, hyperparathyroidism is characterized by hyperabsorption of calcium from the gut which is reminiscent of an over-activity of vitamin D. Finally, recent studies of animals outlined in Section II above indicate that PTH is an important modulator of the biosynthesis of 1,25-$(OH)_2D$. This interrelationship has recently been probed in man by measuring plasma 1,25-$(OH)_2D$ in patients with parathyroid disease.

1. Primary Hyperparathyroidism

As can be seen in Fig. 7, circulating 1,25-$(OH)_2D$ is significantly elevated in patients with primary hyperparathyroidism (Brumbaugh *et al.*, 1974a; Haussler *et al.*, 1976a). This demonstrates the dominant influence of PTH on the biosynthesis of 1,25-$(OH)_2D$, because this elevated level is maintained in the face of hypercalcemia. The enhanced 1,25-$(OH)_2D$ is correlated with the increase in calcium absorption (Haussler *et al.*, 1975) and probably contributes to the hypercalcemia and neph-rolithiasis of this disorder. This is consistent with the concept that PTH acts at the gut only through its effect on vitamin D metabolism. Only surgical removal of the parathyroid adenoma will cause a cessation in the autonomous PTH secretion and return the production of 1,25-(OH)$_2$D to a normal rate.

2. *Hypoparathyroidism*

Hypoparathyroidism, either idiopathic or postsurgical, and pseudohypoparathyroidism are associated with slightly depressed plasma concentrations of 1,25-(OH)$_2$D (Table I, and Haussler *et al.*, 1976a). Thus whether PTH is lacking, as in hypoparathyroidism, or its renal receptor or the subsequent biochemical machinery are missing due to a genetic defect, as in pseudohypoparathyroidism (Drezner *et al.*, 1976), the same effect of suboptimal 1,25-(OH)$_2$D production occurs in the patient. The relative deficiency of 1,25-(OH)$_2$D in hypoparathyroid-ism has been treated by administration of synthetic 1,25-(OH)$_2$D$_3$ or 1α-(OH)D$_3$; serum calcium was successfully raised to normal levels by this therapy (Russell *et al.*, 1974; Kooh *et al.*, 1975). Figure 8 illustrates serum calcium improvement in a typical case of hypoparathyroidism treated with up to 1 μg of 1,25-(OH)$_2$D$_3$ per day (Haussler, Lightner and Nu-gent, unpublished results). Therefore, until PTH is routinely available

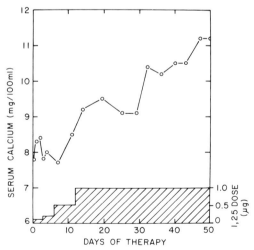

Fig. 8. Serum calcium response to 1,25-(OH)$_2$D$_3$ (1,25) in a 6-year old male with idiopathic hypoparathyroidism. The patient was receiving 10 gm of calcium carbonate per day during the entire course of the therapy, and prior to treatment was shown to be resistant to therapy with up to 300,000 I.U. vitamin D$_2$ per day.

for these patients, therapy with 1,25-$(OH)_2D_3$ is an efficacious method for maintaining normal serum calcium concentrations.

F. Nutritional Osteomalacia

Classic vitamin D-deficient rickets and osteomalacia are rare in modern societies. Pathologic effects are obviously caused by a simple lack of the vitamin and its active metabolites. These facts have been verified in animals by a recent study of Hughes *et al.* (1977) in which it was shown that chicks raised for 3 weeks on a vitamin D-deficient diet had undetectable levels of 25-(OH)D and 1,25-$(OH)_2D$, coincident with classic signs of rickets. Measurement of several cases of adult nutritional osteomalacia (Table I) confirms that the hormonal metabolite is strikingly lower than normal. This is just what one would expect and contrasts with anticonvulsant-induced osteomalacia where the circulating hormone is normal. Although vitamin D itself is an acceptable therapeutic agent in nutritional osteomalacia, the more active metabolites and analogues have been found to be effective at extremely low doses (Bordier *et al.*, 1974).

G. Vitamin D-Resistant Rickets

Marked hypophosphatemia occurs in X-linked vitamin D-resistant rickets, and the primary lesion in this disorder is thought to be deficient phosphate conservation at the kidney (Glorieux *et al.*, 1972). Vitamin D and PTH involvement in this disorder have been controversial. Work by Arnaud *et al.* (1971) strongly suggests that PTH is normal in untreated vitamin D-resistant rickets, and as reported by Haussler *et al.* (1976a), 1,25-$(OH)_2D$ is also in the normal range in these patients (Table I). In support of vitamin D-resistant rickets not being a 1,25-$(OH)_2D$ deficiency disease, Brickman *et al.* (1973) have found that 1,25-$(OH)_2D_3$ is ineffective therapeutically when administered to such patients. Since plasma 1,25-$(OH)_2D$ is normal, it is apparent that the hypophosphatemia which is the hallmark of this disorder is the cause of the rickets. This disorder would thus be more appropriately termed familial hypophosphatemic rickets.

H. Osteoporosis

Osteoporosis is the most common generalized disorder of bone. It is characterized by too little calcified bone and is apparently the end result of a number of disease states which affect the skeleton. The disease is rare in young adults, and its incidence rises sharply in the sixth decade in women and the seventh in men. It is especially prevalent in post-menopausal women and can occasionally occur in young patients without apparent cause, where it is termed juvenile osteoporosis. It is generally accepted that osteoporosis results from bone mineral resorption exceeding new bone formation. Although the etiology is probably multifactorial, vitamin D therapy has been reported to be effective in several clinical studies, especially those involving juvenile osteoporosis. M. R. Haussler, and B. E. C. Nordin (unpublished) have recently measured circulating $1,25\text{-}(OH)_2D$ in juvenile and adult osteoporosis. The results are included in Table I and demonstrate that levels in both types of osteoporosis are within the normal adult range, but age-matched controls are needed for comparison with the juvenile osteoporotics. These findings show that osteoporosis is not caused by a simple deficiency in the hormonal form of vitamin D, but rather must result from a complex imbalance in the factors regulating bone mineral.

I. Idiopathic Hypercalciuria

Thirty percent of all patients with recurrent calcium containing kidney stones have excessive urinary calcium excretion. Most of these patients have hyperabsorption of calcium from the intestine (Pak *et al.*, 1974), but exhibit normal or slightly suppressed levels of PTH (Pak *et al.*, 1974; Shen *et al.*, 1975). Hyperabsorption of calcium may result from either increased circulating $1,25\text{-}(OH)_2D$ or from an intestinal lesion, per se. Recent measurements by Kaplan *et al.* (1977) and Shen *et al.* (1975) of $1,25\text{-}(OH)_2D$ in forty cases of idiopathic hypercalciuria are compiled in Table I. It is evident that the entire population of patients displays a significant elevation of circulating $1,25\text{-}(OH)_2D$. In contrast to this is another hyperabsorption disease, sarcoidosis, in which the $1,25\text{-}(OH)_2D$ has been found to be normal (Table I). The increase in $1,25\text{-}(OH)_2D$ in idiopathic hypercalciuria produces the symptoms of this disorder, but the cause of the $1,25\text{-}(OH)_2D$ increase is unknown. One clue is that hypophosphatemia was noted in the original description of idiopathic hypercalciuria by Albright *et al.* (1953), and hypophosphatemia is a known stimulator of $1,25\text{-}(OH)_2D$ production in experimental animals (Hughes *et al.*, 1975). Therefore, one current hypothesis for the etiology of idiopathic hypercalciuria is that the primary lesion is an unexplained phosphate leak at the kidney, which presumably enhances the production of $1,25\text{-}(OH)_2D$ and ultimately produces hyperabsorption of calcium.

V. CALCINOGENIC PLANTS AS A SOURCE OF
1,25-DIHYDROXYVITAMIN D_3

Although the 1,25-$(OH)_2D_3$ hormone has been found in experimental animals and in humans, it has not previously been detected in plants. Yet the ingestion of certain botanical species by grazing animals causes calcinosis and pathological features similar to hypervitaminosis D (**Wasserman, 1975**). These animals are usually hypercalcemic and hyperphosphatemic with extensive soft tissue calcification, resulting in stiffness of limbs, emaciation, and possibly death. One such calcinogenic plant species found in South American countries is *Solanum malacoxylon* (*S.m.*). An aqueous extract of *S.m.* has been shown to mimic the biological properties of 1,25-$(OH)_2D_3$ (Wasserman, 1975). Numerous findings clearly demonstrate that the vitamin D-active substance in *S.m.* is at least a functional analogue of 1,25-$(OH)_2D_3$, not requiring metabolic activation in the kidney. In contrast to these biological similarities is a marked chemical difference between the *S.m.* factor, which is water-soluble and

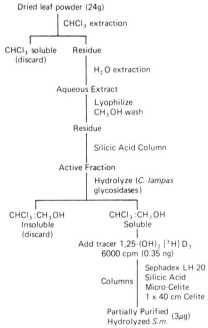

Fig. 9. Hydrolysis by *C. lampas* glycosidases and purification of the lipophilic fragment of the active calcinogenic factor from *S. malacoxylon.* Adapted from Haussler *et al.* (1976b), by courtesy of Pergamon Press.

has an apparent molecular weight in excess of 1000 (Humphreys, 1973), and 1,25-$(OH)_2D_3$, which is preferentially soluble in organic solvents and has a molecular weight of 416 (Holick *et al.*, 1971). Therefore, the identification of the active *S.m.* principle and its comparison with the animal hormone was of considerable interest. Preliminary characterization of the *S.m.* factor suggested that it was a sterol with attached glycosidic moieties (Peterlik and Wasserman, 1975). The factor could be hydrolyzed *in vitro* by β-glucosidase or *in vivo* by the chick to yield a biologically active compound which is soluble in organic solvents. This lipophilic substance was found to be strikingly similar to the 1,25-$(OH)_2D_3$ hormone, both in its chromatographic mobility and in its ability

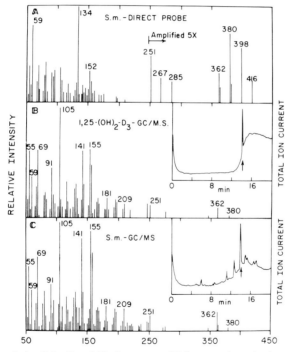

Fig. 10.   Analysis of the lipophilic fragment of *Solanum malacoxylon* by gas chromatography and mass spectrometry. (A) Direct probe mass spectrum of 1 μg of purified hydrolyzed *S.m.* (B) Gas chromatogram/mass spectrum and 1 μg of synthetic 1,25-$(OH)_2D_3$. (Inset) Gas chromatographic trace; arrow shows peak fraction which was characterized by mass spectrometry. (C) Gas chromatogram/mass spectrum of 2 μg of purified hydrolyzed *S.m.* (Inset) Gas chromatographic trace; arrow shows peak fraction which was characterized by mass spectrometry. Reprinted from Wasserman *et al.* (1976), by courtesy of the American Association for the Advancement of Science. Copyright 1976 by the American Association for the Advancement of Science.

to compete with radioactive 1,25-(OH)$_2$D$_3$ for binding to the specific intestinal receptor protein (Peterlik *et al.*, 1976; Haussler *et al.*, 1976b). Very recently, the active calcinogenic factor of *Solanum malacoxylon* has been isolated and identified by physical and chemical means as a 1,25-(OH)$_2$D$_3$-glycoside (Haussler *et al.*, 1976b; Wasserman *et al.*, 1976). Figure 9 illustrates the scheme utilized by Haussler, Wasserman and their associates to extract and purify the active principle. The critical factors in this purification scheme include the hydrolysis of the water-soluble factor with a mixed glycosidase preparation from the sea worm, *Charonia lampas*, and purification of the liberated sterol by a procedure similar to that used by Hughes *et al.* (1976) to isolate 1,25-(OH)$_2$D$_3$ from plasma. Identification of the compound was accomplished by direct probe mass spectrometry and coupled gas chromatography/mass spectrometry (Wasserman *et al.*, 1976). Figure 10 depicts these results and indicates that the active *S.m.* principle is 1,25-(OH)$_2$D$_3$. The most compelling evidence is the coincident migration of the *S.m.* fragment with 1,25-(OH)$_2$D$_3$ on gas chromatography, and the identical mass spectra of the resulting peaks (Fig. 10B and C).

It must be emphasized that, since Haussler *et al.* (1976b) and Wasserman *et al.* (1976) used glycosidic cleavage to isolate 1,25-(OH)$_2$D$_3$ from *S.m.*, in the native plant this hormone is linked to one or more carbohydrate moieties. Therefore, as is depicted in Fig. 11, the naturally occurring form of this principle is a 1,25-(OH)$_2$D$_3$-glycoside. More work is necessary to define the composition of the carbohydrate(s) linked to the sterol and to determine the position(s) of conjugation. Even if there is a

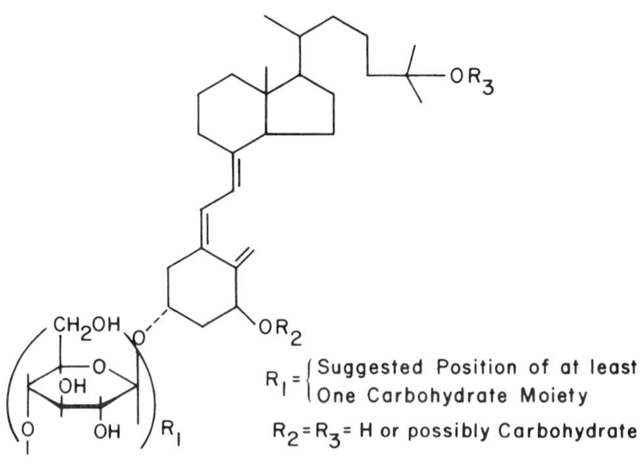

$R_1 = \begin{cases} \text{Suggested Position of at least} \\ \text{One Carbohydrate Moiety} \end{cases}$

$R_2 = R_3 = $ H or possibly Carbohydrate

Fig. 11. 1,25-(OH)$_2$D$_3$-glycoside: Possible structure of the calcinogenic principle as it exists in *Solanum malacoxylon*.

family of calcinogenic compounds with varying carbohydrate sequences, it appears that the common active unit is the 1,25-(OH)$_2$D$_3$ hormone. This is supported by the fact that oral administration of *S.m.* to chicks rapidly produces significant plasma 1,25-(OH)$_2$D$_3$ (Peterlik *et al.*, 1976), a finding which also implies that animals possess endogenous glycosidases for hydrolyzing the native factor or that hydrolysis is due to intestinal microbial action. The reason for the existence of such calcinogenic factors remains unknown. On one hand, they may play a role in the mineral metabolism of the plants, while on the other, they may serve some survival function in the plant's ecosystem. The discovery of 1,25-(OH)$_2$D$_3$ glycoside in *Solanum malacoxylon* raises the question of whether this sterol hormone is present in other calcinogenic plants, such as *Cestrum diurnum* which is found in the southeastern United States. Finally, as outlined earlier in this chapter, 1,25-(OH)$_2$D$_3$ has emerged as an important therapeutic agent in disorders such as renal osteodystrophy and hypoparathyroidism. It is possible that the water-soluble 1,25-(OH)$_2$D$_3$-glycosides of calcinogenic plants may offer some advantages over the native sterol hormone in the treatment of such clinical conditions of defective 1,25-(OH)$_2$D biosynthesis.

VI. PERSPECTIVES IN FUTURE VITAMIN D RESEARCH

In spite of the incredible list of discoveries that have been made in the last 10 years in the area of vitamin D research, there remain a number of significant questions to be answered. The elucidation of the new metabolic pathway for vitamin D and focus on the renal 1α-hydroxylase enzyme raise the question of what physiologic modulators act at the 1α-hydroxylase to affect the biosynthesis of the 1,25-(OH)$_2$D hormone during times of calcium and phosphorus stress. Especially important in this context is the characterization of the physiologic loops which function in states such as active growth, pregnancy, and lactation. The new frontier in the regulation of the 1α-hydroxylase may in fact turn out to be the interaction of pituitary, hypothalamic or other brain factors with this important vitamin D-metabolizing enzyme. Moreover, it will be a challenge for biochemists to delineate the molecular mode of action of these various humoral factors in controlling the kidney 1α-hydroxylase. Finally, the balance of the metabolic pathway for vitamin D must be worked out and special attention must be paid to the mode of excretion of the D-vitamins. The significance of 1,24,25-(OH)$_3$D in humans must also be studied and an assay for this potentially important metabolite should be devised.

In terms of the cellular mode of action of 1,25-(OH)$_2$D in the intestine, two areas which will undoubtedly see active future research are: (1) isolation of nuclear mRNA for CaBP and mRNA's for other proteins specifically induced by the hormone, and (2) the identification of these proteins and their reconstruction into a functional calcium transporting complex in model membranes. In addition, little or no work has been done on the mode of action of 1,25-(OH)$_2$D in other target tissues, such as bone and kidney.

Although the major defects in vitamin D metabolism, whether they be drug or disease related, appear to be elucidated at least in a qualitative sense, the subtler details of these disorders require more investigation. For instance, the degree of renal failure in kidney patients should be correlated with the relative impairment of 1,25-(OH)$_2$D biosynthesis. Also measurement of 1,25-(OH)$_2$D in a larger sample of patients with renal stone disease may help to identify subtypes of idiopathic hypercalciuria. Experimental therapy with vitamin D metabolites and analogues should continue at a rapid pace, but hopefully these clinical studies will be coupled with assessment of circulating active D-vitamins before and after treatment. Based upon the advances in vitamin D research already recorded plus the projected progress of the next few years, the successful treatment for many metabolic bone diseases appears to be on the near horizon.

REFERENCES

Albright, F., Henneman, P. H., Benedict, P. H., and Forbes, A. P. (1953). Idiopathic hypercalciuria. *Proc. R. Soc. Med.* **46**, 1077–1081.
Arnaud, C., Glorieux, F., and Scriver, C. R. (1971). Serum parathyroid hormone in X-linked hypophosphatemia. *Science* **173**, 845–847.
Belsey, R., DeLuca, H. F., and Potts, J. T. (1971). Competitive binding assay for vitamin D and 25-OH vitamin D. *J. Clin. Endocrinol. Metab.* 33, 554–557.
Bhattacharyya, M. H., and DeLuca, H. F. (1974). Subcellular location of rat liver calciferol-25-hydroxylase. *Arch. Biochem. Biophys.* **160**, 58–62.
Björkhem, I., and Holmberg, I. (1976). A novel specific assay of 25-hydroxyvitamin D$_3$. *Clin. Chim. Acta* **68**, 215–221.
Blunt, J. W., DeLuca, H. F., and Schnoes, H. K. (1968). 25-Hydroxycholecalciferol. A biologically active metabolite of vitamin D$_3$. *Biochemistry* **7**, 3317–3322.
Bordier, P., Pechet, M. M., Hesse, R., Marie, P., and Rasmussen, H. (1974). Response of adult patients with osteomalacia to treatment with crystalline 1α-hydroxy vitamin D$_3$. *N. Engl. J. Med.* **291**, 866–871.
Boyle, I. T., Gray, R. W., and DeLuca, H. F. (1971). Regulation by calcium of *in vivo* synthesis of 1,25-dihydroxycholecalciferol and 21,25-dihydroxycholecalciferol. *Proc. Natl. Acad. Sci. U.S.A.* **58**, 2131–3134.

Brickman, A. S., Coburn, J. W., and Norman, A. W. (1972). Action of 1,25-dihydroxycholecalciferol, a potent kidney-produced metabolite of vitamin D_3, in uremic man. *N. Engl. J. Med.* **287,** 891–895.

Brickman, A. S., Coburn, J. W., Kurokawa, K., Bethune, J. E., and Norman, A. W. (1973). Actions of 1,25-dihydroxycholecalciferol in patients with hypophosphatemic, vitamin D-resistant rickets. *N. Engl. J. Med.* **289,** 495–498.

Brickman, A. S., Sherrard, D. J., Jowsey, J., Singer, F. R., Baylink, D. J., Maloney, N., Massry, S. G., Norman, A. W., and Coburn, J. W. (1974). 1,25-Dihydroxycholecalciferol. *Arch. Intern. Med.* **134,** 883–888.

Brumbaugh, P. F., and Haussler, M. R. (1973). $1\alpha,25$-Dihydroxyvitamin D_3 receptor: Competitive binding of vitamin D analogs. *Life Sci.* **13,** 1737–1746.

Brumbaugh, P. F., and Haussler, M. R. (1974a). $1\alpha,25$-Dihydroxycholecalciferol receptors in intestine. I. Association of $1\alpha,25$-dihydroxycholecalciferol with intestinal chromatin. *J. Biol. Chem.* **249,** 1251–1257.

Brumbaugh, P. F., and Haussler, M. R. (1974b). $1\alpha,25$-Dihydroxycholecalciferol receptors in intestine. II. Temperature-dependent transfer of the hormone to chromatin via a specific cytosol receptor. *J. Biol. Chem.* **249,** 1258–1262.

Brumbaugh, P. F., and Haussler, M. R. (1975). Specific binding of 1,25-dihydroxycholecalciferol to nuclear components of chick intestine. *J. Biol. Chem.* **250,** 1588–1594.

Brumbaugh, P. F., Haussler, D. H., Bressler, R., and Haussler, M. R. (1974a). Radioreceptor assay for $1\alpha,25$-dihydroxyvitamin D_3. *Science* **183,** 1089–1091.

Brumbaugh, P. F., Haussler, D. H., Bursac, K. M., and Haussler, M. R. (1974b). Filter assay for $1\alpha,25$-dihydroxyvitamin D_3. Utilization of the hormone's target tissue chromatin receptor. *Biochemistry* **13,** 4091–4097.

Brumbaugh, P. F., Hughes, M. R., and Haussler, M. R. (1975). Cytoplasmic and nuclear binding components for $1\alpha,25$-dihydroxyvitamin D_3 in chick parathyroid glands. *Proc. Natl. Acad. Sci. U.S.A.* **72,** 4871–4875.

Chaplin, H., Clark, L. D., and Roes, M. W. (1951). Vitamin D intoxication. *Am. J. Med. Sci.* **221,** 369–378.

Christiansen, C., Rodbro, P., and Mogens, L. (1973). Effect of vitamin D on bone mineral mass in normal subjects and in epileptic patients on anticonvulsants: A controlled therapeutic trial. *Br. Med. J.* **2,** 208–209.

Copp, D. H. (1968). Parathyroid hormone, calcitonin and calcium homeostasis. *Parathyroid Horm. Thyrocalcitonin (Calcitonin), Proc. Parathyroid Cont., 3rd, 1967* (R. V. Talmage and L. F. Belanger, Excerpta Med. Found. Int. Congr. Ser. No. 159, pp. 25–39.

Corradino, R. A. (1973a). 1,25-Dihydroxycholecalciferol: Inhibition of action in organ-cultured intestine by actinomycin D and α-amanitin. *Nature (London)* **243,** 41–42.

Corradino, R. A. (1973b). Embryonic chick intestine in organ culture *J. Cell Biol.* **58,** 64–78.

Corradino, R. A. (1976). Diphenylhydantoin: Direct inhibition of the vitamin D_3-mediated calcium absorptive mechanism in organ cultured duodenum. *Biochem. Pharmacol.* **25,** 863–864.

Corradino, R. A., Fullmer, C. S., and Wasserman, R. H. (1976). Embryonic chick intestine in organ culture: Stimulation of calcium transport by exogenous vitamin D-induced calcium-binding protein. *Arch. Biochem. Biophys.* **174,** 738–743.

Counts, S. J., Baylink, D. J., Shen, F. H., Sherrard, D. J., and Hickman, R. O. (1975). Vitamin D intoxication in an anephric child. *Ann. Intern. Med.* **82,** 196–200.

DeLuca, H. F. (1971). The role of vitamin D and its relationship to parathyroid hormone and calcitonin. *Recent Prog. Horm. Res.* **27,** 479–516.

DeLuca, H. F. (1974). Vitamin D: The vitamin and the hormone. *Fed. Proc., Fed. Am. Soc. Exp. Biol.* **33,** 2211–2219.
DeLuca, H. F. (1976). Recent advances in our understanding of the metabolism of vitamin D and its regulation. *Clin. Endocrinol. (Oxford)* **5,** 97s–108s.
Drezner, M. K., Neelon, F. A., Haussler, M. R., McPherson, H. T., and Lebovitz, H. E. (1976). 1,25-Dihydroxycholecalciferol deficiency: The probable cause of hypocalcemia and metabolic bone disease in pseudohypoparathyroidism. *J. Clin. Endocrinol. Metab.* **42,** 621–628.
Eisman, J. A., DeLuca, H. F., and Kream, B. E. (1976). Intestinal 1,25-dihydroxyvitamin D_3 binding protein: Use in a competitive binding assay. *Fed. Proc., Fed. Am. Soc. Exp. Biol.* **35,** 1718 (abstr.).
Emtage, J. S., Lawson, D. E. M., and Kodicek, E. (1973). Vitamin D-induced synthesis of mRNA for calcium binding protein. *Nature (London)* **246,** 100–101.
Fraser, D. R., and Kodicek, E. (1970). Unique biosynthesis by kidney of a biologically active vitamin D metabolite. *Nature (London)* **228,** 764–766.
Fraser, D., Kooh, S. W., Kind, H. P., Holick, M. F., Tanaka, Y., and DeLuca, H. F. (1973). Pathogenesis of hereditary vitamin-D-dependent rickets. *N. Engl. J. Med.* **289,** 817–822.
Garabedian, M., Holick, M. F., DeLuca, H. F., and Boyle, I. T. (1972). Control of 25-hydroxycholecalciferol metabolism by parathroid glands. *Proc. Natl. Acad. Sci. U.S.A.* **69,** 1673–1676.
Ghazarian, J. G., Jefcoate, C. R., Knutson, J. C., Orme-Johnson, W. H., and DeLuca, H. F. (1974). Mitochondrial cytochrome *P*-450. *J. Biol. Chem.* **249,** 3026–3033.
Glorieux, F. H., Scriver, C. R., Reade, T. M., Goldman, H., and Roseborough, A. (1972). Use of phosphate and vitamin D to prevent dwarfism and rickets in X-linked hypophosphatemia. *N. Engl. J. Med.* **287,** 481–487.
Haddad, J. G., and Chyu, K. J. (1971). Competitive protein-binding radioassay for 25-hydroxycholecalciferol. *J. Clin. Endocrinol. Metab.* **33,** 992–995.
Hahn, T. J., Hendin, B. A., Scharp, C. R., and Haddad, J. G. (1972). Effect of chronic anticonvulsant therapy on serum 25-hydroxycholecalciferol levels in adults. *N. Engl. J. Med.* **287,** 900–904.
Hahn, T. J., and Avioli, L. V. (1975). Anticonvulsant osteomalacia. *Arch. Intern. Med.* **135,** 997–1000.
Harrison, H. E., and Harrison, H. C. (1975). Rickets then and now. *J. Pediatr.* **87,** 1144–1151.
Haussler, M. R. (1968). The specific association of a vitamin D metabolite with the genome of its target organ *in vivo.* Ph.D. Thesis, University of California, Riverside.
Haussler, M. R. (1974). Vitamin D: Mode of action and biomedical applications. *Nutr. Rev.* **32,** 257–266.
Haussler, M. R., and Rasmussen, H. (1972). The metabolism of vitamin D_3 in the chick. *J. Biol. Chem.* **247,** 2328–2335.
Haussler, M. R., Myrtle, J. F., and Norman, A. W. (1968). The association of a metabolite of vitamin D_3 with intestinal mucosa chromatin *in vivo. J. Biol. Chem.* **243,** 4055–4064.
Haussler, M. R., Boyce, D. W., Littledike, E. T., and Rasmussen, H. (1971). A rapidly acting metabolite of vitamin D_3. *Proc. Natl. Acad. Sci. U.S.A.* **68,** 177–181.
Haussler, M. R., Bursac, K. M., Bone, H., and Pak, C. Y. C. (1975). Increased circulating $1\alpha,25$-dihydroxyvitamin D_3 in patients with primary hyperparathyroidism. *Clin. Res.* **23,** 322 (abstr.).
Haussler, M. R., Baylink, D. J., Hughes, M. R., Brumbaugh, P. F., Wergedal, J. E., Shen, F.

H., Nielsen, R. L., Counts, S. J., Bursac, K. M., and McCain, T. A. (1976a). The assay of lα,25-dihydroxyvitamin D$_3$: Physiologic and pathologic modulation of circulating hormone levels. *Clin. Endocrinol. (Oxford)* 5, 151s–165s.

Haussler, M. R., Wasserman, R. H., McCain, T. A., Peterlik, M., Bursac, K. M., and Hughes, M. R. (1976b). 1,25-Dihydroxyvitamin D$_3$ glycoside: Identification of a calcinogenic principle of *Solanum malacoxylon*. *Life Sci.* **18**, 1049–1056.

Henderson, R. G., Ledingham, J. G. G., Oliver, D. O., Small, D. G., Russell, R. G. G., Smith, R., Walton, R. J., Preston, C., Warner, G. T., and Norman, A. W. (1974). Effects of 1,25-dihydroxycholecalciferol on calcium absorption, muscle weakness, and bone disease in chronic renal failure. *Lancet* **1**, 379–384.

Hill, L. F., Mawer, E. B., and Taylor, C. M. (1975). Determination of plasma levels of 1,25-dihydroxycholecalciferol in man. *In* "Vitamin D and Problems Related to Uremic Bone Disease" (A. W. Norman *et al.*, eds.), pp. 755–762. de Gruyter, Berlin.

Holick, M. F., Schnoes, H. K., DeLuca, H. F., Suda, T., and Cousins, R. J. (1971). Isolation and identification of 1,25-dihydroxycholecalciferol. A metabolic of vitamin D active in intestine. *Biochemistry* **10**, 2799–2804.

Holick, M. F., Kleiner-Bossaller, A., Schnoes, H. K., Kasten, P. M., Boyle, I. T., and DeLuca, H. F. (1973). 1,24,25-Trihydroxyvitamin D$_3$. *J. Biol. Chem.* **248**, 6691–6696.

Holmes, A. M., Enoch, B. A., Taylor, J. L., and Jones, M. E. (1973). Occult rickets and osteomalacia amongst the Asian immigrant population. *Q. J. Med.* **42**, 125–149.

Hughes, M. R., Brumbaugh, P. F., Haussler, M. R., Wergedal, J. E., and Baylink, D. J. (1975). Regulation of serum lα,25-dihydroxyvitamin D$_3$ by calcium and phosphate in the rat. *Science* **190**, 578–580.

Hughes, M. R., Baylink, D. J., Jones, P. G., and Haussler, M. R. (1976). Radioligand receptor assay for 25-hydroxyvitamin D$_2$/D$_3$ and 1,25-dihydroxyvitamin D$_2$/D$_3$: Application to hypervitaminosis D. *J. Clin. Invest.* **58**, 61–70.

Hughes, M. R., Baylink, D. J., Gonnerman, W. A., Toverud, S. U., Ramp, W. K., and Haussler, M. R. (1977). Influence of dietary vitamin D$_3$ on the circulating concentration of its active metabolites in the chick and rat. *Endocrinology* **100**, 799–806.

Humphreys, D. J. (1973). Studies on the active principle of *Solanum malacoxylon*. *Nature (London), New Biol.* **246**, 155–157.

Jenkins, M. V., Harris, M., and Wills, M. R. (1974). The effect of phenytoin on parathyroid extract and 25-hydroxycholecalciferol-induced bone resorption: Adenosine 3′,5′-cyclic monophosphate production. *Calcif. Tissue Res.* **16**, 163–167.

Jensen, E. V., and DeSombre, E. R. (1973). Estrogen-receptor interaction. *Science* **182**, 126–134.

Jubiz, W., Haussler, M. R., McCain, T. A., and Tolman, K. G. (1977). Plasma 1,25-dihydroxyvitamin D levels in patients receiving anticonvulsant drugs. *J. Clin. Endocrinol. Metabl.* **44**, 617–621.

Kaplan, R. A., Haussler, M. R., Deftos, L. J., Bone, H., and Pak, C. Y. C. (1977). The role of lα,25-dihydroxycholecalciferol in the mediation of intestinal hyperabsorption of calcium in primary hyperparathyroidism and absorptive hypercalciuria. *J. Clin. Invest.* **59**, 756–760.

Kleiner-Bossaller, A., and DeLuca, H. F. (1974). Formation of 1,24,25-trihydroxyvitamin D$_3$ from 1,25-dihydroxyvitamin D$_3$. *Biochim. Biophys. Acta* **338**, 489–495.

Kooh, S. W., Fraser, D., DeLuca, H. F., Holick, M. F., Belsey, R. E., Clark, M. B., and Murray, T. M. (1975). Treatment of hypoparathyroidism and pseudohypoparathyroidism with metabolites of vitamin D: Evidence for impaired conversion of 25-hydroxyvitamin D to lα,25-dihydroxyvitamin D. *N. Engl. J. Med.* **293**, 840–844.

Koshy, K. T., and VanDerSlik, A. L. (1976). High-pressure liquid chromatographic method for the determination of 25-hydroxycholecalciferol in cow plasma. *Anal Biochem.* **74**, 282–291.

Kumar, R., Harden, D., and DeLuca, H. F. (1976). Metabolism of 1,25-dihydroxyvitamin D₃: Evidence for side-chain oxidation. *Biochemistry* **15**, 2420–2423.

Lawson, D. E. M., Fraser, D. R., Kodicek, E., Morris, H. R., and Williams, D. H. (1971). Identification of 1,25-dihydroxycholecalciferol, a new kidney hormone controlling calcium metabolism. *Nature (London)* **230**, 228–230.

MacIntyre, I., Colston, K. W., Evans, I. M. A., Lopez, E., McAuley, S. J., Piegnoux-Deville, J., Spanos, E., and Szelke, M. (1976). Regulation of vitamin D: An evolutionary view. *Clin. Endocrinol. (Oxford)* **5**, 85s–95s.

McLaughlin, M., Fairney, A., Lester, E., Raggatt, P. R., Brown, D. J., and Wills, M. R. (1974). Seasonal variations in serum 25-hydroxycholecalciferol in healthy people. *Lancet* **1**, 536–538.

McLeroy, V. J., and Schendel, H. E. (1973). Influence of oral contraceptives on ascorbic acid concentrations in healthy, sexually mature women. *Am. J. Clin. Nutr.* **26**, 191–196.

McNutt, K. W., and Haussler, M. R. (1973). Nutritional effectiveness of 1,25-dihydroxycholecalciferol in preventing rickets in chicks. *J. Nutr.* **103**, 681–689.

O'Malley, B. W., and Schrader, W. T. (1976). The receptors of steroid hormones. *Sci. Am.* **234**, 32–43.

Pak, C. Y. C., Ohata, M., Lawrence, E. C., and Snyder, W. (1974). The hypercalciurias. *J. Clin. Invest.* **54**, 387–400.

Peterlik, M., and Wasserman, R. H. (1975). 1,25-Dihydroxycholecalciferol-like activity in *Solanum malacoxylon:* Purification and partial characterization. *FEBS Lett.* **56**, 16–19.

Peterlik, M., Bursac, K., Haussler, M. R., Hughes, M. R., and Wasserman, R. H. (1976). Further evidence for the 1,25-dihydroxyvitamin D-like activity of *Solanum malacoxylon. Biochem. Biophys. Res. Commun.* **70**, 797–804.

Pierides, A. M., Simpson, W., Ward, M. K., Ellis, H. A., Dewar, J. H., and Kerr, D. N. S. (1976). Variable response to long-term 1α-hydroxycholecalciferol in haemodialysis osteodystrophy. *Lancet* **1**, 1092–1095.

Ponchon, G., Kennan, A. L., and DeLuca, H. F. (1969). "Activation" of vitamin D by the liver. *J. Clin. Invest.* **48**, 2032–2037.

Preece, M. A., McIntosh, W. B., Tomlinson, S., Ford, J. A., Dunnigan, M. G., and O'Riordan, J. L. H. (1973). Vitamin-D deficiency among Asian immigrants to Britain. *Lancet* **1**, 907–910.

Puschett, J. B., Beck, W. S., and Jelonek, A. (1975). Parathyroid hormone and 25-hydroxy vitamin D₃: Synergistic and antagonistic effects on renal phosphate transport. *Science* **190**, 473–475.

Raisz, L. G., Trummel, C. L., Holick, M. F., and DeLuca, H. R. (1972). 1,25-Dihydroxycholecalciferol: A potent stimulator of bone resorption in tissue culture. *Science* **175**, 768–769.

Rasmussen, H., DeLuca, H. F., Arnaud, C., Hawker, C., and von Stedingk, M. (1963). The relationship between vitamin D and parathyroid hormone. *J. Clin. Invest.* **42**, 1940–1946.

Richards, I. D. G., Sweet, E. M., and Arneil, G. C. (1968). Infantile rickets persists in Glasgow. *Lancet* **1**, 803–805.

Russell, R. G. G., Walton, R. J., Smith, R., Preston, C., Basson, R., Henderson, R. G., and

Norman, A. W. (1974). 1,25-Dihydroxycholecalciferol and 1α-hydroxycholecalciferol in hypoparathryoidism. *Lancet* **2**, 14–17.

Salimpour, R. (1975). Rickets in Tehran study of 200 cases. *Arch. Dis. Child.* **50**, 63–66.

Schaefer, K., Kraft, D., von Herrath, D., and Opitz, A. (1972). Intestinal absorption of vitamin D₃ in epileptic patients and phenobarbital-treated rats. *Epilepsia* **13**, 509–519.

Shen, F., Baylink, D. J., Nielson, R., Hughes, M. R., and Haussler, M. R. (1975). Increased serum 1,25-dihydroxycholecalciferol in patients with idiopathic hypercalciuria. *Clin. Res.* **23**, 423 (abstr.).

Sklan, D., Budowski, P., and Katz, M. (1973). Determination of 25-hydroxycholecalciferol by combined thin layer and gas chromatography. *Anal. Biochem.* **56**, 606–609.

Sotaniemi, E. A., Hakkarainen, K. H., Puranen, J. A., and Lathi, R. O. (1972). Radiologic bone changes and hypocalcemia with anticonvulsant therapy in epilepsy. *Ann Intern. Med.* **77**, 389–394.

Stamp, T. C. B., Round, J. M., Rowe, D. J. F., and Haddad, J. G. (1972). Plasma levels and therapeutic effect of 25-hydroxycholecalciferol in epileptic patients taking anticonvulsant drugs. *Br. Med. J.* **4**, 9–12.

Tanaka, Y., and DeLuca, H. F. (1973). The control of 25-hydroxyvitamin D metabolism by inorganic phosphorus. *Arch. Biochem. Biophys.* **154**, 566–574.

Tanaka, Y., and DeLuca, H. F. (1974). Stimulation of 24,25-dihydroxyvitamin D₃ production by 1,25-dihydroxyvitamin D₃. *Science* **183**, 1198–1200.

Taylor, A. N., Henry, H. L., Hartenbower, D. L., Walling, M. W., Norman, A. W., and Coburn, J. W. (1976). Biological effects of 24,25-dihydroxy-vitamin D₃ in chicks and intact and nephrectomized rats. *Fed. Proc., Fed. Am. Soc. Exp. Biol.* **35**, 339 (abstr.).

Tolman, K. G., Jubiz, W., Sannella, J. J., Madsen, J. A., Belsey, R. E., Goldsmith, R. S., and Freston, J. W. (1975) Osteomalacia associated with anticonvulsant drug therapy in mentally retarded children. *Pediatrics* **56**, 45–51.

Tsai, H. C., and Norman, A. W. (1973). Studies on the mode of action of calciferol. VI: Effect of 1,25-dihydroxy-vitamin D₃ on RNA synthesis in the intestinal mucosa. *Biochem. Biophys. Res. Comm.* **54**, 622–627.

Tsai, H. C., Midgett, R. J., and Norman, A. W. (1973). Studies on calciferol metabolism. *Arch. Biochem. Biophys.* **157**, 339–347.

Tucker, G., Gagnon, R. E., and Haussler, M. R. (1973). Vitamin D-25-hydroxylase: Tissue occurrence and apparent lack of regulation. *Arch. Biochem. Biophys.* **155**, 47–57.

von Herrath, D., Kraft, D., Schaefer, K., and Koeppe, P. (1972). Influence of phenobarbital and diphenylhydantoin on vitamin D metabolism and calcium retention in rats. *Res. Exp. Med.* **158**, 194–204.

Wasserman, R. H. (1975). Active vitamin D-like substances in *Solanum malacoxylon* and other calcinogenic plants. *Nutr. Rev.* **33**, 1–5.

Wasserman, R. H., and Taylor, A. N. (1968). Vitamin D-dependent calcium-binding protein. *J. Biol. Chem.* **243**, 3987–3993.

Wasserman, R. H., Henion, J. D., Haussler, M. R., and McCain, T. A. (1976). Evidence that a calcinogenic factor in *Solanum malacoxylon* is 1,25-dihydroxy-vitamin D₃ glycoside. *Science* **194**, 853–855.

Wertalik, L. F., Metz, E. N., LoBuglio, A. F., and Balcerzak, S. P. (1972). Decreased serum B₁₂ levels with oral contraceptive use. *J. Am. Med. Assoc.* **221**, 1371–1374.

Yeung, D. L., and Chan, P. L. (1975). Effects of a progestogen and a sequential type oral contraceptive on plasma vitamin A, vitamin E, cholesterol and triglycerides. *Am. J. Clin. Nutr.* **28**, 686–691.

Zerwekh, J. E., Haussler, M. R., and Lindell, T. J. (1974a). Rapid enhancement of chick intestinal DNA-dependent RNA polymerase II activity by 1α,25-dihydroxyvitamin D₃, *in vivo. Proc. Natl. Acad. Sci. U.S.A.* **71,** 2337–2341.

Zerwekh, J. E., Brumbaugh, P. F., Haussler, D. H., Cork, D. J., and Haussler, M. R. (1974b). 1α-Hydroxyvitamin D₃. An analog of vitamin D which apparently acts by metabolism to 1α,25-dihydroxyvitamin D₃. *Biochemistry* **13,** 4097–4102.

Zerwekh, J. E., Lindell, T. J., and Haussler, M. R. (1976). Increased intestinal chromatin template activity: Influence of 1α,25-dihydroxyvitamin D₃ and hormone-receptor complexes. *J. Biol. Chem.* **251,** 2388–2394.

27

Toxic Effects of Megadoses of Fat-Soluble Vitamins

LOTTE ARNRICH

I. INTRODUCTION

"Megavitamin" as used in this discussion refers to a vitamin supplement that supplies an amount of the vitamin far in excess of the established recommended allowance. A precise definition is difficult because the magnitude of the excess will vary for each specific vitamin with tolerance of the organism, with form, duration, and route of administration, and with environmental factors.

Generally, excesses in water-soluble vitamins are rapidly excreted, while the fat-soluble vitamins are retained efficiently in the body. This applies specifically to vitamins A and D of which single large doses may be stored in the body for months. Consequently, the presence of the vitamin and its metabolites may have not only physiological but also pharmacological consequences.

Evidence for adverse effects of intakes exceeding recommended amounts by large factors is relatively meager for the tocopherols and for the vitamin K group. In contrast, documentation regarding toxicities of preformed vitamin A (retinol) and the readily available forms of vitamin D (ergocalciferol and cholecalciferol) has accumulated over several decades and is extensive.

Interest in health problems associated with massive doses of fat-soluble vitamins has gained new impetus because of (1) a surge in the practice of self-dosing with massive amounts of vitamins, (2) controversies regarding the legal aspects of unlimited access to people of high-potency preparations, and (3) the need for emergency measures for massive dosing of vitamin A for children in the developing world.

Understanding of the pathogenesis of hypervitaminoses A and D has benefited from new information such as that related to the transport mechanism of vitamin A via retinol-binding protein (RBP) or to recognition of the hydroxylated functional forms of vitamin D. Yet, the basic processes implicated in the toxicity of vitamins are only poorly understood.

The following discussion of hypervitaminoses focuses primarily on vitamin A, and in a limited way on vitamins E and K insofar as knowledge is available. Vitamin D is being dealt with in another section of this symposium, but will be discussed here as vitamin D toxicity relates to vitamin A. Other interactions between vitamins, especially those between vitamins A and E, are considered.

An attempt has been made to concentrate on relatively recent clinical and experimental data, since a number of comprehensive reviews of the older literature are available (Ostwald and Briggs, 1966; Sebrell and Harris, 1967, 1971, 1972; Hayes and Hegsted, 1973).

II. HYPERVITAMINOSIS A

Most cases of hypervitaminosis A in humans have resulted from consumption of livers high in vitamin A (polar bear, seal, halibut) or of high-potency vitamin A preparations. Clinical manifestations vary between acute intoxications, usually transitory, and chronic hyper-vitaminosis.

An exhaustive review of 517 cases on record at time of publication (Körner and Völlm, 1975) indicated less current concern with the inci-dence of acute than of chronic toxicity, although 75% of cases reported over a period of 4 decades had been classified as acute. Clinico-experimentally-induced acute toxicity in young children, the principal victims, has been on the decline for the last 15 years as a result of change in medical practice.

Of current interest is chronic hypervitaminosis A, which in the survey of Körner and Völlm (1975) was attributable almost equally to medical prescriptions and self-medication. Doses varied from 2000 to 60,000 IU/kg body weight and, duration of administration, from 41 to 3600 days.

Principal manifestations of chronic hypervitaminosis A include des-quamation of epidermis and mucous membranes, disorders of bone tissue and skeletal structures, elevation of cerebrospinal fluid pressure, hepatomegaly, and associated subjective symptoms as well as biochemical changes.

The following discussion highlights selected topics related to the pathology of hypervitaminosis A in man and presents supporting evi-dence in experimental animals and isolated biological systems.

A. Skeletal Tissue

Lesions of skeletal structures in chronic hypervitaminosis A have long been recognized in children and adults. Of the numerous clinical defects and subjective symptoms reported in response to vitamin A toxicity, those related to bone changes appear among the most lasting ones (Hayes and Hegsted, 1973). Permanent bone malformations, however, seem relatively rare (Ruby and Mital, 1974). Bone abnormalities de-scribed in young children include premature closure of the epiphyseal growth plate, retarded growth of long bones, and cortical thickening. The report of Ruby and Mital (1974) is of particular interest because it follows a child to age 13 who had overdosed with vitamin A for seven months during infancy, leading to subsequent fractures and permanent deformities. The findings corroborate earlier ones from 7 subjects (Pease, 1962). Skeletal damage in most of these cases resulted in flexion contracture, short stature, and length discrepancies in the lower ex-tremities. Epiphyseal irregularities of the vertebrae also were present.

In laboratory animals such as rats, lesions in skeletal tissues and structures are outstanding symptoms in hypervitaminosis A. Spontaneous fractures, thinning of long bones, pelvic girdles, and spinal bones, together with almost complete resorption of fibulae, have been noted (Leelaprute *et al.*, 1973). Microscopically, Haversian canals may be enlarged and appear spongy. Periosteal surfaces tend to show irregular erosion and demineralization.

The extensive *in vitro* experiments by Fell and associates have contributed much to our understanding of the basic mechanism underlying *in vivo* changes in bone with excess vitamin A. In the early phases of this work, cultivation of cartilaginous limb-bone rudiments of chick embryos, pretreated with vitamin A, showed excessive release of acid proteases into the medium, associated with loss of polymeric chondroitin sulfate and degradation of cartilage matrix (Fell and Dingle, 1963). Subsequent studies carried out at the Strangeways Research Laboratories suggested changes in membrane permeability of cells and cell organelles, including lysosomes rich in proteolytic enzymes, due to added vitamin A (Lucy and Dingle, 1964; Fell, 1970). Enhanced proteolytic activity may therefore account for the damage to the bone matrix in hypervitaminosis A. This concept of the membrane-seeking property of retinol has been accepted readily by many investigators and has been used in interpretations of numerous tissue defects in hypervitaminosis A. For example, reduction in longitudinal growth of long bones due to degenerative changes in cartilaginous epiphyseal plates has been proposed as one of the mechanisms operating in bone deformity in experimental animals. In addition, suppressed osteoblastic activity in hypervitaminosis A is considered to be the cause of reduction of appositional bone formation (Clark, 1971).

B. Calcium Metabolism

The reduction in mineral elements caused by excessive resorption of periosteal surfaces and other areas of bone have promoted investigations into bone composition in hypervitaminosis A. Although the well-documented changes with excess vitamin A were present in young rats,—spontaneous fractures, absence of fibulae, reduced bone wall thickness—calcium content per unit weight of bone did not differ from that of untreated controls. Calcium retention, however, was significantly reduced by 65%, resulting in a reduction of total calcium in the body (Khogali, 1966). In human subjects, persistent negative calcium balances in hypervitaminosis A suggested increased mobilization of endogenous calcium (Katz and Tzagournis, 1972). Increased urinary calcium excretions also have been reported in humans (Wieland *et al.*, 1971). The losses in urinary calcium were associated with hypercalcemia, a disorder usually found in hypervitaminosis D, but encountered repeatedly in recent years in human hypervitaminosis A (Wieland et al., 1971; Katz and Tzagournis, 1972). Serum calcium levels as high as 18.9 mg/dl have occurred. The hypercalcemia may be accompanied by generalized skeletal pains in addition to other symptoms of hypervitaminosis A described earlier. Although concurrent high intakes of vitamin D were suspected, but were ruled out, as the possible cause for hypercalcemia in hypervitaminosis A (Frame et al., 1974), it is recognized that, with the availability of multivitamin preparations, both vitamins A and D may be taken in excess, thus making diagnosis difficult (Muenter, 1974).

Metastatic calcification of nonskeletal tissue is another disorder of calcium metabolism encountered in hypervitaminosis A. Calcium deposits in myocardial muscle, kidneys, liver, lungs, and arteries have occurred in rats given large doses of vitamin A (Strebel et al., 1969; Leelaprute et al., 1973). Soft tissue calcification, together with hypercalcemia, seems to occur with excess intakes of both vitamins A and D, although the primary lesions differ. Vitamin D causes dissolution of the mineral phase of bone while excess vitamin A affects the organic matrix. Both types of toxicity seem to result in release of calcium from skeletal tissue. Possible consequences are elevated serum calcium concentrations, abnormal calcium deposits, and excessive urinary calcium losses.

C. Hepatic Pathology and Lipid Metabolism

Hepatomegaly and splenomegaly are encountered frequently in clinical hypervitaminosis A (Körner and Völlm, 1975). Detailed histological examination of liver biopsy samples has revealed lipid deposition, hepatic fibrosis, obstruction of portal blood flow with portal hypertension, and central vein sclerosis (Russell et al., 1974).

In rats alterations in hepatic lipid metabolism due to excess vitamin A included increases in hepatic lipids, especially in triglycerides and possibly in cholesterol (Singh et al., 1969; Mathur et al., 1974; Mallia et al., 1975; Setty and Misra, 1975). Hepatic lipid elevation, however, may not be seen consistently and may be age- and sex-dependent (Ram and Misra, 1975). Elevation of serum free fatty acids (Mathur et al., 1974), indicative of lipolysis in adipose tissue, was associated with reduced uptake of lipid by adipose tissue and heart (Setty and Misra, 1975). Some of these alterations in lipid metabolism have been linked to increased adrenocortical activity because adrenalectomy prevented some of the metabolic effects of hypervitaminosis A, such as mobilization of fatty acid from adipose tissue and increased synthesis of glyceride–glycerol from glucose (Singh et al., 1969).

D. Teratogenesis

Teratogenesis in experimental animals due to hypervitaminosis A has been under study for almost 4 decades. Malformations have been described for all body systems (Shenefelt, 1972). Extent and frequency of occurrence of these are closely related to time of dosing during fetal development. In a systematic study covering the first 14 days of gestation in rats, Morriss (1973) reaffirmed that the central nervous system was affected first during days 4–8, with resulting anencephaly and exencephaly. These malformations were followed in time by eye defects, facial malformations with cleft palate, and finally limb defects. The critical period for most malformations was that coinciding with active organogenesis at about day 8, but the greatest frequency of limb anomalies occurred around day 12. Defects in limb organogenesis seem to be followed by postorganogenic bone growth impediment (Love and Vickers, 1971).

In other species, events following dosing with excess vitamin A seem related similarly to various critical periods in fetal development. Hypervitaminosis A induced in female hamsters during critical periods of organogenesis affected especially vertebrae and kidneys while defects with lack of calcification were predominant when dams were dosed at subsequent periods of gestation (Robens, 1970). It seems that vitamin A in excess acts in fetal development similarly to other teratogenic agents (Shenefelt, 1972).

The mechanism underlying the teratogenic action of vitamin A is still poorly understood. Attempts have been made to ascertain whether vitamin A exerts its teratogenic action primarily on the embryo or secondarily through maternal hypervitaminosis A. With suitable dosage of vitamin A in the medium, cultured embryos developed abnormally, with defects similar to those seen *in vivo* in hypervitaminosis A (Morriss and Steele, 1974). Similarly organ cultures of mouse limb buds grown in media with added vitamin A produced oligodactyly consistent with those seen *in vivo* (Nakamura, 1975). It seems therefore, that the teratogenic action of excess vitamin A is by direct induction in the embryo.

Further insight into the mode of action of vitamin A in teratogenesis comes from detailed studies of changes in ultrastructures of embryos *in vivo* (Morriss, 1973). Membrane swelling and associated irregularities, such as cytoplasmic vacuoles beneath plasma membranes, mitochondrial swelling and condensing, and nuclear membrane swelling were associated with cell death. These subcellular abnormalities seemed to resemble those produced by excess vitamin A on cell structures *in vitro*

(Lucy and Dingle, 1964). However, lysosomal membranes, which seem specifically unstable towards excess vitamin A with resulting release of lysosomal enzymes (Fell and Dingle, 1963), may not be involved in the teratogenesis of vitamin A. The evidence is circumstantial and is based on comparisons of enzymatic activities in embryo, yolk sac, and uterus of rats that had been either ovariectomized or given excess vitamin A (Schultz, 1969). In almost all instances, the lysosomes of the conceptus of the vitamin A-treated dams seemed stable, compared with those of ovariectomized rats.

In most studies related to experimental teratogenesis of vitamin A, doses approximately 100 times or more the requirement of the experimental animal have been used. The equivalent for humans in terms of the recommended allowance would be 500,000 IU. This amount would have to be administered at the crucial period of human fetal organogenesis.

Concern has been expressed about the possibility of teratogenic effects in humans due to indiscriminatory intakes of vitamin A during pregnancy (Morriss, 1973). Others discount reasons for concern because of the large discrepancy in dosage level (Yarington and Stivers, 1974). Prescriptions of 50,000 to 150,000 IU/day for dermatologic disorders are not uncommon (American Academy of Pediatrics, Committee on Drugs and Nutrition, 1974), so that the teratogenic equivalent could be consumed in a few days by a pregnant woman. The renal anomalies of a child born to a mother who had taken excessive amounts of vitamin A during pregnancy may be an isolated incidence (Bernhardt and Dorsey, 1974), but the report indicates that such consequences can be real and that caution against excessive vitamin A intakes during pregnancy is justified.

With the rising interest in prenatal nutritional impact on mental development, it is not surprising that experimental findings have linked maternal hypervitaminosis A to certain aspects of behavior and learning abilities. Defects in body systems of the developing fetus resulting from excess maternal vitamin A intake in rats have been well studied, but little attention has been given to behavioral changes in offspring until recently (Butcher et al., 1972; Hutchings et al., 1973; Vorhees, 1974). The dosage selected for the pregnant rats (100,000 IU/kg) was less than that considered teratogenic for the central nervous system, but the gestational period chosen for dosing coincided with maximal susceptibility of the central nervous system (Butcher et al., 1972). Offspring had malformations that did not interfere with swimming ability in preliminary training, but behavioral performances in a water-filled T-maze were significantly poorer than those of controls. Since learning impairment was not modified by cross-fostering, the defects were attributed to *in utero* excess of vitamin A.

Long lasting behavioral changes in offspring could also be elicited in rats with intakes below 100,000 IU/kg (Vorhees, 1974). With maternal vitamin A doses of 40,000 IU/kg or less, offspring did not differ physically from controls when testing began. Neither could analysis of open field activity differentiate between offspring of treated and untreated dams. All experimental groups, regardless of dosage, however, showed decreased avoidance and discrimination acquisition. With a teratogenic dose of 300,000 IU/kg and treatment of dams at an advanced stage of pregnancy (days 14, 15) auditory discrimination was impaired in the offspring. These defects were associated with overall reduction in brain size and obvious microcephaly (Hutchings *et al.*, 1973). With an even later treatment period of the dams, however, learning abilities of the offspring were similar to those of controls (Hutchings and Gaston, 1974).

These reports of changes in behavior and learning ability of young whose mothers had received subteratogenic amounts of vitamin A emphasize the danger of overdosing during pregnancy. In the absence of detectable damage to the physical development of the young, changes may be produced in the central nervous system even with transitory exposure of the maternal organism to excess vitamin A. These alterations could have serious consequences for the offspring in later life.

E.   Transport of Retinol in Hypervitaminosis A

The recently acquired understanding of the transport mechanism of retinol has helped to differentiate between physiological and potentially toxic effects of vitamin A in the body. It had been noted that retinol, previously bound *in vivo* to protein, was less toxic to organ cultures *in vitro* than was retinol added directly to the medium (Fell and Mellanby, 1952). After the identification of retinol-binding protein (RBP), which binds retinol specifically at a 1:1 molar ratio, the earlier experiments were confirmed (Dingle *et al.*, 1972). Retinol bound nonspecifically to serum proteins degraded the extracellular matrix of embryonic skeletal tissue in organ culture while the retinol–RBP complex had no discernible effect.

Goodman and associates (Mallia *et al.*, 1975) have recently reported changes in retinol transport system that may occur in hypervitaminosis A. In instances of massive dosing with vitamin A, the capacity of rat liver to take up retinol seemed to have an upper limit. Furthermore, the concentrations of RBP in both liver and serum were suppressed by as much as 50% with the toxic dose, indicating interference with synthesis of RBP in addition to saturation of available RBP. Because total plasma vitamin A was considerably elevated concomitantly with reduced RBP, the partition of retinol between various protein fractions was determined. The nonlipoprotein fraction of hydrated density (d) greater than 1.21 contained nearly all the RBP. In control animals, 82% of the plasma retinol was unesterified and found in this fraction. In contrast, the nonesterified fraction of plasma vitamin A was reduced to 16% in rats given excess vitamin A while 85% was carried as retinyl esters in lipoproteins d <1.21. It has been suggested that this nonspecifically bound fraction exhibits the damaging surface-active, membrane-seeking properties of vitamin A, resulting in lysosomal instability with the release of lysosomal hydrolases. Goodman (1974) suggested that "Vitamin A toxicity occurs *in vivo* only when the level of vitamin A in the body is such that retinol begins to circulate in plasma, and to be presented to membranes in a form other than bound to RBP."

F. Prophylactic Measures with Massive Doses of Vitamin A

One specific aspect of megavitamin usage should be considered here: the emergency measure of single prophylactic dosing of vitamin A. The practice is under consideration or in operation in parts of the world where blindness due to vitamin A deficiency in young children is a grave problem and where adequate nutrition of vitamin A through diet is at present unrealistic (Srikantia and Reddy, 1970).

On the basis of field trials in India, a single dose of 200,000 IU given every 6 months to children 1–3 years of age has been recommended as a public health measure to prevent vitamin A deficiency (Swaminathan *et al.*, 1970). The national program in operation in certain states of India has been evaluated with generally encouraging results (Vijayaraghauan *et al.*, 1975). However, the possibility that acute toxicity may occur at the time of dosing has been considered. In the trials in India, clinical toxicity occurred rarely (Swaminathan *et al.*, 1970), but a transient increase in urinary excretion of typical lysosomal enzymes was reported in about half of a group of children tested (Reddy and Mohanram, 1971). The efficiency of massive doses with regard to protection also has been questioned. After the excretion of a tracer dose given with a single massive dose, Pereira and Begum (1973) concluded that retention was relatively poor, at about 40%, in seemingly healthy children. This could at best offer protection for 19 weeks only. It was argued that protection would be reduced further if, as is commonly found in children at risk in the developing world, illness and infections were present. In spite of the hazards involved, investigators seem to favor the emergency measure. The benefits derived from even partial protection against blindness associated with vitamin A deficiency far outweigh the disadvantages associated with transient toxic effects in a few children.

III. EXCESS VITAMIN E

Large dietary supplements of vitamin E are being consumed at present and are sold freely without prescription to the general public. The health benefits derived from megadoses of vitamin E remain largely unsubstantiated (National Academy of Sciences, 1973).

Most reviewers of the clinical literature agree that megadoses of vitamin E are essentially nontoxic (Bieri, 1975; Herbert, 1975; Witting, 1975); yet indiscriminate consumption of vitamin E may be unwise, because understanding is limited of possible subclinical and biochemical effects of excessive intakes of vitamin E. Concern about this problem has been expressed repeatedly (Briggs, 1974; Bieri, 1975; Horwitt, 1976).

Side effects due to prolonged consumption of vitamin E in doses from 2 to 12 gm are on record (Hillman, 1957) and have been summarized recently (Hayes and Hegsted, 1973). Symptoms have, for the most part, been subjective and nonspecific. The list includes gastrointestinal disturbances, weakness, fatigue, angular stomatitis, cheilosis, and others. In addition, creatinuria, hypoglycemia, and reduced prothrombin levels have been encountered with high intakes of vitamin E.

Beneficial, as well as deleterious, manifestations of excess vitamin E have occurred in laboratory animals. Large doses of vitamin E have offered protection against toxicity of certain drugs, selenium toxicity, irradiation damage, vitamin A toxicity, and environmental toxic agents. In contrast, vitamin E in excess depressed growth in rats (Corrick, 1969) and chicks (March et al., 1973), interfered with thyroid function and produced hepatic changes, including elevation in total lipids, cholesterol, and fatty acid patterns (Alfin-Slater et al., 1972). Antagonistic interactions between tocopherol in excess and specific aspects of vitamin A metabolism will be discussed later.

Concern has been expressed that vitamin E in excess may interfere with normal coagulation processes, resulting in increased requirement for vitamin K (March et al., 1973). Potentiation by excess tocopherol of anticoagulants used clinically led to studies relative to vitamin E action on vitamin K-dependent coagulation factors (Corrigan and Marcus,

1974). It has been suggested that metabolites of α-tocopherol formed in the body, such as α-tocopherylquinone or hydroquinone, may act as antimetabolites to vitamin K (March *et al.*, 1973). The antivitamin K activity of tocopheryl hydroquinone has recently been described (Rao and Mason, 1975).

IV. TOXICITY OF VITAMIN K

Vitamin K in excess, like vitamin E, is considered to be innocuous (Deutsch, 1966). This generalization probably should be applied to the naturally occurring, fat-soluble forms of the vitamin only. Water-soluble analogues of menadione (K_3), lacking the hydrophobic side chain, have produced side effects, especially in newborn infants (Vest, 1966). The practice of administering large doses of vitamin K_3 analogues to women at time of delivery was developed to meet obstetric complications resulting from hypoprothrombinemia in the newborn. This measure, as well as direct prophylactic dosing with vitamin K of newborns, has caused hemolytic anemia in infants with complications such as hyperbilirubinemia, icterus, and kernicterus. Occasionally, the outcome has been fatal (American Academy of Pediatrics, Committee on Nutrition, 1961). Premature infants seem especially vulnerable to overdosing with vitamin K (Allison, 1955).

Mechanisms underlying hemolytic anemia with its clinical consequences have been explored in newborn and adult rats. Water-soluble analogues of menadione seemed to act as oxidizing hemolysins on erythrocytes (Wynn, 1963). Formation of methemoglobin by menadione supports this concept. The work with newborn rats suggests that the excess bilirubin, produced as a consequence of hemolysis, places a special burden on the immature liver because conjugation with glucuronide for bilirubin elimination is an essential hepatic process that functions at a low level in the newborn. In addition, competition between vitamin K analogues and bilirubin for the available conjugation mechanism may further decrease the body's ability to reduce the bilirubin excess.

The danger of complications arising from vitamin K overdosing has led to severe criticism of the prophylactic dosing of women during labor. Furthermore, it is recognized that only moderate doses of vitamin K are effective in as much as the immature liver of the newborn cannot be stimulated to prothrombin synthesis beyond its limited functional capacity (Murphy, 1961). At present, low-dose injections of vitamin K after birth are favored in combating hypoprothrombinemia in the newborn (Snyderman and Holt, 1973).

V. INTERACTIONS IN HYPERVITAMINOSES

A. Vitamins A and D

The pathogenesis of hypervitaminosis D in light of recent research has been covered in another section of this symposium. In addition, comprehensive reviews of the classical literature are available (Sebrell and Harris, 1971; Hayes and Hegsted, 1973; National Academy of Sciences, National Research Council, 1975). This discussion is limited to the interaction of excess vitamin D with excess vitamin A.

The pathological impact of excess vitamin D is primarily related to skeletal tissue and secondarily to soft tissue metastasis. Calcification of organs and vessels follows hypercalcemia, which in turn reflects accentuated physiological functions of vitamin D—stimulation of calcium absorption and mobilization of calcium from bone.

The effect of vitamin A in excess on certain aspects of bone structure and metabolism has been discussed (Section II, A). Primary target in skeletal tissue seems to be the organic matrix so that reduced mineralization occurs secondary to matrix dissolution. Yet, as mentioned earlier, some defects from hypervitaminosis A resemble those seen in vitamin D intoxication— metastatic calcification, occasionally hypercalcemia, and calcinuria. Although bone ash content tends to diminish with excess vitamin D, this parameter seems to remain normal in hypervitaminosis A. In short, although different in etiology, pathological changes seen with each vitamin in excess have certain similarities. One might expect that the two nutrients would act synergistically. Reports, however, indicate an antagonistic interaction.

The interaction between the two vitamins A and D was noted early (Morgan et al., 1937). Synthetic vitamin A was not available at that time, but the results have since been confirmed in general with pure preparations in rats (Clark and Bassett, 1962; Bélanger and Clark, 1967) and in chicks (Taylor et al., 1968). In the early study by Morgan and associates (1937), vitamin A in large excess protected young rats from vitamin D toxicity. The extent of the reversal of toxicity symptoms varied with vitamin A source and was most favorable with the largest doses. In general, large doses of vitamin A restored growth rate almost to normal, reduced hypercalcemia, maintained bone ash concentration, and reduced calcium in kidney, heart, and lung tissue.

In a factorial experiment with both vitamins A and D increasing by tenfold increments from 1 to 1000 of basal level, Taylor et al. (1968) were able to distinguish between three categories of biochemical responses to excess vitamins D and A in chicks: (a) those affected by both vitamins, where antagonism was marked—plasma calcium, phosphorus, and acid phosphatases; (b) those affected by excess vitamin A only—lysosomal enzymes in plasma and packed cell volume; and (c) those that were negative—calcium absorption. Clark and Smith (1964) concluded that the protective effect of vitamin A results from increased mucopolysaccharide and collagen turnover but that vitamin A has no influence on the enhanced calcium absorption in the intestine associated with high intakes of vitamin D.

B. Vitamins A and E

Interactions of vitamin E with vitamin A in its various dietary forms may be synergistic as well as antagonistic, depending on amounts involved, specific chemical forms of vitamin A, points of interaction in the metabolism of vitamin A, and related factors.

The present discussion is limited to instances in which either one or both of the vitamins occur in excess. Stabilization by vitamin E of erythrocytes against lysis caused by vitamin A has been described *in vitro* (Lucy and Dingle, 1964) as well as *in vivo* (Soliman, 1972). The membrane-stabilizing effect of vitamin E on circulating cells is, however, hard to extend to the whole organism for which mitigation of growth depression due to excess vitamin A by vitamin E has been reported (McCuaig and Motzok, 1970; Jenkins and Mitchell, 1975). In a systematic experiment with rats, a wide range of tocopherol intakes was combined with toxic levels of vitamin A. Growth depression caused by vitamin A toxicity could indeed be reversed, but only when the α-tocopherol dose exceeded the rat's requirement by a factor of fiftyfold. In contrast, with excess vitamin E, serum and liver concentrations of retinol were further elevated above the levels associated with hypervitaminosis A alone, thus suggesting a synergistic effect. In some yet unexplained way, vitamin E ameliorated to some extent the pathogenic effects of vitamin A without lowering its concentration in circulation or liver.

The synergism between vitamins A and E has been tested in children with the hope of improving the effectiveness of single-dose prophylactic measures in countries where vitamin A deficiency poses severe health problems (Kusin *et al.*, 1974). A single massive dose of retinyl acetate tagged with trace amounts of [³H]retinol was administered in the presence of different doses of tocopherol. The minimum effective vitamin E dose was 500 mg; with this large supplement, absorption of vitamin A increased by 22% over control values. Overall retention of vitamin A was not changed, however, by high tocopherol intakes because the increase in vitamin A absorption was offset by a similar increase in urinary excretion. Interactions between vitamins A and E seem to affect different points in vitamin A metabolism. Reports of conservation of hepatic stores of vitamin A by vitamin E go back to the early studies of Moore (Davies and Moore, 1941) and have been corroborated by Cawthorne *et al.* (1968). Increased urinary excretion of vitamin A in the presence of large doses of vitamin E is therefore difficult to reconcile with the idea that hepatic stores are protected in the presence of excess tocopherol.

Interactions of a different nature, with physiological intakes of vitamin A or β-carotene, but excessive supplements of DL-α-tocopheryl acetate, have been studied in our laboratory. The approach seemed realistic in view of the current practice of self-dosing with supplements of vitamin E, often exceeding recommended daily intakes by more than fiftyfold. The data extend work reported earlier, which showed an antagonism between vitamin A and tocopherol slightly in excess of the optimum dosage (Johnson and Baumann, 1948).

Utilization of β-carotene, measured after a 4-week feeding period by retinol deposits, was reduced from 15 to 10% as tocopherol supplements were increased from 1 to 10 mg per day. Further increase to 50 mg tocopherol per day virtually blocked the utilization of the carotene supplements for hepatic retinol storage so that the animals differed little from vitamin A-deficient controls (Fig. 1). In additional experiments, the effect of the high tocopherol dose was tested with either retinyl acetate or β-carotene as the source of vitamin A (Fig. 2). Although β-carotene utilization for retinol storage dropped from 22 to 2% of the dose with the increase of the tocopherol supplement from 1 to 50 mg per

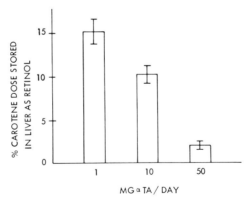

Fig. 1. Percent utilization of dietary β-carotene measured as hepatic retinol. Young, vitamin A-depleted rats were fed 64 μg β-carotene and 1, 10, or 50 mg DL-α-Tocopheryl acetate (αTA) daily for 28 days.

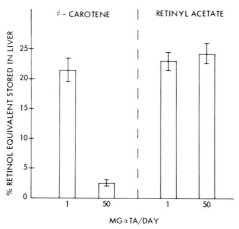

Fig. 2. Percent utilization of retinol equivalents of dietary β-carotene or retinyl acetate. Young, vitamin A-depleted rats were fed 78 μg β-carotene or 38 μg retinyl acetate with 1 or 50 mg DL-α-Tocopheryl acetate (αTA) daily for 28 days.

day, utilization of the retinyl acetate supplement was unaffected by excess tocopherol. The data strongly suggest that tocopherol interacts with β-carotene in metabolic steps that occur preceding the formation of retinol. These would be confined to the small intestine since, in the rat, the intestinal mucosa is the principal site of the conversion process. Indirect measures of the overall conversion (namely, fecal losses of un-

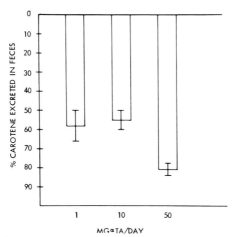

Fig. 3. Percent of β-carotene dose excreted in feces. Young, vitamin A-depleted rats were fed 65 μg β-carotene and 1, 10, or 50 mg DL-α-Tocopheryl acetate (α TA) daily for 5 days.

766   Lotte Arnrich

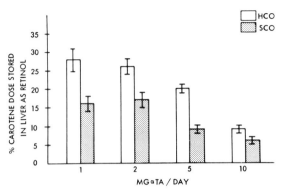

Fig. 4. Percent utilization of dietary β-carotene measured as hepatic retinol. Young, vitamin A-depleted rats were fed 72 μg β-carotene and 1, 2, 5, or 10 mg DL-α-Tocopheryl acetate (αTA) daily for 28 days. Dietary fat was either hydrogenated coconut oil (HCO) or stripped corn oil (SCO).

converted β-carotene) lend support to the hypothesis that blocking of intestinal processes of β-carotene metabolism by excess tocopherol may be of significance. In our experiments, daily fecal losses of β-carotene increased from 58 to 81% of the dose with the high tocopherol supplement (Fig. 3).

The mechanism underlying the inhibition of β-carotene utilization by large amounts of tocopherol is not understood. If, as has been suggested, tocopherol acts as an antioxidant (High, 1956) it may inhibit the activity of the specific dioxygenase, which cleaves β-carotene to form retinol in the intestinal mucosal cell (Olson and Hayaishi, 1965). Proof for this mechanism is lacking at present. Indeed, the finding that substitution of stripped corn oil high in polyunsaturated fatty acids for hydrogenated coconut oil suppressed β-carotene utilization at each progressive step of tocopherol supplementation (Fig. 4) does not support the antioxidant hypothesis.

Extrapolation of the findings reported here to man are not justified without further study. The results suggest, however, that biochemical changes may occur with indiscriminately high intakes of a vitamin that seem to be innocuous from a clinical standpoint. The concern has been expressed with regard to the vitamin A and E relationship (Bieri, 1973).

VI. RESEARCH NEEDS

Research needs related to toxicities of megadoses of fat-soluble vitamins fall into three major categories: those pertaining to (1) basic mechanisms underlying toxic manifestations and associated physico-chemical phenomena; (2) interactions of pharmacological doses of these vitamins or their metabolites with other nutrients; (3) delineations of upper limits of vitamin intakes in quantities and dosing periods relative to possible benefits derived from megadoses.

The following specific areas need research input:

(a) In hypervitaminosis A, a delineation between physiological functions and pharmacological effects, related primarily to membrane stability, is needed. Although much information is available on the pathogenesis of vitamin A in skeletal tissue, data on effects of excess vitamin A in intermediary metabolism are just beginning to accumulate.

(b) Teratogenic consequences of large doses of vitamin A on the central nervous system need further study. Teratogenic effects of large excesses of vitamin E have attracted little attention so far. Epidemiological data in humans with regard to teratogenic consequences of megadoses of fat-soluble vitamins and their interrelationships are lacking.

(c) Interactions in nutrient utilization and in modifications of nutrient requirements with excessive intakes of vitamins, especially vitamins A and E, need to be explored. Experiments with vitamin E, based on intakes corresponding to present-day megadose practices, are needed.

(d) Well-controlled studies related to health benefits of megadoses of vitamins are required either to substantiate or refute claims. Where benefits are indicated, recommendations for upper limits of dose over time are needed for sound counseling by professionals and for intelligent decisions by those of the public who are practicing self-medication.

REFERENCES

Alfin-Slater, R. B., Aftergood, L., and Kishineff, S. (1972). Investigations on hypervitaminosis E in rats. *Nutr., Proc. Int. Congr., 9th, 1972* Abstracts. p. 191.

Allison, A. C. (1955). Danger of vitamin K to newborn. *Lancet* **268,** 669.

American Academy of Pediatrics, Committee on Drugs and on Nutrition. (1974). The use and abuse of vitamin A. *Nutr. Rev.* **32,** S41–S43.

American Academy of Pediatrics, Committee on Nutrition. (1961). Vitamin K compounds and the water-soluble analogues. Use in therapy and prophylaxis in pediatrics. *Pediatrics* **28,** 501–507.

Bélanger, L. F., and Clark, I. (1967). Alpharadiographic and histological observations on the skeletal effects of hypervitaminoses A and D in the rat. *Anat. Rec.* **158,** 443–452.

Bernhardt, I. B., and Dorsey, D. J. (1974). Hypervitaminosis A and congenital renal anomalies in a human infant. *Obstet. Gynecol.* **43,** 750–755.

Bieri, J. G. (1973). Effect of excessive vitamins C and E on vitamin A status. *Am. J. Clin. Nutr.* **26,** 382–383.

Bieri, J. G. (1975). Vitamin E. *Nutr. Rev.* **33**, 161–167.

Briggs, M. H. (1974). Vitamin E in clinical medicine. *Lancet* **1**, 220.

Butcher, R. E., Brunner, R. L., Roth, T., and Kimmel, C. A. (1972). A learning impairment associated with maternal hypervitaminosis A in rats. *Life Sci.* **11**, Part I, 141–145.

Cawthorne, M. A., Bunyan, J., Diplock, A. T., Murrell, E. A., and Green, J. (1968). On the relationship between vitamin A and vitamin E in the rat. *Br. J. Nutr.* **22**, 133–143.

Clark, I., and Bassett, C. A. L. (1962). The amelioration of hypervitaminosis D in rats with vitamin A. *J. Exp. Med.* **115**, 147–155.

Clark, I., and Smith, M. R. (1964). Effects of hypervitaminosis A and D on skeletal metabolism. *J. Biol. Chem.* **239**, 1266–1271.

Clark, L. (1971). Hypervitaminosis A: A review. *Aust. Vet. J.* **47**, 568–571.

Corrick, J. A. (1969). Growth and reproduction of albino rats as affected by various excessive levels of dietary vitamin E. *Diss. Abstr. B* **29**, 2249B.

Corrigan, J. J., and Marcus, F. I. (1974). Coagulopathy associated with vitamin E ingestion. *J. Am. Med. Assoc.* **230**, 1300–1301.

Davies, A. W., and Moore, T. (1941). Interaction of vitamins A and E. *Nature (London)* **147**, 794–796.

Deutsch, E. (1966). Vitamin K in medical practice: Adult. *Vitam. Horm. (N.Y.)* **24**, 665–680.

Dingle, J. T., Fell, H. B., and Goodman, D. S. (1972). The effect of retinol and of retinol-binding protein on embryonic skeletal tissue in organ culture. *J. Cell. Sci.* **11**, 393–402.

Fell, H. B. (1970). The direct action of vitamin A on skeletal tissue in vitro. *In* "The Fat Soluble Vitamins" (H. F. DeLuca and J. W. Suttie, eds.), pp. 187–202. Univ. of Wisconsin Press, Madison.

Fell, H. B., and Dingle, J. T. (1963). Studies on the mode of action of excess vitamin A. 6. Lysosomal protease and the degradation of cartilage matrix. *Biochem. J.* **87**, 403–408.

Fell, H. B., and Mellanby, E. (1952). The effect of hypervitaminosis A on embryonic limb-bones cultivated *in vitro*. *J. Physiol (London)* **116**, 320–349.

Frame, B., Jackson, C. E., Reynolds, W. A., and Umphrey, J. E. (1974). Hypercalcemia and skeletal effects in chronic hypervitaminosis A. *Ann. Intern. Med.* **80**, 44–48.

Goodman, DeW. S. (1974). Vitamin A transport and retinol binding protein metabolism. *Vitam. Horm. (N.Y.)* **32**, 167–180.

Hayes, K. C., and Hegsted, C. M. (1973). Toxicity of the vitamins. *In* "Toxicants Occuring Naturally in Foods" Subcommittee on naturally occuring toxicants in foods (F. M. Strong, chairman), pp. 235–253. Nat. Acad. Sci.

Herbert, V. (1975). The rationale of massive-dose vitamin therapy. (Megavitamin therapy: Hot fictions versus cold facts.) *Proc.—West Hemisphere Nutr. Cong.*, 4th, 1974 pp. 84–91.

High, E. G. (1956). Further antioxidant studies concerned with the metabolism of carotene and vitamin A. *Arch. Biochem. Biophys.* **60**, 456–562.

Hillman, R. W. (1957). Tocopherol excess in man: Creatinuria associated with prolonged ingestion. *Am. J. Clin. Nutr.* **5**, 597–600.

Horwitt, M. K. (1976). Vitamin E: A reexamination. *Am. J. Clin. Nutr.* **29**, 569–578.

Hutchings, D. E., and Gaston, J. (1974). The effects of vitamin A excess administered during the mid-fetal period on learning and development in rat offspring. *Dev. Psychobiol.* **7**, 225–233.

Hutchings, D. E., Gibbon, J., and Kaufman, M. A. (1973). Maternal vitamin A excess during the early fetal period: Effects on learning and development in the offspring. *Dev. Psychobiol.* **6**, 445–457.

Jenkins, M. Y., and Mitchell, G. V. (1975). Influence of excess vitamin E on vitamin A toxicity in rats. *J. Nutr.* **105,** 1600–1606.

Johnson, R. M., and Baumann, C. A. (1948). The effect of alpha-tocopherol on the utilization of carotene by the rat. *J. Biol. Chem.* **175,** 811–816.

Katz, C. M., and Tzagournis, M. (1972). Chronic adult hypervitaminosis A with hypercalcemia. *Metab., Clin. Exp.* **21,** 1171–1176.

Khogali, A. (1966). Bone strength and calcium retention of rats in hypervitaminosis A. *Q. J. Exp. Physiol. Cogn. Med. Sci.* **51,** 120–129.

Körner, W. F., and Völlm, J. (1975). New aspects of the tolerance of retinol in humans. *Int. J. Vitam. Nutr. Res.* **45,** 363–372.

Kusin, J. A., Reddy, V., and Sivakumar, B. (1974). Vitamin E supplements and the absorption of a massive dose of vitamin A. *Am. J. Clin. Nutr.* **27,** 774–776.

Leelaprute, V., Boonpucknavig, V., Bhamarapravati, N., and Weerapradist, W. (1973). Hypervitaminosis A in rats. Varying responses due to different forms, doses and routes of administration. *Arch. Pathol.* **96,** 5–9.

Love, A. M., and Vickers, T. H. (1971). Hypervitaminosis A dysmelia in rats. *Br. J. Exp. Pathol.* **52,** 656–668.

Lucy, J. A., and Dingle, J. T. (1964). Fat-soluble vitamins and biological membranes. *Nature (London)* **204,** 156–160.

McCuaig, L. W., and Motzok, I. (1970). Excessive dietary vitamin E: Its alleviation of hypervitaminosis and lack of toxicity. *Poult. Sci.* **49,** 1050–1052.

Mallia, A. K., Smith, J. E., and Goodman, DeW. S. (1975). Metabolism of retinol-binding protein and vitamin A during hypervitaminosis A in the rat. *J. Lipid Res.* **16,** 180–188.

March, B. E., Wong, E., Seier, L., Sim, J., and Biely, J. (1973). Hypervitaminosis E in the chick. *J. Nutr.* **103,** 371–377.

Mathur, A. K., Ramanathan, R., and Misra, U. K. (1974). Effect of feeding excess of vitamin A and vitamin C on liver, plasma and adrenal lipids of rats. *Int. J. Vitam. Nutr. Res.* **44,** 19–25.

Morgan, A. F., Kimmel, L., and Hawkins, N. C. (1937). A comparison of the hypervitaminoses induced by irradiated ergosterol and fish liver oil concentrates. *J. Biol. Chem.* **120,** 85–102.

Morriss, G. M. (1973). The ultrastructural effects of excess maternal vitamin A on the primitive streak stage rat embryo. *J. Embryol. Exp. Morphol.* **30,** 219–242.

Morriss, G. M., and Steele, C. E. (1974). The effect of excess vitamin A on the development of rat embryos in culture. *J. Embryol. Exp. Morphol.* **32,** 505–514.

Muenter, M. D. (1974). Hypervitaminosis A. *Ann. Intern. Med.* **80,** 105–106.

Murphy, J. J. (1961). Thromboplastin formation in premature and fullterm infants during the first months of life. *Ann. Paediatr.* **196,** 122–129.

Nakamura, H. (1975). Analysis of limb anomalies induced *in vitro* by vitamin A (retinol) in mice. *Teratology* **12,** 61–70.

National Academy of Sciences. (1973). Supplementation of human diets with vitamin E. *Nutr. Rev.* **31,** 327–328.

National Academy of Sciences, National Research Council. (1975). Hazards of overuse of vitamin D. *Nutr. Rev.* **33,** 61–62.

Olson, J. A., and Hayaishi, O. (1965). The enzymatic cleavage of β-carotene into vitamin A by soluble enzymes of rat liver and intestine. *Proc. Natl. Acad. Sci. U.S.A.* **54,** 1364–1370.

Ostwald, R., and Briggs, G. M. (1966). Toxicity of the vitamins. *Natl. Acad. Sci. Publ.* **1354,** 183–220.

Pease, C. N. (1962). Focal retardation and arrest of growth of bones due to vitamin A intoxication. *J. Am. Med. Assoc.* **182,** 980–985.

Pereira, S. M., and Begum, A. (1973). Retention of a single oral massive dose of vitamin A. *Clin. Sci. Mol. Med.* **45,** 233–237.

Ram, G. C., and Misra, U. K. (1975). RNA synthesis in liver nuclei of young rats fed varying amounts of vitamin A. *Int. J. Vitam. Nutr. Res.* **45,** 124–128.

Rao, G. H., and Mason, K. E. (1975). Antisterility and antivitamin K activity of D-α-tocopherol hydroquinone in the vitamin E-deficient female rat. *J. Nutr.* **105,** 495–498.

Reddy, V., and Mohanram, M. (1971). Urinary excretion of lysosomal enzymes in hypovitaminosis and hypervitaminosis A in children. *Int. J. Vitam. Nutr. Res.* **41,** 321–326.

Robens, J. F. (1970). Teratogenic effects of hypervitaminosis in the hamster and the guinea pig. *Toxicol. Appl. Pharmacol.* **16,** 88–99.

Ruby, L. K., and Mital, M. H. (1974). Skeletal deformities following chronic hypervitaminosis A. *J. Bone Joint Surg., Am. Vol.* **56,** 1283–1287.

Russell, R. M., Boyer, J. L., Bagheri, S. A., and Hruban, Z. (1974). Hepatic injury from chronic hypervitaminosis A resulting in portal hypertension and ascites. *N. Engl. J. Med.* **291,** 435–440.

Schultz, R. L. (1969). Effects of ovariectomy and hypervitaminosis A on lysosomes of the rat conceptus. *Teratology* **2,** 283–296.

Sebrell, W. H., Jr., and Harris, R. S. (1967). "The Vitamins," Vol. 1. Academic Press, New York.

Sebrell, W. H., Jr., and Harris, R. S. (1971). "The Vitamins," Vol. 3. Academic Press, New York.

Sebrell, W. H., Jr., and Harris, R. S. (1972). "The Vitamins," Vol. 5. Academic Press, New York.

Setty, O. H., and Misra, U. K. (1975). Uptake of plasma lipids by extrahepatic tissues of vitamin A fed rats. *Int. J. Vitam. Nutr. Res.* **45,** 107–112.

Shenefelt, R. E. (1972). Gross congenital malformations. Animal model: Treatment of various species with a large dose of vitamin A at known stages of pregnancy. *Am. J. Pathol.* **66,** 589–592.

Singh, V. N., Singh, M., and Venkitasubramanian, T. A. (1969). Early effects of feeding excess vitamin A: Mechanism of fatty liver production in rats. *J. Lipid Res.* **10,** 395–401.

Snyderman, S. E., and Holt, L. E. (1973). Nutrition in infancy and adolescence. *In* "Modern Nutrition in Health and Disease" (R. S. Goodhart and M. E. Shils, eds.), pp. 659–680. Lea & Febiger, Philadelphia, Pennsylvania.

Soliman, M. K. (1972). Vitamin-A-Überdosierung. II. Zytologische and biochemische Veränderungen im Blut von mit hohen Dosen Vitamin A bzw. α-Tocopherol behandelten Ratten. *Int. J. Vitam. Nutr. Res.* **42,** 576–582.

Srikantia, S. G., and Reddy, V. (1970). Effect of a single massive dose of vitamin A on serum and liver levels of the vitamin. *Am. J. Clin. Nutr.* **23,** 114–118.

Strebel, R. F., Girerd, R. J., and Wagner, B. M. (1969). Cardiovascular calcification in rats with hypervitaminosis A. *Arch. Pathol.* **87,** 290–297.

Swaminathan, M. C., Susheela, T. P., and Thimmayamma, B. V. S. (1970). Field prophylactic trial with a single annual oral massive dose of vitamin A. *Am. J. Clin. Nutr.* **23,** 119–122.

Taylor, T. G., Morris, K. M. L., and Kirkley, J. (1968). Effects of dietary excesses of vitamins A and D on some constituents of the blood of chicks. *Br. J. Nutr.* **22,** 713–721.

Vest, M. (1966). Vitamin K in medical practice: Pediatrics. *Vitam. Horm. (N.Y.)* **24**, 649–663.

Vijayaraghauan, K., Naidu, A. N., Rao, N. P., and Srikantia, S. G. (1975). A simple method to evaluate the massive dose vitamin A prophylaxis program in preschool children. *Am. J. Clin. Nutr.* **28**, 1189–1193.

Vorhees, C. V. (1974). Some behavioral effects of maternal hypervitaminosis A in rats. *Teratology* **10**, 269–274.

Wieland, R. G., Hendricks, F. H., Amat, F. L., Gutierrez, L., and Jones, J. C. (1971). Hypervitaminosis A with hypercalcaemia. *Lancet* **1**, 698.

Witting, L. A. (1975). Vitamin E as a food additive. *J. Am. Oil Chem. Soc.* **52**, 64–68.

Wynn, R. M. (1963). Relationship of menadiol tetrasodium diphosphate (Synkayvite) to bilirubinemia and hemolysis in the adult and newborn rat. *Am. J. Obstet. Gynecol.* **86**, 495–503.

Yarington, C. T., Jr., and Stivers, F. E. (1974). Lathyrogenic effects of vitamin A in the rat embryo. *Laryngoscope* **84**, 1310–1315.

28

Diet and Drug Therapy of Hyperlipoproteinemia

GUSTAV SCHONFELD and JOSEPH L. WITZTUM

I. INTRODUCTION

Atherosclerotic cardiovascular disease is the leading cause of death in the Western world. Atherosclerosis can involve all of the major arteries of the body, producing lesions in the walls of blood vessels, which may result in partial or complete occlusions of the lumens of the involved vessel. Weakening of arterial walls may also occur leading to aneurysmal dilatations. The overall effect is interference with the flow of arterial blood to vital organs, and the production of symptoms which involve most of the major organ systems of the body including the central nervous system, the heart, the intestines, the kidneys, and the extremities (Table I). Although the initiating causes and the factors which lead to the

TABLE I
Some Atherosclerotic Syndromes[a]

Artery	Syndrome
Carotid or basilar	Transient ischemic attack
	Cerebrovascular accident (stroke)
	Amaurosis fugax
Coronary	Angina pectoris
	Myocardial infarct
	Arrhythmia
	Heart failure
Mesenteric	Abdominal angina
	Intestinal infarction
Renal	Renovascular ischemia and hyper-
	tension
	Renal infarct
Aorto–iliac	Buttock claudication
	Impotence
	Aneurysm
Femoral–popliteal	Lower extremity claudication
	Gangrene

[a] The above are some of the most frequently seen syndromes due to partial or complete occlusions of arteries by atherosclerosis.

progression of the atherosclerotic process have not been completely delineated, it is clear that certain human populations have a greater propensity for developing clinical atherosclerosis than do others. The factors which put people at higher than usual risk include high blood pressure, cigarette smoking, and hypercholesterolemia (and other kinds of hyperlipoproteinemia). The strong connection between hyperlipoproteinemia and atherosclerosis, and the hope that atherosclerosis may be prevented by the treatment of hyperlipoproteinemia represents some practical motivation for research into the causes of hyperlipoproteinemia. It is also the prime rationale for the treatment of hyperlipoproteinemia in man. This chapter will review some of the evidence which connects hyperlipoproteinemia with atherosclerosis, present the rationale and methods for diet and drug therapy, and present some of the results of therapy in man.

II. ATHEROSCLEROSIS AND HYPERLIPOPROTEINEMIA

Four sorts of evidence establish the connection between hyperlipoproteinemia and atherosclerosis, particularly atherosclerotic cardiovascular disease. These may be divided into epidemiologic, genetic, experimental, and therapeutic. The epidemiologic evidence is illustrated by the following studies.

A seven-nation survey (Fig. 1) in which the average dietary intake of saturated fatty acids is strongly correlated with serum cholesterol levels, and serum cholesterol levels in turn are strongly correlated with rates of fatal and nonfatal myocardial infarction (Stamler, 1975). The weakness of this and similar studies lies in the fact that factors other than greater dietary intakes of saturated fatty acids and serum cholesterol separately or together could have contributed to the differences in the cardiovascular events. This objection was overcome by studies of ethnically similar groups which live in different environments. Two ethnic groups have been particularly well studied in this regard: Men of Japanese origin who live in Hawaii and Japan, and Yemenite Jews. It is well established that the diets in Japan contain less cholesterol and more polyunsaturated fats than those eaten in Hawaii (Keys *et al.*, 1958). Similarly the dietary habits of Yemenite Jews recently arriving in Israel differ greatly from those who have lived in Israel for 20 years or more (Toor, 1957). In each case, the intake of diets high in saturated fats and in cholesterol was positively correlated with serum cholesterol levels and with cardiovascular event rates (Fig. 2).

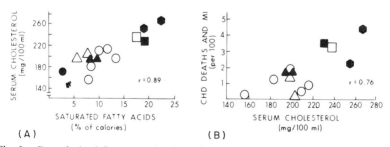

(A)   (B)

Fig. 1. Data derived from examination of 12,000 middle-aged males in seven countries. Each geometric design represents a cohort from one country. A. Relationship between median serum cholesterol and average percent of dietary calories desired from saturated fat; B. Relationship between median serum cholesterol and age standardized 5-year incidence rate for fatal and nonfatal coronary heart disease. □ United States; ● Finland; ■ Netherlands; ▲ Italy; ○ Yugoslavia; △ Greece; ● Japan. Data adapted from seven-country study as reported by Stamler (1975).

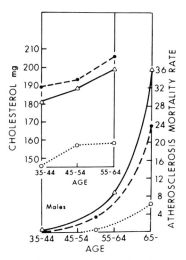

Fig. 2. Atherosclerosis mortality rate (per 1000 inhabitants per year) for three male cohorts in Israel during the years 1953–1955. △, European Jews, ●, Early Yemenite immigrants (immigrants of over 20 years), ○, Recent Yemenite immigrants (less than 5 years). The mortality rate was four times higher for early immigrants. In the inset are the cholesterol levels (in mg/dl) for the same three cohorts. Redrawn from Toor (1957).

Perhaps the most convincing epidemiologic evidence comes from prospective studies. In these large studies, unselected individuals are examined at the beginning of the project and at regular intervals thereafter to ascertain what factors those people who develop myocardial infarctions or other coronary events share in common. One such study is the Framingham Study (Fig. 3) in which approximately 5000 individuals have been followed for over 20 years. These data clearly show a strong relationship between the levels of serum cholesterol at the beginning of the study and the subsequent development of cardiovascular events (Kannel *et al.*, 1971). Similar data on smoking and high blood pressure have established these too as independent coronary "risk-factors" (Stamler, 1975).

Recent studies have shown that low density lipoprotein (LDL)-cholesterol is at least as good a discriminator of coronary risk as is total cholesterol. Thus LDL is implicated as a possible causal factor in atherosclerosis. On the other hand, high density lipoprotein (HDL)-cholesterol is negatively correlated with coronary risk (Fig. 4) (Rhoads *et al.*, 1976) leading some to suggest that HDL may have a "protective" effect (Miller and Miller, 1975).

The genetic evidence of the atherosclerosis–cholesterol connection was obtained from studies of probands and families with hyperlipo-

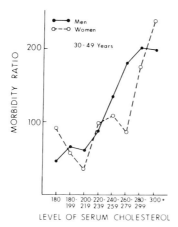

Fig. 3. Risk of coronary heart disease (over 14 years) versus cholesterol level at initial examination in men and women age 30–49 at entry as determined in the Framingham Study. Note that for men in particular, no critical level of cholesterol was observed, rather the risk increased proportionately to the cholesterol level. Adapted from Kannel *et al.*, (1971).

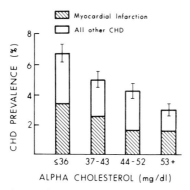

Fig. 4. Estimated prevalence of coronary heart disease (CHD) according to quantities of HDL (alpha) cholesterol. This study is part of the Honolulu Heart Study which is prospectively following Hawaiian men of Japanese ancestry. These statistics are based on a selected sample of 1,859 men age 50–72 years. In this population, CHD was significantly correlated with total and LDL (beta) cholesterol, but not with triglycerides. The inverse relationship between alpha cholesterol and CHD was independent of total and beta cholesterol and obesity. Adapted from Rhoads *et al.*, (1976).

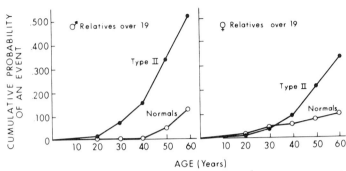

Fig. 5. Life table analysis of Coronary Artery Disease (CAD) as determined by analysis of 1,023 relatives of 116 kindred with familial Type II hyperlipoprotemia. By age 60, males with Type II had a 50% chance of having CAD, a fivefold increased risk compared to their normolipemic male relatives. The increased risk was detectable as early as the third decade of life. Though not so dramatic, hypercholesterolemic females were also at increased risk. Adapted from Stone *et al.*, (1974).

proteinemia (Fig. 5). Affected male members of families with monogenic hypercholesterolemia developed coronary heart disease approximately five times more frequently than did the nonaffected males. Affected females developed coronary heart disease at approximately three times the rates of the nonaffected women (Stone *et al.*, 1974).

Atherosclerosis has been produced experimentally in many species. The experimental models most relevant to human disease are those of the nonhuman primates. Lesions may be produced in these animals with a fair degree of predictability. The most florid lesions are produced by the induction of vascular injury by a variety of techniques, combined with the feeding of high cholesterol, high saturated fat diets which result in hyperlipoproteinemia. However, even dietary hyperlipoproteinemia alone without injury is followed by the appearance of atherosclerotic lesions (Ross and Glomset, 1976; Kritchevsky, 1975).

The work of several groups has provided a plausible role for lipoproteins both in the production and perpetuation of lesions (Ross and Harker, 1976). According to this concept atherogenesis begins with an injury to the endothelial layer of the vessel wall (Fig. 6-1). The injury may be mechanical (wall stress), immunologic (immune complex + complement), or chemical (hyperlipoproteinemia per se, homocystinemia), but however produced, the injury exposes the subendothelial surfaces to circulating blood (Fig. 6-2). Platelets in blood adhere to and become activated by these denuded surfaces (Fig. 6-3). The activation results in

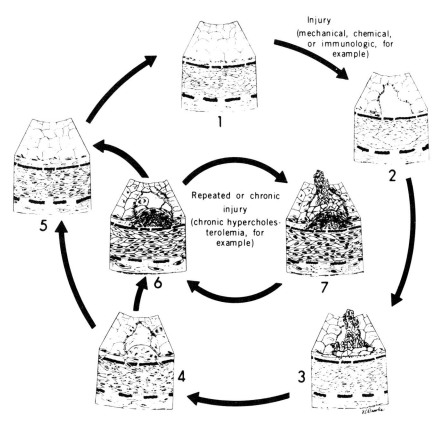

Fig. 6. Proposed scheme of the origin and perpetuation of atherosclerosis as suggested by Ross and Harker. According to this concept, hypercholesterolemia is atherogenic because it produces an initial injury (step 1), is a smooth muscle cell mitogen (step 4), and by virtue of its continuous presence maintains this destructive cycle (step 7). A more complete discussion of this theory can be found in the text. Published with permission of the editors. Ross and Harker (1976).

the release of a platelet factor, a mitogenic protein, which stimulates the proliferation of arterial smooth muscle cells and their migration from the media into the intimal layers of the artery (Fig. 6-4). The platelet factor is thought to be the most important mitogen, but plasma LDL also is or contains a mitogen for arterial smooth muscle cells. Thus, hyperlipoproteinemia alone may produce endothelial injury, and may also participate in the proliferative response.

In the normolipemic primate, the increased wall thickness, which follows mechanical injury, remains for a few months. But then lesions regress to the point where, after about one year, the vessel has regained its original appearance (Fig. 6-5). But severe or continuing injury or hyperlipidemia may result in the progressive enlargement of lesions (Fig. 6-6,7) and lesions may become sufficiently "advanced" to make regression unlikely.

Hyperlipoproteinemia per se may interfere with regression by overwhelming the capacity of the lysosomal system of the arterial smooth muscle cells to hydrolyze cholesterol esters. This could lead to the progressive accumulation of cholesterol esters by cells and their conversion to "foam cells."

Indeed, the vessels of animals after 8-10 months of experimentally induced hypercholesterolemia (without mechanical injury) contain atheromatous lesions which approach the severity of lesions seen in the mechanically injured, hypercholesterolemic animal (Ross and Harker, 1976). From the above analysis, it is clear that elevated levels of lipoproteins could be instrumental in atherogenesis at each of the major stages of lesion development: (a) injury, (b) cell proliferation, and (c) lesion regression.

The fourth kind of evidence linking hyperlipidemia with atherosclerosis comes from attempts at reversing the atherosclerotic process by lowering the level of lipids in blood. These attempts have used diets or drugs, both in man and experimental animals. The evidence for reversibility in animals is quite strong (Armstrong, 1976). Similar data are hard to come by in man because at the present time all reliable methods for evaluating blood vessel anatomy require direct catheterization of those arterial beds to be examined. The performance of "invasive" procedures on asymptomatic individuals may be hard to justify on moral grounds. For this reason, therapeutic trials in man use clinical "end points" such as the occurrence of angina pectoris, myocardial infarction, or sudden death as indices for the success or failure of therapeutic interventions. These end points are at best insensitive and indirect indicators of the effectiveness of any preventive or therapeutic interventions on the progression or regression of arterial lesions. This is because the connection between clinical symptoms and the anatomic status of lesions is not entirely clear. For example, symptoms could develop in individuals even though the appearance of vessels may not have changed or conversely, lesions can enlarge appreciably without producing symptoms.

In spite of these difficulties, some (Leren, 1966 Rinzler, 1968; Dayton et al., 1969; Miettinen et al., 1972) but not all (Rose et al., 1965; Medical Research Council, 1968; Frantz et al., 1975) studies have shown that dietary measures for lowering blood lipids are effective in preventing either the first (Table II) or subsequent myocardial infarctions in men.

TABLE II
Finnish "Diet-Heart" Study[a]

	Control diet		Therapeutic diet	
	Cholesterol	Death rate	Cholesterol	Death rate
Hospital N	266	13.0	217	5.7
Hospital K	268	15.2	234	7.5
Pooled death rates	—	14.1	—	6.6 ($p<0.002$)

[a] Effect of a long-term (12-year) dietary trial with a cholesterol lowering diet on mortality from coronary heart disease (CHD). Two Finnish mental hospitals were used. From 1959–1965 all patients in hospital N received the therapeutic diet (soybean "filled" skim milk, and substitution for butter of a highly unsaturated margarine, diet P/S ratio was 1.4–1.8) while patients in hospital K received a control diet (P/S ratio of 0.2–0.3). From 1965–1971 the diets were reversed. The pooled results for males are given in this table. Cholesterol values are mean serum cholesterol in mg/dl. Death rates are adjusted death rates from coronary heart disease in man; deaths/1000 person-years. Adopted from Miettinen *et al.* (1972).

Several drugs have been tried for the prevention of second myocardial infarctions. The results have been disappointing in regard to preventing deaths from new coronary heart disease events (Dewar, 1971; Oliver, 1971; Stamler, 1975). These studies were carried out with subjects not selected for hyperlipoproteinemia. But these negative results cannot be extrapolated to efforts at primary prevention particularly in younger age groups with lipid disorders. In fact, studies are currently in progress to evaluate the effects of cholesterol lowering on the development of coronary events in subjects with hypercholesterolemia. In a few isolated cases where estimates of blood flow or angiographic examinations of vessel anatomy have been possible, regression of lesions have been demonstrated (Zelis *et al.*, 1970; Starzl *et al.*, 1974). Indeed, as mentioned above, it is the dual hope of inducing regression of existing atherosclerotic lesions and the prevention of new lesions which provides the cardinal reasons for the treatment of human hyperlipoproteinemia. The other reasons for therapy are the amelioration of the symptoms associated with the hyperlipoproteinemic state itself.

III. HYPERLIPOPROTEINEMIA

The hyperlipoproteinemias comprise a large group of heterogeneous disorders the classification of which is at the moment in a state of flux. The classification currently in widest use is a descriptive one, that uses

TABLE III
The Lipoproteins of Human Plasma[a]

Density class	Density range (gm/ml)	Flotation range (S_f)	Electrophoretic mobility	Lipoprotein family	Particles found in density class
Chylomicrons	0.95–0.97	>400	origin	LpA LpB LpC	Exogenous particles from gut; Large endogenous particles from liver
VLDL	0.95–1.006	20–400	α_2-globulin ("pre-beta")	LpB LpC LpE	Endogenous particles from liver; small exogenous particles from gut; chylomicron remnants; Type III β-VLDL
LDL	1.006–1.063	0–20	β-globulin	LpB LpC LpD	Degradation products of VLDL: Abnormal LDL in Type IV. Lp(a)
Lp(a)	1.060–1.090	0–4	α_2-globulin ("pre-beta")	LpB Lp(a) Albumin	HDL$_1$; Lp(a)
HDL	1.063–1.21	F1–10	α_1-globulin	LpC LpA LpD	Lp(a)

[a] The density and electrophoretic nomenclatures are based on "operational" considerations, whereas the "lipoprotein family" is a conceptual classification which holds that each lipoprotein family is defined by its characteristic apolipoprotein, e.g., lipoprotein A (LpA) is the family containing apolipoprotein A (ApoA), LpB is the family containing ApoB. According to this theory, each density or electrophoretic class may contain one or more of the lipoprotein families free or complexed to each other. Lp(a) is also called "sinking pre-beta" since it migrates in the pre-beta position, but it is found in the HDL density class. The function of this lipoprotein is unknown, but it is at times confused with pre-beta VLDL. Lipoproteins are isolated from plasma by ultracentrifugation at various densities. The "density cuts" may contain partially catabolized particles arising from gut and/or liver depending on the dietary intake, time since last meal, and the health status of the

abnormalities in the levels of plasma lipoproteins (Table III) as the basis for classification. During the past few years a marked improvement in the understanding of the physiology of lipid transport and in the genetics of hyperlipoproteinemia has taken place. These developments have started a trend toward the classification of the hyperlipoproteinemias on the basis of their pathophysiology. In this section we shall briefly discuss lipoprotein physiology and hyperlipoproteinemia. Several excellent reviews have been published recently (Eisenberg, 1976; Jackson et al., 1976).

The major lipids of plasma—cholesterol, triglycerides, and phospholipids—do not circulate free, but are bound to specific apolipoproteins (Table IV) forming the large complex macromolecules called the lipoproteins. Lipoproteins are classified by their behaviors in the ultracentrifuge or by their electrophoretic mobilities. There is also a classification based on the concept of lipoprotein families (Table III). Under the electron microscope, lipoproteins isolated from plasma appear as spheres, and spectroscopic studies have revealed that the nonpolar lipids—triglycerides and cholesterol esters—form the core of the spherical particles, whereas the more polar compounds—apoproteins and phospholipids—are disposed close to or on the outer surface. Utilizing this structure, lipoproteins can transport water-insoluble lipids through plasma water. The apoproteins, in addition to being structural components of the lipoproteins, also are important as modulators of lipoprotein metabolism (Table V).

Chylomicrons are formed in the intestine. Ingested fat which consists of about 95% triglyceride and 5% cholesterol is emulsified with bile acids and hydrolyzed by pancreatic lipases. The resulting free fatty acids, monoglycerides, and free cholesterol are absorbed across the brush border membrane of the intestinal absorbtive cell. Inside the cell, the lipids are re-esterified and the resulting triglycerides and cholesterol esters are combined with small amounts of phospholipids and specific apolipoproteins to form chylomicrons, which contain 95% triglyceride by weight. These exit the absorptive cells and enter the circulation via the lymphatic system.

Walls of arteries contain an enzyme complex called lipoprotein lipase which hydrolyzes the chylomicron triglycerides, producing fatty acids and glycerol. Fatty acids enter the various tissues where they may be used as sources of energy or stored as triglycerides. During the "fed state" a large proportion of the dietary fatty acids enter the adipose tissue, whereas in the "fasted state" fatty acids may enter muscle, e.g., the heart, preferentially. Chylomicrons depleted of triglycerides are called "remnants". The remnant is taken up by the liver where its cholesterol

TABLE IV
The Apoprotein Contents of Human Lipoproteins[a]

Density class	ApoA		ApoB (R-ser)	ApoC			Lp(a)	ApoD (ApoA-III)	ApoE (Arginine-rich)
	A-I (R-gln I)	A-II (R-gln II)		C-I (R-ser)	C-II (R-glu)	C-III (R-ala)			
Chylomicrons	trace	trace	5–10	←	60–70	→			
VLDL	<1	trace	37 (20–60)	3	6	40		ND	12 (7–15)
LDL	ND	ND	>80		<10			+	trace
Lp(a)	ND	ND	65		ND		20	—	—
HDL	65–70	20–25	ND		5–10			1–2	ND

[a] Numbers represent % of total apoprotein mass. +, Identified by disc gel electrophoresis or immunologically; no quantitative estimates available. ND, none detected. The chemistry of ApoB is not completely defined. It may represent two or more proteins. ApoE also consists of ~4 uncharacterized subunits. VLDL subclasses vary in apoprotein composition The S_f 100–400 subfraction contains 20% ApoB, 7% arginine-rich and 70% ApoC. S_f 20–50 contains 60% ApoB, 15% arginine-rich and 25% ApoC. S_f 50–100 has an intermediate apoprotein composition. Lp(a) contains albumin (~15%) in addition to ApoB and the specific Lp(a) apoprotein.

TABLE V
Physiologic Functions of Apoproteins

Apoprotein	Physiologic function	Pathophysiologic role
A-I	Activation of lecithin: cholesteryl acyltransferase (LCAT)	Reduced to 1–2% of normal levels in hypoalphalipoproteinemia (Tangier disease); A-I deficiency may lead to decreased "reverse transport" of cholesterol, and the deposition of cholesteryl esters in the tissues of Tangier disease patients
A-II	Binds lipids avidly, structural role in HDL	Reduced to <10% of normal in Tangier disease
B	Essential in transporting lipids from gut and liver in chylomicrons and VLDL	Reduced to <10% of normal levels in abetalipoproteinemia, these patients have extremely low levels of blood lipids, probably due to lack of secretion of VLDL and chylomicrons
C-I	Activation of LCAT, activation of lipoprotein lipase (LPL_{C-1})	Unknown
C-II	Activation of LPL	C-II and C-III together modulate LPL activity *in vitro*; absence of C-II and disturbed C-II/C-III ratios have been noted in some cases of hypertriglyceridemia (Types IV and V)
C-III	Inhibition of C-II activation of LPL	
D (thin-line peptide)	Unknown	Unknown
E-I E-II E-III (arginine-rich apoproteins)	Unknown, may serve as a recognition marker between lipoproteins and cells	E-I and E-II increased and E-III absent or decreased in the VLDL of patients with dysbetalipoproteinemia (Type III); ApoE increased in the lipoproteins of animals fed a high cholesterol diet
Lp(a)	Unknown	Unknown

(which is primarily of dietary origin) serves to regulate hepatic cholesterol synthesis. In normal man a fat-containing meal produces peak
chylomicronemia within 3–4 hours and chylomicrons disappear from
plasma by 8–12 hours.

The triglycerides circulating in plasma in addition to arising from gut
may also enter plasma from the liver. This organ utilizes free fatty acids
taken up from plasma or fatty acids synthesized *de novo* from carbohydrates or alcohol to form triglycerides. Hepatic triglyceride is combined
with cholesterol, phospholipids, and apoproteins and secreted as very
low density lipoprotein (VLDL). In plasma the triglycerides of VLDL are
hydrolyzed by lipoprotein lipase making free fatty acids and glycerol
available to peripheral tissues. The triglyceride-depleted VLDL particle
has been called an intermediate density lipoprotein (IDL). The further
intravascular processing of IDL results in the formation of LDL. It is
thought that in man LDL derives from the metabolism of VLDL (and
perhaps chylomicrons). In other species of animals LDL may be secreted
by the liver directly. The LDL may be taken up by specific adsorptive
endocytosis into a variety of tissues including the arterial smooth muscle
cell. (This may play an important role in atherogenesis.) Thus, the final
disassembly of the LDL particle is an intracellular process, the net result
of which is the transport of cholesterol from the liver to peripheral
tissues ("forward" transport).

The last class of lipoproteins, HDL, is secreted by liver and probably
by the intestine as well. HDL seems to be secreted as a simple particle
consisting of phospholipids and one or two apolipoproteins, and then
acquires other apoproteins and lipids in plasma following secretion.
HDL has important functions in the metabolism of the other lipoproteins and in the transport of cholesterol from the peripheral tissues to
the liver ("reverse" transport). This is needed because the cholesterol
nucleus is not degraded by mammalian cells. Thus, LDL and HDL may
have the combined function of maintaining the cellular balance of
cholesterol, LDL bringing cholesterol and HDL removing it. It is possible to envision that high levels of LDL accompanied by low levels of HDL
could be atherogenic, and that the opposite combination could decrease
the risk of atherosclerosis. This hypothesis has good epidemiologic support as noted above.

In clinical practice, hyperlipidemia (elevations of plasma triglycerides,
cholesterol, or both) is recognized first. Hyperlipidemia is then converted to hyperlipoproteinemia to make a specific diagnosis.

Hyperlipidemia is diagnosed when plasma levels of cholesterol or triglycerides or both are elevated under well-defined conditions. Since the
time of the last meal greatly influences lipid and lipoprotein levels, nor-

mal lipid values have been defined in the fasting state. Therefore, samples of blood must be drawn after 12–14 hours of fasting. Diet and drugs also affect lipoproteins; therefore, subjects should not be eating any atypical diets nor be taking any medications known to alter lipoprotein levels. Because acute illnesses may also change lipid levels, diagnosis of lipoprotein disorders should be delayed until any acute illness has abated. Finally, it is useful to draw more than one baseline blood sample (e.g., three samples 2–4 weeks apart) to assess the degree of spontaneous fluctuation in any individual before any therapy is begun. It is clear from Table VI that the levels of both cholesterol and triglycerides are strongly related to age and to sex. Hypercholesterolemia can be defined as any value above the ninety-fifth percentile for the appropriate age and sex of the patient. However, it is worth distinguishing "normal" values derived

TABLE VI
Cholesterol and Triglycerides[a]

	Males		Females	
Age	Mean	95th percentile	Mean	95th percentile
Cholesterol				
10–14	165	205	165	205
15–19	150	200	165	220
20–29	180	235	180	235
30–39	205	270	190	250
40–49	215	280	210	285
50–59	215	280	220	310
Triglycerides				
10–14	65	145	75	150
15–19	80	160	75	150
20–29	105	250	90	210
30–39	130	300	100	225
40–49	140	380	110	240
50–59	140	330	120	260

[a] Data based on analysis of 1000 subjects. Each cell had more than 50 subjects. Values were obtained by the Autoanalyzer II procedure on extracted plasma. Less specific methods, using unextracted serum such as the SMA-12 procedure may give values 15–25% higher. We consider cholesterol values above the ninety-fifth percentile to represent hypercholesterolemia, but arbitrarily consider TG values above 200 mg/dl to represent hypertriglyceridemia. (G. Schonfeld, G. Weidman, and J. L. Witztum, unpublished observations).

TABLE VII
Hyperlipoproteinemia According to NIH Criteria[a]

| Lipoprotein phenotype | Abnormality | | | Causes of secondary hyperlipoproteinemia |
	Ultracentrifugal nomenclature	Electrophoretic nomenclature	
I	Hyperchylomicronemia	Chylomicron band	Uncontrolled diabetes, dysglobulinemias (especially systemic lupus erythematosus), hypothyroidism
IIA	LDL increased	Increased beta band	Porphyria, hypothyroidism, biliary obstruction, nephrosis, dysglobulinemias (especially myeloma), pregnancy
IIB	LDL plus VLDL increased	Increased beta and pre-beta bands	Same as for IIA
III	Accumulation of "Remnants" or IDL (degradation products of chylomicrons and/or VLDL)	"Floating beta" "Broad beta"	Hypothyroidism, alcoholism, dysglobulinemias, uncontrolled diabetes
IV	VLDL increased	Increased pre-beta	Lipodystrophy, diabetes, alcohol intake, glucocorticoids, chronic renal disease, estrogens, pregnancy, glycogen storage disease
V	VLDL and chylomicrons increased	Increased pre-beta and chylomicron bands	Alcoholism, pancreatitis, dysglobulinemias, uncontrolled diabetes.

[a] Hyperlipoproteinemias are defined by the elevations of individual classes of lipoproteins. The elevations may be "primary," or secondary to other diseases

by statistical calculations from "ideal" values derived by risk factor analysis. In the case of cholesterol, "ideal" values would probably be closer to 200 mg/dl than to the ninety-fifth percentile values. The same ninety-fifth percentile criteria are applied in the case of hypertriglyceridemia in subjects below the age of 20. However, on the basis of risk factor analysis, most workers in the field consider triglyceride levels above 200 mg/dl to be undesirably high. This criterion is therefore arbitrarily applied to the age groups above 20 years. If hyperlipidemia is present, one needs to distinguish between primary and secondary causes (Table VII). The latter consists of a variety of disorders which are accompanied by disturbances in lipid or lipoprotein metabolism. In these cases, the lipoprotein abnormalities usually regress with the treatment of the primary disorder.

With hyperlipidemia having been diagnosed, it is useful to know which lipoproteins are responsible for the elevations of the lipids because, as stated before, the currently most widely accepted classification of lipid disorders (primary and secondary) is based on elevations of specific classes of lipoproteins in plasma (Table VII). For this classification, it is necessary to quantify the lipoproteins levels in plasma. Several methods are available. The most accurate one measures the lipid contents of individual lipoprotein fractions by a combination of chemical, ultracentrifugal and precipitation techniques. However, this is a relatively laborious and expensive procedure which is used primarily in research. More simplified schemes have been devised for estimating the lipoprotein classes in plasma for clinical practice. The earliest and best known of these is lipoprotein electrophoresis. From a knowledge of the plasma cholesterol and triglyceride levels and the lipoprotein electrophoresis, one can estimate which lipoproteins are increased and whether lipoproteins of abnormal mobility are present. It is also possible to identify chylomicrons or the presence of abnormal amounts of VLDL by the inspection of plasma which has been kept at 4°C for 16–24 hours. In fact, the diagnosis of over 80% of the patients as to phenotype (according to the NIH criteria) can be made simply from knowing the plasma triglyceride and cholesterol levels and from an inspection of plasma (Table VIII). However, Types I and III hyperlipoproteinemia can be diagnosed with certainty only by the use of special techniques. In addition to the lipoprotein abnormalities, the hyperlipoproteinemias are associated with signs and symptoms involving many organ systems (Table IX); these may be useful aids in making a diagnosis.

The value of the phenotypic classification of primary hyperlipoproteinemia has been questioned recently on several grounds: (a) the apparent phenotype of any individual may change with diet or therapy,

TABLE VIII
Practical Approach to Phenotyping[a]

Lipids	Plasma	Type
Chol high, TG normal	Clear	Type IIA
Chol high, TG > 200–400	Chylomicrons absent Plasma clear to turbid	LDL chol < 190 → Type IV LDL chol > 190 → Type IIB (Type III suspect)
Chol high, TG 400–1000	Chylomicrons absent Plasma turbid	→ Type IV
	Chylomicrons present Plasma turbid	→ Type V (Suspect Type III)
Chol high, TG > 1000	Chylomicrons present Plasma turbid	→ Type V
	Chylomicrons present Plasma clear	→ Type I
Chol normal, TG high	Chylomicrons absent Plasma turbid	Type IV

[a] When plasma triglycerides are less than 400 mg/dl, LDL-cholesterol (in mg/dl) may be estimated from the formula: VLDL-cholesterol = total cholesterol -[(TG/5 + 45] where TG/5 is an estimate of VLDL-cholesterol.

confusing both patient and doctor; (b) not all of the phenotypes correspond to genetic entities (e.g., Types IIb, IV, and V); (c) some of the phenotypes are heterogeneous with respect to symptomatology and prognosis; and (d) therapy is not yet specific enough to warrant the many subdivisions. The objections are valid but the phenotyping system remains useful, provided it is remembered that the classification is but a shorthand method for describing the hyperlipoproteinemia and that phenotyping must be done under the strict conditions specified above. Results of therapy are followed by estimating triglyceride and cholesterol levels. Therefore, phenotyping of treated patients is unnecessary and may be misleading.

Other classifications of the hyperlipidemias are being attempted based on current understanding of the pathophysiology and genetics of hyperlipoproteinemias (one example is shown in Table X). The primary hyperlipoproteinemias for which the pathophysiology has been worked out reasonably well include (1) lipoprotein lipase deficiency (Type I); (2)

defective-LDL hypercholesterolemia (Type II); (3) LDL-receptor deficient or defective monogenic hypercholesterolemia (Type II); (4) broad Beta disease (Type III), a disorder of apolipoprotein E; and (5) ApoCII deficient hypertriglyceridemia (Type V). Perhaps 10% or less of patients with hyperlipoproteinemia fall into these well-defined categories. There remain large populations of patients with (6) primary hypertriglyceridemia (Type IV), (7) primary hypercholesterolemia (Type IIa),

TABLE IX
Presenting Complaints in Primary Hyperlipoproteinemia

	Pathology
Skin	Eruptive xanthoma—Types I and V
	Palmar xanthoma—Type III
	Xanthelasma—Types II and III
	Tuberous and tendinous xanthoma—
	Types II and III
Eye	Lipemia retinalis—Type V
	Arcus corneae—all types
ENT	Yellow plaques on buccal mucosa—
	Type II
Pulmonary	None described
Heart	Coronary artery disease—Types II-V,
	particularly Type II
Gastrointestinal	Pancreatitis—Types I and V
	Abdominal pain—Types I and V
	Hepatosplenomegaly—Types I and V
Renal	Renovascular disease—Types II and III
Neuromuscular	Peripheral neuropathy—Type V
Rheumatologic	Fibrositis-arthritis involving particu-
	larly ankles and Achilles tendon—
	Type II
	Migratory polyarthritis—Type V
Extremities	Intermittent claudication—Types II-IV,
	particularly Type III

TABLE X
Pathogenetic Classification of Primary and Secondary Hyperlipoproteinemias: Putative Mechanisms and Metabolic Consequences[a]

Name of condition	Abnormal rates of production	Associated clinical condition
Secondary hyperlipoproteinemias		
Type II	Overproduction of VLDL and increased VLDL conversion to LDL	Nephrosis
Type IV	VLDL overproduction, alcohol stimulation of lipid synthesis	Alcoholism
	VLDL overproduction, part of general response of liver to urinary losses of protein	Nephrosis
	Mixed picture, some patients overproduce VLDL, others have slow clearance	Diabetes mellitus
	Hepatic overproduction of VLDL, decreased fat cell LPL	Corticosteroid therapy
	The shunting of glucose 6-P toward glycolysis and fatty acid synthesis, results in increased hepatic VLDL production	Glycogenosis, Type I (von Gierke)
Hyperlipoproteinemia of pregnancy	Levels of all lipoproteins increase, hepatic triacylglycerol synthesis and VLDL output are increased	Pregnancy and estrogen therapy
Hyperlipoproteinemia of obesity	Enhanced secretion of VLDL	Mild (105% ideal body weight) to severe obesity

Name of condition	Defective lipoproteins	Associated clinical condition
*Hyperbetalipoproteinemia (Type II)	Defective LDL which is not "recognized" by cells leading to deficient LDL catabolism and accumu-	Familial; accelerated atherosclerosis

Name of condition	Abnormal catabolism	Associated clinical condition
Primary dysbetalipoproteinemia (Type III)	Deficiency of ApoC-III and increased ApoE-I and ApoE-II in VLDL; abnormal catabolism of remnants, accumulation of abnormal βVLDL	Familial; accelerated atherosclerosis
*Hyperchylomicronemia-hyperprebetalipoproteinemia (primary Type V)	Decreased ApoC-I and ApoC-II activatable lipoprotein lipase; decreased ratios of ApoC-II/ApoC-III; chylomicrons not hydrolyzed by normal postheparin lipase; low lipase activity and/or abnormal activation of lipase; deficient VLDL and chylomicron catabolism; accumulation of VLDL and chylomicrons	Possible familial; glucose intolerance, pancreatitis, eruptive xanthoma
Hyperlipoproteinemia of liver disease (Lp-X)	Production and release of abnormal LDL, called Lp-X, by liver	Obstructive jaundice
Hyperlipoproteinemia of paraproteinemia (secondary Type V)	Formation of abnormal lipoprotein substrates in plasma because of complexing of paraprotein with lipoproteins, results in high VLDL and chylomicron levels	Consequences of hyperchylomicronemia, e.g., pancreatitis, eruptive xanthoma
*Primary hyperchylomicronemia (Type I)	Lipoprotein lipase deficiency; absent ApoC-I activatable lipase and decreased ApoC-II activated lipase; deficient chylomicron catabolism, accumulation of chylomicrons	Hepatosplenomegaly, abdominal pain, eruptive xanthoma, pancreatitis
*Primary hyperbetalipoproteinemia (Type II)	Deficient, or defective cellular receptors for LDL leading to deficient catabolism of LDL; disturbed regulation of cholesterol synthesis; accumulation of LDL	Severe atherosclerosis in early life, familial
Secondary Type IV or Type V hyperlipoproteinemia of renal disease	Lipoprotein lipase deficiency, or inhibition, delayed clearance of VLDL	Uremic syndrome, accelerated atherosclerosis

TABLE X, *continued*

Name of condition	Abnormal rates of production	Associated clinical condition
Hyperlipoproteinemia of lupus erythematosus (secondary Type I or Type V)	Circulating antiheparin; interference with lipoprotein lipase release or with lipase–lipoprotein interaction	Syndrome of clinical lupus erythematosus
Hyperlipoproteinemia of hypothyroidism (secondary Type II or Type III)	Diminished lipid synthesis in liver, also lower activities and rates of synthesis of lipoprotein lipase in adipose tissue leading to slowed clearance and accumulation of LDL in plasma	Syndrome of hypothyroidism
Diabetic lipemia (secondary Type V)	Deficient tissue synthesis and/or activation of lipoprotein lipase; deficient catabolism of VLDL and chylomicrons	Clinical complications of diabetes mellitus including atherosclerosis

Name of condition	Unknown and mixed etiologies	Associated clinical condition
*Primary hyperprebeta-lipoproteinemia (Type IV)	Overproduction of VLDL and/or deficient catabolism; accumulation of VLDL, mixed etiology, none well defined.	Glucose intolerance, obesity, hyperuremia, hypertension
Hyperlipoproteinemia of porphyria (secondary Type II)	Excess accumulation of LDL, etiology unknown	Syndrome of porphyria
Hyperalphalipoproteinemia		Longevity, decreased prevalence of atherosclerosis

a Primary hyperlipoproteinemias are preceded by an asterisk.

and (8) primary elevations of both lipids (Types IIb, IV, and V). In some instances the hypertriglyceridemia (Types IV and V) is due to the over-production of VLDL; in other cases, it is due to the poor clearance of lipoproteins from plasma. The molecular bases of these kinetic defects are not known. Patients with primary hypertriglyceridemia may come from families with "familial hypertriglyceridemia", or from families with " combined or multiple phenotype hyperlipidemia"; these families contain individuals with Type II, IV, and V hyperlipoproteinemias. Obviously, more work is needed in the metabolism and genetics of the primary hypertriglyceridemias. The large groups of patients with isolated hypercholesterolemia, or "mixed" hyperlipidemia, also comprise heterogeneous populations in terms of metabolism and/or genetics, e.g., in addition to monogenic (LDL-receptor negative) hypercholesterolemia, there are patients with "sporadic" and "polygenic" hypercholesterolemia, and also "familial combined hyperlipidemia".

Although the descriptive and pathophysiologic classifications serve to increase our understanding of the primary hyperlipoproteinemias, they provide us with more information than we need for therapy at the present time. As will be seen, for a practical approach it is sufficient to know whether the disorder consists primarily of elevations of triglycerides or cholesterol or both and whether chylomicrons are present.

IV. DIETARY THERAPY OF HYPERLIPOPROTEINEMIA

It is well recognized that age, sex, and heredity may play major, if not dominant, roles in determining plasma lipid levels. That the diets of populations are also important can be appreciated from the previously cited observations on Japanese men in Hawaii, the United States, and Japan; and the studies of long-term Yemenite immigrants to Israel who have higher cholesterol values than the new immigrants (Fig. 2). In addition, vegetarian groups consistently have lower cholesterol values than appropriately matched controls (West and Hayes, 1968) and within such groups lipid values correlate well with the degree of adherence to the vegetarian diet (Sacks et al., 1975). Two issues have to be addressed with regard to the relationship of diet and plasma cholesterol levels. First, what steps can be taken to lower the cholesterol levels of Western populations should this be deemed desirable? Second, how are subjects with definite hyperlipoproteinemia to be treated? If the goal is to achieve ideal lipid values in large populations (e.g., cholesterol and triglyceride values each of 200 mg/dl or less in adults) then dietary manipulation is the only practical way of achieving this goal, given that 20–40% of

Americans are estimated as having values above these "ideals". For the subjects with distinct hyperlipoproteinemia, combined diet and drug therapy is feasible.

A. Dietary Factors Affecting Cholesterol Levels

Plasma cholesterol is affected by three classes of dietary fats: cholesterol, and saturated, and unsaturated fatty acids. Although there is controversy over the relative importance of each of these types of fat in affecting plasma cholesterol levels, there is concensus that diets rich in cholesterol and saturated fats elevate plasma cholesterol levels while diets rich in polyunsaturated fatty acids and restricted in cholesterol lower plasma cholesterol levels.

1. *Dietary Cholesterol*

Previously it was thought that there was an *absolute* limit on the ability of the intestine to absorb dietary cholesterol, but more recent studies have shown that instead there is a proportionate increase in cholesterol absorption such that ~37% of dietary cholesterol is absorbed over a wide range of cholesterol intakes (400–1200 mg/day) (Kudchodkar *et al.*, 1973). This is strikingly different from the almost 100% absorption of unlimited quantities of dietary fatty acids (Borgstom, 1974).

The limited absorption of cholesterol dampens the influence of dietary cholesterol on plasma cholesterol, nevertheless an effect is easily demonstrated particularly when diets without any cholesterol are compared with identical diets rich in the sterol. More significantly, even within the range of typical dietary intakes (600–800 mg cholesterol/day) each increment of 100 mg of cholesterol/1000 kcal of diet results in an average increase of serum cholesterol by 12 mg/dl (Mattson *et al.*, 1972). This increase appears to hold true whether the accompanying dietary fat is saturated or polyunsaturated (Anderson *et al.*, 1976). Larger increases in plasma cholesterol with cholesterol feeding are prevented by limited intestinal absorption, by the re-excretion of cholesterol in bile as the unchanged sterol or as bile acids (Nestel and Poyser, 1976) and by the suppressant effect of dietary cholesterol on hepatic cholesterol synthesis (Bhattathiry and Siperstein, 1963), mediated by the remnant lipoproteins as described previously (Nervi and Dietschy, 1975).

2. *Polyunsaturated Fats*

Of equal, if not greater practical importance in determining plasma cholesterol levels is the degree of saturation of dietary fat. That saturated fat raises, and unsaturated lowers plasma cholesterol levels has been repeatedly documented in epidemiological studies (Fig. 1) and in elegant, experimental work using formula diets on metabolic wards (Spritz *et al.*, 1965; Conner *et al.*, 1969). It is remarkable that when people are given diets which contain saturated fats, but virtually no cholesterol, the isocaloric substitution of polyunsaturated fats for saturated fat will produce a 20% lowering of plasma cholesterol levels. Thus, depression of cholesterol levels by polyunsaturated fats appears to be independent of the presence of dietary cholesterol (Anderson *et al.*, 1976). The case is similar for the elevation of plasma cholesterol by saturated fat. Since the cholesterol raising effect of saturated fatty acids (S) is twice as great as the cholesterol lowering effect of polyunsaturated fatty acids (P), dietary fats with P/S ratios of 2 can be isocalorically substituted for each other without significant changes in serum cholesterol (Grande *et al.*, 1972).

The mechanisms by which saturated fat affects cholesterol levels are not known. One possibility is by increasing the net flux of fatty acids to the liver, which in turn induces increased cholesterol synthesis (Bortz, 1974). The mechanism by which polyunsaturates lower cholesterol is also not defined. Recent investigations have found that when patients were changed from normal or "saturated" to "polyunsaturated" diets, plasma cholesterol levels fell and the excretion of fecal sterols increased (Connor *et al.*, 1969; Nestel *et al.*, 1973, 1975; Grundy, 1975). Earlier studies found similar fecal sterol excretions on both kinds of fat diets in spite of significant cholesterol lowering in plasma by the unsaturated fat diet (Spritz *et al.*, 1965; Grundy and Ahrens, 1970). This is an important difference since the recent findings suggest that polyunsaturates increase the biliary excretion of cholesterol (or bile acids) and thus drain cholesterol from the body. The earlier studies raise the possibility that polyunsaturates lower cholesterol merely by redistributing cholesterol between plasma and tissue compartments. The differences in the studies may reflect the heterogeneity of patients studied.

Other mechanisms for the effects of polyunsaturated fats have been proposed. One is that they increase LDL removal from plasma (Levy, 1972). Another interesting proposal is based on the observation that on polyunsaturated fat diets the fatty acids esterified to cholesterol tend to be polyunsaturated. Polyunsaturated fatty acids have greater "bulkiness" (steric hindrance) than do saturated fatty acid. Thus, cholesterol esters containing polyunsaturated fatty acids are larger and less of them could be accommodated per LDL particle (Spritz and Mishkel, 1969). This could result in lower plasma cholesterol levels. The failure to find a single explanation for the effect of cholesterol lowering by polyunsaturates probably stems from the heterogeneity of subjects studied. It is also possible that polyunsaturates produce changes at multiple metabolically important sites.

Not as widely appreciated as the cholesterol response to polyunsaturated fat diets is the fall of plasma triglycerides in some subjects on these diets (Grundy, 1975; Nestel et al., 1975). This may be due to inhibited VLDL synthesis and/or increased triglyceride clearance (Nestel et al., 1975; Nestel and Barter, 1971).

In sum, dietary cholesterol makes significant contributions to the plasma cholesterol levels of most subjects. Therefore, significant decreases in plasma cholesterol could be achieved by decreasing the cholesterol contents of American diets. For example, decreasing cholesterol intake from 800 mg to less than 100 mg/day and keeping everything else equal could cause a 30–40 mg/dl lowering. However, it is unlikely that many patients, much less whole populations, could follow such extremely restrictive diets. Changes in P/S ratio also affect plasma cholesterol levels and an increase of this ratio from the American diet average <0.3 to ~2.0 is an effective and reasonably convenient way to achieve modest cholesterol lowering. Thus most workers favor diets that combine moderate restriction of dietary cholesterol (to ~300 mg/day) with increases in the P/S ratio to near 2. Such diets cause a 25% reduction of serum cholesterol in healthy young adults under controlled conditions (Levy, 1972) and a 7–16% reduction when applied to a variety of free living or semi-confined populations of adults (Wilson et al., 1971; Ahrens, 1976). The effect of total caloric intake is of relatively minor importance in determining plasma cholesterol (in contrast to its major importance in hypertriglyceridemia). However, subjects who are obese, and who have associated hypertriglyceridemia (e.g., Type IIb), may experience significant cholesterol drops with caloric restriction (Leelarthaepin et al., 1974; Lisch et al., 1974).

The Los Angeles V.A. dietary trial, during which a control diet and a high polyunsaturated diet were fed to two groups of old veterans, resulted in a reduction of cardiovascular deaths in those on the experimental diet. However, questions were raised about the safety of such diets because increased numbers of deaths due to carcinoma were also noted in the group eating the experimental diet (Pearce and Dayton, 1971). To answer these doubts, reviews of the 13-year trial of the Diet Heart Study in New York City and of other dietary trials were carried out. These failed to find any increases in cancer rates (Ederer et al., 1971; Singman et al., 1973).

There is also a report that there was an increased incidence of gallstones in groups eating polyunsaturated diets (Sturdevant et al., 1973) and experimental evidence exists that such diets do increase the lithogenicity of the bile in some but not all patients (Grundy, 1975). However, the Finnish Diet Study failed to find any difference in gallstone incidence between control and experimental groups (Miettinen et al., 1976). Nevertheless, it is possible that high polyunsaturated diets may lead to increased incidence of gallstones, especially in obese subjects in whom increased lithogenicity already exists.

Based on the considerations of safety, cholesterol lowering efficacy, and potential for coronary prevention, it is the recommendation of the Nutrition Committee of the American Heart Association that moderate cholesterol lowering diets (cholesterol 300 mg/day, P/S ratio ~2.0) can and should be followed by most adult Americans. Use of diets with higher P/S ratios should be reserved for specific therapeutic applications.

Most experts feel if prevention of atherosclerosis by dietary modification is to be maximally effective, dietary changes should be instituted at an early age, especially in those children at high risk. Several studies show the feasibility and marked responsiveness of adolescents and children (McGandy et al., 1972; Stein et al., 1975). Since the formula diets now being consumed by 80% of normal infants are also low in cholesterol and relatively rich in polyunsaturates, one might question that such diets in infancy would lead to higher cholesterol levels later in life due to failure of development of the regulatory mechanisms which maintain plasma cholesterol levels within acceptable ranges. However, the plasma cholesterol levels of infants 1 year of age are not influenced by the antecedent diet experience of the infants, implying that restrictions of cholesterol intake even during the first weeks or months of life do not adversely affect subsequent ability to maintain cholesterol homeostasis (Glueck et al., 1972).

If it is indeed deemed important that the mean cholesterol level of the Western peoples should be lowered (and this is still a hotly debated issue) a variety of voluntary approaches are available to individuals for the construction of cholesterol lowering diets. One can reduce intakes of animal fats, organ foods, milk products, egg-yolks, and shrimp, and increase the intake of vegetable oils, fish, and fowl. For those not wishing to give up beef and veal, a "soft-fat" meat, containing large amounts of unsaturated fats has been developed (Hodges et al., 1975; Nestel et al., 1973). However, this beef is available only to experimenters. Commercial marketing will probably depend on costs and demand. Literature and professional help are also readily available at most affiliates of the American Heart Association.

Most diet studies to date have involved the use of personal contacts between health professionals and the study subjects. A recent study demonstrates that significant dietary changes lasting at least 2 years, as determined by self reporting, can be brought about in large general populations without personal professional counseling by the use of mass-media education campaigns. In the Stanford Heart Disease Prevention Program 20–40% reductions in cholesterol and saturated fat consumption were obtained in whole communities (Stern *et al.*, 1976). Optimal results were obtained by the combined use of media and personal contacts. It is not known whether this approach will serve to maintain populations on cholesterol lowering diets over long periods of time in the face of habits and the countervailing educational campaigns of those who disagree with this approach to coronary prevention.

The diet therapy of subjects with primary hypercholesterolemia (Types IIa and IIb) follows the principles listed above. Results of such therapy in adults and children are given in Figs. 7–10.

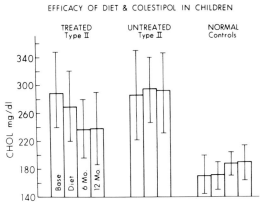

Fig. 7. Effects of diet and colestipol resin therapy in children (ages 5–15) with familial Type II hyperlipoproteinemia. The children were divided into three groups. "Treated" (N = 7): children who were judged to have good adherence by independent observers (parents, M.D.'s, and dietitians). After baseline period, an NIH Type IIA diet (cholesterol restricted to 300 mg/day, P/S ratio ~2) was prescribed. After 3 months, colestipol-HCl (20 gm/day) was begun. "Untreated" (N = 7): judged to have minimal adherence to diet or medication taking and exhibited poor clinic attendance as well. "Normal (N = 7): normolipemic siblings of the treated and untreated groups. They received no diet or medication. Three lipid determinations were made on all subjects at monthly intervals for the baseline and dietary periods, and three observations at bimonthly intervals on drug therapy. The three lipid analyses of each period were used for calculations. Each bar and bracket represents the group mean and SD. Cholesterol values remained unchanged in the untreated and control groups. Modest reductions with diet and drug therapy were achieved. Even in the "treated group" adherence to both diet and drug was suboptimal (Schwarz, Alpers, and Schonfeld, unpublished observations).

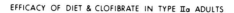

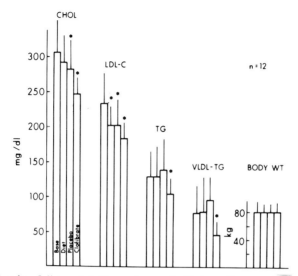

Fig. 8. Results of diet and clofibrate therapy in IIa hyperlipoproteinemia. All patients had primary Type IIa. After three baseline visits at 3–4 week intervals, an NIH type IIa diet (cholesterol intake ~300 mg/day and P/S ratio of ~2) was given to the patients by a trained dietitian. Three followup visits for lipid analysis were done. Clofibrate and/or placebo were then given for 6 months each in a double-blind crossover design. Patients were seen at 2-month intervals. The three lipid analyses of each period were used for calculations. Each bar represents the mean and SD for the group. Clofibrate was effective in lowering both total and LDL-Chol, as well as VLDL–TG levels. Asterisk: means versus baseline period significantly different by paired t-test ($p \leq 0.02$) (J. L. Witztum and G. Schonfeld, unpublished observations).

B. Dietary Factors Affecting Triglyceride Levels

As noted previously, plasma triglyceride may be due to intestinal (chylomicrons) or hepatic (VLDL) lipoproteins. Since chylomicrons are normally cleared from the plasma 8–12 hours after a meal, their presence in fasting plasma (Types I and V) indicates a deficient clearing mechanism for dietary triglycerides. For such individuals, diet therapy is aimed at reducing the exogenous fat load so that the circulating chylomicron levels will be reduced. This includes all dietary triglyceride, both saturated and polyunsaturated. The exceptions are glycerides containing "medium-chain" fatty acids (less than 12 carbons). These glycerides are absorbed directly into the portal vein and are taken up by the liver. "Medium-chain triglycerides" may be used as fat supplements in individuals with severe fat intolerance (Levy, 1972).

802

Gustav Schonfeld and Joseph L. Witztum

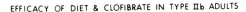

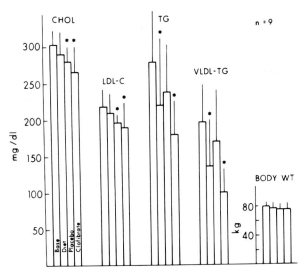

Fig. 9. Results of diet and clofibrate therapy in IIb hyperlipoproteinemia. All patients had primary Type IIb. The protocol was identical to that described in the legend for Fig. 9 except an NIH Type IIb diet was prescribed (similar to IIa except it restricts carbohydrate to 40% of calories). The effect of clofibrate was more pronounced on VLDL–TG levels in these patients, though modest reductions in cholesterol also occurred. Asterisk: means versus baseline significantly different by paired t-test ($p \leq 0.05$) (G. Schonfeld and J. L. Witztum, unpublished observations).

Fasting chylomicronemia is rare in subjects with hypertriglyceridemia, therefore most triglyceride elevations are due to excess VLDL. In contrast to the relatively simple relationship between chylomicrons and dietary fat, many factors affect VLDL levels, including obesity, caloric excess, high carbohydrate diets, and alcohol consumption. The relative potency of each of these factors is debated, but clearly all of them lead to higher VLDL levels in some patients.

Even mildly overweight individuals, who would not be thought to be obese by current standards (e.g., 105% of ideal body weight), have elevated plasma triglycerides compared to lean controls (Blacket et al., 1975). Since minor degrees of obesity are very common in our affluent society, this may be the most common reason for hypertriglyceridemia. Obesity is associated with accelerated VLDL secretion (Robertson et al., 1973; Witztum and Schonfeld, 1976) probably due to the accompanying hyperinsulinemia which stimulates hepatic triglyceride synthesis and secretion (Nikkilä, 1969). Even modest weight loss is accompanied by

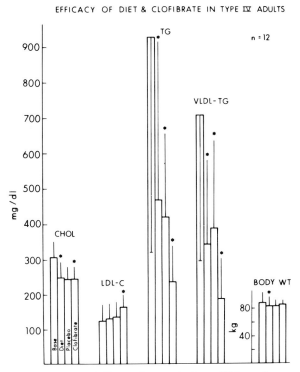

Fig. 10. Results of diet and clofibrate therapy in Type IV hyperlipoproteinemia. All patients had primary Type IV. Protocol was identical to that described in the legend for Fig. 9 except an NIH Type IV diet was prescribed (carbohydrates restricted to 45% of calories with restriction of simple sugars and alcohol). Significant reductions in total TG as well as VLDL–TG were observed, though a significant increase in LDL–Chol was observed in the group (G. Schonfeld and J. L. Witztum, unpublished observations). Asterisk: means versus baseline period significantly different by paired t-test ($p \leqslant 0.01$).

marked falls in triglycerides and lower levels will be maintained as long as the new low weight is held.

Total intake of calories is important in regulating VLDL levels. Subjects fed hypercaloric diets over a few days experienced marked increases in their plasma triglycerides even before they had gained any weight. This phenomonen was associated with both increased triglyceride synthesis and delayed clearance. In a reverse experiment, acute reductions in caloric intake resulted in dramatic falls in the triglyceride levels of most subjects. This effect could be related to increased clearance and reduced synthesis (Nestel *et al.*, 1970). (It is because of these acute fluctuations in triglyceride levels that blood lipids should not be

measured for diagnosing hyperlipoproteinemia while changes are occurring in caloric intake or body weight.)

High carbohydrate diets induce VLDL–triglyceride elevations in normals and in patients with hyperlipidemia (Glueck *et al.*, 1969; Ahrens *et
al.*, 1957). The magnitude of the response is in general related to initial
triglyceride levels (Reaven *et al.*, 1967). Thus, a high carbohydrate diet
may cause a 2.5-fold increase of plasma triglycerides in most subjects.
But the same diet may cause a disproportionately greater elevation in
some "carbohydrate sensitive" individuals. The initial VLDL rise in all
subjects is due to increased rates of VLDL secretion probably by liver
alone (Quarfordt *et al.*, 1970; Schonfeld and Pfleger, 1971). This is followed in most subjects by increased levels of activators of lipoprotein
lipase (Schonfeld *et al.*, 1976) which lead to greater triglyceride clearance

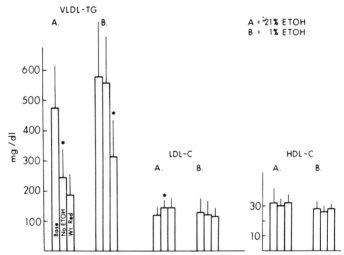

Fig. 11. Effect of abstinence from dietary ethanol on plasma lipoprotein lipid levels.
Sixteen patients with hypertriglyceridemia were studied. Ethanol represented 10–50%
(average 21%) of the total daily caloric intake of eight of these individuals (Group A). The
other eight had virtually no ethanol consumption (Group B). Groups were alike in mean
age, sex, adiposity and race. Each subject had three lipoprotein lipid determinations during the baseline (6–8 weeks) and again during each of the dietary periods. Results represent group means based on the above average values. Bar = 1 SD.
VLDL–triglycerides (TG) fell during ethanol abstinence in Group A. Since Group B
were ethanol abstainers from the start, their values remained unchanged. Body weights
were not significantly changed during this period. Both groups experienced drops in
VLDL–triglycerides on weight reduction. Mean weight losses were 4.9 and 4.4 kg for
Groups A and B, respectively (J. L. Witztum and G. Schonfeld, unpublished observation).

TABLE XI

Diet and Drug Therapy in Type III Hyperlipoproteinemia[a,b]

	Date	Total triglycerides	VLDL	LDL	HDL	Total cholesterol	VLDL	LDL	HDL
Case #1[c]									
Baseline	4/18/74	715	622	50	18	515	308	152	31
Baseline	5/30/74	924	850	47	17	404	251	142	28
On diet—2 months	7/11/74	203	147	34	12	268	66	149	37
On diet—3 months (7.5 kg wt loss)	8/12/74	172	118	32	5	207	43	113	44
Case #2[d]									
Baseline	3/13/73	439	336	60	25	436	175	168	43
Baseline	4/11/73	560	430	52	26	495	300	162	41
Diet	5/2/73	302	220	61	15	515	176	263	51
Diet	6/6/73	286	199	59	15	486	143	264	48
On clofibrate—3 months	9/12/73	113	61	28	9	235	33	106	75
On clofibrate—5 months	2/11/74	100	64	25	12	226	35	83	113
Case #3[e]									
Baseline	2/9/76	541	—	—	—	291	—	—	27
Baseline	5/21/76	904	772	53	27	445	286	83	27
On diet—1 month	8/12/76	283	208	41	22	207	80	97	33
On diet—3 months	10/21/76	72	—	—	—	153	—	—	—
Off diet, increased alcohol intake	11/18/76	827	745	43	24	319	185	100	27

[a] All values in mg/dl.

[b] All diets given are NIH-Type III (ratio of protein:CHO:fat = 20:40:40 with cholesterol ~300 mg/day, P/S ~2, restricted sweets and alcohol). IBW, ideal body weight. (J. Witztum and G. Schonfeld, unpublished observations.)

[c] Case #1: 36 years, male; tuboeruptive xanthoma on elbows, 120% IBW, asymptomatic.

[d] Case #2: 47 years, female; palmar xanthoma, tuboeruptive xanthoma on elbows, xantholasma at time of initial visits, 115% IBW. All lesions cleared after 1 year of therapy. Sister has Type III hyperlipoproteinemia.

[e] Case #3: 40 years, male; asymptomatic, 100% IBW, moderate drinker (6–12 beers/week).

TABLE XII
Diet and Drug Therapy in Type V Hyperlipoproteinemia[a,b]

	Date	Total triglycerides	VLDL	LDL	HDL	Total cholesterol	VLDL	LDL	HDL
Case #1[c]									
Baseline	4/13/76	2866	2670	52	38	570	438	54	14
On Type V diet	5/21/76	5096	—	—	—	495	—	—	—
On Type V diet	7/8/76	1725	1431	37	18	300	185	22	78
On northindrone acetate-5mg									
1 week	7/15/76	2202	—	—	—	341	—	—	—
1 month	8/10/76	3096	—	—	—	380	—	—	—
On clofibrate—1 month	9/28/76	799	718	37	9	244	105	110	23
On clofibrate—3 months	11/11/76	1134	—	—	—	291	—	—	—
Case #2[d]									
Baseline	11/8/76	7671	7250	174	19	1014	925	106	14
On diet 2 weeks—off alcohol	11/22/76	301	241	65	12	358	102	239	24
On diet 1 month—off alcohol	12/6/76	216	145	74	19	232	48	161	27

Case #3[e]

Baseline	3/13/76	8820	—	—	—	1030	—	—	—
Baseline	3/25/76	2673	2590	110	33	850	705	101	14
Diet and insulin	4/1/76	829	738	106	14	535	297	205	19
Diet and insulin	5/6/76	245	173	28	11	208	236	126	33
8 kg weight loss	8/26/76	131	87	34	9	234	18	170	33
Gained 4 kg	9/30/76	253	198	42	11	275	43	192	30

[a] All values in mg/dl.

[b] All diets are NIH-Type V (fats 30% or less of calories, CHO 50%, no alcohol), IBW = ideal body weight. (J. L. Witztum and G. Schonfeld, unpublished observations).

[c] Case #1: 58 years, male; insulin requiring diabetic in good control, 120% IBW, frequent episodes abdominal pain. Myocardial infarction 10 years ago.

[d] Case #2: 44 years, male; presented with lipemia retinalis and eruptive xanthoma—asymptomatic, 90% IBW, normal OGTT, modest alcohol intake (6 beers/week).

[e] Case #3: 35 years, male; newly discovered diabetic out of control, 122% IBW, lipemia retinalis.

rates and a new steady state at higher levels of plasma triglycerides. "Carbohydrate sensitive" individuals may not be able as efficiently to increase their VLDL–triglyceride catabolic rates to meet the diet induced greater influx of VLDL. This may be due to impaired adaptation of the ApoC-activators (Carlson and Ballantyne, 1976). Such subjects could have unusually high responses to carbohydrate diets.

The degree of triglyceride elevation is also dependent on the type of dietary carbohydrate. Simple sugars, such as sucrose, cause greater rises than do starches (Nestel *et al.*, 1970). A most interesting observation is that the dietary carbohydrate must be taken orally to produce the triglyceride elevation. Isocaloric carbohydrate loads given intravenously have no triglyceride raising effects (DenBesten *et al.*, 1973). This raises the interesting possibility that an intestinal "messenger" may be important in stimulating hepatic VLDL production or that the gut itself contributes to the plasma triglyceride response. Of course, it is also possible that the smaller dose of carbohydrate delivered directly to the liver by the intravenous route affected the results of this study.

In sum, triglyceride elevations not due to chylomicrons (Types IIb, III, and IV) can be treated by combinations of reduction of ideal body weight, reduced carbohydrate intake, and the avoidance of simple sugars and alcohol. Therapy is tailored to the individual patient. It is our experience (see Figs. 9–11, Tables XI and XII) that in the vast majority of patients with hypertriglyceridemia, dietary therapy *alone* will reduce triglyceride levels toward normal values, in some cases dramatically. Other investigators have reported similar experiences. Thus reduction in mean plasma triglyceride levels from 273 mg/dl to 126 mg/dl was achieved and sustained in twenty men over a 10-month period by weight reduction alone (body weights fell by 7 kg from 107% of ideal, low weights were maintained by the ingestion of 75% of original calories) (Blacket *et al.*, 1975). In another study, an isocaloric low carbohydrate (30% of calories) modification of the American Heart Association prudent diet reduced triglyceride levels by 37% (from 258 mg/dl to 162 mg/dl in a group of thirteen nonobese patients without affecting their body weights (Hulley *et al.*, 1972). Even simple communication techniques can bring about triglyceride reductions (40–50%) in large groups of men (Smith *et al.*, 1976).

V. DRUG THERAPY

Drug therapy in hyperlipoproteinemia is reserved for those patients whose dietary response is deemed suboptimal and where lowering of lipoprotein levels is thought to be important. The latter group consists of patients who are symptomatic from their hyperlipoproteinemia or who are at particularly high risk for the development of vascular disease by virtue of family history or due to the presence of other coronary risk factors. Diet therapy is continued as drugs are added because the effects of the two modalities are frequently additive.

Drugs may be divided into those that are effective in (a) the hyper-cholesterolemias, (b) the hypertriglyceridemias, and (c) those that are effective in both. Several excellent reviews have been published recently (Levy *et al.*, 1974; Bencze, 1975; Yeshurun and Gotto, 1976).

A. Cholesterol (LDL) Lowering Drugs

1. *Cholestyramine and Colestipol-HCl*

The current drugs of choice for treatment of hypercholesterolemia (Type II) are both anionic polymeric resins which bind bile acids in the

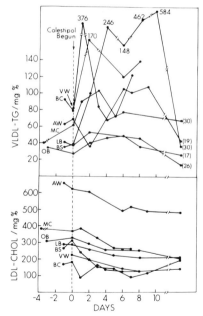

Fig. 12. Time course of the changes in VLDL–TG and LDL–Chol following initiation of therapy with the bile sequestrant, colestipol-HCl (20 gm/day). Note that in all subjects there was an initial sharp rise in VLDL–TG levels, while LDL–Chol was falling, but the TG elevations were transient and returned to baseline values in every case. The number in parentheses refers to the number of days after initiation of therapy that this measurement was made. Witztum *et al.*, (1976).

intestine. With usual therapeutic doses the net excretion of bile acids in stool is increased severalfold. This is followed by enhanced hepatic cholesterol and bile acid synthesis (Havel and Kane, 1973). The greater movement of sterols from liver to bile and out of the body is associated with higher rates of production of VLDL and greater fractional rates of catabolism of plasma LDL (Langer *et al.*, 1969). Thus there is an increased flux of VLDL and LDL through the plasma. The biochemical mechanisms which underlie the associations between hepatic cholesterol–bile acid synthesis and VLDL–LDL metabolism are not clear, but the results of therapy are a variable elevation of VLDL–cholesterol and triglyceride levels and a persistent 25–35% lowering of plasma LDL cholesterol levels in children and in adults (Figs. 7 and 12 and Table XIII).

TABLE XIII
Effect of Long-Term Treatment with Colestipol on Lipoprotein Lipids[a]

	Before (mg/dl)	After (mg/dl)	P
Total cholesterol	345 ± 66	258 ± 63	<0.001
Total triglyceride	121 ± 37	133 ± 39	NS
VLDL–Chol	13.5 ± 6.3	15.8 ± 7.9	NS
VLDL–TG	65.4 ± 30.8	83.2 ± 35.2	NS
$\dfrac{\text{VLDL–TG}}{\text{VLDL–Chol}}$	5.41 ± 2.45	5.46 ± 0.84	NS
LDL–Chol	277 ± 67	188 ± 53	<0.001
LDL–TG	38.1 ± 9.9	32.6 ± 8.7	<0.01
$\dfrac{\text{LDL–TG}}{\text{LDL–Chol}}$	0.14 ± .03	0.18 ± 0.06	<.005
HDL–Chol	50.6 ± 13.7	51.2 ± 16.3	NS
HDL–TG	9.7 ± 3.7	10.6 ± 4.7	NS
$\dfrac{\text{HDL–TG}}{\text{HDL-Chol}}$	0.20 ± .07	0.21 ± 0.06	NS

[a] "Before" data represent the mean of three determinations, made at monthly intervals before therapy, on each of twelve subjects. "After" data include the mean of three consecutive determinations done after the longest period of therapy for that patient (between a minimum of 3 and a maximum of 12 months). The mean of the three observations for each period for each of the twelve patients was used to calculate the mean ± SD for the value of each lipoprotein and for the TG/Chol ratio of each lipoprotein. Statistics were by paired Students *t*-test (Witztum *et al.*, 1976).

The major advantages of the bile acid binding resins for clinical practice are their effectiveness in lowering plasma cholesterol and the fact that they are "nonsystemic", i.e., they are not absorbed from the gut. The latter attribute greatly limits their potential for producing allergic or toxic reactions. In fact, side effects are limited to local effects produced by the bulkiness of the drugs, e.g., bloating and constipation. No serious side effects have been reported. Cholestyramine and colestipol may interfere with the absorption of certain drugs (e.g., digoxin or thyroxine) or nutrients (e.g., fat-soluble vitamins, iron). Problems may be avoided by taking other medications 1–2 hours before the resins are ingested.

2. β–Sitosterol

β-Sitosterol, a plant sterol preparation which also contains small amounts of campesterol and stigmasterol lowers plasma cholesterol on the average of about 10% without appreciably affecting triglycerides. It probably acts by competitively inhibiting the absorption of cholesterol from the gut lumen (Kudchodkar *et al.*, 1976), without more than 1–2% of the dietary β-sitosterol itself being absorbed. This preparation has the advantage of being virtually nonsystemic but large doses of it produce mild diarrhea in some people. The major disadvantage of β-sitosterol is its relatively low efficacy. In addition, some infants and rare adults do absorb large amounts (20–30%) of dietary plant sterols and appreciable amounts of plant sterols are found in plasmas of these subjects. In adults with β-sitosterolemia, xanthoma-containing plant sterols have been found (Shulman *et al.*, 1976). The drug is not widely used at the present time.

3. D-Thyroxine

D-Thyroxine, the dextro isomer of the natural thyroid hormone is an effective LDL–cholesterol lowering agent which probably acts by increasing the catabolism of LDL (Table X). Effects on plasma triglycerides are small and variable. Its use is limited to young subjects with Type IIa hypercholesterolemia who have no heart disease and whose progress can be adequately monitored by medical personnel. It is contraindicated in anyone with known heart disease. These caveats are prompted by the experience of the Coronary Drug Project wherein those survivors of myocardial infarctions treated with D-thyroxine experienced an excess number of deaths compared with similar subjects treated with placebo or other medications (Coronary Drug Project Research Group, 1972).

Cholestyramine, β-sitosterol, and D-thyroxine have been approved by the Food and Drug Administration for use in the treatment of hypercholesterolemia. Colestipol is now approved. The drugs to be discussed below have been approved for other medical indications and have been used experimentally in the treatment of hypercholesterolemia. Since FDA has not approved these drugs in the treatment of hypercholesterolemia, they are to be considered as experimental drugs with respect to hypercholesterolemia.

4. *p-Aminosalicylic Acid (PAS)*

p-Aminosalicylic acid, an antituberculosis drug, was originally noted to reduce cholesterol levels in patients with tuberculosis. Since that time, 15–30% decreases in plasma cholesterol have been routinely achieved by several investigators (Barter *et al.*, 1974). Triglycerides are also decreased by approximately 10%. The usefulness of the older preparations of PAS was severely limited due to the side effects of nausea, vomiting, and diarrhea. A newer preparation (PAS-C) seems to be without these side effects. PAS-C deserves further consideration as a cholesterol lowering preparation. Its mode of action is unknown.

5. *Neomycin*

Neomycin, a polyene antibiotic when ingested orally in smaller than usual antibiotic doses (1–1.5 versus 6–8 gm/day) lowers cholesterol by ~20%. Triglyceride levels are not changed (Samuel *et al.*, 1967). The hypocholesterolemic effects may be due to production of cholesterol malabsorption either by interference with micellar solubilization or mucosal transport (Sedaghat *et al.*, 1975). The drug is as effective in lowering plasma cholesterol levels as are the bile acid-binding resins, but it produces abdominal discomfort and diarrhea in 10% of those taking it for hypercholesterolemia. These side effects are reversible at reduced dosages. But the use of neomycin has probably been limited for other reasons. The drug is absorbed from the gut only to a very limited extent (2–3% of oral dose), but the systemic toxicities of neomycin are irreversible otic and renal damage. Although these toxic manifestations have not been reported with the reduced oral doses used in hypercholesterolemia, clinicians nevertheless have been cautious. This is a wise course at the present time, when the risk to benefit ratio of cholesterol lowering by this means is unknown.

B. Triglyceride (VLDL) Lowering Drugs

1. *Clofibrate*

Clofibrate is probably the most widely used medication for the treatment of hyperlipoproteinemia. This is in part because, in contrast with the resins which are bulky powders, clofibrate is a capsule which is easy and convenient for the patient to take. It is relatively free of side effects, modestly effective in Type II, moderately effective in Type IV, and very effective in Type III hyperlipoproteinemia (Figs. 9–11, Tables XI and XII). Clofibrate lowers primarily VLDL levels and works best when used in conjunction with diet. In fact, poor adherence to diet can result in large elevations of VLDL even when adherence to drug therapy is adequate. One undesired effect of clofibrate is a rise of LDL levels as VLDL levels are falling. This happens most often in patients with Type IV hyperlipoproteinemia and may require an adjustment of diet or the addition of an anticholesterol drug (Fig. 11) (Rose *et al.*, 1976).

In animal and in *in vitro* experiments clofibrate decreases lipolysis in adipose tissue, diminishes fatty acid and triglyceride synthesis in liver, and reduces hepatic secretion of VLDL. These data suggest that at least in animals (primarily the rat) clofibrate lowers plasma lipids by decreasing VLDL input into plasma. However, experiments in man have not demonstrated inhibition of VLDL secretion. Instead, in man, clofibrate therapy is followed by increased activity of lipoprotein lipase and increased fecal excretion of bile acids. These results are more compatible with enhanced rates of lipoprotein catabolism (Havel and Kane, 1973). The molecular bases underlying these effects in man are not known.

Clofibrate is a systemic drug and several side effects have been reported. The most frequent is a mild elevation of hepatic enzymes in blood which seems to have no deleterious effects. Other side effects include cardiac arrhythmias and a myopathic syndrome which occurs primarily in persons with chronic renal disease. Drug interactions particularly with anticoagulants and the reduced dosage requirements in subjects with renal disease are well known (Yeshurun and Gotto, 1976).

2. Nicotinic Acid

Nicotinic acid and its derivatives are potent depressants of plasma triglyceride (VLDL and chylomicron) levels particularly in Types III and V hyperlipoproteinemia where decrements of 50–90% in plasma triglycerides have been obtained. Nicotinic acid has also been used in Types IIb and IV hyperlipoproteinemia with approximately 25% decrements in triglyceride and in Type IIa hyperlipoproteinemia where triglyceride and cholesterol levels fall by approximately 10% each (Yeshurun and Gotto, 1976).

The considerations which keep this group of medications from being "first line" drugs relate to the fact that they are systemic and have unpleasant and potentially serious side effects. The former includes flushing, itching, dry skin, acanthosis nigricans, nausea, and diarrhea; and the latter, hyperglycemia, hyperuricemia, and hepatic toxicity. It should be noted that the serious side effects are unusual and reversible, and the mild ones can be avoided or overcome by the administration of the drugs at slowly increasing increments until therapeutic doses are reached. The mode of action of nicotinic acid is unknown. In the rat it is a powerful inhibitor of lipolysis in adipose tissue and it also decreases hepatic cholesterol and triglyceride synthesis. Its mode of action in man is controversial. Some workers feel that its primary effect like that in the rat is to inhibit VLDL secretion by liver; others feel that its major effect is to increase the catabolism of VLDL and chylomicrons (Bencze, 1975).

3. Progestational and Anabolic Steroids

Progestational and anabolic steroids have been used only experimentally in the treatment of hypertriglyceridemia, particularly Type V disease, in a limited number of cases (Glueck, 1971; Glueck *et al.*, 1971). In the subjects 30–50% decreases in triglycerides have been obtained and the therapeutic effect has been accompanied by increased activities in postheparin lipoprotein lipase. No deleterious effects have been recorded. This approach to the therapy of hypertriglyceridemia deserves further experimental exploration.

VI. RESEARCH NEEDS

From the above review it is obvious that a great deal remains to be learned about the etiologies of the hyperlipoproteinemias. In this respect, the studies of this group of disorders is comparable to that of hypertension—the etiology of ~10% of the cases is known, the rest remain "primary" or "essential". It may be expected from what is known about hyperlipoproteinemias, hypertension, and metabolic diseases in general that etiologic defects will be found to be related to synthesis, assembly, catabolism, and regulation. Diverse genetic mechanisms may also be involved. Thus, a broadly based research effort continues to be necessary.

Another area where much basic information is being collected is atherogenesis and lesion regression. Important work includes (a) diet studies in man and experimental animals, (b) examination of the biology of arterial cells in tissue culture, including the interactions of cells with blood platelets and lipoproteins, (c) assessment of the physical state of lipids in atheromatous lesions at various stages of development. Much work remains to be done in all of these areas. For example, it is essential to know how arterial cells handle lipids and lipoproteins, specifically how cholesterol accumulates in cells and whether anything can be done to interfere with this process. It would also be important to know how lipids and other materials accumulate in the extracellular portions of arteries and whether anything can be done to prevent this or to mobilize lipids already deposited.

A third area is therapy. Current attempts in this area are centered on demonstrating that therapy is efficacious in preventing or delaying coronary events. It may be necessary to apply such trials to populations with defined disorders of lipoprotein metabolism. Pharmacologic science also needs to devise more efficacious cholesterol lowering drugs which have fewer unpleasant side effects.

REFERENCES

Ahrens, E. H. Jr. (1976. The management of hyperlipidemia: Whether, rather than how. *Ann. Intern. Med.* **85,** 87–93.

Ahrens, E. H., Jr., Insull, W., Jr., Blomstrand, R., Hirsch, J., Tsaltas, T. T., and Peterson, M. L. (1957). The influence of dietary fats on serum-lipid levels in man. *Lancet* **1,** 944–953.

Anderson, J. T., Grande, F., and Keys, A. (1976). Independence of the effects of cholesterol and degree of saturation of the fat in the diet on serum cholesterol in man. *Am. J. Clin. Nutr.* **29,** 1184–1189.

Armstrong, M. (1976). Regression of atheroscleorsis. *Atheroscler. Rev.* **1,** 137–182.

Barter, P. J., Connor, W. E., Spector, A. A., Armstrong, M., Connor, S. L., and Newman, M. A. (1974). Lowering of serum cholesterol and triglyceride by paraaminosalicylic acid in hyperlipoproteinemia. *Ann. Intern. Med.* **81,** 619–624.

Bencze, W. L. (1975). Hypolipidemic agents *In* "Hypolipidemic Agents" (D. Kritchevesky, ed.), pp. 349–408. Springer-Verlag, Berlin and New York.

Bhattathiry, E., and Siperstein, M. (1963). Feedback control of cholesterol synthesis in man. *J. Clin. Invest.* **42,** 1612–1618.

Blacket, R. B., Leelarthaepin, B., Woodhill, J. M., and Palmer, A. J. (1975). Type-IV hyperlipidaemia and weight-gain after maturity. *Lancet* **2,** 517–520.

Borgström, B. (1974). Fat digestion and absorption. *Biomembranes* **4B,** 555.

Bortz, W. M. (1974). The pathogenesis of hypercholesterolemia. *Ann. Intern. Med.* **80,** 738–746.

Carlson, L. A., and Ballantyne, D. (1976). Changing relative proportions of apolipoproteins CII and CIII of very low density lipoproteins in hypertriglyceridaemia. *Atherosclerosis* **23,** 563–568.

Connor, W. E., Witiak, D. T., Stone, D. B., and Armstrong, M. L. (1969). Cholesterol balance and fecal neutral steroid and bile acid excretion in normal men fed dietary fats of different fatty acid composition. *J. Clin. Invest.* **48,** 1363–1375.

Coronary Drug Project Research Group. (1972). The coronary drug project: Findings leading to further modifications of its protocol with respect to dextrothyroxine. *J. Am. Med. Assoc.* **220,** 996–1008.

Dayton, S., Pearce, M. L., Hashimoto, S., Dixon, W. J., and Tomiyasu, U. (1969). A controlled clinical trial of a diet high in unsaturated fat. *Circulation* **39–40,** Suppl.2, II-1-63.

DenBesten, L., Reyna, R. H., Connor, W. E., and Stegink, L. D. (1973). The different effects on the serum lipids and fecal steroids of high carbohydrate diets given orally or intravenously. *J. Clin. Invest.* **52**, 1384–1393.

Dewar, H. A. (1971). Trial of clofibrate in the treatment of ischaemic heart disease (five-year study by a group of physicians of the Newcastle upon Tyne region). *Br. Med. J.* **4**, 767–775.

Ederer, F., Leren, P., Turpeinen, O., and Frantz, I. D. (1971). Cancer among man on cholesterol-lowering diets. *Lancet* **2**, 203.

Eisenberg, S. (1976). Lipoprotein metabolism and hyperlipemia. *Atheroscler. Rev.* **1**, 23–60.

Frantz, I. D., Dawson, E. A., Kuba, K., Brewer, E., Gatewood, L., and Bartsch, G. (1975). The Minnesota Coronary Survey: Effects of diet on cardiovascular events and deaths. *Circulation* **52**, Suppl. 2, II-4.

Glueck, C. J. (1971). Effects of oxandrolane on plasma triglyceride and PHLA in patients with Types III, IV, and V familial hyperlipoproteinemia. *Metab., Clin. Exp.* **20**, 691.

Glueck, C. J., Levy, R. I., and Fredrickson, D. S. (1969). Immunoreactive insulin, glucose tolerance, and carbohydrate inducibility in Types II, III, IV, and V hyperlipo-proteinemia. *Diabetes* **18**, 739–747.

Glueck, C. J., Levy, R. I., and Fredrickson, D. S. (1971). Norethindrone acetate, posthepa-rin lipolytic activity, and plasma triglycerides in familial types I, III, IV, and V hyperlipoproteinemia. *Ann. Intern. Med.* **75**, 345–352.

Glueck, C. J., Tsang, R., Balistreri, W., and Fallat, R. (1972). Plasma and dietary cholesterol in infancy: Effects of early low or moderate dietary cholesterol intake on subsequent response to increased dietary cholesterol. *Metab., Clin. Exp.* **21**, 1181–1192.

Grande, F., Anderson, J. T., and Keys, A. (1972). Diets of different fatty acid composition producing identical serum cholesterol levels in man. *Am. J. Clin. Nutr.* **25**, 53–60.

Grundy, S. M. (1975). Effects of polyunsaturated fats on lipid metabolism in patients with hypertriglyceridemia. *J. Clin. Invest.* **55**, 269–282.

Grundy, S. M., and Ahrens, E. H. Jr. The effects of unsaturated dietary fats on absorption, excretion, synthesis and distribution of cholesterol in man. *J. Clin. Invest.* **49**, 1135–1152.

Havel, R. J., and Kane, J. P. (1973). Drugs and lipid metabolism. *Annu. Rev. Pharmacol.* **13**, 287–308.

Hodges, R. E., Salel, A. F., Dunkley, W. L., Zelis, R., McDonagh, P. F., Clifford, C., Hobbs, R. K., Smith, L. M., Fan, A., Mason, D. T., and Lykke, C. (1975). Plasma lipid changes in young adult couples consuming polyunsaturated meats and dairy products. *Am. J. Clin. Nutr.* **28**, 1126–1140.

Hulley, S. B., Burrows, M. I., Wilson, W. S., and Nichaman, M. Z. (1972). Lipid and lipoprotein responses of hypertriglyceridaemic out-patients to a low-carbohydrate modification of the A.H.A. fat-controlled diet. *Lancet* **1**, 551–555.

Jackson, R. L., Morrisett, J. D., and Gotto, A. M., Jr. (1976). Lipoprotein structure and metabolism. *Physiol. Rev.* **56**, 259–316.

Kannel, W. B., Castelli, W. P., Gordon, T., and McNamara, P. M. (1971). Serum choles-terol, lipoproteins, and the risk of coronary heart disease: The Framingham Study. *Ann. Intern. Med.* **74**, 1–12.

Keys, A., Kimura, N., Jusukawa, A., Bronte-Stewart, B., Larsen, N., and Keys, M. H. (1958). Lessons from serum cholesterol studies in Japan, Hawaii and Los Angeles. *Ann. Intern. Med.* **48**, 83–94.

Kritchevsky, D. (1975). Animal models for atherosclerosis research. *In* "Hypolipidemic Agents" (D. Kritchevsky, ed.), pp. 215–227. Springer-Verlag, Berlin and New York.

Kudchodkar, B. J., Sodhi, H. S., and Horlick, L. (1973). Absorption of dietary cholesterol in man. *Metabl., Clin. Exp.* **22,** 155-163.

Kudchodkar, B. J., Horlick, L., and Sodhi, H. S. (1976). Effects of plant sterols on cholesterol metabolism in man. *Atherosclerosis* **23,** 239-248.

Langer, T., Levy, R. I., and Fredrickson, D. S. (1969). Dietary and pharmacologic perturbation of beta lipoprotein (βLP) turnover. *Circulation* **40,** III-14.

Leelarthaepin, B., Woodhill, J. M., Palmer, A. J., and Blacket, R. B. (1974). Obesity, diet, and Type-II hyperlipidaemia. *Lancet* **2,** 1217-1221.

Leren, P. (1966). The effect of plasma cholesterol lowering diet in male survivors of myocardial infarction. *Acta Med. Scand., Suppl.* p. 466.

Levy, R. I., moderator. (1972). Dietary and drug treatment of primary hyperlipoproteinemia. *Ann. Intern. Med.* **77,** 267-294.

Levy, R. I., Morganroth, J., and Rifkind, B. M. (1974). Drug therapy: Treatment of hyperlipidemia. *N. Engl. J. Med.* **209,** 1295-1301.

Lisch, H.-J., Bolzano, K., Herbst, M., Sailer, S., Sandhofer, F., and Braunsteiner, H. (1974). Effect of body weight changes on plasma lipids in patients with primary hyperlipoproteinemia. *Atherosclerosis* **19,** 477-484.

McGandy, R. B., Hall, B., Ford, C., and Stare, F. J. (1972). Dietary regulation of blood cholesterol in adolescent males: A pilot study. *Am. J. Clin. Nutr.* **25,** 61-66.

Mattson, F. H., Erickson, B. A., and Kligman, A. M. (1972). Effect of dietary cholesterol on serum cholesterol in man. *Am. J. Clin. Nutr.* **25,** 589-594.

Medical Research Council. (1968). Controlled trial of soya-bean oil in myocardial infarction. *Lancet* **2,** 693-700.

Miettinen, M., Turpeinen, O., Karvonen, M. J., Elosuo, R., and Paavilainen, E. (1972). Effect of cholesterol-lowering diet on mortality from coronary heart disease and other causes. *Lancet* **2,** 835-838.

Miettinen, M., Turpeinen, O., Karvonen, M. J., Paavilainen, E., and Elosuo, R. (1976). Prevalence of cholelithiasis in men and women ingesting a serum-cholesterol-lowering diet. *Ann. Clin. Res.* **8,** 111-116.

Miller, G. J., and Miller, N. E. (1975). Plasma high density lipoprotein concentration and development of ischaemic heart-disease. *Lancet* **1,** 16-19.

Nervi, F. O., and Dietschy, J. M. (1975). Ability of six different lipoprotein fractions to regulate the rate of hepatic cholesterogenesis *in vivo. J. Biol. Chem.* **250,** 8704-8711.

Nestel, P. J., and Barter, P. (1971). Metabolism of palmitic and linoleic acids in man: Differences in turnover and conversion to glycerides. *Clin. Sci.* **40,** 345-350.

Nestel, P. J., and Poyser, A. (1976). Changes in cholesterol synthesis and excretion when cholesterol intake is increased. *Ann. Intern. Med.* **25,** 1591-1599.

Nestel, P. J., Carroll, K. F., and Havenstein, N. (1970). Plasma triglyceride response to carbohydrates, fats and caloric intake. *Metab. Clin. Exp.* **19,** 1-18.

Nestel, P. J., Havenstein, N., Whyte, H. M., Scott, T. W., and Cook, L. J. (1973). Lowering of plasma cholesterol and enhanced sterol excretion with the consumption of polyunsaturated ruminant fats. *N. Engl. J. Med.* **288,** 379-382.

Nestel, P. J., Havenstein, N., Homma, Y., Scott, T. W., and Cook, L. J. (1975). Increased sterol excretion with polyunsaturated fat high cholesterol diets. *Metab., Clin. Exp.* **24,** 189-198.

Nikkilä, E. A. (1969). Control of plasma and liver triglyceride kinetics by carbohydrate metabolism and insulin. *Adv. Lipid Res.* **7,** 63-134.

Oliver, M. R. (1971). Ischaemic heart disease: A secondary prevention trial using clofibrate (a report by a research committee of the Scottish Society of Physicians). *Br. Med. J.* **4,** 775-784.

Pearce, M. L., and Dayton, S. (1971). Incidence of cancer in men on a diet high in polysaturated fats. *Lancet* **1**, 464-467.

Quarfordt, S. H., Frank, A., Shames, D. M., Berman, M., and Steinberg, D. (1970). Very low density lipoprotein triglyceride transport in Type IV hyperlipoproteinemia and the effects of carbohydrate rich diets. *J. Clin. Invest.* **49**, 2281-2297.

Reaven, G. M., Lerner, R. L., Stern, M. P., and Farquhar, J. W. (1967). Role of insulin in endogenous hypertriglyceridemia. *J. Clin. Invest.* **46**, 1756.

Rhoads, G. G., Gulbrandsen, C. L., and Kagan, A. (1976). Serum lipoproteins and coronary heart disease in a population study of Hawaii Japanese men. *N. Engl. J. Med.* **294**, 293-298.

Rinzler, S. (1968). Primary prevention of coronary heart disease by diet. *Bull. N.Y. Acad. Med.* [2] **44**, 936.

Robertson, R. P., Gavareski, D. J., Henderson, J. D., Porte, D., Jr., and Bierman, E. L. (1973). Accelerated triglyceride secretion: A metabolic consequence of obesity. *J. Clin. Invest.* **52**, 1620-1626.

Rose, G. A., Thomson, W. B., and Williams, R. T. (1965). Corn oil in treatment of ischaemic heart disease. *Br. Med. J.* **1**, 1531-1533.

Rose, H. G., Haft, G. K., and Juliano, J. (1976). Clofibrate-induced low density lipoprotein elevation therapeutic implications and treatment by colestipol resin. *Atherosclerosis* **23**, 413-427.

Ross, R., and Glomset, J. A. (1976). The pathogenesis of atherosclerosis. *N. Engl. J. Med.* **295**, 369-425.

Ross, R., and Harker, L. (1976). Hyperlipidemia and atherosclerosis. *Science* **193**, 1094-1100.

Sacks, F. M., Castelli, W. P., Donner, A., and Kass, E. H. (1975). Plasma lipids and lipoproteins in vegetarians and controls. *N. Engl. J. Med.* **292**, 1148-1151.

Samuel, P., Holtzman, C. M., and Goldstein, J. (1967). Long-term reduction of serum cholesterol levels of patients with atherosclerosis by small doses of neomycin. *Circulation* **35**, 938.

Schonfeld, G., and Pfleger, B. (1971). Utilization of exogenous free fatty acids for the production of very low density lipoprotein triglyceride by livers of carbohydrate-fed rats. *J. Lipid Res.* **12**, 614-621.

Schonfeld, G., Weidman, S. W., Witztum, J. L., and Bowen, M. (1976). Alterations in levels and interrelations of plasma apolipoproteins induced by diet. *Metab., Clin. Exp.* **25**, 261-275.

Sedaghat, A., Samuel, P., Crouse, J. R., and Ahrens, A. H., Jr. (1975). Effects of neomycin on absorption synthesis and/or flux of cholesterol in man. *J. Clin. Invest.* **55**, 12.

Shulman, R. S., Bhattacharyya, A. K., Connor, W. E., and Fredrickson, D. S. (1976). β-Sitosteroleia and xanthomatosis. *N. Engl. J. Med.* **294**, 482-483.

Singman, H. S., Archer, M., and Bergner, L. (1973). Cancer mortality and polyunsaturated fatty acids. *Mt. Sinai J. Med. N.Y.* **40**, 677-680.

Smith, L. K., Luepker, R. V., Rothchild, S. S., Gillis, A., Kochman, L., and Warbasse, J. R. (1976). Management of Type IV hyperlipoproteinemia: Evaluation of practical clinical approaches. *Ann. Intern. Med.* **84**, 22-28.

Spritz, N., and Mishkel, M. A. (1969). Effects of dietary fats on plasma lipids and lipoproteins: An hypothesis for the lipid-lowering effect of unsaturated fatty acids. *J. Clin. Invest.* **48**, 78-86.

Spritz, N., Ahrens, E. H., Jr., and Grundy, S. (1965). Sterol balance in man as plasma cholesterol concentrations are altered by exchanges of dietary fats. *J. Clin. Invest.* **44**, 1482-1493.

Stamler, J. (1975). Major coronary risk factors before and after myocardial infarction. *Postgrad. Med.* **57,** 25–30.

Starzl, T. E., Chase, H. P., Putnam, C. W., and Nora, J. J. (1974). Follow-up of patient with portacaval shunt for the treatment of hyperlipidemia. *Lancet* **2,** 714–715.

Stein, E. A., Mendelsohn, D., Fleming, M., Barnard, G. D., Carter, K. J., du Toit, P. S., Hansen, J. D. L., and Bersohn, I. (1975). Lowering of plasma cholesterol levels in free-living adolescent males; use of natural and synthetic polyunsaturated foods to provide balanced fat diets. *Am. J. Clin. Nutr.* **28,** 1204–1216.

Stern, M. P., Farquhar, J. W., Maccoby, N., and Russell, S. H. (1976). Results of a two-year health education campaign on dietary behavior. *Circulation* **54,** 826–833.

Stone, N. J., Levy, R. I., Fredrickson, D. S., and Verter, J. (1974). Coronary artery disease in 116 kindred with familial Type II hyperlipoproteinemia. *Circulation* **49,** 476–488.

Sturdevant, R. A. L., Pearce, M. L., and Dayton, S. (1973). Increased prevalence of cholelithiasis in men ingesting a serum cholesterol-lowering diet. *N. Engl. J. Med.* **288,** 24–28.

Toor, M. (1957). Serum-lipids and atherosclerosis among Yemenite immigrants in Israel. *Lancet* **1,** 1270–1273.

West, R. O., and Hayes, O. B. (1968). Diet and serum cholesterol levels. *Am. J. Clin. Nutr.* **21,** 853–862.

Wilson, W. S., Hulley, S. B., Burrows, M. I., and Nichaman, M. Z. (1971). Serial lipid and lipoprotein responses to the American Heart Association fat-controlled diet. *Am. J. Med.* **51,** 491–503.

Witztum, J. L., and Schonfeld, G. (1976). The hepatic secretion of apoproteins A-I and B (ApoA-I,ApoB) in the rat. *Clin. Res.* **24,** 373A.

Witztum, J. L., Schonfeld, G., and Weidman, S. W. (1976). The effects of colestipol on the metabolism of very-low-density lipoproteins in man. *J. Lab. Clin. Med.* **88,** 1008–1018.

Yeshurun, D., and Gotto, A. M., Jr. (1976). Drug treatment of hyperlipidemia. *Am. J. Med.* **60,** 379–395.

Zelis, R., Mason, D. T., Braunwald, E., and Levy, R. I. (1970). Effects of hyperlipoproteinemia and their treatment on the peripheral circulation. *J. Clin. Invest.* **49,** 1007–1015.

29

Medicinal Uses of Foods

ROBERT M. KARK

I. INTRODUCTION

Man eats nearly everything from sand and earth to the bark of trees, including whole animals with their intestinal contents. Consider, in civilized man, the popularity of sardines, oysters, whitebait, and snails. Among the hunter-food gatherers, such as the Eskimo on King William Land, meat is eaten in the Elizabethan sense. That is, the whole animal is consumed. The gut or "boudins" of buffalo were favorite tidbits of the plain Indians. Grubs, worms, locusts, and bird's nests are also acceptable foods in different societies.

The animal, vegetable, and mineral foods man consumes contain substances with pharmacologic or toxic properties, and we have learned to eschew or have been taught to avoid those which have them in high concentration. Yet, we do eat common foods containing various active chemicals, which we destroy or remove by preparation. The deadly cyanide in cassava, a staple food in the tropics, is removed by careful preparation of the raw root (Food and Nutrition Board, 1973). The root is grated, soaked in water, and allowed to ferment for a few days. Under these conditions, the cyanogen in the cassava is extensively hydrolyzed, and both it and the products of hydrolysis are leached out. There are many plant foods consumed by man which contain toxic cyanogenotic glycosides, such as amygdalin. Among these are choke cherries—the name is descriptive of the toxic effects they have produced—and the seeds or pits of almonds. Incidently, there is absolutely no evidence that amygdalin is a vitamin for man or beast.

Presumably many natural substances in food can be useful drugs in the appropriate setting, if we could only discover their value. We know some well-defined chemicals in foods may be essential to health, can act as a drug in the treatment of disease (and react with other drugs or nutrients) or can be detrimental to health, either acutely or over a long period of time. It all depends on how much is consumed and for how long. Vitamin D_3 is such a chemical.

Consider the plant *Solanum glaucophyllum*, which grows abundantly in the Argentine. When consumed by cattle it produces severe nephrocalcinosis and other findings reminiscent of vitamin D toxicity. The leaf contains huge amounts of a chemical not yet clearly defined which in microgram amounts is as effective as 1α-25-DHCC (1α-25-dihydroxycholecalciferol), the active end product of vitamin D_3 (J. M. Favus and W. Walleing, personal communication). This newly discovered chemical holds promise for the prevention and treatment of rickets: of vitamin D-dependent rickets; of renal osteodystrophy; of senile and other forms of osteoporosis (osteopenia) and of certain aspects of hypoparathyroidism and pseudohypoparathyroidism.

Man also plays Russian roulette with his health or life, when for pleasure, or from hunger, particularly during periods of famine, he eats foods which he knows are toxic. Every year, hundreds of hedonistic Chinese and Japanese die from eating the tails of pufferfish, *Fugu poecileonotous*, and its relatives (Food and Nutrition Board, 1973). Reports from China on intoxications from eating pufferfish date back thousands of years, probably to 2000–3000 BC. The active noxious agent is tetrodotoxin, which is found mainly in the ovaries, liver, intestine, skin, and spawn of the pufferfish, sometimes referred to as blowfish, or globefish, because of their ability to distend their abdomen. About thirty species are distributed worldwide, but the most poisonous species are caught along the coasts of Japan and China. The choice edible species are those that are the most poisonous.

Proficiency in the recognition of the different species of pufferfish and proper evisceration before eating are the best safeguards against poisoning. It is of interest that the Japanese government licenses trained and experienced persons for species identification and removal of the poisonous visceral organs from the fish without contaminating the white tail meat. Obviously, pufferfish poisoning is a public health problem in Japan and nearby areas, since the average number of deaths from eating pufferfish in Japan, over a period of years, is about 100 per year out of 200 reported cases. Over 98% of the deaths occur because of ignorance and carelessness in the handling and preparation of the poisonous species. It is rare that anyone is poisoned from eating the fish in any of the well-managed restaurants employing licensed handlers, but this does happen from time to time.

During famine in India, neurologic disturbances occur and may kill peasants, when they consume the vetch, *Lathyrus satyrus* (Food and Nutrition Board, 1973). In Jamaica, malnourished infants and children die from eating the delightfully tasting ackee apple. As a supplement to an otherwise adequate diet, foods made from vetches and dishes made from the ackee apple usually do not produce ill effects in the healthy. The danger to man arises when these readily available and very inexpensive commodities provide all, or a large proportion of the food consumed. Vetches contain a number of toxic substances. Among these are diaminobutyric acids and aminonitriles. β-Aminopropionitrile produces severe skeletal abnormalities when fed to young rats, and also aortic aneurysms in both rats and chicks. These findings are quite unlike those seen in classical lathyrism which produces a polyneuritic disorder. Thus, there are at least two distinct syndromes associated with eating *Lathyrus* seeds; the classical form should be referred to as neurolathyrism, and the syndrome produced by β-aminopropionitrile as osteolathyrism.

β-Aminopropionitrile and certain other synthetic compounds that produce osteolathyrism appear to exercise their toxic effects by interfering with the formation of cross-linkages between the polypeptide chains in collagen and elastin, thereby weakening the bones and blood vessel walls. While osteolathyrism resulting from the consumption of plant foods does not appear to be a health problem, it is of interest that Marfan's syndrome resembles closely the osteolathyrism produced in experimental animals by β-aminopropionitrile.

The ackee fruit (*Blighia sapida*) of Jamaica grows on a tree 15–25 ft high (Food and Nutrition Board, 1973). The fruit is an extremely popular food. It is said that, in general, the housewife is aware of the health hazard of eating the arilli of the unripe fruit, but nevertheless poisonings occur every now and then when the fruit is not carefully selected.

The fruit contains a water-soluble substance, Hypoglycin (α-amino-β-methylenecyclopropanyl propionic acid) which can cause acute hypoglycemia and is responsible for the often fatal "vomiting sickness" which has been reported so often in children in Jamaica.

Further investigations of the poisonous chemicals in these plants may provide potential agents for the treatment of diseases in man. The animal and biochemical studies initiated in the Department of Orthopedics at the University of Iowa on aminonitriles have already clarified our understanding of the biochemistry and physical chemistry of collagen in health and disease. The investigations on hypoglycin have not yet provided us with a new antidiabetic agent, but have clarified the function of a vitamin, carnitine.

It appears that all foods and beverages contain chemicals inimicable to health, and usually we recognize without too much difficulty the acute toxic effects they produce. Others we consume in such small amounts that they have no immediate ill effects on life and the pursuit of happiness. However, we are beginning to suspect that some foods we eat contain small quantities of substances which may be harmful to health when consumed over a long period of time, and these may produce serious chronic illness.

Aflatoxins (Food and Nutrition Board, 1973) and sodium chloride (Food and Nutrition Board, 1973) are two substances in food which, presumably, produce chronic disease in man. Sodium chloride is considered by many to produce hypertension when consumed in large enough amounts by sensitive individuals who are genetically susceptible. It is thought that the aflatoxins which are synthesized by aspergilli growing on moist peanuts and other foods are the cause of cirrhosis and hepatomas in populations living in hot, humid climates, such as Indonesia and central Africa.

The aspergilli are fungal organisms fascinating both to the mycologist interested in morphological taxonomy and to natural products chemists, who have found them to be sources of many biologically active metabolites. The widespread geographical distribution of these organisms and their presence on several foods as "storage fungi" make them of much concern to scientists and physicians throughout the world.

The first aflatoxins were discovered in the early 1960's after the occurrence of epidemic illness among poultry in England. The outbreaks of "turkey X disease" was caused by aflatoxin contaminating the Brazilian peanut meal used in formulating British poultry rations. During studies of its effects in animals, contaminated peanut meal fed to rats was found to produce primary hepatomas.

Several investigators have reported the presence of aflatoxin or one of its metabolites in urine and milk of peasants in India. Aflatoxin M_1 has been detected in peanut butter samples and in the urine of Filipinos who had eaten contaminated peanut butter. However, there is little direct evidence as to the susceptibility of man to aflatoxins. But geographical and concomitant environmental factors provide presumptive evidence that the relatively high incidence of cirrhosis and primary hepatoma in certain developing countries is associated with environmental exposure to aflatoxins rather than being primarily genetic in origin.

Molds and yeasts also produce liver disease in sheep when grass contaminated with fungal growth is consumed, and torula yeast produces cirrhosis in experimental animals. All of us are beholden to the fungi that produce antibiotics for our use. The question which we now have to ask is whether there is another side of this coin. Are some chronic neurologic and hepatic disorders which occur in man derived from fungal growth in our food and drink?

II. VEGETABLE, ANIMAL, AND MINERAL PRESCRIPTIONS AND USES

Shamans, witchdoctors, seers, and apothecaries have used vegetables, animals, and minerals as food for healing (Coon, 1971; Lee and Devore, 1972). When physicians came into being, they took over the traditional priestly and old wives' medicines and began a systematic search for drugs in vegetables, minerals, and animals. Physic gardens flourished from the fourteenth century onward and even now useful botanicals continue to come to light. The medieval alchemist was transformed into the medically trained research chemist early in the eighteenth century, and the fathers of modern geology and minerology from 1750 on were, in the main, M.D.'s. In those days, it was well nigh impossible to earn a living as a scientist and those so inclined became physicians to support themselves.

A. Vegetables

One reads in the Bible that "The leaves of the tree were for the healing of the nations" (Revelations 22:2) and, of course, the use of plants for healing is as old as man and connected with religion and other arcane matters, such as astrology. All civilized nations have published herbals, and the most famous English herbal is Culpeper's.

Herbals (Arber, 1938) are early botanical books containing descriptions and illustrations of herbs and plants with their properties, chiefly those "virtues" which made them useful to man as medicines and condiments. Most of the herbals were written between 1470 and 1670. Among the famous herbalists were Gaspard Boulin, Hieronymus Bock, and Nicholas Culpeper, a relative of the colonial Governor of Virginia (1682–1683).

Mingled often with painstaking accuracy in their description of plants were fantastic illustrations and many suggestions about the magical power of plants, e.g., astrologic relationships, and the "doctrine of signatures." This latter theory of herb medicines was based on the superficial resemblance of certain plants or plant parts to specific human organs or diseases. The appropriate herbs were used for any disorder of its human counterpart. Thus, certain heart-shaped leaves, like foxglove, were thought to relieve heart disease; the convoluted walnut, brain disease; and the figworts, whose flowers "have deep throats" were given for scrofula* (hence the figwort family named Scrophularaeclae).

Among the well known medicinal usefulness of vegetable foods are the vitamins they synthesize and store, and which have preventative, therapeutic, pharmacologic, and toxic properties.

Not only have scurvy grass, rose hip preserve, and spruce leaves saved the lives of shipwrecked marines, explorers, military garrisons, and towns under siege, but the ascorbic acid these plants contain when given in large amounts has pharmacologic properties, for example, in inducing abortions in animals.

Many natural and synthetic vitamins have been used as pharmacologic agents when given properly in large amounts to treat skin disorders such as pityriasis rubra pilaris, or genetic diseases such as maple syrup urine disease. But they are being used improperly in "mega" doses to treat schizophrenia, myocardial infarcts, coronary artery sclerosis, and many other disorders.

Of course, in "mega" doses, ascorbic acid has also been touted as a means of preventing common colds. There is a feeling among untutored persons, who are not pharmacologists, that if a little is good for you, a lot can be much better, or even work miracles.

"Mega" doses of vitamins are effective in some inborn errors of metabolism (Goodhart and Shils, 1973), such as vitamin D-resistant rickets (up to 100,000 units vitamin D_3 per day); thiamine-responsive maple syrup urine disease (10 mg thiamine hydrochloride per day in infants); methylmalonicacidemia with hyperglycinemia, which responds to 1000 μg of vitamin B_{12}, which is 200 times the normal dosage; homocystinuria in which up to 500 mg of pyridoxine per day may be required to return biochemical and clinical abnormalities to normal, and

---

*"Tuberculosis adenitis of the neck, also known as the King's Evil, which was cured by the magic touch of royalty."

hydroxykynureninuria which responds to 10 mg of niacin per day. In all these disorders, the metabolic pathways which have been disturbed by a genetic enzyme deficiency are corrected by rational use of a drug, even if we call it a vitamin.

Small outbreaks of goiter have been recorded in isolated communities compelled by circumstances to live mainly on cabbage (Rolleston, 1936). And in 1921, A. M. Chesney of John Hopkins showed that rabbits eating cabbage developed goiters (Rolleston, 1936). In 1941, Kennedy and Purvis (Kennedy, 1942) found that rape seed would induce thyroid goiter, and in 1943, Edwin Bennett Astwood discovered that the active agents in cabbage and other members of the brassica family, were thiourea and thiouracil (Astwood, 1943, 1945). They act to block the formation of thyroid hormone by interfering with the binding of circulating iodine into its organic form in the thyroid gland, and Astwood used them successfully to treat Grave's disease. Since then many useful related compounds have been synthesized to treat hyperthyroidism (e.g., propylthiouracil). Astwood's investigations have had a profound effect, not only in the treatment of hyperthyroidism, but also in clarifying the physiologic chemistry of the production of thyroid hormone (Harrison, 1974).

The fungus *Claviceps purpurla* grows on rye and there are well-documented reports of outbreaks of ergot poisoning from the highly toxic alkaloids consumed in rye bread made from contaminated flour. Symptoms are vomiting, diarrhea and abdominal pain, ischemic peripheral gangrene, psychosis, and coma.

Of the many alkaloids extracted from the fungus, ergot and ergotamine are best known. These pharmacologic vasoactive drugs are widely employed—ergotamine in the successful treatment of migraine, and ergot as a uterine stimulant (Harrison, 1974).

The plant silphium (*Birea cyrenaica*) was grown on the heights of Barca in the Roman provence of Tripolitonia by Hebrew slaves and was distributed for consumption as a tranquilizer all over the Mediterranean basin. The whole economy of Libya was dependent on the export of this plant, which was a monopoly. It was so important to the Romans that it was depicted on the obverse of Trajan's coins. About 101 AD, the slaves revolted. They uprooted and destroyed every known silphium plant, and it became extinct overnight. Its only known modern relative is *Thapsia garganica*. As a result of this destruction, Libya became bankrupt and was destroyed by the Turks. What happened to those dependent on silphium to tranquilize them is not known.

Psychotrophic drugs are being used most effectively these days and many plants and foods contain psychotrophic agents, for example, reserpine. We know that nutmeg, parsley, and mace, which are consumed every day all over the world, contain myristicin, which is narcotic, and there are many other goods which contain potentially useful or useful psychotrophic drugs (Food and Nutrition Board, 1973).

Few would disagree with the potential harm to man from alcohol, the best known psychotrophic food. Dr. Salvatore Lucia of California is one of many physicians, from time immemorial, who have written books on the medicinal use of wine. The Wine Advisory Board (1972) of California has produced a sixty-page pamphlet which contains 269 references on publications in scientific and medical journals on the value of wine in the treatment of disease. Since alcohol is metabolized in the body and produces energy without requiring insulin, alcoholic beverages, particularly wine, provide a readily available source of calories for diabetics, who were managed before the discovery of insulin by the Allan treatment which employed a diet rich in wines. This made the diabetics somewhat alcoholic, but prolonged their lives.

Alcohol also relieves the pain of angina, an observation first described by Heberden. It is also effective in some peripheral vascular diseases such as Raynaud's phenomenon. Wilkins noted that when prolonged peripheral vascular dilatation is required, the effects of amyl nitrate, nitroglycerine, and acetylcholine are likely to be too evanescent. On the other hand, 0.5 ml alcohol per kilogram body weight (6 ounces of sherry or port or 10 ounces of table wine) may induce a dilatation of peripheral vessels lasting up to 4 hours.

The Alcohol Center at Yale studies indicated that 4–8 ounces of white unfortified wine relieves emotional tension and obviously this is one of the reasons why so many people consume alcohol. This is particularly true in the elderly where it also acts as a sedative and where it has been found effective in the treatment of malabsorption in old age. Generations of physicians have agreed with the pharmacologist, Gold, in calling "wine, the nurse of old age".

B. Animal

The painting by Bernado Strozzi illustrates the cure of xerophthalmia by vitamin A in fish liver and gall. It depicts the magical relief of Tobit's blindness by the Archangel Raphael ("God Heals"), who applied fish gall and raw liver to Tobit's membrane-covered eyes. The story is told in the Apocrypha as follows:

> Tobias caught a fish, and the angel said, "Open the fish and take the heart and the liver, and the gall and put them up safely," and when they had roasted the fish, they did eat it. And the young man said to the angel, "To what use is the heart and the

liver and the gall of the fish?" And he said to him, "Touching the heart and the liver if any be possessed by a devil, we must make smoke therefore before the man or the woman, and the party shall be no more vexed. As for the gall, it is good to anoint a man that hath whiteness in his eyes, and he shall be healed . . . ." Then said Raphael: "I know Tobit, thy father will open his eyes. Therefore anoint thou his eyes with the gall, and the whiteness shall fall away, and he shall see thee." And Tobit went forth to the door and stumbled, but his son ran and took hold of him and he stroked the gall on his father's eyes. And his eyes began to smart and the whiteness peeled away from the corners of his eyes, and when he saw his son, he fell upon his neck and he wept.

Liver (Harrison, 1974) has been used from time immemorial by the Chinese for the treatment of sprue, particularly so-called tropical sprue, and we all know that Minot and Murphy were the first clinicians in America to receive the Nobel Prize. The award was made in 1929 to Minot and Murphy, and the pathologist, Whipple, for their treatment of patients ill with pernicious anemia with a diet rich in liver. Pernicious anemia has also responded to consumption of dried raw tripe and, indeed, one patient with pernicious anemia was treated by Bethel and Sturgis and improved dramatically following consumption of gelatin capsules containing extracts of his own feces. The bacteria in his colon had synthesized B_{12} which, as we know, is only absorbed in the upper bowel.

Besides liver, dehydrated thyroid, brains, bone marrow, blood, and testes have been used to treat a wide variety of diseases, particularly anemia and endocrine disorders.

While testicular extracts are useful for the treatment of eunuchs and the anemia of chronic renal failure, alas they do not cure most cases of impotence, and they are not aphrodisiacs. Oysters, the horns of narwals, or of rhinoceroses, and a wide variety of other horned animal products, have been used unsuccessfully to try and restore virility. Nor are any plant foods that I know of, such as chocolate, useful.

Since 1892, dried thyroid gland taken orally has been used to treat patients with myxedema (Gull, 1873–1874) and other forms of hypothroidism. In 1769, Thomas Prosser gave an account of the cure of the bronchocele or Derbyshire neck (Rolleston, 1936). He employed a powder containing calcined sponge. In 1820, William Prout in England and Jean François Concidit in France gave iodine extracted from seaweed to cases of goiter with good effect. Murray in 1891 was the first to treat a case of hypothyroidism by injecting an extract of fresh sheep thyroid gland. In the following year, Horwitz, Mackenzie, and Fox independently discovered that thyroid tissue was fully effective when given by mouth (Rolleston, 1936) and Fenwick (1891) reported on its diuretic action in myxedema.

There are an increasing number of endocrine hormones being extracted from animal tissue for the treatment of disease and new useful hormonal drugs can be expected to be discovered, particularly from the hypothalamus. Recently, extracts of the hypothalamus have been found to contain simple polypeptide components. Excess or absence of these compounds produce hypothalamic regulatory disorders. The discovery of these small and powerful hormones has caused a revolution in endocrinology. There is speculation now that they could change the face of psychiatry, because of their effect on mood and behaviour. Thyroid releasing hormone which is found in many parts of the brain, as well as being concentrated in the hypothalamus, appears to be of interest in relation to depression, which it has been reported to relieve (Kastin *et al.*, 1972).

Incidentally, cheeses and other foods, which contain tyramine, produce a marked rise in blood pressure, which can be life-threatening to hypertensive patients taking monamine oxidase inhibitors. Presumably, the tyramine escapes oxidative deamination that would normally occur in the liver and releases norepinephrine in supranormal amounts (Harrison, 1974).

Raw eggs are supposedly popular with opera singers and those who celebrate New Year's Day. Some avidly consume them to the exclusion of all other foods. This unusual and peculiar food fad produces biotin deficiency in man, which is as rare as hen's teeth. The dermatitis and other abnormalities produced are due to the presence of a biotin antimetabolite in the white of egg (Goodhart and Shils, 1973).

C. Mineral

Long before we had flame photometers to measure sodium and potassium, physicians were using barley water or imperial mixture to treat patients. When we look into the ancient medical indications for the use of these two old draughts, we find that they were used for patients whom nowadays we would diagnose as having potassium deficiency. Analysis of barley water reveals a high concentration of potassium, and imperial mixture contains three potassium salts.

Donald McEachern of the Montreal Neurologic Institute used to delight in recalling the history of a patient with recurring weakness who insisted he was cured by drinking O'Keefe's Export-Ale, as indeed, he was. He had periodic paralysis with hypokalemia, and analyses of Canadian beers and ales indicated that O'Keefe's had the highest concentration of potassium of them all, and when taken, completely relieved his symptoms, as did, of course, 10 gm of potassium chloride.

In adynamica episodica hereditaria the serum potassium is elevated or normal. The attacks of muscle weakness are brought on by hunger, relieved by a meal and made worse by potassium (Goodhart and Shils, 1973; Harrison, 1974). Loss of potassium from the body with muscle weakness is associated with excess consumption of licorice (Goodhart and Shils, 1973; Harrison, 1974). This confection contains a steroid, glycyrrhizic acid, which produces sodium retention with edema, as well as hypertension and cardiac enlargement. On the other hand, the muscle weakness of normokalemic familial periodic paralysis can be relieved by intravenous or oral sodium chloride (Goodhart and Shils, 1973), a mineral salt and condiment which appears to be a cause of hypertension (Food and Nutrition Board, 1973; Goodhart and Shils, 1973).

For many years there has been vigorous discussion within (and outside) the literature concerning the possible relationship between a high salt intake and the development of hypertension in man. Excellent reviews and papers by experts suggest that genetically susceptible individuals in a population may indeed develop chronic hypertension as a result of consuming large quantities of sodium from childhood (Food and Nutrition Board, 1973). Moreover, population studies have shown that mild hypertensives consuming more salt than their normotensive neighbors return to normal when their high salt intake was reduced (Morgan *et al.*, 1975).

Two germane papers by Lot Page have demonstrated that low-salt, pre-industrial societies who consume less than 50 mgs of sodium each day, have blood pressures which range about 100/60 mg Hg and *which never increase with age*. Their renin and aldosterone levels are high and they are quite healthy. Apparently, when members of a low-salt primitive Venezuelan tribe moved from their inland forest to the sea, their blood pressures became elevated. Moreover, the Harvard team led by Lot Page studied blood pressures in a number of the Solomon Isles. The native Solomon islanders are slowly being Westernized. The results of the study showed an increase in blood pressure in certain groups of Solomon islanders. This increase was directly related to consumption of the new Western diets which contain much more sodium than the diet they had consumed previously and was not the result of acculturalization and the stresses of the new Western life style.

Meneely showed that the hypertension, and particularly the vascular lesions, in rats consuming large amounts of sodium chloride, could be ameliorated by a high potassium diet. Since then a number of papers have been published suggesting the value of potassium in the prevention and management of hypertension (Food and Nutrition Board, 1973).

With regard to the many trace elements related to disease, Chatin in

1850 was the first to show that iodine could prevent endemic goiter and cretinism. Zinc has been used successfully to treat Egyptian dwarfs and hypogeusic, anosmic underdeveloped children in Denver, who are "picky eaters". Recently it has been used successfully to treat the skin disorder acrodermatitis enteropathica in adults and children. The exact pathophysiology is not known, particularly the relationship of zinc to diodoquin which has been used successfully in the past for treating acrodermatitis enteropathica.

There is evidence accumulating that trivalent chromium might be important in relation to diabetes. Much more fascinating is a single case report beautifully documented of the control of diabetes with alfalfa tea (Rubenstein *et al.*, 1962).

A rather brittle young diabetic was admitted to the hospital in Johannesburg, South Africa. He had had hypoglycemic attacks as well as very high blood sugar levels, but no gross ketonemia, nor ketonuria. He reported that infusions of alfalfa helped him. He was very difficult to control with insulin, and therefore, alfalfa tea was administered. Every time he drank the alfalfa tea, the blood sugar came under control. It was then found that alfalfa has a high manganese content and manganese was infused. Every time this was done, the blood sugar was markedly reduced, sometimes to hypoglycemic levels.

Many other trace elements, as well as other hormones, were tested but none were effective. Later a partial pancreatectomy was done as an islet cell tumor was suspected to be present. None was found in the specimen but the diabetes was much better controlled than before the operation. The nature of the relationship of manganese to diabetes in general, and to this patient in particular, is still obscure, despite the very detailed and exhaustive investigations carried out by Rubenstein *et al.* (1962).

III. DIETS

The use of diets for treatment of disease is as old as agriculture, and much of its use in the past has been based on personal recommendation.

For example, in 1564, William Bullin prescribed the following empiric diet for good health:

> Eate good broth made of chickens, leane Mutton, roste a little partriche, eate light leavened breade; bewar of grosse meates, Beefe, Porke, etc., and salletes, strong wine, Spice, sweete meates, and rawe fruits. I praie you remember this, and drinke your Diacodion at night to reconcile slepe again, and be somewhat laxative.

Since the introduction of synthetic, "purified" diets (total parenteral nutrition and so-called elemental diets) and the use of specific "deficient" diets (gluten-free diet; lactose-deficient diet), physicians have been taking a more scientific look at diets. Old stand bys, such as the Sippy diets for ulcers and the roughage-free diet for diverticulosis, have been discarded and new metabolically tailored diets, such as the alpha ketoacid diet for chronic renal failure, and the phytanic acid-free diet for Refsum's disease are under study. Some new diets, such as the high-bran, high fiber diet which is supposed to prevent cancer of the colon and other ills of Western man, are controversial.

IV. CONCLUSION

While it is true that man is wittingly or unwittingly harmed by some foods he eats, the public in the United States appears to seek a risk-free diet. This is—as with the rest of life—an unrealistic and immature view of the practicalities of the human condition. There is hardly a food which does not contain, albeit in minute amounts, some natural toxic chemicals. It is a pipe dream to long for an acceptable, sterile, nutritionally complete, bland pap, free of any trace of a chemical which is carcinogenic or allergenic or harmful in some other way when concentrated or taken in significant amounts.

It is because of these unrealistic hopes and dreams for perfect health or eternal life that much of the public behaves irrationally in its attitude to food and the blandishments of quacks. It is unfortunate but we must recognize that quacks and empirics will always be with us. Such as Maurice Messegue (1972), the present-day French herbalist, who in his book, relates how he cured Mistinguett's legs (insured for more than a million dollars) with a cabbage poultice to her kidney area and with potions of assorted vegetables and herbs. Thereafter, he became the attendant to President Herriot of France and to many powerful and wealthy businessmen and to the jet set everywhere. Counterbalancing this sad tale is the exciting potential for using enzymes from animal tissues to treat genetic enzyme deficiencies in patients with inborn errors of metabolism.

In Fabry's disease (Goodhart and Shils, 1973; Harrison, 1974; Volk and Schenk, 1976), the absence of the enzyme alpha galactosidase causes an accumulation of glycolipids, mainly galactosylgalactosylglucosyl ceramide in the cells of different organs. This produces angiokeratomas of the skin, neurological disorders, and chronic renal failure.

In 1971 the missing enzyme was restored by transplantation of a healthy kidney to a patient with Fabry's disease and renal failure. This operation was successful, not only as far as renal function was concerned, but also in restoring normality to other organs involved.

Gaucher's disease is an inherited metabolic disorder, the result of a deficiency of the enzyme glucocerebrosidase (Brady *et al.*, 1974). This results in an accumulation of glucocerebrosides in the liver, spleen, and other organs and tissues of affected individuals. Brady treated patients with Gaucher's disease by intravenous administration of the missing enzyme isolated from normal human placenta. This resulted in a marked decrease in the abnormal lipid which had accumulated in the liver and red blood cells of the patient. What was perhaps even more significant was the finding that the effect of the infusion persisted for many months after it was given. This unforeseen result raises hopes for the successful treatment of single or isolated enzyme deficiency disorders. The possibility of eventually using oral replacement is obviously highly speculative but it is food for thought.

All of the above examples of interaction between man and animals and the toxic and pharmacologic compounds in their food indicate the enormous potential for interaction that exists between the synthetic and the natural drugs we employ in medicine. They also indicate the potential that still exists today for finding new and useful drugs in foods as well as the potential for illuminating the study of intermediary metabolism in man by study of the metabolism of useful and toxic drugs in bacteria, fungi, and plants.

REFERENCES

Arber, A. R. (1938). "Herbals, Their Origin and Evolution," 2nd ed. Longmans, Green, New York.
Astwood, E. B. (1943). Treatment of hyperthyroidism with thiourea and thiouracil. *J. Am. Med. Assoc* **122,** 78.
Astwood, E. B. (1945). Some observations on the use of thiobarbital as an antithyroid agent in the treatment of Graves' disease. *J. Clin. Endocrinol.* **5,** 345.
Brady, R. O., Pentchew, P. G., Gal, A. E., Hibbert, S. R., and Dekaban, A. S. (1974). Replacement therapy for inherited enzyme deficiency. *N. Engl. J. Med.* **291,** 989.
Chatin, G. A. (1850). Existence de l'iode dans les plantes d'eau douce. Consequences de ce fait pour la géognoise, la physiologie végétale, la thérapeutique et peut-être pour l'industrie. *C. R. Hebd. Seances Acad. Sci.* **30,** 352.
Coon, C. S. (1971). "The Hunting Peoples." Little, Brown, Boston, Massachusetts.
Fenwick, E. H. (1891). The diuretic action of fresh thyroid juice. *Br. Med. J.* **2,** 789.
Food and Nutrition Board. (1973). "Toxicants Occurring Naturally in Foods." Natl. Acad. Sci., Washington, D.C.

Goodhart, R. S., and Shils, M. E. (1973). "Modern Nutrition in Health and Disease." Lea & Febiger, Philadelphia, Pennsylvania.

Gull, W. W. (1873–1874). On a cretinoid state supervening in adult life in women. *Trans. Clin. Soc. London* **7**, 180.

Harrison, T. R. (1974). "Principles of Internal Medicine." McGraw-Hill (Blakiston), New York.

Kastin, A. J., Fluneusing, R. H., Schalch, D. S., and Anderson, M. S. (1972). Improvement in mental depression with decreased thyrotropin response after administration of thyrotroxin releasing hormone. *Lancet* **2**, 740.

Kennedy, T. H., (1942). *Nature, (London),* **150**, 233.

Lee, R. B., and Devore, I., eds. (1972). "Man The Hunter," Aldine, Chicago, Illinois.

Messegue, M. (1972). "Of Men and Plants." Macmillan, New York.

Morgan, T., Carney, S., and Wilson, M. (1975). Interrelationship in humans between sodium intake and hypertension. *Clin. Exp. Pharmacol. Physiol. Suppl.* **2**, 127.

Murray, G. R. (1891). Note on the treatment of myxoedema by hypodermic injections of an extract of the thyroid gland of a sheep. *Br. Med. J.* **2**, 796.

Rolleston, H. D. (1936). "The Endocrine Organs in Health and Disease, with an Historical Review." Oxford Univ. Press, London and New York.

Rubenstein, A. H., Levin, N. W., and Elliott, G. A. (1962). Manganese induced hypoglycemia. *Lancet* **2**, 1348.

Volk, B. W., and Schenk, L., eds. (1976). "Current Trends in Single Lipidoses." Pergamon, Oxford.

Wine Advisory Board. (1972). "Use of Wine in Medical Practice: (A Summary)." Wine Advisory Board, San Francisco, California.

Author Index

Numbers in italics refer to the pages on which complete references are listed.

A

Aach, R. D., 511, 528, *536*
Abaza, M. A., 225, *238*
Abbey, A., 636, 637, *645*, *647*
Abbott, O. J., 639, *643*
Abbott, S. L., 651, *659*
Abdallah, A. H., 56, 57, 64, *65*, *70*
Abe, M., 170, *184*
Abel, E. L., 63, *65*
Abou Akkada, A. R., 215, 223, 225, *238*
Abramson, R. K., 269, 271, *274*
Acar, J. F., 655, *660*
Acker, D. C., 595, *608*
Ackrill, P., 328, *340*
Adair, E. R., 35, *65*
Adams, F., 320, *340*
Adams, P. W., 142, *147*, 154, 155, 165, 166, 169, 170, 171, *182*, *186*
Adams, W. H., 90, *109*
Adamson, R. H., 508, *538*
Adeyanju, S. A., 595, 596, *604*, *606*
Adir, J., 322, *340*
Adler, J. H., 586, *604*
Aedo, R., 400, 403, *407*
Aerberli, P., 53, *65*
Affrime, M., 448, 449, *472*
Aftergood, L., 760, *767*
Agradi, E., 478, 479, 481, 484, *500*
Agrawal, B. B. L., 707, *712*
Agtarap, A., 640, *643*
Ahlskog, J. E., 26, 28, 45, 46, *65*
Ahmed, F., 172, 176, 177, *182*
Ahrens, E. H., Jr., 122, *129*, 797, 798, 804, 812, *815*, *816*, *818*, *819*

Aitio, A., 268, 270, *274*
Akinlaja, A., 60, 61, *76*
Alberstein, P., 438, *444*
Albert, A., 321, *340*
Albright, F., 739, *744*
Alderson, N. E., 637, *643*
Alexander, M., 214, *238*
Alfin-Slater, R. B., 760, *767*
Algeo, J. W., 593, *607*, 630, 631, *645*
Allen, G., 210, *239*
Allen, G. S., 44, 48, *65*
Allen, R. S., 552, *573*
Allet, B., 655, *659*
Alleyne, G. A., 400, *406*
Allison, A. C., 512, *533*, 761, *767*
Allison, M. J., 193, 204, 205, 207, 210, 211, 214, 219, *244*
Almgren, P. E., 168, *185*
Alperin, J. B., 172, *182*
Al-Rashid, R. A., 373, 383, *395*
Altman, K., 156, *182*
Alvares, A. P., 373, 390, 391, 392, 393, *395*
Aly, H. E., 154, 158, 160, 165, *182*
Amare, M., 507, *536*
Amat, F. L., 754, 755, *771*
Amit, Z., 63, *68*
Anand, B. K., 22, 24, 30, 59, *65*, *66*, *68*, *79*
Ancona, C. V., 426, 427, *441*
Andary, T. J., 689, 700, 705, *714*
Anden, N.-E., 23, *66*
Andersen, A. E., 41, *75*
Anderson, C., 400, *406*
Anderson, E. S., 653, 658, *659*, *661*
Anderson, G. C., 601, *608*

837

Subject Index

A

A4696, 236
AAF, *see* N-2-Fluorenylacetamide
Abortion, induction of, 826
Absorption
  of folate, 86–89
    azulfidine inhibition of, 98
    diphenylhydantoin inhibition of, 94–96
    ethanol inhibition of, 89–94, 101–103
    oral contraceptive agents and, 96–98
  of vitamin B_{12}, 98–99
    p-aminosalicylic acid and, 101
    biguanides and, 103
    colchicine and, 100–101
    ethanol and, 101–103
    neomycin and, 100
    thiamine and, 103–105
Acetaldehyde, 425
  ethanol toxicity and, 426, 438–440
Acetaldehyde syndrome, 333
Acetanilide, metabolism of, ascorbic acid
    and, 348, 349, 357
Acetate, methane production and, 234–235
Acetazolamide, 284
Acetic acid, 619
  methane production and, 227
  in rumen, 238
Acetohydroxamate (AHA), 221–222
Acetone, 476
Acetylation, 309, 313, 315
Acetylcholine, food intake regulation and,
    29
Acetyl-CoA, synthesis of, 313
N-Acetylcysteine, 284
N-Acetylglucosamine, 312
Acetylkynurenine, oral contraceptives and,
    166

Acetylsalicylic acid
  absorption of, food and, 320, 321
  binding to plasma proteins, 448
  mucosal damage and, 280, 281, 282–283,
    285, 288, 292, 293
  in undernourished infants, 400–403
  vitamin needs and, 139
Ac-globulin, 705
  in thrombin formation, 692, 694, 695
Acid, peptic ulcers and, 280
Acidosis, 219
  salicylates and, 403
Acrodermatitis enteropathica, zinc and,
    832
Actinomycin D, 726
Active transport, 85–86
Adenosine triphosphatase, ethanol sup-
    pression of, 94
Adenosine triphosphate citrate lyase, inhi-
    bition of, 55
Adenosylmethionine, 312
Adenyl cyclase, ethanol stimulation of, 94
Adipose tissue
  entered by fatty acids, 783
  free fatty acid release from, 453–454
Adiposity
  food intake regulation and, 34–35
  ventromedial hypothalamus and, 26
Adipsia, brain and, 26–28
Adrenal system
  agents carcinogenic in, 511
  synthetic estrogens and, 599–600
Adrenergic systems, in food intake regula-
    tion, 28–29
Adrenocorticotropin, estrogens and, 599–
    600
  synthetic, 599